# Textbook of Veterinary Orthopaedic Surgery

Hari Prasad Aithal • Amar Pal •
Prakash Kinjavdekar • Abhijit M Pawde

# Textbook of Veterinary Orthopaedic Surgery

Springer

Hari Prasad Aithal
Training and Education Centre
ICAR- Indian Veterinary
Research Institute
Pune, India

Amar Pal
Division of Surgery
ICAR- Indian Veterinary
Research Institute
Bareilly, Uttar Pradesh, India

Prakash Kinjavdekar
Division of Surgery
ICAR- Indian Veterinary
Research Institute
Bareilly, Uttar Pradesh, India

Abhijit M Pawde
Division of Surgery
ICAR- Indian Veterinary
Research Institute
Bareilly, Uttar Pradesh, India

ISBN 978-981-99-2574-2 ISBN 978-981-99-2575-9 (eBook)
https://doi.org/10.1007/978-981-99-2575-9



This Springer imprint is published by the registered company Springer Nature Singapore Pte Ltd.
The registered company address is: 152 Beach Road, #21-01/04 Gateway East, Singapore 189721, Singapore

*Dedicated to*
***Our Families***
*(* for their unwavering Support, Love, and Affection*)*

# Preface

Veterinary orthopedics in recent years has made tremendous advancements, in terms of greater understanding of fracture biology and fixation, and development of versatile techniques and mechanically stable fixation implants. This has resulted in effective treatment of even some of the complicated cases, which are otherwise difficult to manage by conventional methods. Nevertheless, use of most of the advanced techniques is confined to select veterinary institutions and colleges, and only to a few "qualified" veterinary surgeons. While most of the veterinary graduates are well trained and confident of undertaking many soft tissue surgeries, they are less prepared to treat orthopedic conditions such as fractures. Hence, there is a great need to train and infuse confidence among the veterinary graduates and surgeons to treat a variety of fractures and other orthopedic conditions routinely encountered in veterinary practice. The main purpose of publishing this *Textbook of Veterinary Orthopedic Surgery* is to disseminate basic knowledge about veterinary orthopedics among the veterinary professionals and describe in simple terms the basic and advanced techniques of fracture fixation and other treatment modalities both in small and large animals to help veterinary graduates, postgraduates, practicing surgeons, and university teachers and trainers. The textbook can be a ready reckoner for all sorts of veterinary orthopedic problems.

The chapters in the book are dedicated to basic considerations in orthopedics such as structure of bone, types of bone, development and growth of bone, fracture classification, biomechanics and healing, fixation implants, emergency treatment, assessment and first aid of fracture cases, anesthesia and pain management, and timing and selection of fracture fixation techniques. Basic principles of external, internal, and external skeletal fixation techniques have been described in detail. Further different fixation techniques for management of specific fractures in both small and large animals have been elucidated. Some of the recently developed internal fixation and external skeletal fixation implants for large animals have been detailed. Separate chapters have been dedicated to fractures in young, osteoporotic and avian fractures, management of open fractures, bone grafts and scaffolds, complications of fracture fixation, metabolic bone diseases and antebrachial bone deformities, joint luxations, arthritis, common ligament and tendon injuries, and physiotherapy and rehabilitation of veterinary orthopedic patients. Most of the techniques described are those practiced by the authors based on their vast clinical experience. All the sections include an adequate number of sketches, diagrams, or/and photographs to describe almost each and every technique for better understanding.

We are thankful to our colleagues and friends who have provided some quality figures of clinical cases for inclusion in this book. We are also grateful to authors and publishers for granting permission to reproduce some of the published figures. We express our gratitude to our mentor, Dr Gaj Raj Singh, who was an inspiration for our interest in veterinary orthopedics, especially large animal fracture fixation. We take this opportunity to thank our PG students who have helped us in treating the dumb animals and relieving their pain. We are also thankful to our families for their constant support even when we stole their share of time both while doing our clinical practice and also while writing the textbook manuscript. We would also like to remember those patients who selflessly allowed us to "experiment" on them and enable us to learn a lot during our long journey. Thanks are also due to our Directors and Joint Directors of Indian Veterinary Research Institute, who have encouraged and supported us during our entire career. We are also grateful to Springer Nature, and Dr Bhavik Sawhney, Senior Editor-Biomedicine for helping us publish this book. We sincerely hope that our efforts will not go in vain and we will come up to the expectations of our valued readers.

Pune, Maharashtra, India — Hari Prasad Aithal
Bareilly, Uttar Pradesh, India — Amar Pal
Barielly, Uttar Pradesh, India — Prakash Kinjavdekar
Barielly, Uttar Pradesh, India — Abhijit M Pawde

# Contents


**1 Basic Considerations** . . . . . . . . . . 1
1.1 Structure and Types of the Bone . . . . . . . . . . 2
1.1.1 Components of the Bone . . . . . . . . . . 2
1.1.2 Structure of the Bone . . . . . . . . . . 3
1.1.3 Circulation of the Bone . . . . . . . . . . 5
1.2 Bone Development and Growth Regulation . . . . . . . . . . 7
1.2.1 Development of the Bone . . . . . . . . . . 7
1.2.2 Calcium Regulation . . . . . . . . . . 9
1.3 Fracture Biomechanics and Classification . . . . . . . . . . 10
1.3.1 Mechanical Properties of the Bone . . . . . . . . . . 12
1.3.2 Fracture Forces . . . . . . . . . . 13
1.3.3 Classification of Fracture . . . . . . . . . . 15
1.3.4 Incidence of Fractures . . . . . . . . . . 19
1.4 Fracture Healing and Methods to Enhance Healing . . . . . 20
1.4.1 Fracture Healing . . . . . . . . . . 20
1.4.2 Methods to Enhance Fracture Healing . . . . . . . . 22
1.5 Implants Used for Fracture Fixation . . . . . . . . . . 25
1.5.1 Stainless Steel . . . . . . . . . . 26
1.5.2 Titanium . . . . . . . . . . 26
1.5.3 Cobalt-Chrome . . . . . . . . . . 28
1.5.4 Aluminum Alloy . . . . . . . . . . 28
1.5.5 Non-biodegradable Polymers . . . . . . . . . . 28
1.5.6 Biodegradable Metals . . . . . . . . . . 29
1.5.7 Bioresorbable Polymers . . . . . . . . . . 30
1.6 Instrumentation for Fracture Fixation . . . . . . . . . . 31
1.6.1 Basic Instruments (Fig. 1.20) . . . . . . . . . . 32
1.6.2 Instruments for Bone Plating . . . . . . . . . . 32
1.6.3 Instruments for Intramedullary Pinning . . . . . . . . 35
1.6.4 Instruments for Interlocking Nailing . . . . . . . . . . 35
1.6.5 Instruments for Rush Pinning . . . . . . . . . . 36
1.6.6 Instruments for Kuntscher Nailing . . . . . . . . . . 37
1.6.7 Instruments for Bone Stapling . . . . . . . . . . 37
1.6.8 Instruments for Orthopedic Wiring . . . . . . . . . . 37
1.6.9 Instruments for External Skeletal Fixation . . . . . . 38

1.7 Examination of the Animals with Fracture . . . . . . . . . . . . 40
1.7.1 Things we Should Avoid while Examining an Injured Animal . . . . . . . . . . . . . . . . . . . . . . . . . 41
1.8 Emergency Treatment of Fracture and First Aid . . . . . . . . 41
1.9 Anesthesia and Pain Management in Animals with Fracture . . . . . . . . . . . . . . . . . . . . . . . . . . . . . . . . . . 42
1.9.1 Anesthesia in Cattle . . . . . . . . . . . . . . . . . . . . . . 42
1.9.2 Anesthesia in Sheep/Goat . . . . . . . . . . . . . . . . . 44
1.9.3 Anesthesia in Horse . . . . . . . . . . . . . . . . . . . . . . 44
1.9.4 Anesthesia in Pig . . . . . . . . . . . . . . . . . . . . . . . . 45
1.9.5 Anesthesia in Dog . . . . . . . . . . . . . . . . . . . . . . . 46
1.9.6 Anesthesia in Cat . . . . . . . . . . . . . . . . . . . . . . . . 47
1.9.7 Management of Pain . . . . . . . . . . . . . . . . . . . . . 48
1.10 Methods of Fracture Reduction . . . . . . . . . . . . . . . . . . . . 50
1.11 Timing and Selection of Fracture Fixation Technique . . . . 54
1.11.1 Timing of Definitive Fixation . . . . . . . . . . . . . . . 55
1.11.2 Selection of Fixation Technique . . . . . . . . . . . . . 56
1.12 Chapter 1: Sample Questions . . . . . . . . . . . . . . . . . . . . . 58
References . . . . . . . . . . . . . . . . . . . . . . . . . . . . . . . . . . . . . 60

**2 Principles of Fracture Fixation Techniques** . . . . . . . . . . . . . 65
2.1 External Fixation Techniques . . . . . . . . . . . . . . . . . . . . . . 66
2.1.1 Bandages . . . . . . . . . . . . . . . . . . . . . . . . . . . . . . 66
2.1.2 Splints . . . . . . . . . . . . . . . . . . . . . . . . . . . . . . . . 68
2.1.3 Slings . . . . . . . . . . . . . . . . . . . . . . . . . . . . . . . . . 70
2.1.4 Plaster Cast . . . . . . . . . . . . . . . . . . . . . . . . . . . . 70
2.1.5 Fiberglass Cast . . . . . . . . . . . . . . . . . . . . . . . . . 76
2.1.6 Modified Thomas Splints . . . . . . . . . . . . . . . . . . 77
2.1.7 Thomas Splint-Cast Combination . . . . . . . . . . . . 80
2.2 Internal Fixation Techniques . . . . . . . . . . . . . . . . . . . . . . 83
2.2.1 Intramedullary Pin/Nail . . . . . . . . . . . . . . . . . . . 83
2.2.2 Bone Plate and Screw Fixation . . . . . . . . . . . . . . 94
2.2.3 Ancillary Fixation Devices . . . . . . . . . . . . . . . . . 105
2.3 External Skeletal Fixation . . . . . . . . . . . . . . . . . . . . . . . . 111
2.3.1 Indications . . . . . . . . . . . . . . . . . . . . . . . . . . . . . 112
2.3.2 Advantages of ESF . . . . . . . . . . . . . . . . . . . . . . . 112
2.3.3 Disadvantages of ESF . . . . . . . . . . . . . . . . . . . . . 113
2.3.4 Fixator Configurations and Types . . . . . . . . . . . . 113
2.3.5 Biomechanics of ESF . . . . . . . . . . . . . . . . . . . . . 113
2.3.6 Linear External Skeletal Fixation Systems for Small Animals . . . . . . . . . . . . . . . . . . . . . . . . . . . 117
2.3.7 Transfixation Pinning and Casting in Large Animals . . . . . . . . . . . . . . . . . . . . . . . . . . . . . . . 124
2.3.8 Linear External Skeletal Fixation Systems for Large Animals . . . . . . . . . . . . . . . . . . . . . . . . . . . 127
2.3.9 Circular External Skeletal Fixation . . . . . . . . . . . 131
2.3.10 Acrylic- or Epoxy-Pin Fixation Systems . . . . . . . 137
2.3.11 Complications of ESF . . . . . . . . . . . . . . . . . . . . 145
2.4 Chapter 2: Sample Questions . . . . . . . . . . . . . . . . . . . . . 146
References . . . . . . . . . . . . . . . . . . . . . . . . . . . . . . . . . . . . . 147

**3 Management of Specific Fractures in Small Animals** . . . . . . . 155
3.1 Fractures of Scapula . . . . . . . . . . . . . . . . . . . . . . . . . . . . . 156
3.2 Fractures of Humerus . . . . . . . . . . . . . . . . . . . . . . . . . . . . 158
3.2.1 Fractures of the Proximal Humerus . . . . . . . . . . . 158
3.2.2 Diaphyseal Fractures of Humerus . . . . . . . . . . . . 159
3.2.3 Fractures of the Distal Humerus . . . . . . . . . . . . . 161
3.3 Fractures of Radius-Ulna . . . . . . . . . . . . . . . . . . . . . . . . . 165
3.3.1 Fractures of the Proximal end of Radius/Ulna . . . 165
3.3.2 Diaphyseal Fractures of Radius-Ulna . . . . . . . . . 166
3.3.3 Fractures at the Distal Radius and Ulna . . . . . . . 169
3.4 Fractures of Femur . . . . . . . . . . . . . . . . . . . . . . . . . . . . . 171
3.4.1 Femur Head-Neck and Subtrochanteric Fractures . . . . . . . . . . . . . . . . . . . . . . . . . . . . . 173
3.4.2 Femoral Diaphyseal Fractures . . . . . . . . . . . . . . 178
3.4.3 Distal Femoral Fractures . . . . . . . . . . . . . . . . . . 189
3.5 Fractures of Tibia-Fibula . . . . . . . . . . . . . . . . . . . . . . . . . 194
3.5.1 Proximal Physeal Fractures . . . . . . . . . . . . . . . . 194
3.5.2 Diaphyseal Fractures . . . . . . . . . . . . . . . . . . . . . 194
3.5.3 Distal Tibial/Malleolar Fractures . . . . . . . . . . . . 198
3.6 Fractures of Metacarpus and Metatarsus . . . . . . . . . . . . . 199
3.7 Fractures of Mandible . . . . . . . . . . . . . . . . . . . . . . . . . . . 201
3.7.1 External Fixation . . . . . . . . . . . . . . . . . . . . . . . . 204
3.7.2 Internal Fixation . . . . . . . . . . . . . . . . . . . . . . . . 205
3.7.3 External Skeletal Fixation . . . . . . . . . . . . . . . . . 205
3.7.4 Complications and Prognosis . . . . . . . . . . . . . . . 206
3.8 Fractures of Pelvis . . . . . . . . . . . . . . . . . . . . . . . . . . . . . 207
3.8.1 Surgical Approach . . . . . . . . . . . . . . . . . . . . . . . 210
3.8.2 Surgical Management . . . . . . . . . . . . . . . . . . . . 210
3.8.3 Postoperative Care and Complications . . . . . . . . 214
3.9 Fractures of Spine . . . . . . . . . . . . . . . . . . . . . . . . . . . . . . 214
3.9.1 Nonsurgical Stabilization of the Spine . . . . . . . . 215
3.9.2 Surgical Stabilization of the Spine . . . . . . . . . . . 215
3.9.3 Thoracic and Lumbar Fracture/Luxations . . . . . . 215
3.9.4 Reduction and Surgical Fixation . . . . . . . . . . . . . 217
3.9.5 Lumbosacral Fractures . . . . . . . . . . . . . . . . . . . . 222
3.10 Chapter 3: Sample Questions . . . . . . . . . . . . . . . . . . . . . 223
References . . . . . . . . . . . . . . . . . . . . . . . . . . . . . . . . . . . . . 225

**4 Management of Specific Fractures in Large Animals** . . . . . . . 231
4.1 Fractures of Scapula and Humerus . . . . . . . . . . . . . . . . . 232
4.2 Fractures of Radius-Ulna . . . . . . . . . . . . . . . . . . . . . . . . . 234
4.3 Fractures of Femur . . . . . . . . . . . . . . . . . . . . . . . . . . . . . 238
4.4 Fractures of Tibia . . . . . . . . . . . . . . . . . . . . . . . . . . . . . . 243
4.5 Fractures of Metacarpus, Metatarsus, and Phalanges . . . . . 251
4.6 Fractures of Pelvis . . . . . . . . . . . . . . . . . . . . . . . . . . . . . 256
4.7 Fractures of Mandible . . . . . . . . . . . . . . . . . . . . . . . . . . . 257
4.8 Chapter 4: Sample Questions . . . . . . . . . . . . . . . . . . . . . 262
References . . . . . . . . . . . . . . . . . . . . . . . . . . . . . . . . . . . . . 263

5 **Fractures in Young, Osteoporotic, and Avian Bones** . . . . . . . 267
5.1 Fractures in Young Animals . . . . . . . . . . . . . . . . . . . . . . 268
5.1.1 Open Reduction and Internal Fixation . . . . . . . . . 269
5.1.2 Fractures Involving the Growth Plate . . . . . . . . . 276
5.2 Fractures in Osteopenic/Osteoporotic Bones . . . . . . . . . . 277
5.3 Fractures in Avian Bones . . . . . . . . . . . . . . . . . . . . . . . 281
5.3.1 Methods of Fracture Repair . . . . . . . . . . . . . . . . 282
5.4 Chapter 5: Sample Questions . . . . . . . . . . . . . . . . . . . . 286
References . . . . . . . . . . . . . . . . . . . . . . . . . . . . . . . . . . . . . 287

6 **Open Fractures** . . . . . . . . . . . . . . . . . . . . . . . . . . . . . . . . . 289
6.1 Classification of Open Fractures . . . . . . . . . . . . . . . . . . . 290
6.2 Soft Tissue Infection, Osteomyelitis, and Antibiotic Therapy . . . . . . . . . . . . . . . . . . . . . . . . . . . . . . . . . . . . . 290
6.3 Management of Soft Tissue Injuries and Wound Closure . . . . . . . . . . . . . . . . . . . . . . . . . . . . . . . . . . . . 292
6.4 Treatment of Open Fractures . . . . . . . . . . . . . . . . . . . . . 293
6.5 Postoperative Care of Open Fractures . . . . . . . . . . . . . . . 297
6.6 Chapter 6: Sample Questions . . . . . . . . . . . . . . . . . . . . 299
References . . . . . . . . . . . . . . . . . . . . . . . . . . . . . . . . . . . . . 300

7 **Bone Grafts and Scaffolds in Fracture Repair** . . . . . . . . . . . . 303
7.1 Functions of Bone Grafts or Implants . . . . . . . . . . . . . . . 304
7.2 Types of Bone Grafts . . . . . . . . . . . . . . . . . . . . . . . . . . 305
7.2.1 According to Origin . . . . . . . . . . . . . . . . . . . . . 305
7.2.2 According to Composition . . . . . . . . . . . . . . . . . 306
7.3 Processing of Bone Grafts . . . . . . . . . . . . . . . . . . . . . . . 306
7.4 Process of Bone Graft Incorporation . . . . . . . . . . . . . . . . 307
7.5 Bone Substitutes . . . . . . . . . . . . . . . . . . . . . . . . . . . . . 307
7.5.1 Demineralized Bone Matrix . . . . . . . . . . . . . . . . 307
7.5.2 Calcium Phosphate Synthetic Substitutes . . . . . . 307
7.5.3 Synthetic Polymers . . . . . . . . . . . . . . . . . . . . . . 308
7.6 Bone Inducers . . . . . . . . . . . . . . . . . . . . . . . . . . . . . . . 308
7.6.1 Bone Morphogenic Protein (BMP) . . . . . . . . . . . 308
7.6.2 Transforming Growth Factor-β . . . . . . . . . . . . . . 309
7.6.3 Insulin-like Growth Factor . . . . . . . . . . . . . . . . . 309
7.6.4 Growth Hormone . . . . . . . . . . . . . . . . . . . . . . . 309
7.7 Stem Cells . . . . . . . . . . . . . . . . . . . . . . . . . . . . . . . . . 309
7.8 Chapter 7: Sample Questions . . . . . . . . . . . . . . . . . . . . 310
References . . . . . . . . . . . . . . . . . . . . . . . . . . . . . . . . . . . . . 312

8 **Complications of Fracture Fixation** . . . . . . . . . . . . . . . . . . . . 315
8.1 Delayed Union . . . . . . . . . . . . . . . . . . . . . . . . . . . . . . . 317
8.2 Nonunion . . . . . . . . . . . . . . . . . . . . . . . . . . . . . . . . . . 317
8.3 Malunion . . . . . . . . . . . . . . . . . . . . . . . . . . . . . . . . . . 318
8.4 Fixation Failure . . . . . . . . . . . . . . . . . . . . . . . . . . . . . . 318
8.5 Soft Tissue Infection and Osteomyelitis . . . . . . . . . . . . . . 318

8.6 Fracture Disease . . . . . . 320
8.7 Supporting Limb Laminitis . . . . . . 321
8.8 Chapter 8: Sample Questions . . . . . . 324
References . . . . . . 325

**9 Metabolic Bone Diseases** . . . . . . 327
9.1 Nutritional Secondary Hyperparathyroidism . . . . . . 328
9.2 Rickets . . . . . . 329
9.3 Hypertrophic Osteodystrophy . . . . . . 332
9.4 Osteochondrosis . . . . . . 333
9.5 Retained Cartilage Core . . . . . . 335
9.6 Metaphyseal Chondrodysplasia . . . . . . 335
9.7 Panosteitis . . . . . . 336
9.8 Hip Dysplasia . . . . . . 338
9.9 Prevention and Control of Bone Disorders . . . . . . 347
9.10 Chapter 9: Sample Questions . . . . . . 347
References . . . . . . 348

**10 Antebrachial Bone Deformities** . . . . . . 353
10.1 Closure of Distal Ulnar Growth Plate . . . . . . 355
10.2 Closure of Distal Radial Growth Plate . . . . . . 355
10.3 Closure of Proximal Radial Physis . . . . . . 357
10.4 Closure of Both Growth Plates: Distal Radius and Ulna . . . . . . 357
10.5 Postoperative Care, Management, and Prognosis . . . . . . 358
10.6 Chapter 10: Sample Questions . . . . . . 359
References . . . . . . 360

**11 Joint Luxations** . . . . . . 363
11.1 Small Animals . . . . . . 364
11.1.1 Shoulder Luxation . . . . . . 365
11.1.2 Elbow Luxation . . . . . . 368
11.1.3 Carpal Luxation . . . . . . 370
11.1.4 Hip (Coxofemoral) Luxation . . . . . . 373
11.1.5 Stifle Luxation . . . . . . 376
11.1.6 Patellar Luxation . . . . . . 378
11.1.7 Tarsal Luxation . . . . . . 384
11.2 Large Animals . . . . . . 386
11.2.1 Shoulder Luxation . . . . . . 386
11.2.2 Elbow Luxation . . . . . . 386
11.2.3 Coxofemoral Luxation . . . . . . 387
11.2.4 Patellar Luxation . . . . . . 388
11.2.5 Carpal and Tarsal Luxations . . . . . . 391
11.2.6 Metacarpophalangeal and Metatarsophalangeal Luxations . . . . . . 391
11.3 Chapter 11: Sample Questions . . . . . . 392
References . . . . . . 393

**12 Arthritis** . . . 399
12.1 Traumatic Arthritis . . . 400
12.1.1 Clinical Signs . . . 400
12.1.2 Diagnosis . . . 400
12.1.3 Treatment . . . 401
12.2 Septic (Infectious) Arthritis . . . 402
12.2.1 Causes of Infection . . . 402
12.2.2 Clinical Signs . . . 403
12.2.3 Diagnosis . . . 403
12.2.4 Treatment . . . 404
12.2.5 Follow-Up Care, Management, Complications, and Prognosis . . . 406
12.3 Osteoarthritis . . . 406
12.3.1 Pathophysiology . . . 406
12.3.2 Predisposing Factors . . . 408
12.3.3 Clinical Signs . . . 408
12.3.4 Diagnosis . . . 409
12.3.5 Management . . . 410
12.4 Rheumatoid Arthritis . . . 411
12.4.1 Clinical Signs . . . 412
12.4.2 Diagnosis . . . 412
12.4.3 Treatment . . . 412
12.5 Chapter 12: Sample Questions . . . 412
References . . . 413

**13 Common Tendon and Ligament Injuries** . . . 417
13.1 Tendon Injuries . . . 418
13.1.1 Achilles Tendon . . . 418
13.1.2 Superficial and Deep Digital Flexor Tendons . . . 420
13.1.3 Contracted Flexor Tendons . . . 422
13.1.4 Principles and Techniques of Tendon Suturing . . . 423
13.2 Ligament Injuries . . . 425
13.2.1 Cranial Cruciate Ligament . . . 425
13.2.2 Patellar Ligament . . . 431
13.2.3 Collateral Ligaments . . . 431
13.2.4 Postoperative Care and Management of Tendon/ Ligament Injuries . . . 432
13.3 Chapter 13: Sample Questions . . . 433
References . . . 434

**14 Bone Tumors** . . . 439
14.1 Dogs and Cats . . . 440
14.1.1 Clinical Signs . . . 440
14.1.2 Diagnosis . . . 440
14.1.3 Treatment . . . 442
14.1.4 Prognosis . . . 444
14.2 Large Animals . . . 444
14.3 Chapter 14: Sample Questions . . . 444
References . . . 446

**15 Physiotherapy and Rehabilitation of Orthopedic Patients** . . . 449
15.1 Techniques . . . 451
15.1.1 Cryotherapy . . . 451
15.1.2 Thermotherapy . . . 451
15.1.3 Passive Range of Motion . . . 451
15.1.4 Massage . . . 452
15.1.5 Hydrotherapy . . . 452
15.1.6 Therapeutic Exercise . . . 452
15.1.7 Other Modalities . . . 453
15.2 Rehabilitation in Chronic Cases and Muscular Contracture . . . 453
15.3 Assessment and Monitoring . . . 454
15.4 Chapter 15: Sample Questions . . . 455
References . . . 455

**Chapter-Wise Answers for Objective Questions** . . . 457

# About the Authors

**Hari Prasad Aithal** is a Principal Scientist at Training and Education Centre, ICAR-Indian Veterinary Research Institute, Pune (Maharashtra), India. He has earlier served as a Scientist, Senior Scientist, and Principal Scientist in the Division of Surgery at ICAR-IVRI, Izatnagar, Bareilly (Uttar Pradesh) from 1993 to 2015. He has more than 30 years of experience in research, postgraduate teaching, training, clinical practice, and extension activities. His main domain of research had been orthopedic surgery. His significant contribution in developing novel fracture fixation techniques and devices has resulted in awarding six fracture fixation design registrations and one Indian patent. Further, two external fixation systems developed by him for large animals have been commercialized.

As a teacher, he has taught several courses to PG students. He has published more than 280 research/clinical papers in Indian and international scientific journals of repute, with more than 2140 citations. He has organized numerous training programs, especially on fracture fixation techniques, for veterinary graduates, officers, and practitioners. He has been the Associate Editor/Editor/ Executive Editor of the *Indian Journal of Veterinary Surgery* for 20 years. Co-edited two textbooks and several training manuals, monographs, and book chapters. He has also served as a referee to various international journals, including *The Veterinary Journal*, *Veterinary Surgery*, *The Veterinary Record*, *Journal of Veterinary Medicine*, and *Journal of Small Animal Practice*. He has also been conferred with various awards, including Fellow of National Academy of Veterinary Sciences (India), Fellow of Indian Society for Veterinary Surgery, Best Teacher Award from IVRI Deemed University, Best Scientist Award from Indian Veterinary Association, Dr O Ramakrishna Oration Award and Dr Gajraj Singh Lifetime Achievement Award for Excellence in Veterinary Orthopaedic Surgery from Indian Society for Veterinary Surgery, and several best paper presentation and publication awards.

**Amar Pal** presently works as Principal Scientist, Division of Surgery, In-charge Referral Veterinary Polyclinic, and In-charge Anatomy Section at ICAR-Indian Veterinary Research Institute, Izatnagar, Bareilly (Uttar Pradesh), India. He has done pioneering research in veterinary anesthesia, pain management, urolithiasis, orthopedic surgery, and stem cell biology and therapy in animals. He has developed and registered six designs of orthopedic devices for animals and eight mobile apps on veterinary sciences topics. He has also patented one fixation device for long bone fractures in large animals. He has been a recipient of several awards, including Chancellor's Gold Medal, Vice-Chancellor's Gold Medal, Dr RPS Tyagi Oration Award, Ramani Ramchandran Award, Dr. SJ Angelo Award, Dr. AK Bhargava Gold Medal, Vetquinol Gold Medal, Best Teacher Award of the Institute, and many best paper presentation awards. He is a Fellow of the National Academy of Veterinary Sciences, the Indian Society for Veterinary Surgery, and the Indian Society for Advancement of Canine Practice. Dr. Amarpal has published more than 380 research and clinical papers in Indian and international journals of repute. He has also authored/edited three books and contributed several chapters in textbooks. He is also working as Editor-in-Chief of the *Indian Journal of Veterinary Surgery*.

**Prakash Kinjavdekar** is a Principal Scientist in the Division of Surgery at ICAR-Indian Veterinary Research Institute, Izatnagar, Bareilly (Uttar Pradesh), India. Earlier, he has served as Veterinary Assistant Surgeon in the Department of Animal Husbandry Rajasthan (India), Assistant Project Officer in Rajasthan Cooperative Dairy Federation, Scientist and Senior Scientist in the Division of Surgery at ICAR-IVRI, Izatnagar, Bareilly. He is an experienced teacher, researcher, and extension expert with a professional service of more than 31 years in the field of Veterinary Surgery and Radiology. His research interests had been regional anesthesia in ruminants and orthopedic surgery, which were acclaimed widely and referred to in textbooks on Anaesthesiology and Pharmacology. He has been conferred with various prestigious awards, notably SJ Anjelo Memorial Award, Dr. AK Bhargava Memorial Award (thrice), and Prof. SS Mishra Memorial Award for best papers published in different scientific journals, best paper presentation awards (10), and best poster presentation awards. He has served as a referee to several international and national journals. He has published more than 260 research articles in peer-reviewed Indian and international journals and authored or coauthored two books and many book chapters. He is a member of several national scientific societies and is a Fellow of the Indian Society for Veterinary Surgery.

**Abhijit M Pawde** presently works as a Principal Scientist and In-charge, Centre for Wildlife, ICAR-Indian Veterinary Research Institute, Izatnagar (Uttar Pradesh), India. Before joining as a Scientist in the Division of Surgery, he has earlier worked at Equus Stud Farm, Shirgaon, Pune (Maharashtra). Subsequently, he served as Senior Scientist, Principal Scientist, and Co-ordinator, Referral Veterinary Polyclinic, ICAR-IVRI. During 30 years of his illustrious career, he was actively involved in research, teaching, and clinical services. He was associated with several research projects, and his primary interest was in tissue regeneration and reconstruction, acupuncture, and physiotherapy. He has published more than 150 research papers in peer-reviewed Indian and international journals. Dr. Pawde has been honored as Fellow and Surgeon of the Year awards by the Indian Society for Veterinary Surgery. He has also been the recipient of several best paper presentations and best paper publication awards.

# 1 Basic Considerations

**Learning Objectives**

You will be able to understand the following after reading this chapter:

- Structure and types of the bone
- Development of the bone and regulation of bone growth
- Fracture biomechanics and classification of fracture
- Fracture healing (primary and secondary healing), factors affecting healing, and methods to enhance healing
- Implants and instruments used for fracture stabilization
- Examination of animals with fracture, emergency treatment, and first aid
- Anesthesia and pain management in animals with fracture
- Methods of fracture reduction and selection of fracture fixation technique

**Summary**

- Osteoblasts are bone-forming cells and are involved in the synthesis of proteoglycans and collagen fibrils and production of a mineralizable matrix.
- Calcium phosphate crystals deposited in the form of *hydroxyapatite* are the principal inorganic mineral of the bone, comprising about 75% of dry bone.
- The principal blood vessel supplying the bone is the nutrient artery, which enters the medullary cavity through the nutrient foramen and then bifurcates into the ascending and descending branches within the medullary cavity.
- Calcium metabolism is primarily regulated by three major hormones, parathyroid hormone (PTH), calcitonin (CT), and vitamin D.
- Bending, a combination of compression and tension, is one of the most common forces causing a fracture.
- Based on the direction of fracture line with respect to the long axis of the bone, fractures can be classified as transverse, oblique, spiral, comminuted, multiple, etc.
- Primary bone healing occurs directly by the formation of bone tissue, whereas secondary healing is characterized by the formation of cartilaginous or fibrous connective tissue first, which is subsequently replaced by the bone.
- 316L stainless-steel alloys (low carbon steel having chromium) are most widely

(continued)


H. P. Aithal et al., *Textbook of Veterinary Orthopaedic Surgery*,
https://doi.org/10.1007/978-981-99-2575-9_1

used for manufacturing orthopedic implants.

- Classical clinical signs of fracture in animals are acute non-weight-bearing lameness, soft tissue swelling, and crepitation at the site of fracture site; radiographic examination helps in confirmatory diagnosis.
- The initial care and management of an animal with fracture should include stabilization of the injured animal, dressing of the open wound, and immobilization of the fractured limb to prevent continued injury from the broken bone ends.
- Orthopedic procedures for fracture fixation are always painful due to manipulation of the injured bone and surrounding soft tissues; hence, perioperative pain alleviation therapy should be the priority in all cases, and it should be started before the start of surgery and should continue during surgery and postoperative period.
- Open reduction of fracture is indicated along with internal fixation, primarily in fractures with severe comminution and/or overriding of bone segments.
- The extent of soft tissue injury and open wound associated with fractures are important determinants of the timing and technique of surgical fixation.

## 1.1 Structure and Types of the Bone

The bone is a type of dense connective tissue, which forms the body skeleton. The bone acts as levers for muscles and thus helps in locomotion, gives shape to the body, and provides protective cavities for the vital organs [1]. The blood-forming cells present in the medullary cavity of bones help in formation of new blood cells (haemopoietic tissue), and mesenchymal stem cells help in tissue repair. Further, the bone also acts as mineral reservoir that can be drawn upon whenever required. The bone also plays an important role in acid-base balancing of the body. The bone mineral metabolism revolves around the bone tissues and cells, along with biochemical and endocrine reactions [2].

### 1.1.1 Components of the Bone

A bone has three major constituents, including osteogenic cells, organic matrix, and inorganic minerals [3]. The osteogenic cells contain osteoblasts, osteocytes, and osteoclasts (Fig. 1.1). The organic matrix, which forms about one third of the bone mass, contains predominantly collagen and proteoglycans. About two thirds of the bone is made up of minerals comprising of calcium phosphate crystals deposited in the form of hydroxyapatite [$Ca_5(PO_4)_3(OH)$].

#### 1.1.1.1 The Bone Cells

*Osteoblasts*: Osteoblasts develop from undifferentiated mesenchymal stem cells, also called as osteoprogenitor cells, present in the inner (cambium) layer of periosteum and the bone marrow. These bone-forming cells, present mostly on the periosteal and endosteal surfaces of an actively growing bone, are arranged in a monolayer. Osteoblasts can be morphologically diverse, usually cubic, round, flat, or cylindrical. They are relatively large fusiform cells (15–20 μ diameter) with alkaline cytoplasm that is due to the presence of a large number of nucleosomes and rough endoplasmic reticulum in their cytoplasm [4]. The cytoplasm contains a round or oval nuclei, which is lighter staining but bulky with 1–3 nucleoli. The osteoblasts regulate the mineral transport from the extracellular space to the osteoid seam and the site of mineralization. Osteoblasts are involved in the synthesis of proteoglycans and collagen fibrils and production of a mineralizable matrix. The osteoblasts eject the amorphous calcium phosphate into the extracellular space. The alkaline phosphatase produced by the osteoblasts is thought to initiate the process of mineralization. The amorphous calcium phosphate is transformed to crystalline

**Fig. 1.1** Bone cells: mesenchymal cell (**a**), osteoblast (**b**), osteocyte (**c**), and osteoclast (**d**)

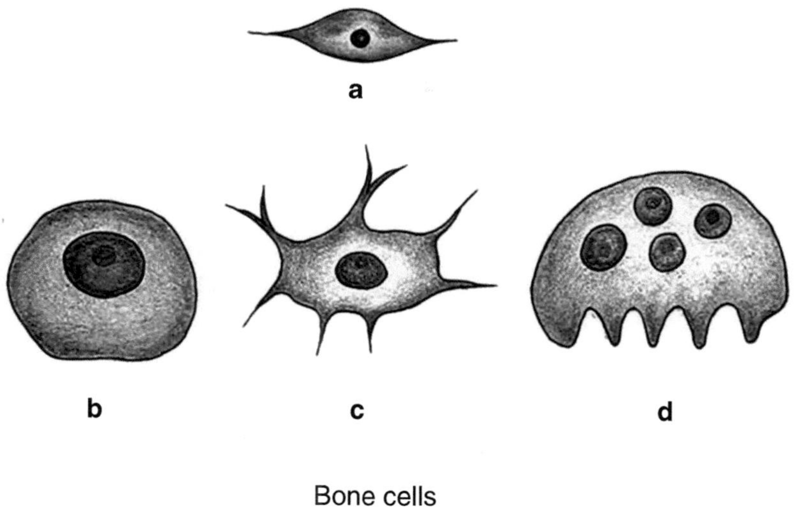


hydroxyapatite both inside and outside the matrix vesicles. When these crystals contact the vesicle membrane, it ruptures, and the exposure of released crystals to a supersaturated solution in the matrix induces their precipitation [5].

*Osteocytes*: About 10% of the osteoblasts get trapped within the lacunae of evolving bone matrix to become osteocytes [6]. They have faintly basophilic cytoplasm and a large oval nucleus with large chromatin granules. Osteocytes are surrounded by mineralized matrix and are interconnected by cytoplasmic processes through a canalicular system [7]. This interconnection of cells regulates the exchange of mineral ions between the extracellular fluid and the bone. Osteocytes are essential to the maintenance of the bone.

*Osteoclasts*: They are the large multinucleated cells found on the bone surfaces [8]. The cytoplasm is pale staining, acidophilic, and foamy. They are essentially seen at the site of remodeling and help in the removal of organic matrix and minerals. Osteoclasts produce acid phosphatase and collagenase, which help in dissolution and removal of the minerals and matrix. The osteoclasts absorb the degraded matrix products by endocytosis and are then ejected into the extracellular space.

#### 1.1.1.2 Organic Matrix

Organic matrix predominantly consists of type 1 collagen (95%) and proteoglycans (4%) and constitutes approximately one third of the bone mass [3]. Bone collagen is capable of calcifying, which is relatively insoluble in salt solutions and weak acids. The mucopolysaccharide (proteoglycan) is an amorphous jelly, which serves as a ground substance for binding of collagen fibers.

#### 1.1.1.3 Inorganic Mineral

The inorganic mineral of the bone, comprising about 75% of dry bone, is calcium phosphate crystals deposited in the form of hydroxyapatite [3]. As mineralization increases, the bone becomes less soluble and stiffer. Bone water is bound to the matrix, which occupies the spaces within the bone, like nutrient canals, the Haversian system, and the ultramicroscopic structures.

### 1.1.2 Structure of the Bone

Although all the bones are made up of the same constituents, the apparent density, porosity, and structure may differ among different bones and also at different locations within a bone. Based on the structure, bones are classified as cortical or compact bone (shaft bones) and cancellous or spongy bone (flat bones and ends of long bones). Based on the shape, the bones are classified as long bones (femur, tibia, humerus, etc.), short bones (carpals and tarsals), and flat bones (skull, pelvis, and ribs).

A typical long bone consists of a diaphysis at the middle and metaphysis and epiphysis on both

**Fig. 1.2** Structure of a long bone

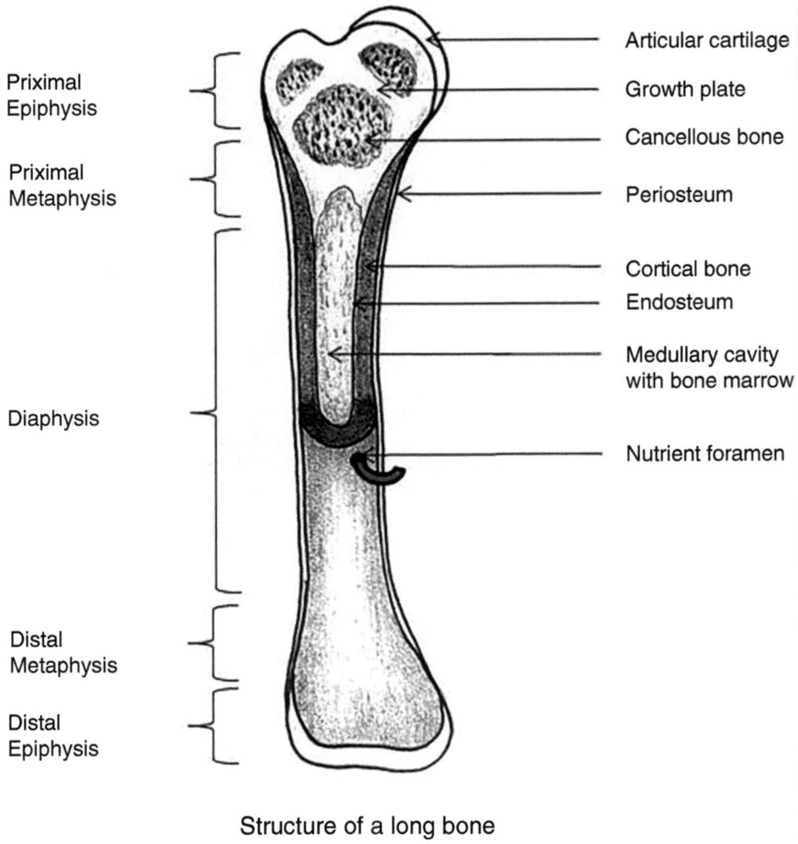


ends (Fig. 1.2). The diaphysis is a hollow tube of cortical bone, its central (medullary) cavity is lined by a layer of endosteum, and it contains the marrow. Haversian canals, which contain nerves and vessels, are distributed longitudinally in the cortex. These canals are surrounded by concentric layers of lamellae (Fig. 1.3). Lamellae have lacunae containing osteocytes, which are interconnected by microscopic channels called canaliculi (Fig. 1.4). The Haversian canals communicate with the medullary cavity through the Volkmann's canals. The basic structural unit of lamellae concentrically arranged around the Haversian canal is called an 'osteon'.

Epiphyseal growth plate (also known as physis) separates the metaphysis from the epiphysis in growing animals. When the animal attains maturity, the growth plate ceases to exist and the epiphysis fuses with the metaphysis. The metaphysis consists of spongy/cancellous bone with a network of fine trabeculae that are interconnected enclosing cavities that contain either hematopoietic (red, in young animals) or fatty (yellow, generally in old animals) marrow. A thin layer of cortical bone extends over the metaphysis. Small and flat bones also have similar spongy structure surrounded by a thin layer of dense bone.

The complete outer surface of the bone is covered by periosteum, except at the ends (joints), which is covered with articular (hyaline) cartilage. Periosteum has an inner cambium layer containing osteoprogenitor cells and an outer fibrous layer attached to the soft tissues surrounding the bone [9]. The osteoprogenitor cells present in the cambium layer multiply and contribute to bone healing during a fracture repair process. Hence, extreme care should be taken to avoid any damage to the periosteum during fracture fixation, especially during bone plate and screw fixation (periosteal stripping is contraindicated).

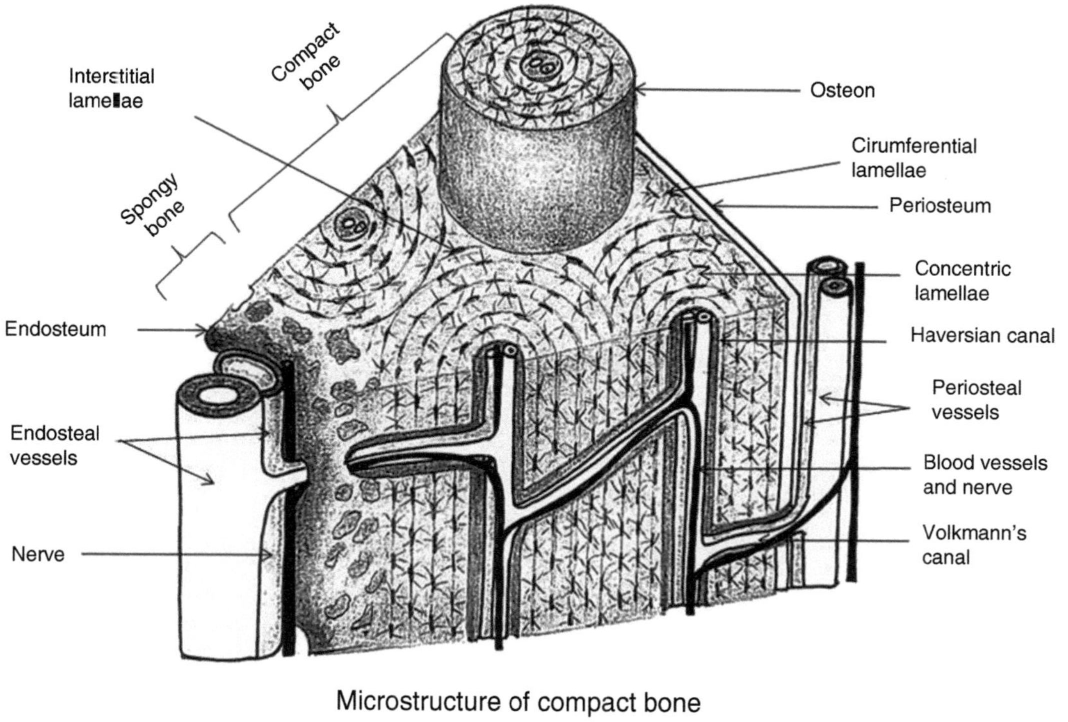


**Fig. 1.3** Microstructure of a compact bone

### 1.1.3 Circulation of the Bone

The bone is richly supplied with blood vessels. The vascular system of a mature long bone has three main components, i.e. afferent vascular system (arteries and arterioles), which carry nutrients; efferent vascular system (veins and venules), which carry waste products; and intermediate vascular system (capillaries in the cancellous bone and vessels in the canals of the cortical bone), which link the afferent and efferent systems [10].

**Fig. 1.4** Microstructure of an osteon

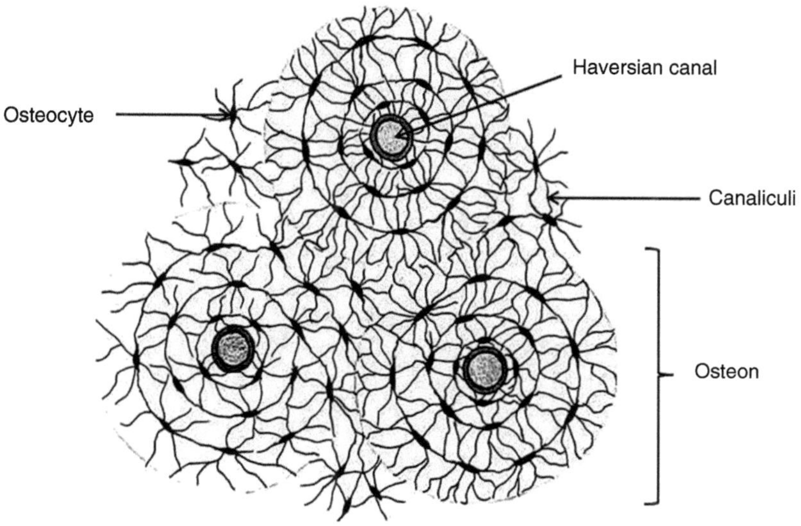

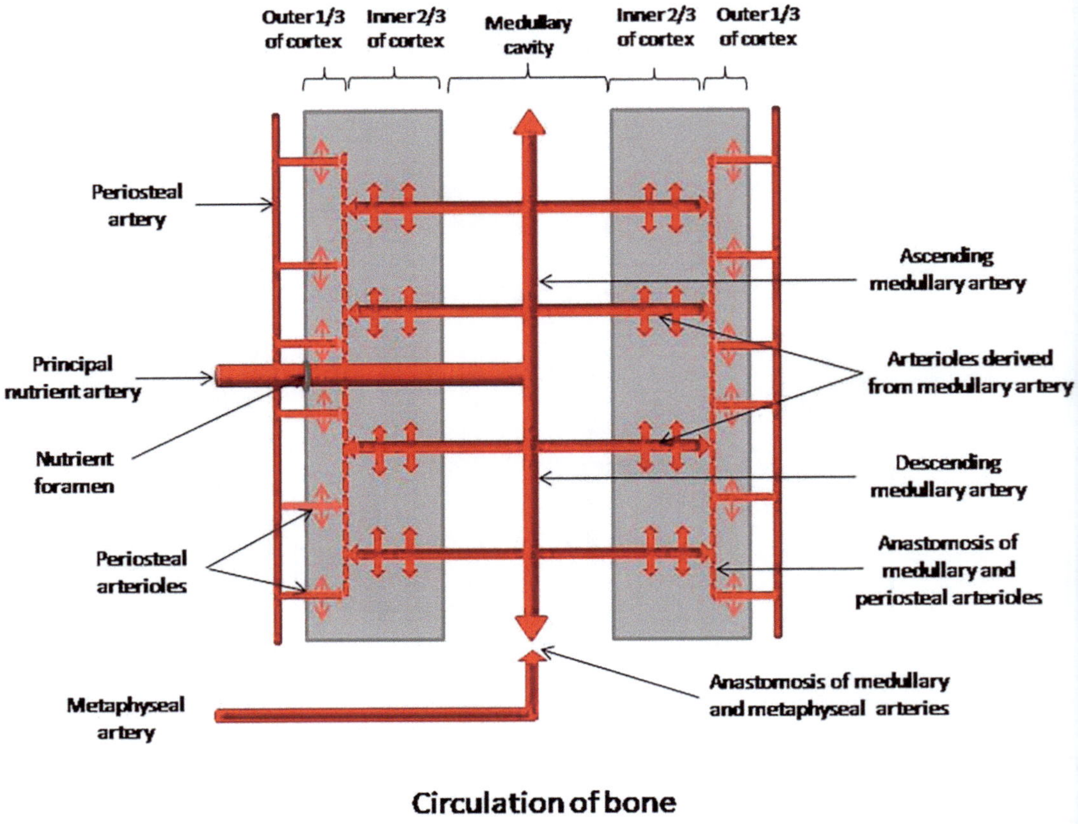


**Fig. 1.5** Circulation of the bone

The principal blood vessel supplying the bone is the nutrient artery, which penetrates the cortex and enters the medullary cavity through the nutrient foramen (Fig. 1.5). The nutrient artery bifurcates into the ascending and descending branches, which further give rise to many arterioles within the medullary cavity [11, 12]. The radiating arteriolar branches enter the endosteal surface of the cortex to supply at least inner two thirds of the cortex (centripetal in nature). Within the cortex, they give rise to branches forming capillaries within the Haversian system; some arterioles traverse the entire cortex to reach and anastomose with the periosteal arterioles. It should be noted that during intramedullary fixation of a long bone fracture, the nutrient artery, the major blood vessel supplying the bone, is most likely to get damaged completely. In such circumstances, the periosteal and metaphyseal arteries play a predominant role by compensating the vascular supply.

The second major vessels supplying the bone are metaphyseal arteries, which are multiple in number and enter the entire periosteal surface of the proximal and distal metaphyses. In young ones, metaphyses, epiphyses, and diaphysis have separate blood supply. Hence, more care should be exercised while treating metaphyseal and epiphyseal fractures in young animals; the techniques which would cause least damage to the epiphyseal plate and epiphyseal vessels should be preferred. In adults (after the fusion of epiphyseal plate), the metaphyseal vessels and the arteriolar branches of nutrient artery anastomose.

The periosteal arterioles originating from the surrounding soft tissues provide circulation to the outer one third of the bone cortex. Periosteal circulation plays a prominent role during fracture healing [13]. Hence, during fracture fixation, soft tissues around the fracture site should be handled carefully to minimize traumatic damage, and also, as far as possible, the soft tissues should not be detached from the bony cortex. The role of periosteal blood supply is also very important as an auxiliary source of blood flow to the entire cortex when there is interruption of supply from the intramedullary nutrient artery, as in the case of intramedullary fixation.

Major venous drainage (efferent vascular system) from a long bone includes metaphyseal vessels, which are a part of periosteal venous system. The cortical venous channels drain into the periosteal venules, which join the veins draining the muscles. A central venous sinus present in the medullary cavity receives transverse venous channels that transport blood from the sinusoids and then emerges from the diaphysis through the nutrient canal as the nutrient vein.

The blood vessels linking the afferent and efferent vascular systems constitute the intermediate vascular system. It comprises the vessels present in rigid canals within the compact long bone. These vessels carry the nutrients to the osteocytes through the canalicular system. The longitudinally directed channels in the Haversian canals are capable of carrying the blood for 1–2 mm length. Therefore, they have vascular connections with the medullary artery all along their course. The retraction of these vessels in the event of a fracture leads to avascular necrosis of bone ends.

## 1.2 Bone Development and Growth Regulation

### 1.2.1 Development of the Bone

The development of the bone starts in the embryonic stage from the mesenchymal tissue, which is a diffuse, loose cellular tissue present between the ectoderm and endoderm. Apart from the bone, other connective tissue structures such as the cartilage, fascia, tendon, ligament, etc. are also developed from differentiation of mesenchymal cells as per the need, condition, and local environment. In early stages of development, the skeletal structures appear as dense concentration of mesenchymal cells that tend to take the shape of the particular bones. Bones are developed either by endochondral or intramembranous ossification [14, 15]. In endochondral ossification, the bone is formed from a model of hyaline cartilage (e.g. long bones), whereas in intramembranous ossification, the bone is directly formed from connective tissue cells (e.g. bones of calvarium).

In endochondral ossification, mesenchymal cells differentiate into chondroblasts, forming a cartilagenous model of the bone, which increases in length and width by interstitial as well as appositional growth (Fig. 1.6). The process involves proliferation, maturation, and enlargement of chondrocytes forming the intercellular substance. The earliest chondrocytes at the center of the model mature, enlarge, and secrete alkaline phosphatase into the intercellular substance. As the cartilagenous cells mature and hypertrophy, and the matrix gets mineralized, the diffusion of nutrients to the chondrocytes is impeded causing cell death. The calcified matrix in the center of the model then disintegrates to form cavities. Simultaneously, vascular buds from the periosteum enter into the disintegrating cartilagenous area, bringing about mononuclear cells and mesenchymal stem cells, which translate into chondroclasts, osteoclasts, and osteoblasts. The ossification generally starts first at the middle of the cartilage model, known as 'primary ossification center' [16]. The process of resorption and replacement of cartilage by newly formed bone (cancellous type) continues along the length. The cancellous bone in the central part is resorbed to form a marrow or medullary cavity, which gets filled up with the myeloid tissue. At the same time, two more ossification centers develop one each in proximal and distal epiphysis replacing the cartilage. The process of endochondral ossification extends peripherally but does not replace all the cartilage; a portion remains on the surface as articular cartilage. Another transverse layer of the cartilage is retained between the epiphysis and metaphysis, which is called the physeal plate or growth plate. As the process of ossification proceeds from both ends, the bone continues

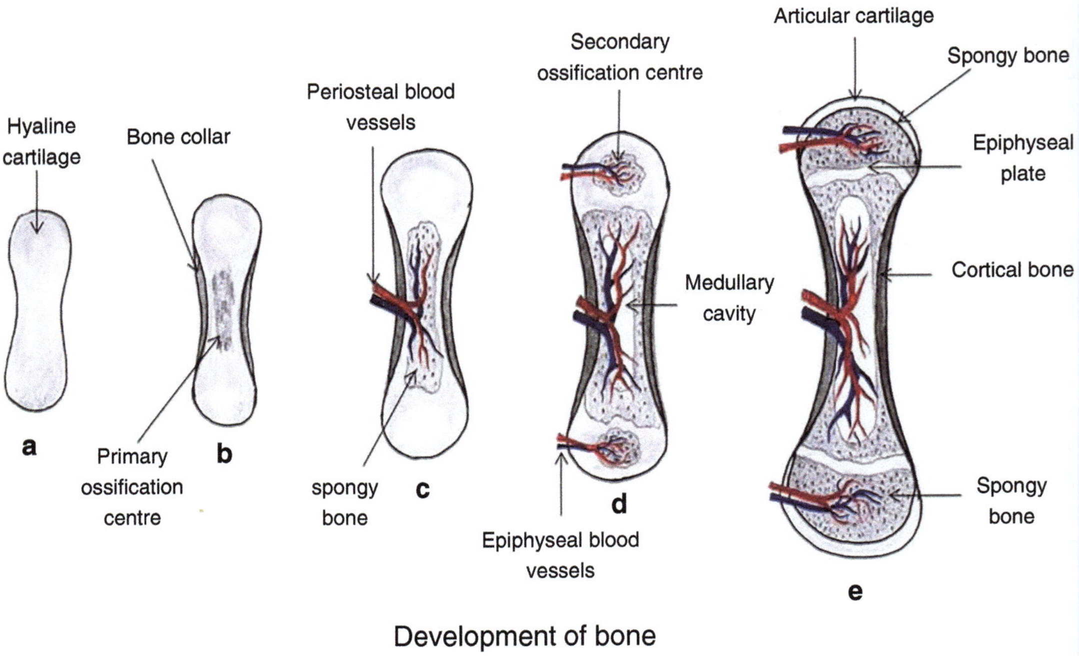


**Fig. 1.6** Development of a long bone (endochondral ossification): (**a**) cartilage model; (**b**) periosteal ossification and calcification of the cartilage at the mid-diaphysis (primary ossification center); (**c**) invasion of vascular mesenchyme, resorption of calcified cartilage, and laying down of new bone on either side; (**d**) further progress in vascular proliferation and laying down of the new bone and appearance of secondary ossification centers at the epiphyseal ends; and (**e**) growth of the bone by ossification from the diaphyseal and epiphyseal ossification centers. Note: cartilaginous growth plate (epiphyseal plate) separating the diaphysis and epiphysis in growing bone

to grow in length at the epiphyseal end through the epiphyseal plate, which remains active throughout the growing period by producing cartilage cells that in turn are replaced by bone cells. The longitudinal growth stops when the animal attains puberty; at that point of time, the growth plate ceases to exist as the metaphyseal and diaphyseal bones fuse together. Circumferential growth continues from the cambium layer of the periosteum by deposition of new bone.

The newly formed (woven) bone contains irregularly arranged bony spicules with more number of cells. The osteoclasts cut a hole in the bone (cutting cone), which progress longitudinally along the course of the vessel, producing the resorption cavity. Osteoblasts align on the walls and secrete concentric layers of mucopolysaccharides to fill the cavity leaving a small central (Haversian) canal that contains vessels and nerves. This process leads to the formation of true osteons with Haversian system. The osteogenic cells continue to add the bone to the surface and thus producing strong compact bony wall.

The bone directly formed from the mesenchymal model of flat bones is called intramembranous bone (e.g. cranial and facial). Intramembranous ossification begins when a cluster of mesenchymal cells directly differentiate into osteoblasts. These osteoblasts begin secreting the intercellular substance and get enclosed to become osteocytes. The actively secreting osteoblasts line the surface of the newly formed spicules of the bone, which continue to grow in a radial manner producing bony scaffold of trabeculae (cancellous bone). The spaces contained within the scaffolding trabeculae enclose the vascular myeloid tissue. The continued deposition of fresh bone lamellae on the trabeculae and appositional bone growth at the surface form the compact bone of inner and outer cortices. The surface connective tissue becomes the periosteum. Thus, a flat bone is formed as a layer of cancellous bone and marrow between the plates of compact bone.

## 1.2.2 Calcium Regulation

Calcium ion present in the bone is not only an essential structural component of the skeleton but also acts as mineral reservoir. It plays a vital role in many basic biological reactions such as enzyme activity, blood coagulation, muscle contraction, neuronal excitability, hormone release, and membrane permeability and is essential for maintenance of blood calcium level. Therefore, the exact control of calcium ion concentration in the skeleton as well as extracellular fluid is vital to the health of human beings and animals. This is possible through intake of balanced diet containing optimum levels of minerals and vitamins and endocrine control mechanisms involving primarily the three major hormones, parathyroid hormone (PTH), calcitonin (CT), and vitamin D [17–19].

### 1.2.2.1 Dietary Calcium and Phosphorus

The skeleton of the embryo first presents as a structure made of cartilage. At birth, only the middle part and the ends of the cartilage templates of long bones are ossified. Most of the bone growth (ossification and calcification) occurs in the early stage of animal's life through endochondral ossification; hence, mineral nutrition has to meet the increased demand of growing period, i.e. up to the age of about 1 year. Impaired supply of calcium, phosphorus, trace minerals, or vitamins may lead to skeletal abnormalities.

In growing dogs, calcium intake through the diet has to be maintained as per the growth rate and the age, starting with 550 mg/kg body weight daily after weaning, 300 mg during 5–6 months, and 140 mg/kg during 7–12 months, with an adequate Ca:P ratio of 1.2–1.5:1.0. Balanced diet formulation should have adequate minerals, which is important to ensure normal bone formation, and maintain the electrolyte balance and acid-base equilibrium. Vitamin D, which regulates calcium absorption and skeletal mineralization, is recommended at 20 IU/kg body weight/day for growth.

### 1.2.2.2 Calcium-Regulating Hormones

*Parathyroid hormone* (PTH) is released by chief cells of the parathyroid gland as a response to lowered blood calcium ion concentration (Fig. 1.7). Blood phosphorus level has no direct control over the synthesis and secretion of PTH; however, an elevated blood phosphorus level may indirectly lead to parathyroid gland stimulation as it can lower the blood calcium level.

PTH helps to mobilize calcium ions from the skeletal reserve into the extracellular fluid (ECF). In the kidney, it reduces absorption of phosphate leading to phosphaturia. Further, it increases urinary excretion of $K^+$ and increases $Ca^+$ absorption. It also regulates the conversion of 25-hydroxycholecalciferol to bioactive 1, 25 Di OH-CC and other metabolites of vitamin D.

Prolonged reduction in the dietary intake of calcium or imbalance in the calcium-phosphorus ratio in the diet in growing animals leads to hypocalcaemia, which stimulates the parathyroid gland, leading to secondary hyperparathyroidism. In such a condition, there will be progressive depletion of minerals from the skeleton causing osteopenia/osteoporosis and may lead to pathological bone fractures.

*Calcitonin* (CT) is secreted by C cells of the thyroid gland. The increased concentration of calcium ion in the plasma and ECF enhances the secretion and release of CT. The release of CT causes hypocalcaemia by temporarily inhibiting the PTH-stimulated bone resorption. CT also brings about hypophosphataemia by increasing the movement of phosphate from the plasma into the soft tissues and bone and also due to inhibition of bone resorption. The action of CT does not depend on vitamin D.

*Vitamin D (cholecalciferol)* is normally ingested only in small quantities in the diet but largely synthesized in the epidermis through precursor molecules like 7-dehydrocholesterol, the reaction catalyzed by UV irradiation (Fig. 1.8). The cholecalciferol is transmitted from the skin

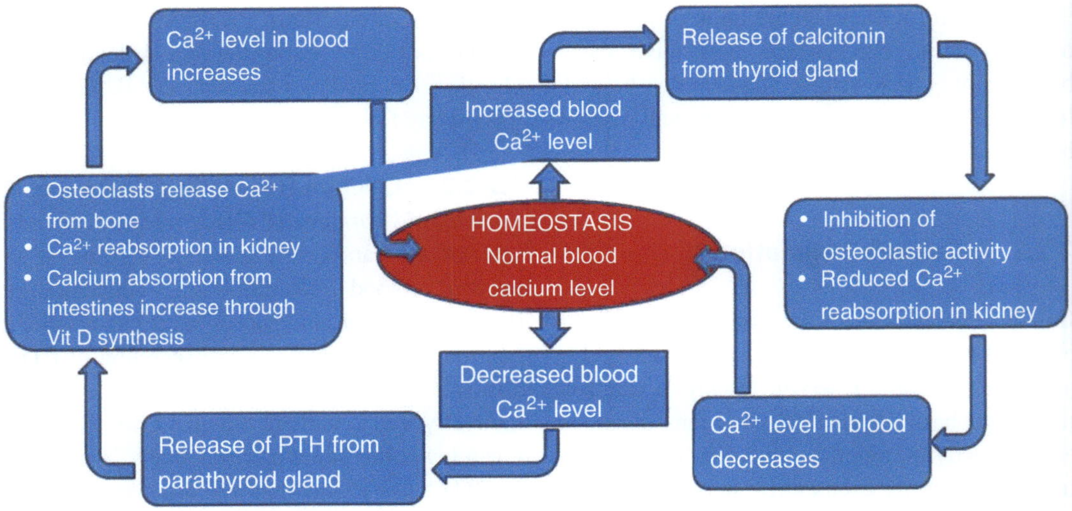


**Fig. 1.7** Calcium homeostasis: decreased calcium level in the blood stimulates the parathyroid gland to release PTH, which in turn helps maintain blood calcium level by its action on the bone (increased osteoclastic activity), the kidney (increased reabsorption of calcium), and the intestines (calcium absorption); increased blood calcium level releases calcitonin from the thyroid gland, which helps decrease blood calcium level by its action on the bone (inhibit osteoclastic activity) and the kidney (reduced calcium reabsorption)

into the blood through vitamin D-binding protein. Unlike many other mammals, dogs and cats are unable to synthesize vitamin D through cutaneous sun exposure, and therefore, they are dependent on its dietary intake [20]. Cholecalciferol gets converted to 25-hydroxycholecalciferol (25 OH-CC) in the liver with the help of an enzyme calciferol-25-hydroxylase. 25-OH-CC gets metabolized to an active form 1, 25, dihydroxycholecalciferol; the process is catalyzed by 25-OH-CC 1α-hydroxylase enzyme in the kidney. The formation of 1, 25-DiOH-CC is accelerated by PTH and low blood $Ca^+$ and $P^+$ levels but suppressed by high blood $P^+$ levels. However, a negative feedback exists whereby vitamin D metabolites decrease PTH secretion and thereby reduce the formation of 1, 25-DiOH-CC. During growth, somatotropin may also enhance the activity of 1α-hydroxylase.

Vitamin D helps in the absorption of calcium and phosphorus from the intestinal mucosa, thereby maintains sufficient levels of $Ca^+$ and $P^+$ in the ECF, and helps in mineralization of the bone matrix [20]. In growing animals, vitamin D is essential for mineralization of physeal (growth plate) cartilage and thereby longitudinal growth of bone. Vitamin D deficiency leads to a condition called rickets, wherein the physeal cartilage fails to mineralize and ossify leading to broadening of the physis (unhindered multiplication of cartilage tissue), weakening of long bones, and stunted growth. In adults, it is required for osteoclastic resorption and calcium mobilization from the bone. In the kidneys, vitamin D stimulates the tubular resorption of calcium. In chronic kidney disease, failure to form active form of vitamin D results in a condition called 'renal rickets', wherein there is softening of the facial bones, leading to 'rubber jaw' condition.

## 1.3 Fracture Biomechanics and Classification

In recent years, several advances have taken place in the area of fracture repair, which were mostly attributed to greater research focus on surgical anatomy, physiology, and biomechanics related to the skeletal system and fracture fixation. An orthopedic surgeon needs to better understand the

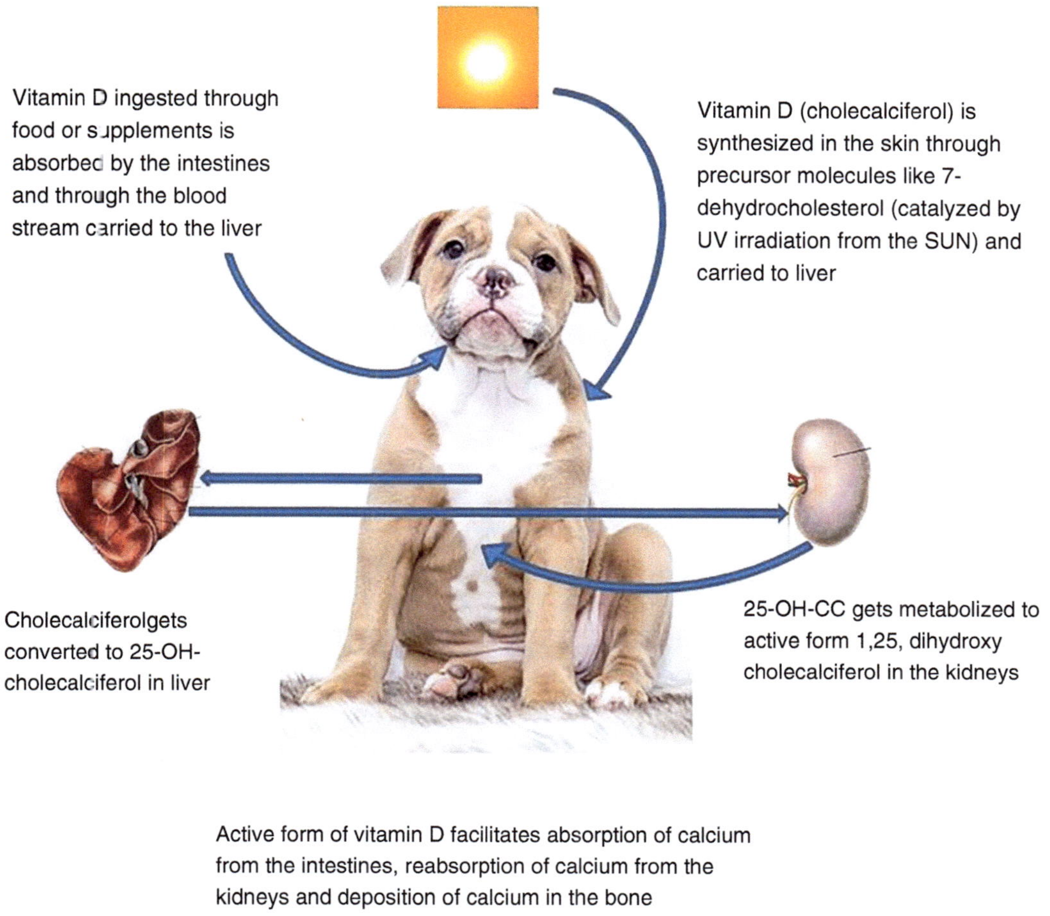


**Fig. 1.8** Illustration detailing the role of vitamin D in calcium metabolism and homeostasis

fracture biology, the principles of implant use, and the bone's response to those implants, rather than simply learning a specific technique for a particular fracture. As *Prof. R.J. Boudrieau* puts it, fracture repair has now become more of a 'science' than an 'art' [21].

Basic understanding of biomechanics related to normal bone, fracture etiology, treatment, and implants used for fracture immobilization helps in better assessment and management of fractures [22, 23]. Force, a basic concept of mechanics, is anything that tends to change the state of a structure with respect to motion or its conformation. When force is applied to a bone, it results in deformation of its structure and generation of internal forces within. The intensity of internal force (force per unit area) at any given point and plane is called as stress, and the deformation (change in unit length) resulting from this internal force is called strain. The stress-strain curve (representing an object's material properties) is similar to that of the force-deformation curve (representing an object's structural properties) and has elastic and plastic regions, a yield point and a failure point or ultimate strength (Fig. 1.9). Each increment of stress/load applied to an object is accompanied by a corresponding change in length, i.e. strain. The bone acts as a linear elastic solid in this region of the stress-strain curve; the slope of the linear elastic region is called as Young's modulus of elasticity.

The mechanical behavior of the bone as well as the fixation implants can be described using two important parameters, i.e. modulus or

**Fig. 1.9** Typical stress-strain curve of a long bone

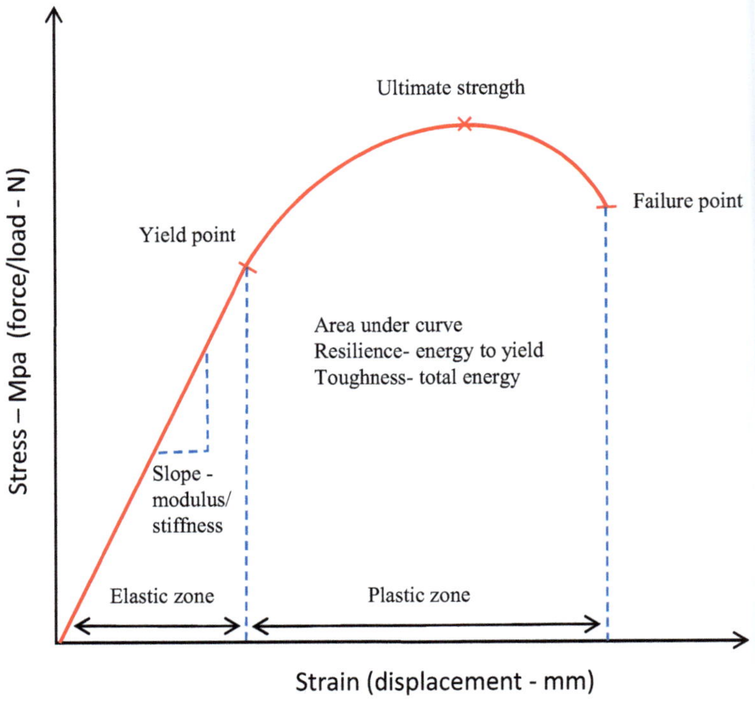


stiffness and strength. The modulus is a measure of the amount of elastic deformation an object undergoes when subjected to loads. Low modulus materials are likely to deform more than high modulus materials when subjected to similar loads. Strength is the ability of a material to sustain the applied load prior to its failure.

### 1.3.1 Mechanical Properties of the Bone

There are several factors which influence the mechanical properties of the bone [22]:

1. *Bone density*: The apparent density (mass of tissue per unit volume) of the bone (g/ml) is directly related to its mineral content and porosity. Porosity varies from 5% to 30% in cortical bone and 30 to 90% in cancellous bone. Apparent density, porosity, and mineralization all have a significant effect on the stress-strain behavior of a bone. Even a little change in the apparent density of the bone will lead to significant difference in the modulus and strength. Generally, it is difficult to radiographically visualize a change until the bone density is altered by 30–50%; hence, one can imagine the magnitude of change in the stiffness and strength of the bone which is apparently osteopenic.
2. *Age of bone*: The bones of immature/young animals have the ability to absorb more energy and elastically deform before failure; hence, greenstick/folding fractures are often seen in such bones. As the age advances, the bone tissue becomes stiffer and stronger. Advanced aging results in decline in bone strength and stiffness (due to increased porosity) as well as energy-absorbing capacity (due to increased collagen cross linking and mineralization); hence, more comminuted fractures occur due to brittleness of the bone.
3. *Mode of loading*: Long bones owing to orthotopic placement are stronger along their long axis and weaker perpendicular to the axis. Thus, a long bone is strongest under

compression, weak under bending, and weakest under tension. Compressive strength of cancellous bone is lower than that of cortical bone.
4. *Rate of loading*: A bone when subjected to sudden or rapid stress exhibits higher elastic modulus and ultimate strength than when subjected to slow or gradual loading over a period of time. The materials whose mechanical characteristics depend on the rate of applied strain, such as the bone, are called viscoelastic.
5. *Direction of loading*: The bone is anisotrophic in nature, i.e. its material properties differ in different directions. Long bones can better resist stresses applied along their longitudinal axis (along the osteonal orientation) than perpendicular to their axis. Further, long bone when loaded in a direction perpendicular to their long axis is more likely to fail in brittle (crackly) manner with little plastic deformation. Hence, when a dog's limb is hit hard by a stick, it is more likely to result in comminuted fracture.

The bone is constantly subjected to different types of loads, in the form of weight bearing or otherwise. As per the functional requirement, the bone undergoes remodeling continuously to change its shape and internal architecture depending on the applied load (Wolff's law). The ends of long bones made of cancellous bone are adopted to absorb the energy and compressive stress generated by weight bearing and distribute them to the rest of the bone. The metaphyseal region is made thicker than other regions to compensate for the weakness of cancellous bone against compressive stress. Smaller diameter in the middle of the long bone reduces the strain in bending and increases its ability to elastic/plastic deformation without leading to a fracture. As age advances, the cortices of long bones become thinner and weaker, but nature compensates it by increasing the outer diameter. A cylindrical shape is better able to resist torsional forces, and a square shape is ideal for resisting bending forces applied along its sides; therefore, the shape of a long bone is a combination of square, triangular, and round, based on the forces they are subjected to. Similarly, the diaphysis of long bone is tubular, which is better able to resist torsional and bending stresses than a solid cylinder. Thus, the shapes of different long bones are ideally designed to uniformly resist different forces applied in all directions.

### 1.3.2 Fracture Forces

The bone has inherent capacity to resist the applied load, sudden overloading, or sustained loading, but over a period of time, these may cause injury and result in the breakage of bone, a fracture. Fracture pattern (type) is characteristic to the applied load, and its understanding would give an insight into the nature of trauma and could be useful in fracture management. There are five basic forces which may act to cause a fracture (Fig. 1.10). During a trauma, however, it is generally a combination of forces acting simultaneously to cause a fracture [22, 23]:

1. *Compression*: Compression occurs when two apposing forces approach one another on the same plane. When a load is applied along the bone, the plane perpendicular to the load experiences maximum compressive stress; hence, normally a transverse fracture is anticipated. However, due to anisotropic nature of the bone, fracture occurs obliquely along the lines of generated shear stress. Fractures produced by compression stress are often seen at the metaphyseal region of long bones as impacted fracture (fracture is visible as a line of increased bone density) and also as compression fracture in the vertebrae (characteristically shortened vertebra as compared to adjoining vertebrae). Such fractures are common when an animal suddenly jumps/falls from a height.
2. *Tension*: Tension fracture occurs when two opposing forces act on the bone through one plane. Maximum tensile stress occurs along the plane perpendicular to the applied load resulting in pulling out of osteons leading to

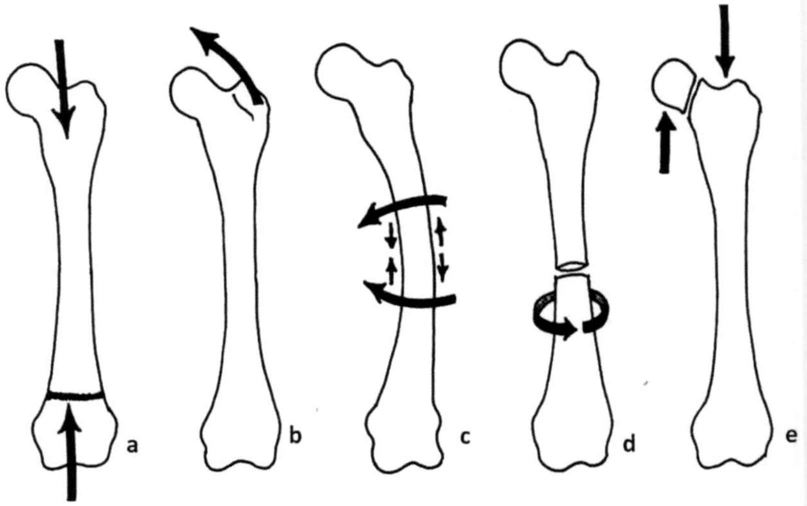


**Fig. 1.10** Fracture forces: (**a**) compression, (**b**) tension, (**c**) bending, (**d**) torsion, and (**e**) shear

a transverse fracture. Sudden pull/stretch from the attached tendon results in tensile force, causing avulsion of bony prominences (usually at traction apophyses), especially in young age where there is incomplete bony fusion at the growth plate. Common sites of avulsion fracture are tuber calcis, olecranon process, and tibial tuberosity, which can be diagnosed by the presence of widening/gaping at the growth plate (wider and irregular radiolucent line) and loss of outer contour of the bony prominence.

3. *Bending*: Bending, a combination of compression and tension, is one of the most common forces causing a fracture. When a bending force overcomes the elastic limit of the bone, a crack develops in the cortex opposite to the applied force (convex/tension side) that gradually continues toward the opposite cortex (concave/compression side) leading to a complete fracture. The fractures caused by bending force are generally short oblique or transverse. Such fractures can occur in different long bones when an animal suddenly falls or jumps from a height or suddenly steps into a dig or hole while running. In hindlimbs, fractures due to bending stress occur more frequently around the stifle joint (distal femur and proximal tibia), and in forelimbs, it is frequently seen at the distal radius-ulna.
4. *Shearing*: When a force transmitted along the axis of a bone acts on a portion of the same bone that lies peripheral to the long axis, it may shear off a portion of the bone. A shearing force can also be transmitted across the joint to other bones. The fracture line caused by the shearing forces is parallel to the direction of the force. Such fractures generally occur during fall/jump from a height. If the animal lands on forelimbs, the axial compression forces are transmitted up along the antebrachium leading to shearing off of the lateral condyle of the humerus. When an animal happens to land on the hindlimb during a fall, it sometimes may cause shearing off of the femoral head and neck.
5. *Torsion*: When a bone is twisted along its long axis, in situations when one end of a bone is fixed and other end is forced to rotate, the bone will be generally subjected to torsional force. The bone subjected to torsional loading leads to spiral fracture due to the combined effects of both shear and tensile stresses. Such fractures are more often seen in the tibia and humerus.

When a bone is loaded, it absorbs the kinetic energy; and upon further loading to failure, the stored energy is released and dissipated through breaking of the bone. In case of a minor trauma, simple two-piece fracture may occur releasing only little amount of energy, whereas during a major trauma (rapid loading with high strain), the bone absorbs greater energy, and sudden release of energy results in comminution (splintering) of the bone with extensive soft tissue injuries. Comminuted fractures are usually caused by complex loading modes and hence result in diverse and complicated fracture patterns. When a bone is subjected to repetitive suboptimal cyclic loads well below that necessary to produce failure by a single load application, the resulting fracture is called a fatigue or stress fracture. Changes in the bone structure or density (as in neoplasia, osteoporosis, secondary hyperparathyroidism, etc.) may also act as stress risers and cause pathological bone fractures when subjected to loads well below the optimal load required to cause a fracture in otherwise normal situations. Stress concentration may also occur when there is elastic modulus mismatch between the bone and implant. Such fractures are generally seen in the diaphysis at the end of the rigid bone plate or a cemented prosthesis. Hence, very rigid implant fixation should be avoided especially in osteoporotic bones, and also, the implant (e.g. a bone plate) should span the whole length of the bone to evenly distribute the stress and avoid stress concentration at the bone-implant junction.

### 1.3.3 Classification of Fracture

'A classification is useful only if it considers the severity of the bone lesion and serves as a basis for treatment and for evaluation of the results' *Maurice E Müller* [24]. Proper classification of fracture not only helps the surgeon to decide the technique of fracture fixation to be used but also predict the possible outcome. Fractures can be classified in many ways.

Based on the connection of fracture site with the outside environment, fracture can be classified as simple (closed) or compound (open). A simple fracture has intact skin, and hence, it is not directly exposed to the environment, whereas a compound fracture is exposed to the outside environment through an open wound in the skin.

Based on the extent of fracture line, a fracture can be classified as incomplete or complete. An incomplete greenstick fracture is more common in immature bones under bending stress. The cortex under the tension side (convex) fractures completely, while the cortex under the compression side (concave) remains intact. In a complete fracture, there will be complete loss of bony continuity with separation and frequently overriding of bone segments.

Based on the direction of fracture line with respect to the long axis of the bone, fracture can be classified as transverse, when the fracture line is transverse to the long axis of the bone (commonly results from bending stress); oblique, fracture line is oblique to the long axis of the bone (generally results from bending stress with axial compression); spiral, fracture line spirals along the long axis of the bone (generally results from rotational or torsion forces); comminuted, two or more fracture lines interconnect to form at least three fracture fragments (generally results from high-energy trauma like automobile accidents); and multiple, two or more fracture lines exist, but they do not interconnect leading to three or more fracture fragments, i.e. two or more separate fractures in the same bone (Fig. 1.11).

Based on the type and extent of deviation/displacement of fracture segments, fracture can be called as impacted fracture, when a cortical fragment is forced/impacted into a cancellous segment (occurs due to compression force at the junction of the diaphysis and metaphysis of long bones); compression fracture, cancellous bone collapses and compresses upon itself (usually occurs in vertebral bodies); and avulsion fracture, a part of the bone (generally apophysis) is torn/avulsed away due to powerful pull of a muscle/tendon attached to it.

Based on its location, fracture can be classified as diaphyseal fracture, at the proximal, middle or distal third of the diaphysis; metaphyseal fracture, either proximal or distal metaphyseal; epiphyseal fracture, either proximal or distal; fracture of the epiphyseal plate, can be proximal or distal epiphyseal plate fracture, which can further be classified as Salter-Harris type I (separation of the epiphysis from the metaphysis at the physeal plate), Salter-Harris type II (separation of a small piece of the metaphyseal bone along with

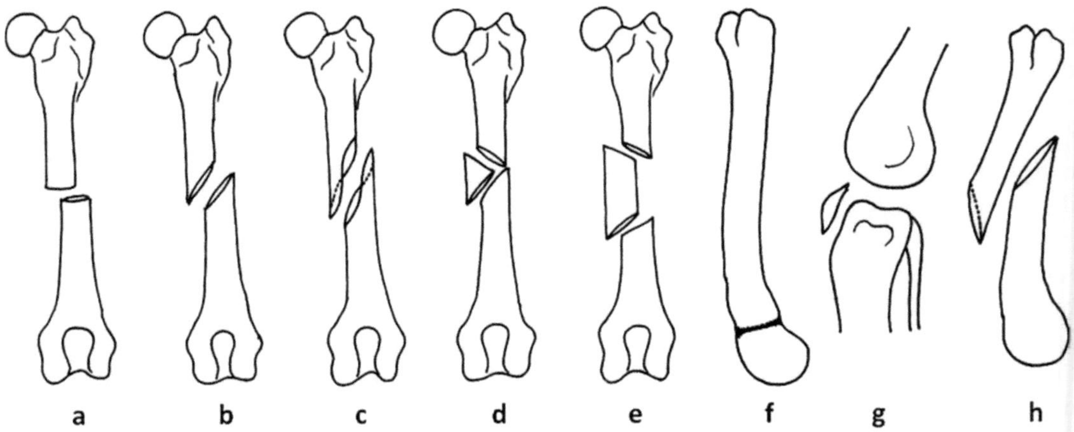


**Fig. 1.11** Fracture types: (**a**) transverse, (**b**) oblique, (**c**) spiral, (**d**) comminuted, (**e**) multiple, (**f**) impacted, (**g**) avulsion, and (**h**) overriding fracture

the epiphysis from the metaphysis at the physeal plate), Salter-Harris type III (fracture of the epiphysis and physeal plate without affecting the metaphysis), Salter-Harris type IV (fracture involving the epiphysis, physeal plate and metaphysis), and Salter-Harris type V (impaction of the physeal plate with the metaphysis driven into the epiphysis) (Fig. 1.12); condylar fracture, a fracture of the metaphysis, physis, and epiphysis together is called as condylar fracture and commonly occurs in immature animals and affects the distal ends of the humerus, femur, and proximal tibia (if both condyles are fractured and separated from the shaft, it is called as supracondylar fracture, and if a fracture occurs separating the medial and lateral condyles, it is called as intercondylar fracture); and articular fracture, a fracture involving the subchondral bone and articular cartilage.

*AO/OTA classification*: A comprehensive system of fracture classification has been developed by the AO (Arbeitsgemeinschaft für Osteosynthesefragen) Foundation or the Association of the Study of Internal Fixation (ASIF) group and the Orthopaedic Trauma Association (OTA). In this system, a fracture is classified based on the extent of severity and complexity of the fracture, difficulty in treatment, and worsening prognosis. The system includes a five-element alphanumeric code, which allows for a detailed and consistent description of a fracture using specific terminology [25].

In AO classification, the first digit denotes the bone: 1, humerus; 2, radius/ulna; 3, femur; 4, tibia/fibula; etc. The second digit denotes the fractured bone segment: 1, proximal end; 2, diaphyseal; 3, distal end; and 4, malleolar (precisely, the proximal and distal end segments are defined as a square having same length sides equal to the widest part of the epiphysis/metaphysis, and between them is the diaphysis) (Fig. 1.13).

Alphabetical letters A, B, and C describe the fracture morphology; for diaphyseal fractures, they denote simple, no comminution of bone segments (A); wedge, comminuted fragments, but contact between the main bone segments restores bone length after reduction (B); and multifragmentary, multiple fracture lines not connected to each other with many fracture fragments (C); for proximal and distal end fractures, they denote extra-articular (A), partial articular (B), and complete articular (C). Morphologically, each type is further divided into 2–3

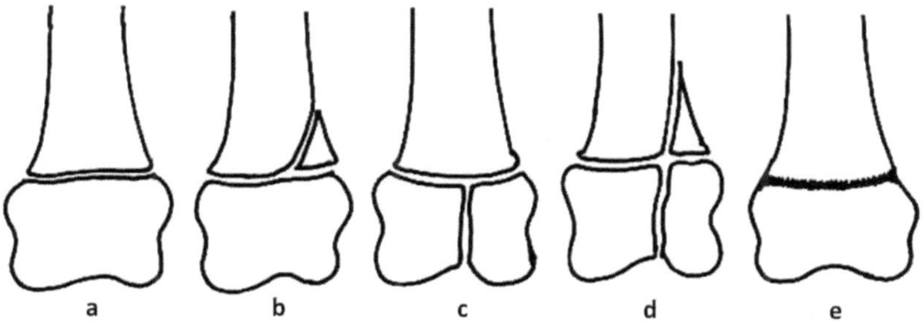


**Fig. 1.12** Salter-Harris classification of epiphyseal fractures: type I (**a**), type II (**b**), type III (**c**), type IV (**d**), and type V (**e**) fractures

groups as per the increasing severity and complexity of fracture, difficulty in treatment, and the prognosis. Based on fracture pattern, diaphyseal simple fractures (A) are further classified as spiral (1), oblique (2), and transverse (3) (Fig. 1.14); wedge fractures (B) are classified as intact (2) and fragmentary (3) (Fig. 1.15); and multifragmentary fractures (C) are classified as intact segmental (2) and fragmentary segmental (3) (Fig. 1.16). End segment fractures can be extra-articular, partial articular, or complete articular (Fig. 1.17). Proximal and distal end extra-articular fractures (A) are classified as avulsion (1), simple (2), and wedge or multifragmentary (3); partial articular fractures (B) are classified as simple (1), split

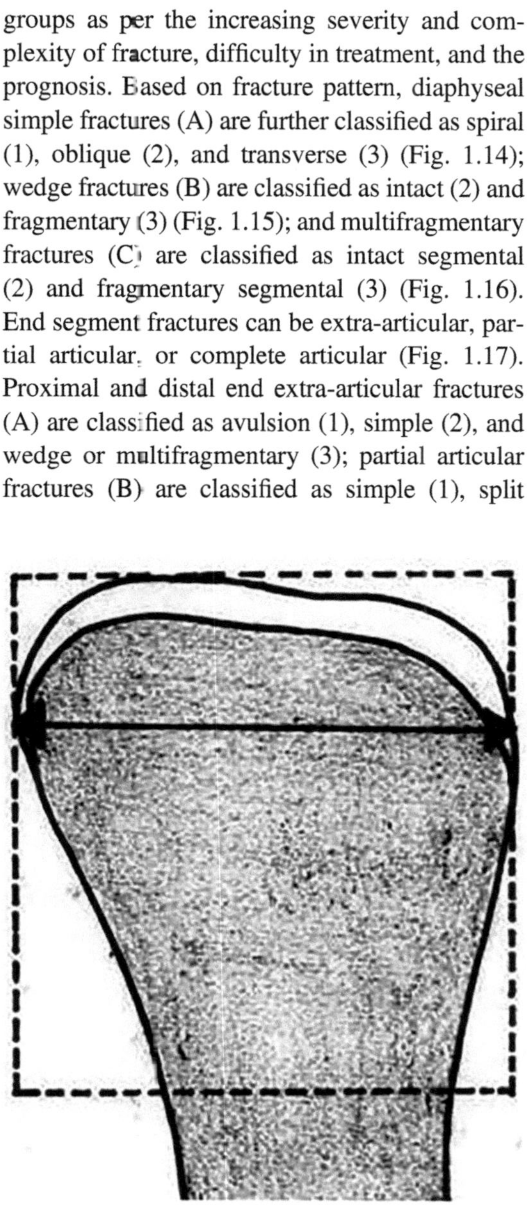

**Fig. 1.13** AO classification of fracture: definition of proximal (1), diaphyseal (2), or distal end (3) segment

and/or depression (2), and fragmentary (3); and complete articular fractures (C) are classified based on articular fracture pattern as simple (1) and multifragmentary (2). Complete articular fractures (C) are subgrouped based on the metaphyseal fracture pattern as simple articular with simple metaphyseal (1), simple articular with multifragmentary metaphyseal (2), and multifragmentary articular with multifragmentary metaphyseal (3).

Some exceptions have been described for the proximal end fractures of the humerus and femur. Simple proximal humeral fractures involving one tuberosity or the metaphysis and proximal femoral fractures involving the trochanter are classified as type A. The partial articular type does not exist in the humerus or femur. Proximal humeral fracture involving one tuberosity and the metaphysis and the proximal femoral fracture involving the femoral neck are classified as type B. Proximal humeral articular fractures involving the humeral neck and fractures involving the femoral head are type C.

For detailed description of the fracture morphology, displacement, location, and associated injuries if any that are general to most fractures, the universal modifiers (such as non-displaced, displaced, impaction, non-impaction, dislocation, etc.) have been described, which are optional. Universal modifiers may be added to the end of the fracture code within square brackets [ ]. Similarly, the fracture qualifications are descriptive terms of fracture morphology or location that are specific to each fracture and are applied as asterisk as a lower case letter within a round bracket () to the end of the fracture code.

*Alphanumeric structure of the AO/OTA classification can be summarized as:*

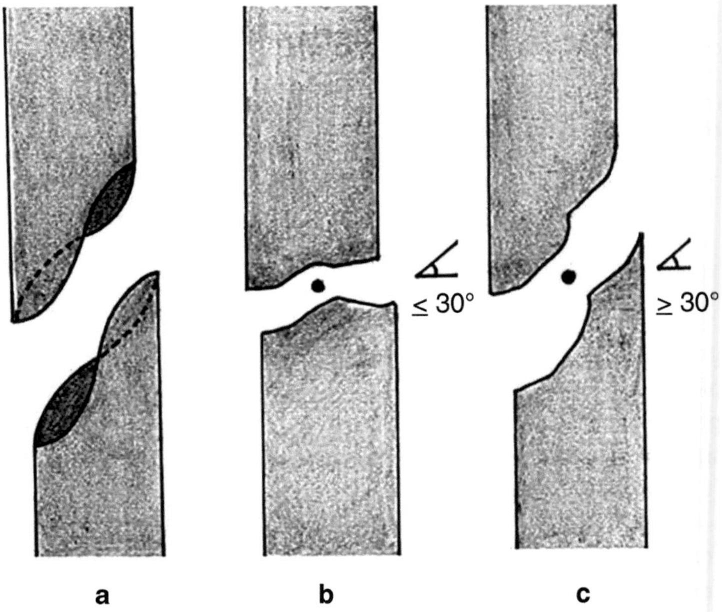


**Fig. 1.14** AO classification of simple diaphyseal fractures based on fracture pattern: spiral (1), oblique (2), and transverse (3)

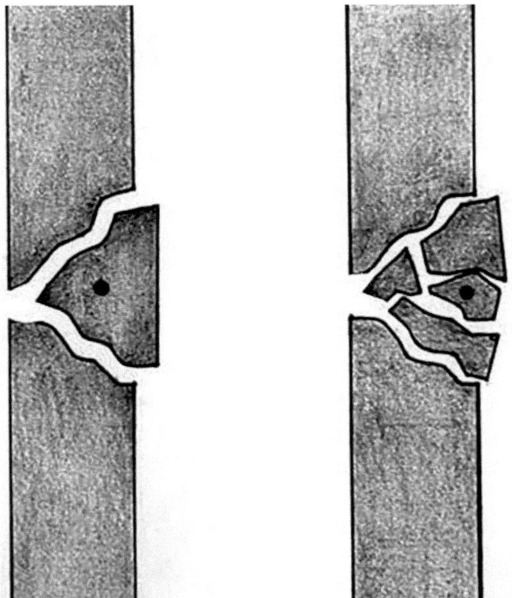


**Fig. 1.15** AO classification of wedge fractures: intact (1) and fragmentary (2)

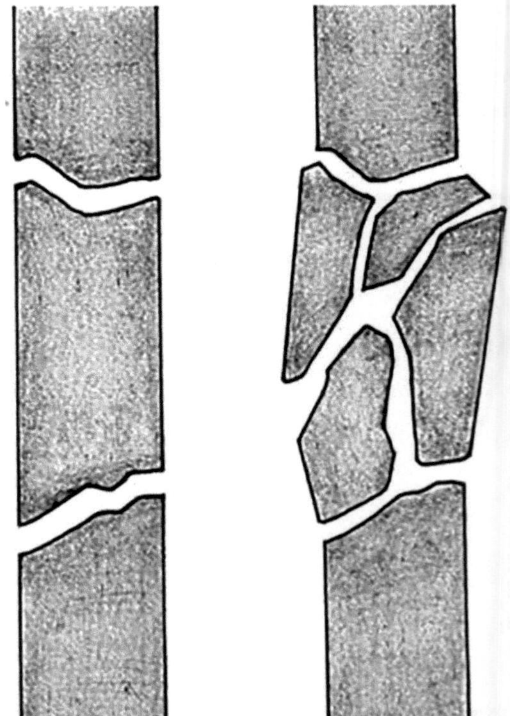


**Fig. 1.16** AO classification of multifragmentary fractures: intact segmental (1) and fragmentary segmental (2)

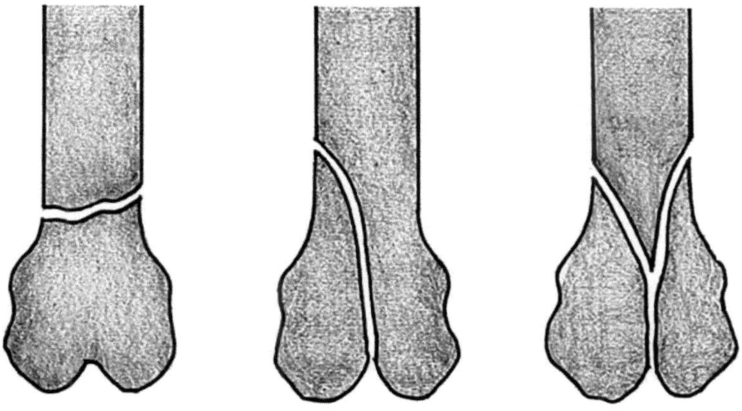


**Fig. 1.17** AO classification of end segment fractures: extracapsular (**a**), partial articular (**b**), and complete articular (**c**)

| Localization | | Morphology | | | | | |
|---|---|---|---|---|---|---|---|
| Bone | Location | Type | Group | . | Subgroup | (Qualifications) | [Universal modifiers] |
| 1/2/3/4/... | 1/2/3/ (4) | A/B/C | 1/2/3 | . | 1/2/3 | | |

Hence, in the example

| | | | | | |
|---|---|---|---|---|---|
| 3 | 3 | C | 2 | . | 3 |

Complete classification is given as 3, femur; 3, distal segment; C, complete articular; 2, multifragmentary; 3, multifragmentary articular with multifragmentary metaphyseal.

Hence, the above alphanumeric code can be read as 'multifragmentary complete articular with multifragmentary metaphyseal fracture of the distal femur'.

### 1.3.4 Incidence of Fractures

The fractures of long bones are common in both small and large animals [26, 27]. In dogs and cats, fractures are more frequent in hind quarters; the femur is the most commonly affected bone (about 30%), followed by the radius/ulna, tibia/fibula, and humerus. Fractures of metacarpals and metatarsals are also often seen. Fractures are caused mostly due to automobile accidents and falls/jumps from height. Hind quarter is more commonly trapped during road traffic accidents. Fractures due to jump/fall are generally centered around the stifle (middle/distal femur and proximal tibia) in hindlimbs and around the carpus (distal radius/ulna or proximal metacarpals) in forelimbs [28]. Automobile accidents generally lead to open comminuted fractures, whereas low-energy falls more often result in simple two-segment closed fractures [29].

In large animals, metacarpal and metatarsal fractures are more frequent (about 50%), followed by that of the tibia and radius/ulna. Fractures of the femur, humerus, pelvis, and phalanges are less common. The cause of fracture is mostly an automobile accident; in young calves and foals, they often occur due to trauma during dystocia or handling. In large animals, fractures are more often open and comminuted in nature. Heavy weight of animals and inadequate care during the immediate post-traumatic period lead to compounding of fractures, more often leading to gross contamination of open wounds.

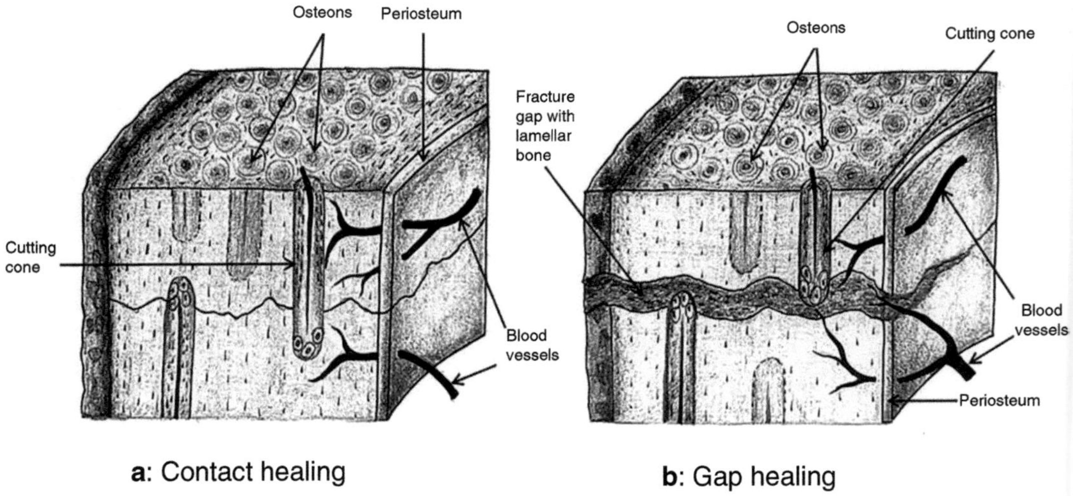


**Fig. 1.18** Types of primary bone healing: (**a**) contact healing and (**b**) gap healing

## 1.4 Fracture Healing and Methods to Enhance Healing

### 1.4.1 Fracture Healing

In contrast to the healing of a soft tissue wound by the formation of fibrous tissue scar, fracture of the bone heals by regeneration, i.e. by the formation of the original bone tissue itself. The healed bone can resume 100% of its original strength and function. Fracture healing is characterized by the presence of necrotic bone, the propagation of osteoprogenitor cells, and the growth of granulation tissue through the callus into almost perfectly reconstructed bone.

Fracture heals either by primary healing or by secondary healing [30]. Primary healing refers to the union between the fracture segments directly by the formation of bone tissue. Secondary healing is characterized by the formation of cartilaginous or fibrous connective tissue first, which subsequently becomes mineralized and replaced by the bone.

*Primary healing* occurs either by 'contact' healing or 'gap' healing (Fig. 1.18). If there is no gap that exists between the fracture segments, contact healing occurs by infiltration of cutter cones of osteoclasts forming longitudinal resporption cavities that forward crossing the fracture line [31]. The resorption cavities mature into crossing osteons by a process identical to Haversian remodeling. Crossing osteons mature by filling the osteonal lamellar bone that unites the two segments. Bony union and Haversian remodeling occur simultaneously. Gap healing occurs when there is a small gap between the fracture segments, which are rigidly fixed. Vascular loops from the medullary vascular system accompanying osteoprogenitor cells grow into the fracture gap and differentiate into osteoblasts. The osteoblasts deposit layers of lamellar bone on the surfaces of the two bone segments until they are united. In larger gaps, the gap is first subdivided into multiple smaller compartments by the formation of woven bone, subsequently filled with concentric layers of the lamellar bone. Once the fracture gap is filled with bone, subsequently Haversian remodeling follows.

Primary healing is facilitated by anatomical bony reduction, complete stability at the fracture site without any micromotion, and interfragmentary compression. Periosteal and endosteal callus is absent as proper reduction and rigid stabilization eliminate the biological signals responsible for recruitment of cells, which contribute to callus formation. Resorption and replacement of necrotic fracture ends do not occur; the avascular bone is revascularized by new vessels that grow into existing intracortical vascular channels. Primary bone union generally

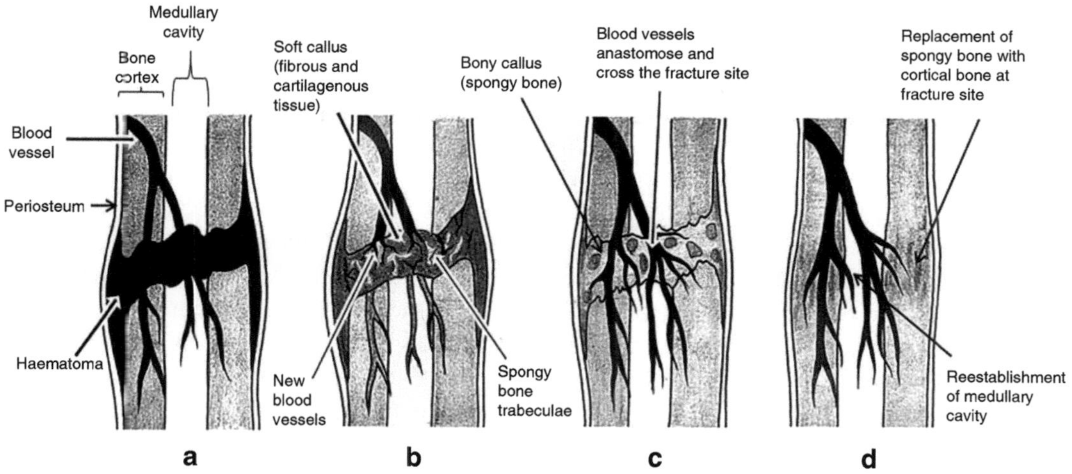


**Fig. 1.19** Stages of secondary bone healing: (**a**) haematoma formation, (**b**) fibrocartilaginous callus formation, (**c**) bony callus formation, and (**d**) bone remodeling

takes longer time than secondary bone union. Further, the bone undergoing primary union is mechanically weaker than secondary union, especially in the initial stages of healing process. In fact, a fracture undergoing secondary healing is considerably stronger than a fracture undergoing primary healing during the early period of the healing process due to its greater cross-sectional fracture callus area. Hence, wherever rigid immobilization of fracture segments is provided using internal fixation techniques such as locking compression bone plating in small animals, the external callus formation is negligible, and fracture healing takes relatively more time, and hence, the implants should be retained for longer period as compared to less rigid intramedullary pins. In large animals, however, it is generally not possible to achieve motionless rigid immobilization and thus primary bone union.

*Secondary healing*: Secondary healing occurs generally in the majority of fractures immobilized with less rigid (semi-rigid) fixation. Secondary healing is characterized by three different phases: inflammatory, reparative, and remodeling (Fig. 1.19) [32].

*Inflammatory phase* is initiated soon after a fracture is sustained. Extensive hemorrhage occurs from the ruptured blood vessels in the torn periosteum, disrupted cortex and medullary cavity, and adjacent soft tissues. Ischaemic necrosis of the bone and other tissues occurs at the fracture site. Subsequently, a fibrin clot is formed, and inflammatory exudates accumulate at the fracture site. There will be transient increase in the extraosseous blood supply that brings along osteoclast progenitor cells, which affect the disposal of necrotic bone and help in callus formation. Sprouting of new blood vessels and the proliferation of fibroblasts begin at the periphery of the clot. By third or fourth day, after the occurrence of a fracture, repair by granulation tissue commences.

*Reparative phase* begins when the signs of acute inflammation subside and the fracture site is bridged by a mass of tissue composed of new blood vessels, fibrous tissue, cartilage, and woven bone, which is called as 'callus'. The callus formed around the fracture segments is known as 'external or periosteal' callus, and that formed between the segments and within the marrow cavity is known as 'internal or endosteal' callus. The callus tissue is derived from the proliferation of pluripotential mesenchymal cells, the osteogenic layer of periosteum, endosteum, and marrow cavity. The nature and amount of callus tissue are determined by several factors such as the relative rapidity/speed with which a callus forms, the amount of movement at the fracture site, and the age and species of the animal involved. In rapidly growing callus, neovascularization cannot keep pace with cellular proliferation, whereas excessive motion at the fracture site may result in severance of blood vessels; in both cases, vascular supply is compromised, which favor chondrocytic differentiation and cartilage formation. The necrotic bone at the fracture end is removed by getting incorporated within the developing callus, reabsorbed by osteoclasts, or encased by a fibrous capsule. Reparative phase ends at a stage where the fracture is strong enough to qualify as clinically healed fracture.

*Remodeling phase* is characterized by a slow change in the shape of the fracture callus and bone. Osteoclastic resorption of redundant trabeculae of woven bone occurs simultaneously along with deposition of new structural trabeculae of lamellar bone in a functionally more advantageous orientation/location (Wolff's law). Eventually, the compact bone of the cortex is slowly restored to its normal osteonal architecture, and the medullary cavity is reestablished.

Several factors influence the fracture healing, such as general health and age of the animal, fracture site and morphology, the extent of soft tissue trauma, adequacy of local vascular supply, presence or absence of bacterial contamination, use of anti-inflammatory drugs, and the degree of movement at the fracture site [33]. Healing occurs relatively faster in young animals, and as age advances, healing delays. Fractures at the metaphyseal region of long bones heal faster than the fractures at the diaphysis due to abundant vascular supply and cells present in the cancellous bone. Long oblique fractures heal quicker than comminuted fractures if same level of fixation rigidity is provided. Fractures stabilized with rigid fixation with compression between the bone segments heal faster than those fractures constantly subjected to tensile force (avulsion fractures). Soft tissue trauma and vascular compromise at the fracture site delay healing as well as contamination of open wound. While micromotion at the fracture site favors early callus formation and bone healing, excessive movement disrupts the invasion of vascular supply and delays fracture healing. The use of anti-inflammatory drugs to reduce pain due to inflammation at the fracture site is debatable. Most commonly used non-steroidal anti-inflammatory drugs (NSAIDs), COX-1 and COX-2 inhibitors, may be useful in reducing pain and preventing further damage, but they may delay fracture healing. Prostaglandin-induced inflammation is beneficial for the fracture healing, and cyclooxygenase enzymes play an important role. Hence, the use of NSAIDs such as aspirin, ibuprofen, meloxicam, indomethacin, etodolac, nabumetone, and naproxen is not generally advocated for fracture pain relief. Alternatively, acetaminophen can be given alone or along with narcotics such as codeine to help reduce the pain of fracture. Further, prolonged used of these drugs should be avoided.

### 1.4.2 Methods to Enhance Fracture Healing

Bone repairs by itself and fracture repair process are spontaneous and natural. However, several factors can influence greatly the quality and speed of the bone healing process.

#### 1.4.2.1 Nutrition

Nutritional supply is needed in each stage of the fracture healing process both in human beings and animals [34, 35]. The complete process of healing requires considerable amount of energy, which is normally met through the dietary intake of calories. For healing to occur, it is essential to synthesize new proteins; hence, adequate supply of amino acids derived from dietary proteins is crucial. Also, the release of free radicals during the fracture trauma can cause oxidative stress.

*Energy*: Fracture healing requires more energy than one might normally expect. In traumatic fracture, metabolic demand increases instantly and thus increased caloric demand up to three times the normal. If this increased energy demand is not met, the healing process can be hampered.

*Protein*: Proteins and minerals are the building blocks of the skeletal tissue [36, 37]. Protein constitutes about half of the bone volume; and for a fracture to heal, a new protein matrix has to be synthesized. Hence, adequate protein supplementation in the diet is essential. Further, protein supplementation may increase the availability of growth factors such as insulin-like growth factor-1 (IGF-1), which can positively impact the overall immune response, bone regeneration, and skeletal integrity. Studies have proved that the intake of protein accelerates fracture healing. The benefits of protein supplementation are more important in those patients with malnutrition or low baseline protein intake. Amino acids such as lysine, arginine, proline, glycine, cysteine, and glutamine are important for fracture healing. Lysine aids in bone regeneration and healing by enhancing calcium absorption and calcium deposition in the bone matrix.

*Minerals*: About 70% of the bone is made up of minerals, including calcium, phosphorus, magnesium, silicon, and zinc. Fracture healing requires specific key minerals. *Calcium and phosphorus*: Calcium and phosphorus are the major bone minerals present in the form of calcium hydroxyapatite crystals. The development and repair of bone tissue require adequate calcium and phosphorus. It is known that fracture can heal normally without dietary supplementation of calcium; but during the early stages of healing, calcium is drawn from the skeleton and additional supply of calcium is beneficial. However, the intake of unusually high minerals may not speed up fracture healing. As calcium absorption and deposition in the bone are dependent on availability of vitamin D, optimum levels of vitamin D along with calcium have to be supplemented daily to achieve best fracture healing [38, 39]. Though phosphorus is adequately present in the normal diet (often more), old patients and those on low protein diets may need additional phosphorus for aiding synthesis of new bone.

*Zinc*: A large number of enzymes involved in cell proliferation requires zinc for their functioning. Supplementation of zinc helps stimulate fracture healing by enhancing bone protein production and callus formation.

*Copper*: Copper helps in the formation of bone collagen and thus essential for bone healing. The requirement of both copper and zinc is proportional to the extent of trauma; as the severity increases, the demand rises.

*Silicon*: Silica, bioactive silicon, is known to play a significant role in the synthesis of bone collagen and augment the effects of calcium and vitamin D3.

*Vitamins*: Vitamins are important as they act as catalysts in many biochemical reactions involving bone regeneration. Several vitamins including vitamin C, D, K, and B play critical roles during fracture healing [38–41]. *Vitamin C* is necessary for bone collagen synthesis, and it also has antioxidant and anti-inflammatory properties. Studies proved that higher vitamin C resulted in a stronger fracture callus. *Vitamin D* regulates calcium absorption and vitamin D deficiency makes less calcium available for fracture healing. Studies have shown suboptimal fracture healing with low vitamin D levels and accelerated callus mineralization and bone healing with administration of vitamin D. Further, vitamin D along with vitamin K is also known to stimulate the stem cells at the fracture site to become osteoblasts. *Vitamin K* on the other hand is needed for the formation of osteocalcin and is essential for biochemical processes involving deposition of calcium in the bone. Vitamin K also helps reducing calcium loss in the urine and thus conserves calcium and enhances fracture healing. *Vitamin B6* deficiency increases the occurrence of fractures and delays fracture healing, and it is known to modulate the effects of vitamin K.

*Anti-inflammatory nutrients*: During the fracture of a bone, the tightly bound collagen strands in the bone are broken, which interact with oxygen-yielding oxygen radical metabolites releasing free radicals. These free radicals further break down the bone collagen and accelerate bone turnover. Several antioxidants such as vitamin E, vitamin C, lycopene, and alpha-lipoic acid were found useful in reducing the destructive effect of oxygen free radicals and improving fracture healing [42].

Many standard NSAIDs, which inhibit the COX-1 and COX-2 enzymes, relieve the pain, but they are known to delay the healing. Contrarily, several nutrients are known to minimize the inflammation and pain and also hasten the fracture healing process. Vitamin C, bioflavonoids, flavonols (quercetin, proanthocyanidins), and omega-3 fatty acids decrease the inflammation and accelerate the healing. Furthermore, the proteolytic enzymes such as bromelain and trypsin are found to reduce inflammation, oedema, and pain in fracture cases.

The bone is a composite tissue requiring numerous nutrients; hence, supplementation of important but a comprehensive range of nutrients may produce more desirable effect on bone healing. Human studies have proved that supplementation of complex multi-nutrients containing proteins, carbohydrates, minerals, and vitamins has shortened the healing time and decreased the mortality in fracture patients, which may hold true to animal patients too.

#### 1.4.2.2 Anabolic Steroids

Several studies report better bone mass density and prevention of osteoporosis in patients treated with anabolic steroids nandrolone decanoate. The role of anabolic steroids in fracture healing is inconclusive. However, several studies have shown better fracture healing with an increased osteoblastic activity and periosteal bone formation and prevention of osteoporosis with administration of anabolic steroids [43–45].

#### 1.4.2.3 Herbal/Homeopathic Drugs

Traditionally, herbal drugs have been used to accelerate fracture healing in several parts of the world. Among them, comfrey (*Symphytum uplandics x.*), commonly cultivated in Europe, used in the form of an infusion has shown beneficial effect on fracture healing. Arnica (*Arnica montana*) is another reportedly useful herb, but it should be used with caution as large dose can be poisonous. *Horsetail grass*, an herb high in silicon, when boiled and fed has shown to speed up fracture healing in early stages. The herb *Cissus quadrangularis* (widely known as *hadjod*, *asthisamharaka*, *veldt grape*, *devil's backbone*, *adamant creeper*, and *pirandai*) has been studied extensively for its fracture-healing benefits [46]. Alcoholic extract of bamboo (*Bambusa arundinacea*) buds has also been shown to accelerate fracture healing in experimental animals [47]. Some of the traditional Chinese herbal medicines have also been reported to be effective in reducing the pain, swelling, and soreness of fracture and also accelerate fracture healing.

Homeopathic medicines used in fracture repair comprise arnica as an anti-trauma medication soon after the fracture, symphytum (comfrey) for reducing inflammation and pain and enhance bone healing, and *Calcarea phosphorica* for non-healing fractures. Studies have shown that a combination of symphytum and *Calcarea phosphorica* was beneficial to enhance bone mineral density, especially in osteoporotic bones.

#### 1.4.2.4 Exercise

Exercise is an important way to accelerate fracture healing [48]. It has been seen to increase the synthesis of matrix and alter its composition, organization, and mechanical properties of a healing bone. Further, exercise increases blood circulation at the fracture site ensuring an adequate flow of nutrients and thus hasten fracture healing. In animal patients, postoperative care, management, and controlled exercise are difficult; however, they should be encouraged to walk and use the fractured limb as early as possible after bone fixation. This will not only 'exercise' the limb but also allow compression between the fracture segments, which favors early new bone (callus) formation and healing. However, undue stress on the broken bone should be avoided; excess/unrestricted fracture site movement could delay healing and lead to complications. Hence, one should ensure that rigid fixation is achieved at the fracture site before allowing the animal to use the repaired limb.

#### 1.4.2.5 Other Physiotherapy Modalities

Several non-invasive alternate treatment modalities such as ultrasound therapy, electrical and electromagnetic stimulation, and acupuncture therapy have been used to stimulate bone healing, especially in delayed union and non-union fractures.

*Ultrasound therapy*: Low-intensity pulsed ultrasound (LIPUS) has been used therapeutically and shown to significantly enhance fracture healing [49, 50]. However, the exact mechanism of osteoinduction is still not properly understood. The studies have shown ultrasound treatment resulting in accelerated osteoblastic activity and multiplication of cells leading to an early and increased callus formation at the fracture site. Further, LIPUS has been suggested to upregulate the receptor activity of neurotransmitters at the fracture site, thereby accelerating bone healing.

*Electrical and electromagnetic stimulation*: Electrical stimulation has been used since long to accelerate fracture healing [51–54]. Early report of electrical stimulation for bone healing dates back to the 1840s, and subsequently, several reports were published narrating the effects of electricity on bone growth and healing. Electrical stimulation has shown to hasten the bone healing in different conditions such as fresh fractures and delayed or non-union fractures and to improve the efficacy of bone grafts, etc. Direct current (DC) is known to work by an electrochemical reaction at the cathode, capacitive coupling (CC) by enhancing multiplication and differentiation of the osteoblasts through its effect on molecular pathways and growth factors, and inductive coupling (IC) results in enhanced differentiation and proliferation of osteoblasts by altering of growth factors, gene expression, and transmembrane signaling. IC and CC upregulate calcium and thus help in bone mineralization and healing. All modes of electric stimulation upregulate the growth factor synthesis, leading to increased proliferation and differentiation of bone cells, thus resulting in enhanced callus formation and maturation.

The use of magnets to enhance bone healing has been proposed by many researchers; the purpose is to improve circulation and thus enhance the delivery of nutrients to the fractured bone [55]. Though the use of static magnets is probably not useful to help a bone to heal faster, there is evidence of beneficial effect of using pulsed electromagnetic fields (PEMF) as a method of bone stimulation. A number of devices were developed to produce electromagnetic fields at the fracture site. The principle of PEMF application is similar to inductive coupling; an electric field (secondary) is generated in the bone through the electric current produced in a coil (by an external field generator). Usually, a range of 1–100 mV/cm electric fields are produced in the bone by applying 0.1–20 G magnetic fields. The effect of electromagnetic stimulation of the bone is believed to be similar to mechanical loading. PEMF have been shown to activate the extracellular matrix protein synthesis and directly influence the synthesis of proteins regulating gene transcription. They are also known to regulate various membrane receptors such as PTH, insulin, IGF-2, LDL, and calcitonin receptors and secretion of many growth factors including bone BMPs 2 and 4 and TGF-beta by stimulation of osteoblasts.

*Acupuncture*: Acupuncture, a non-conventional healing modality, was also used to accelerate fracture healing in both human beings and animals [54]. It has been shown to facilitate faster reductions in swelling and pain, improve range of motion, and promote bone healing. The studies have indicated that acupuncture significantly improves outcomes of patients with bone fractures. Currently, there are no randomized clinical trials to conclusively prove the beneficial effects of acupuncture stimulation on bone healing; however, many small animal and human trials suggest its possible beneficial effects in bone remodeling and increase in testosterone in rats and estradiol levels in postmenopausal women.

## 1.5 Implants Used for Fracture Fixation

Several implants are being used in orthopedics, for a variety of purposes, namely, for fixation of fractures (like plates, screws, wires, rods and nails, external skeletal fixators) and for replacement of joint (hip and stifle joints) and limb, etc. Most of these implants are not made from pure metals but from specially produced metal alloys [56, 57]. Orthopedic implants manufactured from the metal alloys are solidified crystal solutions that are molded to desired size and shaped by melting and allowing cooling. The alloy used to develop orthopedic implants has to be very strong, i.e. it should not bend or break under heavy loading but should not be too stiff to avoid stress protection of the bone and must be well tolerated by the tissues (biocompatible). To achieve optimum mechanical characteristics, the alloy must not contain impurities, the crystal (grain) size should be uniform, and the structure must be free of voids.

All the implants must be wear or corrosion resistant. Metallic surfaces in contact with body fluids tend to corrode. There are several causes for the corrosion of metals implanted within the body. The reduction of pH at the implant site (to about 5.3–5.6) because of the surgical trauma and the decrease in oxygen concentration due to the presence of microbes and the crevices between different parts of the implant may contribute to corrosion. The most common materials currently used to manufacture orthopedic implants such as stainless steel, titanium, and cobalt-chrome are known biocompatible, but the best tolerated is titanium in pure form.

Even though the orthopedic implants can withstand corrosion, still the corrosion can occur when two diverse metals/alloys make contact and when there is metal-on-metal contact (like in plate and screws or total hip joints). As the metal surfaces dissolve releasing metal particles such as cobalt, chromium, and titanium, their concentration in the blood circulation may increase causing health concerns. Nevertheless, till date, it is unproven that these trace metals can cause any pathological changes or induce tumor in patients. While the toxic studies in human patients are inconclusive, it may be less relevant in animal patients due to their shorter lifespan. As the orthopedic implants developed from corrosion-resistant steel and other metal alloys are not ferromagnetic, MRI can be used to examine the patients.

### 1.5.1 Stainless Steel

Stainless-steel alloys are most widely used for manufacturing orthopedic implants worldwide (>50% of implants) [58]. Stainless steel is a typically low-carbon steel having chromium. More elements like molybdenum, nickel, and nitrogen are added along with chromium to increase the desirable characteristics of the steel alloy including corrosion resistance, and impurities including non-metallic components are reduced to improve the qualities for implantation. For the development of orthopedic implants, the stainless-steel type that is mostly used is 316L (Table 1.1). M/S Sherman surgical stainless-steel alloys discovered the 316L stainless steel having iron, chromium, and nickel in different proportions. The letter 'L' indicates low carbon (≤0.03%), which avoids carbide precipitation. When steel is heated to high temperatures (800–1600 °F), carbon precipitates, which combines with the chromium promoting corrosion. By minimizing the amount of carbon, corrosion can be controlled. The low carbon in surgical stainless steel reduces corrosion, adverse tissue reactions, and metal allergies. Nevertheless, when implanted within the body, even the 316L stainless steel may corrode in areas under considerable stress and oxygen depletion (like at screw-plate intersections); hence, they are advisable for use only as temporary fixation implants, like bone plates, rods, wires, screws, etc.

Almost all the orthopedic devices developed using stainless steel for implantations inside the body are generally of type 316L; L grades, however, are more expensive. The properties of the steel alloy can also be varied based on the heat treatment (annealing, softer materials; cold working, strong and hard materials). Relatively, high-carbon-containing stainless-steel types, with sufficient strength and low cost, may be preferred for the development of other accessory orthopedic instruments and external fixator components, which lie outside the body (need not be as inert and corrosion resistant as implantable devices). Mild steel, which is readily available, sufficiently strong, and economical, has been used to develop external components of circular fixators (with nickel coating) for use in large animals.

### 1.5.2 Titanium

Titanium and its alloys are employed in medical engineering since long [59]. Apart from bone fixation implants such as nails, plates, nuts and screws, and external fixator components, they

**Table 1.1** Characteristics of metals and alloys used for bone fixation [57]

| Metal/alloy | Mechanical properties Elastic modulus (GPa) | Yield strength (MPa) | Material properties |
|---|---|---|---|
| Stainless steel (316 L) | 190 | 200–250 | Biocompatible, resistant to corrosion, cost-effective |
| Titanium alloys | 55–100 | 530–900 | Low density, excellent corrosion resistance, osteointegration |
| Co-Cr alloys | 220–230 | 275–1585 | Superior mechanical properties, corrosion, and wear resistance |

have been used to develop joint prosthetic devices, dental implants and prosthetics, cardiac instruments, casings for pacemakers and valves, etc.

High strength, low weight, excellent corrosion resistance (with respect to pitting and stress corrosion cracking), and total biocompatibility make titanium an ideal material for implantation (Table 1.2). Titanium is non-magnetic and has low electric conductivity, and hence, it is safe for use with implanted electronic devices. The density of titanium alloys is more (60% heavier) than aluminum alloys but lesser (40% lighter) than that of stainless steel. Titanium is quite resilient (15–25% elongation) and has a high tensile strength (30 ksi, 207 Mpa). Due to the combined effects of modest weight and great strength, titanium alloys have higher strength-to-weight ratio (about 30% greater) than steel or aluminum alloys. The elastic modulus is almost similar among stainless-steel, aluminum, and titanium alloy materials.

The alloys used for fabrication of a fixation implant should not be much stiffer than the bone itself. If the stiffness of the implant is more, the shielded bone can lose its substance and becomes weak (stress protection). Hence, metal alloys used to develop an implant should have stiffness almost similar to the bone. As titanium alloys' stiffness is close to that of the bone (lowest among all implant alloys), it is preferred for bone fixation, especially in osteoporotic bones. However, high cost of titanium implants limits their use in animal patients in routine clinical practice.

Many newer alloy materials are being investigated for the development of implants having ideal mechanical and biological properties. Ti-15Mo is a comparably new alloy with superior mechanical properties (notch sensitivity and reverse bending) offering better implant designs. Similarly, metal alloys with 'shape memory effect' (alloys that can deform when cold and return to normal shape when heated), also called as shape memory metal/alloy or smart metal/alloy, sound attractive for implant manufacturing. However, presently available memory metals/alloys have not been used as implants due to their hardness, difficulty to machine, and high cost. Nitinol, a shape memory Ti alloy with low elastic modulus and stiffness, has a great potential as a fixation implant, especially in osteoporotic bones. Nitinol foam, made from nickel commercially pure titanium (cpTi) powder, has elastic modulus similar to subchondral bone and interconnecting pores (40–80% porosity); hence, there is a possibility of its use as solid sponges to provide adequate purchase for screws in osteoporotic/spongy bone. Super elastic nitinol appears

**Table 1.2** Comparative mechanical characteristics of different alloys used in orthopedic applications

| Characteristics | S-steel | Titanium | Cobalt-chrome |
|---|---|---|---|
| Stiffness | High | Low | Medium |
| Strength | Medium | High | Medium |
| Corrosion resistance | Low | High | Medium |
| Biocompatibility | Low | High | Medium |

promising for specific applications like spinal deformity corrections.

### 1.5.3 Cobalt-Chrome

Cobalt-chrome alloys are non-precious alloys, first introduced in dentistry in the 1930s. They do not cause systemic toxic reactions because the corrosion is low and the released ions are essential elements (cobalt and chromium are part of the enzyme system). Chromium and molybdenum are critical for corrosion resistance; a minimum of 20% chromium content make the alloy corrosion resistant (by forming oxide layers) and hence biocompatible. The carbon content is restricted to less than 0.02% to avert possible precipitation of carbide (leading to brittleness) during welding. Nickel content of less than 0.1% is considered nickel-free and standard, as it is usually impossible to separate nickel from cobalt completely. Each alloy has its specific features and is used for definite purposes. Cobalt-chrome (Co–Cr) alloys have been recommended for surgical implant applications as they are highly resistant to corrosion and thus for fatigue and cracking; but they are prone to failure due to fatigue fracture. Cobalt-chrome alloy is mostly used to develop joint prostheses; however, poor fabricability and high costs have made Co-based alloys currently unsuitable for routine use in bone fixation implants.

### 1.5.4 Aluminum Alloy

Aluminum alloy (aluminum 7075-T6), apart from stainless steel and titanium, has been used extensively for construction of external fixator components due to their high strength-to-weight ratios. Aluminum is light (Sp.gr 2.7), weighting about 1/2 to 1/3 of stainless steel (Sp.gr 7.9). These alloys, however, are susceptible to corrosion in chloride environments and may lead to fixator failure, if not taken proper care.

Although the metallic implants have desirable mechanical properties for use in orthopedic applications, once implanted, there are possibilities of corrosion and eroding of metals releasing metal particles/ions causing inflammation, a sign of reduced biocompatibility and tissue toxicity. Further, as the metals and bone have significantly different elastic moduli and tensile strength, it can often cause stress protection of the neighboring bone resulting in osteoporosis. Hence, recent innovations are focused on the use of polymeric materials, which are less rigid, more elastic, and useful, in achieving better outcomes.

### 1.5.5 Non-biodegradable Polymers

Polyaryletherketone polymers such as polyetheretherketone (PEEK) and polyetherketoneketone (PEKK) are biocompatible radiolucent thermoplastics that can be easily sterilized [60]. Unlike metals, they do not corrode. They are non-magnetic and therefore MRI compatible. The tensile strength of these polymers is quite reasonable (PEEK, 90–100 MPa), but it can be enhanced by carbon reinforcement. However, the problem with carbon reinforcement is the release of microfibers after wear/fretting/breakage of the implant over a period of time (due to reduction in bonding strength between the polymer and the fibers). These polymers have high chemical resistance; but as they are hydrophobic, they need to be subjected to surface modification/coating before implantation. The use of these polymers in orthopedic applications is limited by their high costs, and currently, they are used in spinal surgery for fusion of the vertebrae.

Bone plates and screws fabricated from carbon fiber (CF)-reinforced PEEK polymers can increase the fatigue life of the implanted device. Carbon-reinforced PEEK polymers have several advantages compared to conventional metals. Carbon-reinforced PEEK has an elastic modulus (3.5 GPa) closer to that of the bone (cortical bone, 12–20 GPa; cancellous bone, 1 GPa) than metals (stainless steel, 230 GPa; titanium, 106–155 GPa), which provide an excellent loading condition to stimulate bone healing and decrease the stress shielding. Bone healing is improved by using the CF PEEK polymer as its stiffness is more similar to the bone than metals. Further, it is easier to remove the CF PEEK plate than a metal plate due to less bone growth around the implant. PEEK is increasingly becoming the material of choice in trauma fixation devices, sports medicine, and oncology. Advancements in PEEK implants featuring antimicrobial properties may reduce the likelihood of infection around the implantation site. Currently, though several such implants are available for use, the main disadvantage is their inability to be contoured at the time of surgery. Further, like metallic implants, they cannot degenerate and are retained in the body permanently; hence, a second surgery may be needed to remove the implants.

Carbon fiber-reinforced polymer composites have been used as implants for fracture fixation [61] and for development of external fixator components such as circular rings (Ilizarov fixator). Unlike stainless steel, titanium, or aluminum, carbon fiber composite is radiolucent, which allows radiographic examination of the fracture site. The carbon fiber component is about 1.5 times lighter than the metallic equivalent. Carbon fiber rings are less stiff than stainless-steel rings, but they can withstand adequate loads. Experimental studies comparing the stainless-steel tubes and carbon fiber rods have proved that during bending, the carbon fiber rods were 15% stiffer and were able to sustain higher loads than stainless-steel tubes.

Ideally, an implant should have mechanical properties (like strength, elastic modulus, and hardness) comparable with the natural bone to allow early weight bearing and functional use of the limb without weakening or displacement of bone segments. It should promote osteosynthesis (osteoinduction and osteoconduction) without causing any inflammatory response or toxicity. Further, it is also desired that an implant is progressively broken down within the body and dissolved slowly and completely after the complete bone healing. Various materials have been researched for the development of such 'ideal' bone fixation devices and have been tested for their clinical usage. These materials are of different types such as metals or metal alloys, ceramics, polymers, or composites. While ceramics have limited application as a fixation device (used extensively for filling of bone defects), metals and metal alloys, polymers, and composites are being tested as bone fixation implants.

### 1.5.6 Biodegradable Metals

Due to their biosafety and biodegradability, Mg, Fe, Zn, and their alloys are being investigated as bone implant materials [62–65]. The advantage with Mg and Mg alloys is that their densities and elastic moduli are similar to that of the natural bone, but their disadvantage is quick degradation in physiological environments resulting in untimely loss of implant strength. Fe and Fe alloys have excellent mechanical properties, but they degrade very slowly to be ideal bone implants. On the other hand, Zn and Zn alloys have suitable degradation rates; however, their main constraints are poor strength and ductility for their applications in bone repair. Efforts are being made to improve the deficiencies by alloying, heat treatment, and surface modification of these biodegradable metals.

Mg alloys are 'revolutionary' biodegradable metal materials, which can be used in orthopedic applications, as they are biocompatible, are biodegradable, and have acceptable mechanical properties. Mg, primarily stored in the bone tissue, is an essential element required for many metabolic processes. Mg released from corrosion of Mg alloy implants is readily eliminated in the urine and therefore does not cause any complications. The mechanical properties of Mg alloys are akin to bone. They are lightweight, having density (1.7–1.9 g/cm) and elastic modulus (45 GPa) very close or similar to that of the cortical bone (density, 1.75 g/cm; modulus, 3–20 GPa), and thus protect from stress shielding (normally seen with stainless steel). Hence, Mg alloys are expected to become ideal load-bearing orthopedic implants.

Although significant progress has been made in research on Mg alloys as bone implants over the past 20–25 years, there have been challenges for their use in bone fixation. More extensive studies are underway to improve the mechanical properties and evaluate in vivo degradation and biocompatibility of Mg alloys. Efforts are being made to develop Mg alloys with controllable degradation through processing control and bionic coating (biofunctional alloy). Works focusing on angiogenesis of Mg-based implants are also under way. The development of the next-generation superior performance Mg alloys may play an important role for their use as bone fixation implants in the future.

### 1.5.7 Bioresorbable Polymers

Biodegradable and resorbable polymeric implants are considered as an effective alternate bone fixation system over metallic implants [59, 66]. They have several advantages as the implants need not be removed after the osseous healing and they are radiolucent and without the problems of corrosion and accumulation of metal in tissues. Stress protection is also of less concern as the load is gradually transferred to the bone as the implants degrade. Several bioresorbable polymers such as polyglycolic acid or polyglycolide (PGA), polylactic acid or polylactide (PLA), polylactide-co-glycolide (PLGA), polydioxanone (PDS), propylene (PP), polysulphone (PS), and polycarbonate (PC) have been used in orthopedic applications (Table 1.3). However, PGA, PLA, and their co-polymers have been studied more extensively due to their superior strength. The molecular weight and crystallinity of a polymer determine its mechanical properties, i.e. polymers with higher degree of crystallinity are stronger and degrade slower. Hence, by altering the molecular weight and crystallinity, the mechanical strength of a polymeric implant can be optimized.

#### 1.5.7.1 Polyglycolide (PGA)

PGA was the first bioresorbable polymer used to develop augmented pins, plates, and screws for bone fixation. It is a hard and crystalline material having molecular weight of 20,000–145,000 and a melting point of 224–230 °C. When implanted, it is degraded by hydrolysis; its mechanical strength is reduced within 6 weeks, and it is completely resorbed within a few months depending on the molecular weight, crystallinity, and size and shape of the material. The main drawback of PGA implants has been early degradation (and loss of mechanical strength) and adverse tissue reactions (2.0–46.7%), which have discouraged the widespread use of PGA implants in favor of PLA having lower rate of degradation and tissue reaction. PGA implants have been used mostly for fixation of fractures in soft cancellous bones.

#### 1.5.7.2 Polylactide (PLA)

PLA is an amorphous to semi-crystalline and highly crystalline thermoplastic polymer having molecular weights of 180,000–530,000, a melting point of 130–180 °C. Several distinct forms of polylactide exist; depending on the L and D configuration, they are called as poly-L-lactide (PLLA) and poly-DL-lactide (PDLLA). Degradation of PLA also occurs by hydrolysis. Biodegradation of PDLA is slower (more resistant to hydrolysis) than for PLA due to the higher crystallinity of PDLA. Physically, blending of PLLA with PDLA maximizes temperature stability.

PLLA interference screws and plates have been used successfully for the repair of skeletal fractures. Much of the PLLA research focusing on veterinary applications has been done in rabbits. PLLA and PDLLA (poly-DL-lactide) have shown desirable characteristics (well tolerance like stainless steel and slow resorption with complete degradation occurring in about 36 months) for use in high-strength fracture fixation, even though they are not strong enough for use in load-bearing bones (PDLLA is less strong than PLLA). Further, a large number of patients with PLLA implants have reported foreign body reactions (aseptic soft tissue reactions) caused by the decaying PLA particles. Nevertheless, in comparison with PGA (6 months), the time for complete resorption of PLA is considerably longer (up to 5 years), and hence, currently, PLLA is more often used to manufacture resorbable orthopedic implants.

**Table 1.3** Mechanical properties of different polymers used for biomedical applications [57]

| | Tensile strength (MPa) | | Flexural strength (MPa) | | Tensile moduli (GPa) | |
|---|---|---|---|---|---|---|
| Polymer | UR | R | UR | R | UR | R |
| PLA | 11.4–72 | 200 | 45–145 | 89.6–412 | 0.6–4 | 6–29.9 |
| PDLLA | 45.5 | – | – | 70–174 | 3.2 | – |
| PLLA | 60.3 | – | 109 | 193 | 3.7 | – |
| PGA | 57 | 250 | – | 370 | 6.5 | – |
| PLGA | 40 | 290 | 150 | 190 | 1.4–2.8 | – |
| PCL | 19.3 | 22.5 | – | – | 0.34 | – |
| PELA | 3.8–16.1 | – | – | – | 0.11 | – |
| Bone | 50–150 | – | 130–180 | – | 12–18 | – |

*R*, reinforced; *UR*, un-reinforced

#### 1.5.7.3 Co-polymers

A complete range of PLGA polymers can be prepared by combining PGA and PLA; both L- and DL-lactides are used for co-polymerization. Co-polymerization of crystalline PGA with PLA results in increased rates of hydration and hydrolysis. By varying the ratio of monomers (glycolide to lactide) in a composition, the properties of a co-polymer (including degradation time) can be controlled [57, 67]. Generally, higher glycolide content results in faster degradation.

As on today, bioresorbable polymeric implants are mainly used to stabilize fractures of the facial bones, foot and ankle, and knee; wrist and hand injuries; in spinal reconstructive surgery; and in pediatric orthopedics.

There has been a significant improvement in biomaterials used in manufacturing bone fixation implants, and the approach has been changed from bioinert stabilizers to bioactive and biodegradable healing promoters. Due to their mechanical strength and low cost, specific classes of bioinert metals such as stainless-steel and titanium alloys are used in routine clinical practice. Nevertheless, bioresorbable implants having significant advantages over these traditional metal implants can make effective fixation devices. Magnesium alloy, a biodegradable metal, which has almost similar density as that of the bone, has been studied to function as an osteoconductive and biodegradable implant material in load-bearing applications; however, there is a need to control the high rate of degradation before it can see the light of load-bearing applications. The bioresorbable polymers and composites are particularly appealing as their development and properties are comparable to host the bone. Innovations in the design and fabrication methods of composite materials have raised the expectations of developing improved implants with better properties. Despite decades of research, no suitable implant that fully meets all the requirements for bone fixation has been developed, and a large gap still exists between the present treatment modalities and ideal clinical situation. There is a need to take a large leap toward the development of high-performance tissue engineered devices to fulfill the criteria required for an ideal bone fixation.

## 1.6 Instrumentation for Fracture Fixation

The basic material used for making the orthopedic implants is austenitic stainless-steel type AISI 316, which is highly resistant to corrosion. It contains 17.5% chromium, 12% nickel, 2.5% molybdenum, <3% silicon and manganese, and <0.06% carbon, and the remainder is iron. If greater strength and hardness are required, i.e. for tools like drills and screwdrivers, a stainless chromium steel is used, which is relatively less corrosion resistant. To obtain smooth surface (passive layer), the implants are polished mechanically, chemically, and electrolytically.

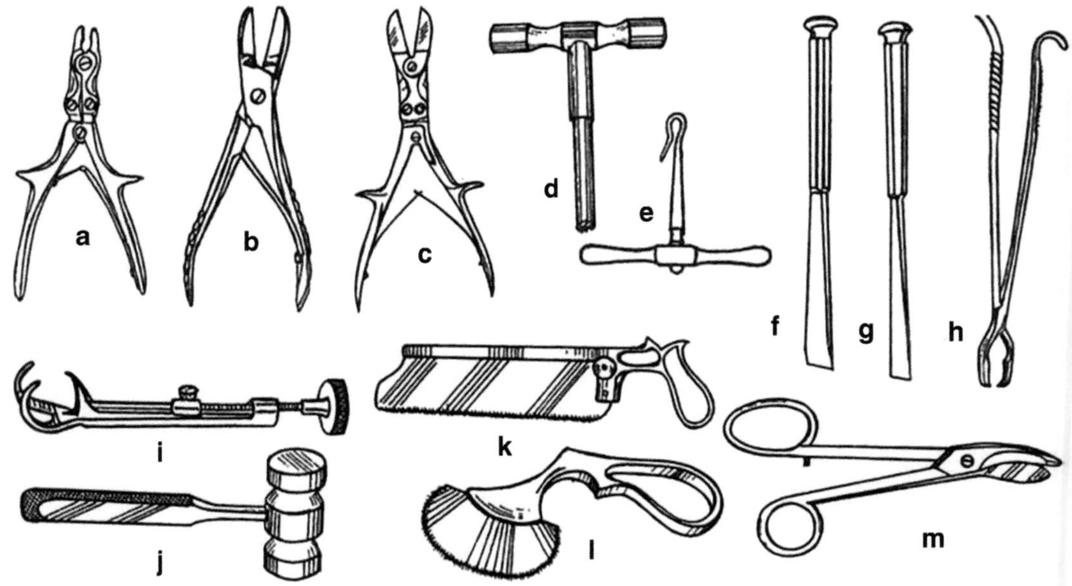


**Fig. 1.20** Basic orthopedic instruments: (**a**) rongeur, (**b, c**) bone-cutting forceps, (**d**) trephine, (**e**) Gigli wire saw, (**f**) chisel, (**g**) osteotome, (**h**) bone-holding forceps, (**i**) Lowman bone clamp, (**j**) bone mallet, (**k**) amputation saw, (**l**) Engel plaster saw, and (**m**) Bolers plaster shears

## 1.6.1 Basic Instruments (Fig. 1.20)

*Rongeurs*: Are forceps with cupped heavy tips, used to remove small pieces of the bone or to break larger bone pieces. They are also used to cut the bone edges.

*Bone-cutting forceps*: Have paired chisel-like tips for sharp cutting of the bone.

*Trephines*: Used to drill holes in the bone.

*Gigli wire saw*: Used for sharp cutting of the bone.

*Chisel*: Cutting instrument with the tip beveled at one surface.

*Osteotome*: Cutting instrument with the tip beveled at both surfaces.

*Bone-holding forceps*: Can be handheld or self-retained. Used to manipulate and hold fractured segments and bone plates.

*Lowman bone clamp*: Used to hold the bone segments and plates.

*Bone curette (Burns)*: Used to 'curette' the bony mass.

*Bone hammer (mallet)*: Used to hammer the instruments like chisel, nails, drivers, etc.

*Amputation saw*: Used to cut the bone during amputation of the limbs.

*Engel plaster saw*: Helps to cut the plaster cast.

*Bolers plaster shears*: Also used to extract the plaster cast; it has the advantage of protecting the skin from any trauma while cutting the plaster.

*Electric saw*: Used to cut the bone (osteotomy/ostectomy), plaster cast, etc.

## 1.6.2 Instruments for Bone Plating

*Screws (cortex screw, cancellous screw, locking screw)*: Cancellous screws have a wider thread and a steeper pitch than cortex screws. Cancellous screws have better holding power in the soft/loosely packed bone, while cortex screws have better holding power in the dense/compact bone. Locking screws have threads at the base of the screw, which help in getting locked with the threaded screw holes present in the locking compression plates. Screws can be fully threaded or half threaded. Half or incomplete threaded screws are used as lag screws to bring compression between the bone segments.

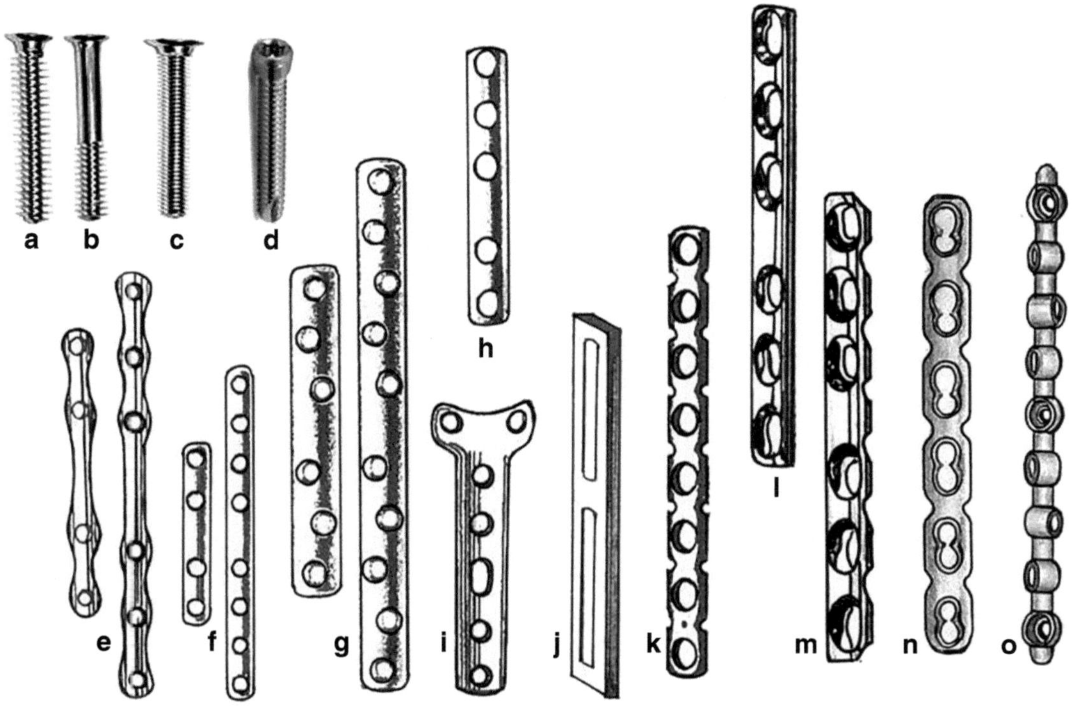


**Fig. 1.21** Bone screws and plates: (**a**) fully threaded cancellous screw, (**b**) lag screw, (c) cortical screw, (d) locking screw, (e) Sherman bone plate, (f) Venable bone plate, (g) heavy-duty bone plate, (h) mini plate, (i) small fragment T-plate, (j) Eggers bone plate, (k) reconstruction plate, (l) dynamic compression plate, (m) limited contact dynamic compression plate, (n) locking compression plate, and (o) String of pearl locking plate

*Bone plates*: There are several types of bone plates (Fig. 1.21).

*Sherman bone plates*: They have constrictions between the screw holes and hence are weak, and their use is limited to small bones, especially in small dogs and cats.

*Venable bone plates*: No constrictions between screw holes and consequently the plates are strong and ideal for veterinary fixations.

*Eggers bone plates*: Have long slots in the plate; hence, screws can be fixed at adjustable distance, not in common use.

*Williams spinal plates*: Are curved and have serrated edges, which help to stabilize the spinal processes.

*Heavy-duty bone plates*: Are very strong and are used as buttress plates, more often in large animal fixations.

*Small fragment T-plates*: Available in different shapes, like 'T' plates, angled plates, etc. Useful for immobilization of pelvic and mandibular fractures and also metaphyseal/epiphyseal fractures of the long bones.

*Mini plates*: Suitable for fixation of radius-ulna fractures in small breeds of dogs and cats. They are also useful for fixation of metacarpal or metatarsal fractures in dogs. 1.5–2.0 mm cortex screws are generally used.

*Reconstruction plates*: Are flexible and can be contoured to any shape and cut to desired length. They are relatively weaker, used normally in pelvic and mandibular fractures and often in metaphyseal/epiphyseal fractures of the long bones.

*Dynamic compression plates*: Screw holes are designed as per the spherical gliding principle. Insertion of screw eccentrically and tightening the screw against the hemi-cylindrical slope of the screw hole displace the plate away from the

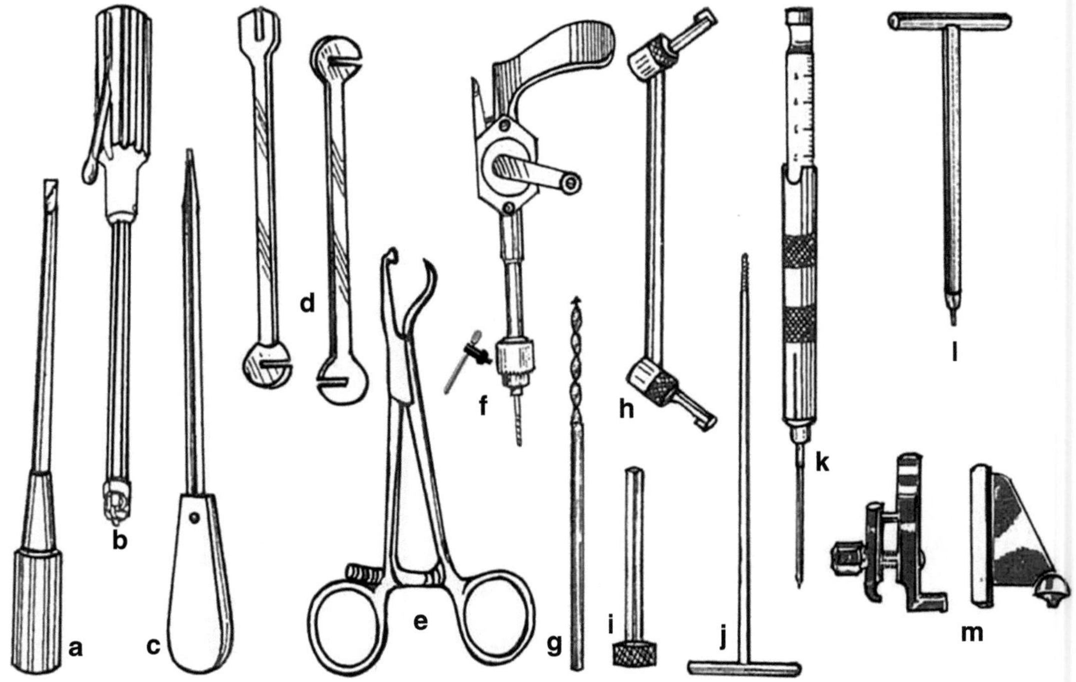


**Fig. 1.22** Instruments for bone plating: (a) Lane screwdriver, (b) Williams screwdriver, (c) screwdriver with hexagonal tip, (d) plate benders, (e) plate-holding forceps, (f) universal bone drill and key, (g) twist drill/drill bit, (h) drill guide, (i) drill sleeve, (j) tap, (k) depth gauge, (l) counter sink, and (m) compression device with special sleeve

fracture line resulting in compression of bone segments at the fracture site.

*Limited contact dynamic compression plates (LCDCP)*: Have undercut beneath each screw hole and between adjacent screw holes, which help to reduce the contact between the plate and the bone surface and in turn minimize the stress shielding and vascular compromise.

*Locking compression plates (LCP)*: Have combi-holes (have threaded and non-threaded part), which allow threaded screws to fix into the plate and function as a fixed-angle device and also allow placement of traditional non-locking screws.

*String of pearl (SOP) locking plates*: Uses cortical screws as locking screws and can be contoured in six degrees of freedom and hence can be bent and twisted to contour to the shape of the bone. It can be used in a variety of fractures such as long bone, pelvic, acetabular, and spinal fractures.

#### 1.6.2.1 Screwdrivers (Fig. 1.22)

*Lane screwdriver*: Simple screwdriver with chisel tip.

*Williams screwdriver*: The lever of the handle operates the locking and releasing device holding the screw. Provides better grip than Lane screwdriver and avoid slipping.

*Screwdriver with hexagonal tip*: Fits accurately into the recessed head (hexagonal shape) of the screws (2.7, 3.5, and 4.5 mm) and allows easy insertion and extraction of the screw without slipping and causing injury. It is more commonly used nowadays.

*Plate benders*: Used to bend and contour the plate to the shape of the bone.

*Plate-holding forceps*: Used to hold the plate snugly.

*Universal bone drill and key*: Used to drill hole in the bone with the help of a drill bit.

*Twist drills/bits*: Sharp edges on the surface helps to 'cut' holes in the bone.

*Drill sleeve*: Ensures proper alignment of holes drilled in the proximal and distal bone cortex. It also protects the drill bit from breakage. It also ensures that the hole is drilled exactly at the center of the hole in the plate and helps to keep the drill bit and the plate apart from each other.

*Drill guide*: Guides drilling a hole in the desired position and prevents drilling a hole very close to the fracture line. Eccentric drill guide is used to drill eccentric holes during compression plating. A special drill guide is used in locking compression plate, which gets locked with the threaded hole and ensures accurate alignment of the drill hole with the threaded screw hole.

*Tap*: Used to cut thread in the drilled hole. Tapping prevents binding of the screw at the distal cortex causing it to strip the bone.

*Measuring scale*: Used to measure the length of the screw.

*Depth gauge*: Used to measure the depth of the drilled hole.

*Counter sink*: Used to make a conical depression in the bone to receive the screw head.

*Orthopedic scale*:- For comparing the bit size with the size of the screw.

*Compression device*: Used to bring compression between the bone segments when standard normal bone plate is used; more useful in large animal fixations.

*Special drill sleeve for compression device*: Ensures the proper distance between the screw hole of the compression device and the last screw hole of the bone plate.

*Periosteal elevator (Bard-Parker)*: Used to strip/separate the periosteum.

### 1.6.3 Instruments for Intramedullary Pinning (Fig. 1.23)

*Steinmann pins*: Most widely used round intramedullary devices, commonly range from 1.5 mm to 6 mm in diameter and are available with trocar, chisel, and threaded trocar points, and can be pointed at one or both ends. Pins with both pointed ends are used during retrograde pinning, and pins with one end pointed (another end blunt) are used in normograde pinning.

*Kirschner wires*: Small trocar pointed steel pins that range in diameter from 0.8 mm to 1.5 mm. Used in a manner similar to that of Steinmann pins. Flexibility permits it to follow the contour of a curving medullary cavity or to be inserted at an angle through the sides of a bone (in condylar/supracondylar fractures). Also useful for tension band wiring and external skeletal fixation.

*Jacob's chuck key*: Used to insert intramedullary pins.

*Berbecker Steinmann pin cutter*: Helps to cut the extra length of pins.

### 1.6.4 Instruments for Interlocking Nailing (Fig. 1.24)

*Interlocking nail*: Is an intramedullary nail which can be secured (locked) in position by proximal and/or distal transfixing screws/bolts, to help prevent rotation of bone segment and collapse at the fracture site. Interlocking nails for dogs range in diameter from 6 mm to 8 mm; for large animals, 10 mm to 18 mm diameter nails may be required. For fixation in the tibia, angled nail is more ideal.

*Curved awl*: Is a long, pointed steel spike used for piercing the cortex to introduce the nail.

*Reamer*: Helps to ream the medullary cavity before fixation of the nail.

*Jig and accessories*

*Jig*: Is an aiming device, having multiple holes corresponding to the holes in the interlocking nail. It guides drilling of holes and fixation of bolts in the bone cortex through the nail.

*Slide hammer*: Attached to the nail and helps to introduce or retract the nail.

*Attachment screw*: Helps attachment of interlocking nail to the jig.

*Insertion tool*: Snugly fixes the nail to the jig and thus helps proper alignment of nail holes with that of the jig.

*Fixation bolts/screws*: Can be smooth (bolt) or threaded (screw), used for transfixing the nail with the bone cortex at the proximal and distal ends.

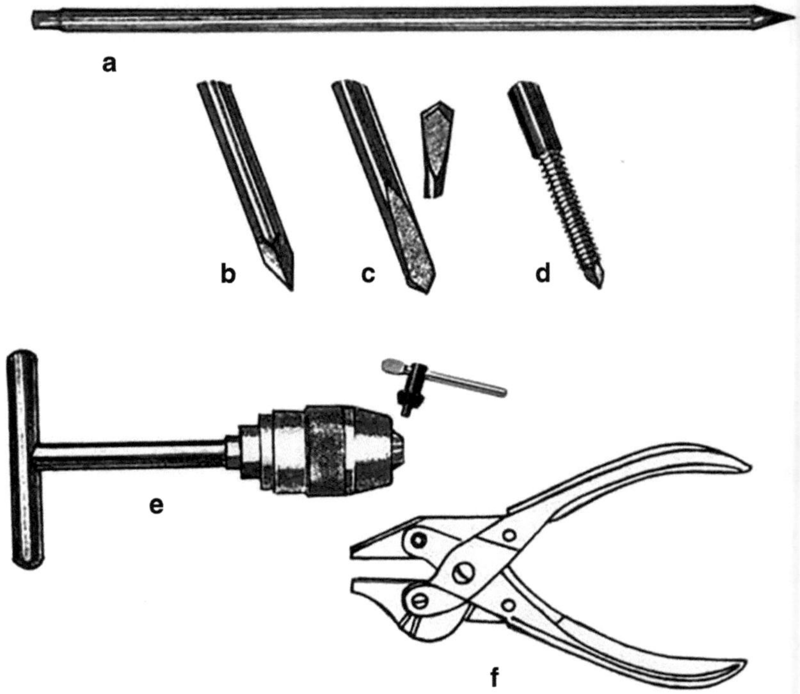


**Fig. 1.23** Instruments for intramedullary pinning: (a) Steinmann pin, (b) trocar point pin tip, (c) chisel point pin tip, (d) end threaded pin with trocar point, (e) Jacob's chuck key, and (f) Berbecker Steinmann pin cutter

*Miscellaneous* instruments: Bone drill (manual/electric) and key, depth gauge, trocar, guide sleeve, tap sleeve, drill guide, drill bits, screwdriver, etc.

### 1.6.5 Instruments for Rush Pinning (Fig. 1.25)

*Rush pins*: Specially designed round, elastic stainless-steel pins, which have a hooked end

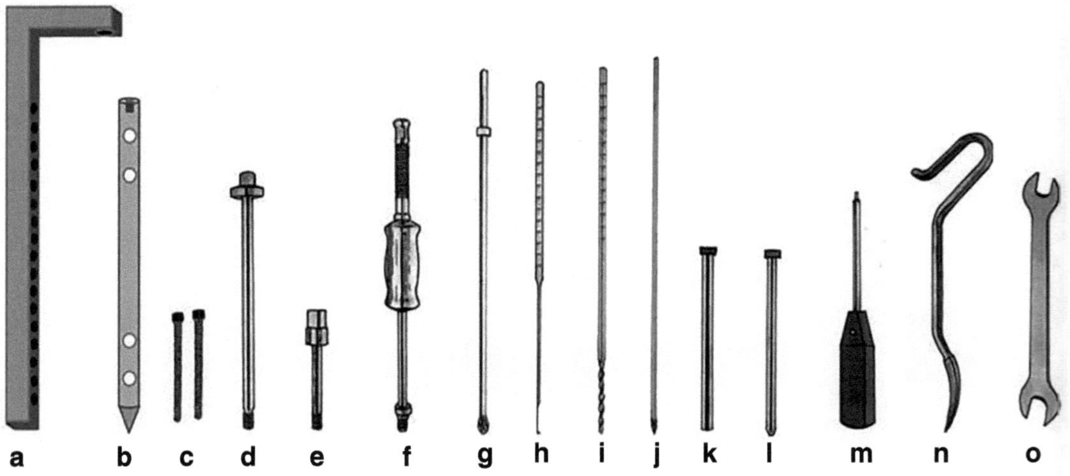


**Fig. 1.24** Instruments for interlocking nail fixation: (a) jig, (b) interlocking nail, (c) fixation bolt, (d) attachment screw, (e) nail adapter bolt, (f) slide hammer, (g) medullary reamer, (h) depth gauge, (i) twist drill, (j) guide wire, (k, l) drill sleeve, (m) hexagonal screwdriver, (n) curved awl, and (o) wrench

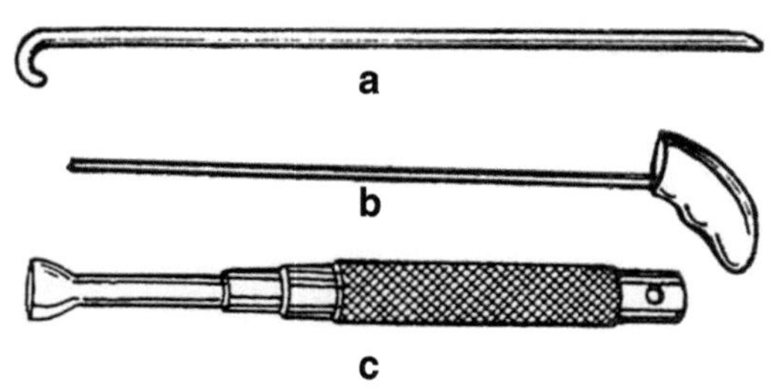


**Fig. 1.25** Instruments for Rush pinning: (a) Rush pin, (b) Rush pin reamer, and (c) Rush pin driver

that is used to drive and seat the pin into the bone and a boat-shaped end that bounces off the inner cortex of the bone as it is inserted. Available in diameter ranging from 2.5 mm to 6 mm. Used mostly in supracondylar femoral fracture fixation.

*Rush IM pin reamer*: Special type of bone reamer used during fixation of a Rush pin.

*Rush IM pin driver*: Used to insert the Rush pins.

### 1.6.6 Instruments for Kuntscher Nailing (Fig. 1.26)

*Kuntscher nails*: Are clover leaf or V-shaped hollow nails, ranging in diameter from 2 mm to 20 mm. One end of the nail is sharpened for impaction, and at the other end, there is a hole to engage an extractor hook. K-nails allow direct contact along the medullary cavity in at least three places, which provides rotational stability to fixation.

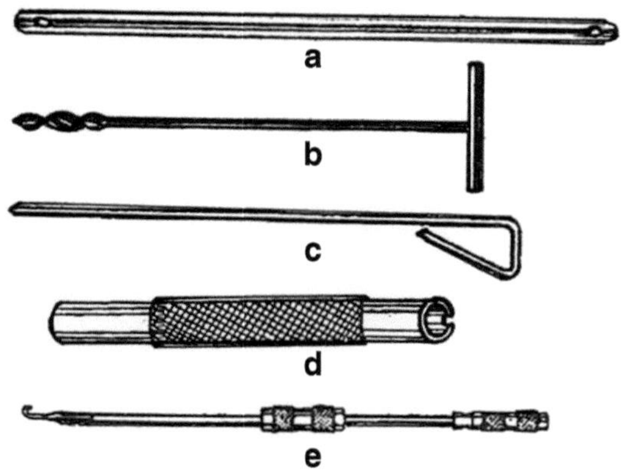


**Fig. 1.26** Instruments for K-nailing: (a) K-nail, (b) medullary reamer, (c) guide wire, (d) K-nail driver, and (e) K-nail extractor

*Medullary canal reamer*: Used to ream the medullary cavity before K-nailing. Due to reaming, the medullary canal becomes more uniform in diameter for greater contact of the nail.

*Guide pin*: Used to guide the K-nail into the medullary cavity. Also helps to measure the length of the medullary cavity to select K-nail of desired length.

*K-nail driver*: Used to drive the K-nail into the medullary cavity. At one end, it has a notch which helps to seat on the nail, whereas the other end is hammered to drive the nail.

*Mallet*: Helps to hammer the nail.

*K-nail extractor*: The hook present at one end of a long rod is engaged into the hole present in K-nail, and the other end is hammered to facilitate easy extraction of the nail.

### 1.6.7 Instruments for Bone Stapling (Fig. 1.27)

*Staples*: 'U'-shaped stainless-steel wires, pointed at both ends. Used mainly to fix metaphyseal/epiphyseal/chip fractures. Commonly used along with other primary fixation devices.

*Staple starter*: Helps to mark the depressions in the bone for proper seating of staples before they are driven into the bone.

*Staple driver*: Helps to secure and insert the staples.

*Staple extractor*: It has an elevated edge at one end, which helps for easy extraction of staples by inserting it between the bone and the staple.

### 1.6.8 Instruments for Orthopedic Wiring (Fig. 1.28)

*Orthopedic wire*: Is a flexible monofilament stainless-steel wire that is most commonly used in combination with some other primary internal fixation techniques, such as IM pins, bone plates, etc. Available in sizes ranging from 16 to 28 gauges.

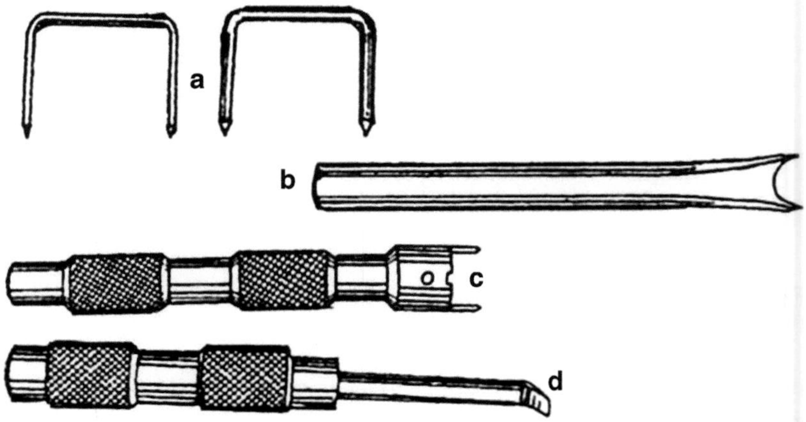


**Fig. 1.27** Instruments for staple fixation: (a) staples, (b) staple starter, (c) staple driver, and (d) staple extractor

*Wire-tightening forceps*: Helps to tighten the wire, so that uniform interfragmentary compression can be achieved at the fracture site.

*Wire twister*: Helps to achieve uniform twisting of both ends of the wire and properly secure while doing full cerclage or hemicerclage wiring.

*Wire cutter*: Used to cut the stainless-steel wires.

*Wire passer*: Mainly used to pass wires around the fractured bone. It helps firmly grip and control the passage of wire without injuring the nerves, vessels, and soft tissues.

### 1.6.9 Instruments for External Skeletal Fixation (Fig. 1.29)

*Fixation pins*: Can be half or full pins and smooth or threaded pins. Threaded pins can be of positive profile (if the core diameter is consistent between smooth and threaded regions) or negative profile (core diameter of the threaded section is smaller than the diameter of the smooth section), and it can be completely threaded or centrally/end threaded.

*Thomson beaded pin*: Used in circular ESF, the presence of a bead in the pin helps to align the

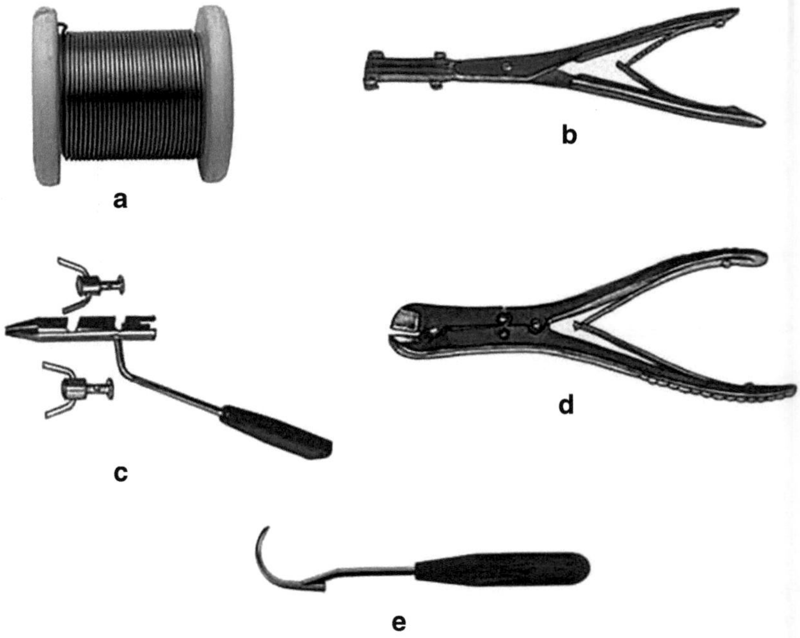


**Fig. 1.28** Instruments for orthopedic wiring: (a) orthopedic wire, (b) wire-tightening forceps, (c) wire twister, (d) wire cutter, and (e) wire passer

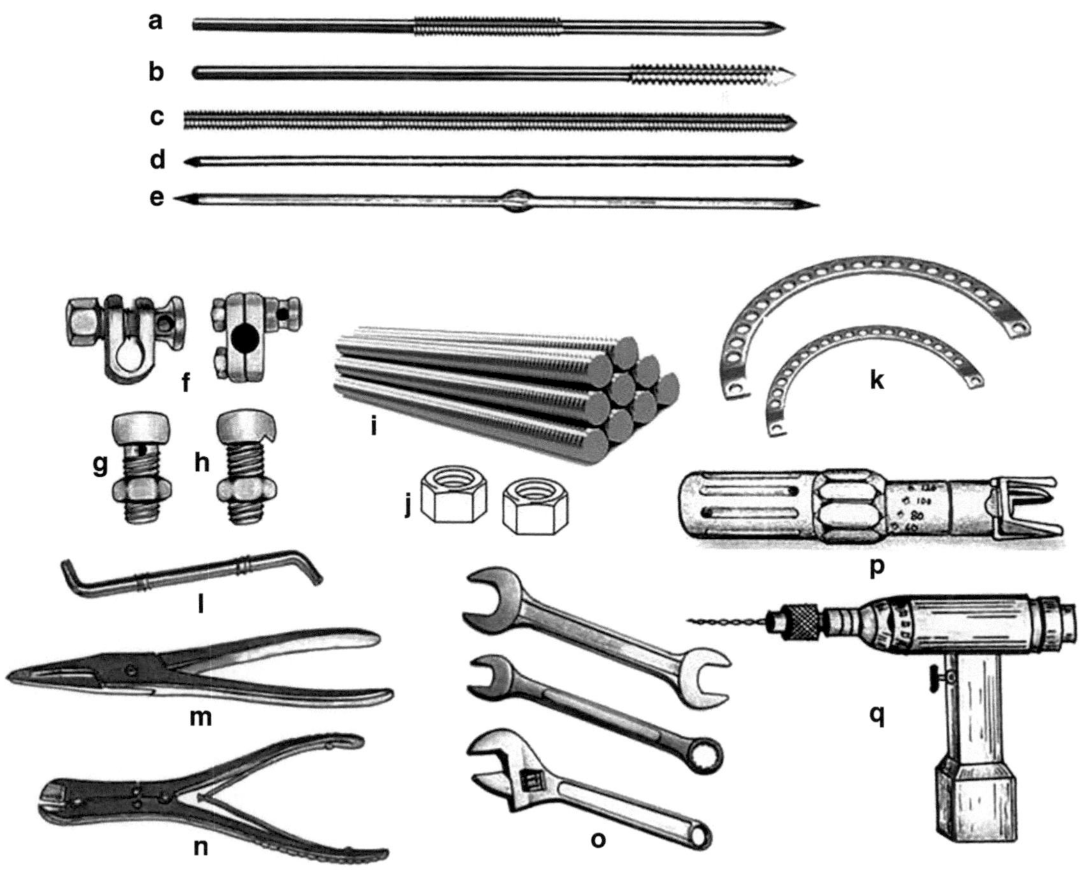


**Fig. 1.29** Instruments for external skeletal fixation: (a) centrally threaded pin, (b) end threaded pin, (c) fully threaded pin, (d) K-wire, (e) Olive (beaded) wire, (f) fixation clamps for linear fixation device, (g, h) cannulated and slotted fixation bolt for circular fixation, (i) threaded rods, (j) nuts, (k) half rings for circular fixation, (l) K-wire bender, (m) pin/wire bender, (n) pin cutter, (o) wrench, (p) wire tensioner, and (q) electric drill

bone segments by pulling the bone segments to a required position. It will also help to prevent translation (movement) of bone segments after bone fixation.

*External connectors*: Are either linear side bars (in linear fixation systems) or circular rings connected through threaded rods (in circular fixation systems). External connectors can be made from different materials such as stainless steel, mild steel, aluminum, carbon fiber, or epoxy.

*Linkage devices*: Clamps (connects the fixation pins to side bars and also connects side bars in linear fixation systems) and fixation bolts, either cannulated or slotted (for joining fixation pins to the rings in circular external fixation systems).

*Nuts and wrenches*: For tightening and loosening the fixation bolts and external connectors/rings.

*Wire tensioner*: Used to apply tension along the transfixation pin before fixing them to the circular fixator; there are many types of wire tensioners available.

*Pin bender/cutter*: To bend or cut the extra length pins.

*Electric drill*: For insertion of transfixation pins.

## 1.7 Examination of the Animals with Fracture

A comprehensive clinical examination of the animal suspected of having a fracture should be carried out before deciding the treatment [68]. Localization and diagnosis of a complete fracture of a long bone are relatively easy by simple clinical examination. Incomplete fractures sometime pose a challenge to examine and correctly diagnose. Lameness is the foremost clinical sign of a fracture. It is always advised to observe the injured animal first from a distance, without attracting the attention of the patient. Observe the animal shifting its weight at a stance or while sitting. It will tend to subtly shift its weight away from its painful limb/s during standing; if both pelvic limbs are injured, it may prefer to sit. Injured animals, especially cattle which are recumbent, should be allowed to remain recumbent during the physical examination. Often, there is a sudden weight shift to the front limbs as the animal attempts to sit or rise. Similarly, a weight shift away from a single uncomfortable limb can be quite evident while sitting.

Animals with complete fractures of the limbs have acute non-weight-bearing lameness (carrying of the limb). There can also be shortening of the affected limb with bending or deformity at the injured site. Based on the site of bending/bowing of the bone, fracture can be localized. Some special fractures may show specific signs. For instance, fracture at the femoral head/neck along with dislocation of the hip joint may result in hyperextension of the stifle joint, whereas in diaphyseal fractures of the humerus (especially at the distal third), knuckling of the paw/digits may be seen due to involvement of the radial nerve.

Soft tissue swelling at the site of fracture is another classical sign, which helps in fracture localization. Soft tissue swelling is more pronounced in fractures of the proximal limb bones (femur/humerus), though it may also be noticed in lower limb fractures. Comminutions of bone fragments generate more heat and hence profound soft tissue swelling. Also, in fractures near the joint or in intra-articular fractures, swelling is generally more, like in cases of fractures near the femoral condyles. The presence or absence of soft tissue swelling sometimes may help to differentiate between a fracture and a joint dislocation, as in case of a luxation of the femoral head and fracture of the femoral head/neck. Soft tissue swelling may not be apparent in old fractures, wherein acute stage of inflammation would have subsided.

Some animals often become recumbent after a trauma, and any attempts to make the animal stand may fail. It is also not advisable to make repeated attempts to lift the animal without proper application of splints and bandages, especially large animals, as it may further damage the injured limb. In such cases, multiple trauma/fractures should be suspected. There could be bilateral limb fractures, pelvic fractures, or spinal fracture. Urinary and fecal incontinence and flaccidity of the tail/hind quarter may be observed in cases of spinal fractures.

Close physical examination of a fractured animal should be undertaken carefully, when the patient is relaxed and comfortable, and the animal may also be sedated (particularly large ruminants) before undertaking examination. The patient may be examined while in standing or recumbent position, whichever is comfortable to the animal. Palpation at the suspected site of fracture may reveal crepitation of bone fragments. However, excessive maneuvering of the fracture site should be avoided, as it may elicit pain response and the animal may get excited. While examining an aggressive or tense animal, we should also make sure to protect ourselves from getting injured.

Radiographic examination confirms the presence or absence of a bone fracture. It also helps to find the type of fracture and its exact location, which ultimately help the surgeon to plan surgical fixation. It is always advisable to make two orthogonal radiographic views for definitive diagnosis of a fracture. If only one view is made, then it should be medio-lateral or latero-medial view for the limb bones, lateral view for the spine, and ventro-dorsal view for the pelvis. Generally, a plain radiograph is sufficient to confirm a bone fracture; however, more advanced techniques such as digital radiography or CT scan would be more accurate, especially to detect occult fractures. In recent years, these techniques are being frequently used in small animal practice, though they are still beyond the reach for large animal use.

### 1.7.1 Things we Should Avoid while Examining an Injured Animal

- Making sudden noise and movements.
- Performing excessive maneuvering and manipulations to detect fracture site crepitus.
- Making excessive attempts to make the animal stand, especially a recumbent large animal.
- Forcing a fractured animal to move before stabilizing with splints and bandages.
- Rush to sedate the animal and perform radiography.
- Rush to undertake definitive surgical fixation.

## 1.8 Emergency Treatment of Fracture and First Aid

The initial care and management of an injured animal are critical, which largely decide the outcome of the case. Before attempting any definitive treatment of a fracture, the patient should be given first aid and emergency treatment, when required [69, 70]. The animal met with an automobile accident or any other trauma must be first rescued from the site. As an injured animal is likely to get excited and there are more chances of further injury at the fracture site, it is all more important to secure the animal. A thorough physical examination of the animal should be carried out, and life-threatening injury should be dealt first. One should ensure that the airway is clear and any external hemorrhage is controlled. Hemorrhage generally does not require a tourniquet to control; small bleeding can be controlled adequately by firm bandaging. Life-threatening hemorrhage may often be seen due to laceration of a major artery. Only if profuse arterial bleeding persists, the need for a tourniquet may arise. If a tourniquet is applied, ensure that it is removed as early as possible. Multiple injuries sometime may be life-threatening, especially if the thoracic part is involved with rib fractures causing flail chest and pneumo-/haemo-thorax. In such cases, emergency care should be provided first. Administration of drugs such as corticosteroids may be beneficial. Assessment of the state of hydration, cardiopulmonary, and shock status is important, and if needed, they should be taken care on priority by administering either blood or plasma expanders/colloid solutions. Normal saline or Ringer's solution though cannot replace blood may help improve circulation.

Once it is ensured that the animal is physiologically stable, any open wound is covered with a clean dressing, and an attempt should be made to immobilize the fractured limb to make the animal comfortable and prevent continued injury from the broken bone ends. If the animal is recumbent, especially a large animal, it should not be disturbed till the physical examination done and the limb immobilized. Only then, an attempt should be made to get the animal stand and allowed to move. Allowing the animal to move before splinting the limb may prove disastrous as it may lead to compounding of a simple fracture [71]. In general, a fracture below the elbow or stifle may be temporarily immobilized using splints or casts. Proximal fractures do not require any immobilization as there is sufficient soft tissue coverage to protect the broken bone. Further, it is not possible to immobilize a fracture in the humerus/femur through external cooptation, especially in large animals. Any such attempt may result in 'fulcrum effect' at the fracture site leading to more soft tissue damage.

The external stabilization of the fractured limb can be done using either splints and bandage or a cast. If an open wound is present, it should be thoroughly cleaned with any antiseptic solution and bandage applied before splinting. In small animals, single lightweight splint made of PVC pipe or a cardboard is enough, and in large animals, at least two strong splints made of bamboo/PVC pipe are placed one at the caudal aspect and another at the cranial/lateral aspect of the limb, and bandage should be applied firmly after placing adequate padding. The joints proximal and distal to the fractured bone should be included in the cooptation, and it should extend from the joint above the fracture and below up to the level of the paw/sole. In large animals, it is desirable to immobilize the whole limb extending from the stifle/elbow up to the sole to provide greater stability.

Administration of anti-inflammatory analgesic drug/s should be initiated as early as possible. This can help in reducing the pain and discomfort to the animal and controlling inflammatory swelling and oedema and hence facilitate surgical fixation of fracture. However, administration of analgesics prior to adequate immobilization of the fractured limb may decrease the pain sensitivity, which may allow unrestricted movement of the broken bone leading to further injury to the animal. Tranquilizers or hypnotics, which also depress CNS and sedate the animal and reduce body movements, may be used especially in vicious animals. A broad-spectrum antibiotic is required if the fracture is open and contaminated. This should continue till definitive fracture fixation is done.

Once stabilized, the animal should be taken to a referral hospital with adequate facility to undertake surgical fixation of fracture. It is relatively easy to carry a small animal, but a greater care is needed to transport a large animal orthopedic patient. The animal should be tranquilized/sedated and properly secured on soft bedding with the fractured limb held upwards. Care should also be exercised while loading and unloading the animal.

## 1.9 Anesthesia and Pain Management in Animals with Fracture

Fracture of the bone is a very painful condition. Further, it is always associated with certain level of soft tissue injury. Thus, maneuvering the fracture fragments even with closed methods would result in excessive pain to the animal. Therefore, anesthesia and effective analgesia are an essential component of any operation conducted in relation to management of bone fracture. A large variety of anesthetic techniques are available for practice in animals [72–78]. However, the choice of the technique for a particular situation may be dictated by several considerations like the species of the animal, the bone involved, the availability of the facility, preferences of the attending veterinarian, etc. Here, we have listed some of the common techniques of anesthesia and analgesia that may be used in orthopedic cases.

### 1.9.1 Anesthesia in Cattle

#### 1.9.1.1 General Anesthetic Techniques

1. **Injectable anesthetics:** Anesthesia can be induced after casting the animal on a hydraulic table in lateral recumbency. The use of indwelling catheter (10–14 gauge; 10–15 cm long) is preferable for intravenous injections to avoid perivascular injection of irritant drugs and for supplemental injections.
   (a) *Ketamine*: Premedication with diazepam, xylazine, acepromazine, or medetomidine produces quiet, smooth anesthetic induction with good muscle relaxation and deep sedation.
   Xylazine, 0.1-0.2 mg/kg body weight i.m.; 0.05–0.1 mg/kg body weight i.v. and ketamine, 2-5 mg/kg body weight i.v. or i.m.; duration of anesthesia, 15–30 min.
   Diazepam, 0.2 mg/kg and ketamine, 5 mg/kg body weight i.v.; duration of anesthesia, 15 min.
   Medetomidine, 0.02 mg/kg body weight and ketamine, 0.5-1.0 mg/kg body weight i.v.; duration of anesthesia, 30 min.
   (b) *Propofol*: A costly drug used in large animals but is a good general anesthetic agent.
   Dose, 5–6 mg/kg body weight i.v.; duration of anesthesia, 4–9 min; recovery, smooth.
   (c) *Tiletamine and zolazepam:* Produces hypoxia when the animal is restrained in dorsal recumbency., 4 mg/kg body weight i.m. and zolazepam, 0.1 mg/kg body weight i.m.; duration of anesthesia, 70 min; recovery, 130 min.

2. **Inhalation anesthetics:** Anesthesia can be induced initially through a mask using a small animal circle system in small ruminants. In large animals, induction is preferably done by an injectable agent after premedication with diazepam (0.1 mg/kg body weight), butorphanol (0.05–0.1 mg/kg body weight), and xylazine (0.02 mg/kg body weight). Endotracheal intubation is then done with or without a laryngoscope. The cuff is inflated, and the tube is secured, and inhalation anesthesia is used for maintenance of anesthesia for a desired period.
   (a) *Halothane*: Used with a precision vaporizer along with oxygen 1–2% is required for maintenance; recovery is rapid.
   (b) *Isoflurane*: Similar effects as that of halothane but recovery is more rapid.

#### 1.9.1.2 Local/Regional Anesthetic Techniques

The technique involves the use of local anesthetics and other drugs to produce desensitization over a limited body area.

##### Anesthetics Used for Local/Regional Analgesia

1. *Local anesthetics*: Lidocaine (2%) is the most commonly used local anesthetic having a shorter onset and longer duration of action than procaine. Bupivacaine (0.5%) and ropivacaine (0.75%) are more potent than lidocaine and mepivacaine and have longer duration of action. Side effects occur on absorption through systemic circulation and produce hypotension on epidural administration due to sympathetic blockade. Respiratory depression occurs from CNS activity.
2. *Alpha-2 agonists*: Produce slower onset and longer duration of regional analgesia than local anesthetics by stimulation of alpha-2-adrenergic receptors in the brain and spinal cord. Sedation, hypotension, bradycardia, decreased secretions, and GIT motility are due to systemic absorption through the venous sinuses of the spinal cord. Xylazine (0.05–0.1 mg/kg body weight), detomidine (60–100 μg/kg body weight), medetomidine (30–60 μg/kg body weight), and romifidine (50 μg/kg body weight) can be used along with lidocaine in order to increase the potency and duration of anesthesia produced by lidocaine.
3. *Opioid analgesics*: Produce analgesia by acting via μ, δ, and κ receptors located in the spinal cord and prevent the release of substance P. Meperidine (1 mg/kg body weight) and buprenorphine (1 mg/kg body weight) have higher potency and longer duration of action than local anesthetics. Produce side effects such as respiratory depression, pruritis, and urinary retention.
4. *NMDA antagonists*: Ketamine produces local analgesia by the antagonism of NMDA receptors. Ketamine (2–3.5 mg/kg body weight) after epidural/spinal administration produces short duration of regional analgesia and cardiac and respiratory stimulation after systemic absorption.
5. *Combination of different drugs*: Combinations of local anesthetic and opioids, local anesthetic and alpha-2 adrenergic agonists, and alpha-2-agonists and ketamine have been used in clinical settings, wherein the doses of drugs used in combination are relatively lower than an individual drug administration, and hence, the side effects are relatively less. They produce synergistic action and longer duration of regional analgesia than that produced by either agent used alone.

##### Techniques of Local/Regional Anesthesia

1. *Infiltration analgesia*: The nerve endings at the actual site of surgery are blocked by lidocaine (0.5–2%) or bupivacaine (0.125–0.5%). An intradermal weal is made with a hypodermic needle. Subcutaneous tissues are then infiltrated, and injection is made after ascertaining that the needle has not entered a blood vessel. As the needle is gradually withdrawn, the anesthetic solution is injected along the length (about 1 mL of anesthetic solution for every cm length).

2. *Regional nerve blocks*: Regional nerves are blocked by fanwise injections of local anesthetics in the tissues on their way to the surgical site. An inverted 'L' block is made by two linear infiltrations by incorporating the whole thickness of the abdominal wall in the flank region. Ring block of the extremities is done through a transverse plane in a circular fashion. Conduction in the sensory nerves is blocked by local anesthetic without touching the operative field.
3. *Intravenous regional analgesia (IVRA)*: A tourniquet is tied on the proximal side of the limb to occlude the arterial supply. Local analgesic solution is then injected intravenously through a needle. Analgesia of the lower extremity up to the level of the tourniquet is effected very rapidly and also wears off rapidly after releasing the tourniquet.
4. *Epidural/spinal analgesia*:

Injection of local analgesic solution into the spinal canal paralyzes the spinal nerves. Epidural injections are made by deposition of analgesics on the dura mater and spinal injections by depositing the solution into the CSF. Caudal block is made by injections in the sacrococcygeal or intercoccygeal space for analgesia of the tail, perineum, vulva, vagina, and caudal thigh region. The needle is inserted between the first and second coccygeal vertebrae or between last sacral and first coccygeal vertebrae. It is advanced ventrally and cranially at 15° angle to enter the neural canal. 5–10 mL of local anesthetic drug is then injected (Table 1.4). The onset of effect occurs within a minute and analgesia persists for an hour. Cranial block is made by injections in the lumbosacral or lumbar epidural space. Lumbar epidural block produces analgesia of the posterior thoracic region, flank, and ventral abdominal region. The motor fibers of the hindlimbs are unaffected. In lumbosacral block, the entire thigh region, posterior flank, perineum, inguinal region, ventral abdomen, hindlimbs, and digits are affected. For these injections, a long spinal needle (14 gauge, 12 cm long) with short bevel is needed. The needle is passed between the two vertebrae and the neural canal is entered through the interarcuate ligament. Analgesic solution is injected which enters freely. If CSF comes out through the hub, then the needle is slightly withdrawn and injection is made.

### 1.9.2 Anesthesia in Sheep/Goat

#### 1.9.2.1 General Anesthetic Techniques

1. **Injectable anesthetics:** Orthopedic surgery is best performed under inhalation anesthesia, using injectable anesthetics as induction agents, and for intubation. However, injectable anesthetics for induction and maintenance of anesthesia can be used (Table 1.5), but prolonged use may cause hypoxaemia. The use of preanesthetics may reduce the dose of anesthetic and shorten recovery time.
2. **Inhalation anesthetics:** Sevoflurane and isoflurane are the most commonly used inhalation anesthetics for better control and rapid recovery. Anesthetic breathing system used for dogs may be utilized for sheep and goats. After anesthetic induction and intubation, isoflurane may be set at 2.0–2.5% with oxygen flow rate of 1–2 L/min.

**Local/regional anesthetics:** Drugs used and techniques are similar to those used in cattle.

### 1.9.3 Anesthesia in Horse

#### 1.9.3.1 General Anesthetic Techniques

1. **Intravenous techniques***:* There are a number of possible combinations of drugs suitable for anesthetic induction (Table 1.6). The choice depends upon the health status of the horse, facilities available, and on the individual preference on their use.
2. **Inhalation agents**: These agents are mainly used for maintenance of anesthesia.
   (a) *Halothane*: Halothane causes dose-dependent decrease in arterial blood pressure and cardiac output and increase in central venous pressure but produces anesthesia without toxicity and causes depression of reflexes and smooth

**Table 1.4** Drugs used for epidural/spinal analgesia in cattle

| Sl. no. | Drug | Onset (min) | Duration (h) | Standing (h) |
|---|---|---|---|---|
| 1. | Lidocaine (2%) with adrenaline 1 mL/5 kg body weight | 25 | 2 | 3.5–5.0 |
| 2. | Bupivacaine 0.5% or 0.75% 1 mL/4 kg body weight | 45 | 4–6 | 8–12 |
| 3. | Xylazine (0.05 mg/kg body weght) with ketamine (2.5 mg/kg body weight) | <5 | 1 | 2–3 |

recovery. Anesthesia can be maintained with 0.7–1.3% of halothane in oxygen. Recovery takes place 0.5–1 h after termination of administration.

(b) *Isoflurane*: Effects are similar to halothane. Other drugs used are enflurane, sevoflurane, and desflurane.

#### 1.9.3.2 Local/Regional Anesthetic Techniques

1. **Local anesthesia**: The important local anesthetic techniques for orthopedic surgery in horse include different regional nerve blocks of the head, forelimbs, and hindlimbs.
2. **Epidural analgesia:** Caudal epidural analgesia is performed between the first and second coccygeal vertebrae. The depression between the first and second coccygeal dorsal spinous process can be palpated about 2.5 cm cranial to the onset of the tail. The epidural needle is inserted at the caudal portion of the first intercoccygeal space directing cranioventrally at an angle of about 30 degrees. 10 mL of 2% lidocaine is sufficient to produce caudal analgesia.

### 1.9.4 Anesthesia in Pig

#### 1.9.4.1 General Anesthesia

In pigs, 6–8 h of fasting and 2 h of deprivation of water is sufficient. Premedication with atropine 0.3–2.4 mg body weight (total dose) i.m. or i.v. or glycopyrrolate 0.2–2.0 mg (total dose) based on animal's body weight will be sufficient to control salivation. Azaperone is the most widely used sedative in pigs (dose 1–8 mg/kg body weight, i.m.). Intravenous injections can be made through auricular veins on the external ear flap. For large quantities of fluids, jugular vein should be catheterized under general anesthesia. The anterior vena cava can be catheterized by restraining the animal on its back with fully extended neck and head in handing down position and forelegs pulled backwards. A 5–7.5 cm long needle is inserted through the skin in the depression lateral to the cranial angle of the sternum and the angle between the first rib and trachea. The needle is then pushed toward an imaginary central point between the scapulae until the vena cava is pierced and blood starts oozing out. A fine plastic catheter should be threaded through the needle. Intubation is difficult in pigs as the larynx is set to an angle to the trachea.

**Table 1.5** Drugs used for general anesthesia in sheep and goats

| Sl. no. | Drugs | Dosage (mg/kg body weight); route of administration | Duration | Remarks |
|---|---|---|---|---|
| 1 | Diazepam + ketamine | 0.2–0.3, i.v. + 5.0–7.5, i.v. | 10–15 min | Butorphanol 0.1 mg/kg body weight may be added |
| 2 | Xylazine + ketamine | 0.1, i.m. + 6.0, i.v./11.0, i.m. | 30 min | Additional ketamine can be added to prolong the time |
| 3 | Xylazine+ tiletamine-zolazepam | 0.1, i.m. + 4.0, i.v. | 45–60 min | Higher dose of xylazine may cause apnoea |
| 4 | Propofol | 4.0, i.v. | Duration is short but can be increased by incremental dose | Quality of anesthesia can be improved by preanesthetics |

**Table 1.6** Combination of different drugs used for induction of general anesthesia intravenously in horses

| Premedicants (mg/kg body weight); route of administration | Induction agents (mg/kg body weight); route of administration | Maintenance agents (increment doses in mg/kg body weight); route of administration |
|---|---|---|
| Acepromazine 0.03–0.05, i.v. | Ketamine 2–2.2, i.v. | Ketamine 1.0, i.v. |
| Xylazine 0.5, i.v. | Ketamine 2–2.2, i.v. | Do -, |
| Detomidine 0.01, i.v. | Ketamine 2–2.2, i.v. | Do -. |
| Xylazine 1.0, i.v. | Ketamine 2–2.2 mg/kg, i.v. | Xylazine 0.5 and ketamine 1.0, i.v. |
| Detomidine 0.01, i.v. | Ketamine 2–2.2, i.v. | Ketamine 1.0, i.v. |
| Romifidine 0.08–0.12, i.v. | Ketamine 2–2.2, i.v. | Romifidine 0.02–0.04 and ketamine 1.0, i.v. |
| Acepromazine 0.03–0.05, i.v. | Guaifenesin 25–50, i.v. followed by ketamine 1.0, i.v. | Ketamine 1.0, i.v. |
| Xylazine 0.5–1.0/detomidine 0.01/romifidine 0.08, i.v. | Guaifenesin 25–50, i.v. followed by ketamine 1.0, i.v. | Ketamine 1.0, i.v. |
| Xylazine 1.0/detomidine 0.01–0.02/romifidine 0.08/kg, i.v. | Guaifenesin 15–30, i.v. followed by ketamine 1.5–2.0, i.v. | Ketamine 1.0, i.v. |

#### 1.9.4.2 Intravenous Techniques

- Azaperone 2 mg/kg body weight i.m.; 20 min later, metomidate 3.3 mg/kg body weight, i.v.
- Azaperone 2 mg/kg body weight, i.m.; 20 min later, thiopental i.v. till effect (5 mg/kg body weight or less).
- Ketamine 20 mg/kg body weight, i.m.
- Xylazine 1 mg/kg body weight, i.m. followed by 15 min later ketamine 2–5 mg/kg body weight, i.v.
- Diazepam 1–2 mg/kg body weight, i.v. followed by ketamine 10–15 mg/kg body weight, i.v.
- Ketamine 2 mg and xylazine 1 mg per mL of 5% guaifenesin is given at 0.6–1.0 mL/kg body weight for induction, and anesthesia can be maintained at 2.2 mL/kg body weight/h

### 1.9.5 Anesthesia in Dog

**Preanesthetic medication:** It usually involves administration of anticholinergic, sedative, and analgesic drugs (Table 1.7).

*Anticholinergic drugs*: To limit bradycardia and to prevent salivation.

1. Atropine sulfate, 0.04 mg/kg body weight, s.c., i.m., or i.v.; onset 20 min; duration 1.5 h.
2. Glycopyrrolate, decreases gastric acidity, causes lesser increase in heart rate as compared to atropine sulfate, and is advantageous in animals with tachycardia. It may be given at 0.01 mg/kg body weight i.m. or 0.005 mg/kg body weight i.v.; onset 40 min; duration 2–4 h.

**Intravenous anesthesia***:* Intravenous agents are used either as sole anesthetic agents or as induction agents for anesthesia to be maintained with inhalation agents.

Sites: The most common site is the cephalic vein, but the lateral saphenous vein, femoral vein, jugular vein, and in anesthetized animal lingual vein may also be used.

**Anesthetic Agents** *Ketamine*: It should not be given as sole anesthetic agent in dogs as it causes excessive muscle tone and spontaneous muscle activity. Anticholinergics should be used to prevent salivation. Xylazine 1 mg/kg body weight i.m. followed 10–15 min later by ketamine 5 mg/kg body weight or combination of medetomidine 0.04 mg/kg body weight i.m. followed 15 min later by i.v. ketamine 3–4 mg/kg body weight makes good anesthetic choice for short surgeries. Diazepam 0.25–0.5 mg/kg body weight i.v. followed 10 min later by ketamine 5 mg/kg body weight i.v. can also be given.

*Propofol*: It is a free-flowing water in oil emulsion. It is a rapidly acting agent producing anesthesia for short duration. It is given intravenously only, but perivascular injection does not produce tissue necrosis. It can be used as a sole anesthetic agent (6–8 mg/kg, i.v.), but due to its very short duration of action, it is used with wide range of preanesthetics and injectable and inhalation

**Table 1.7** Different sedative/analgesic drugs, such as opioids, phenothiazines, benzodiazepines, and alpha-2 adrenergic agonists used in dogs

| Classification of drug | Name of drug | Dose of drug (mg/kg body weight); route of administration | Comments and precautions |
|---|---|---|---|
| Phenothiazines | Acepromazine | 0.05–0.1, i.m. | To be avoided in animals with severe blood loss or hypotension and in dogs with history of seizures and when myelography is scheduled |
| Alpha-2 agonists | Xylazine | 0.5–2.0, i.m. or 0.5–1.0, i.v. | Retching and vomiting, marked sedation; dose of anesthetics is reduced; induction of anesthesia is slowed; risk of anesthetic overdose |
| | Medetomidine | 0.02–0.04, i.m. or 0.01–0.02, i.v. | Profound sedation, severely reduced dose |
| | Romifidine | 0.04–0.08, i.m. | Reduced dose of ketamine up to 4 mg/kg body weight |
| Opioids | Butorphanol | 0.2–0.4, i.m. or i.v. | Onset of action 10–15 min |
| | Pethidine | 3.0–4.0, i.m. | Onset of action in 20 min |
| | Oxymorphone | 0.05–0.20, i.m. or i.v. | Max. dose 5 mg, may initiate vomiting/panting |
| | Buprenorphine | 0.006–0.01 | Onset time is 30–40 min |
| Benzodiazepines | Diazepam | 0.2–0.5, i.v. | Poorly absorbed on i.m. injection |
| | Midazolam | 0.1–0.2, i.m. | Two times more potent than diazepam and more useful for i.m. injection |

anesthetic agents. The common combinations are acepromazine (0.03–0.05 mg/kg body weight, i.m.) + propofol (4–5 mg/kg body weight, i.v.); acepromazine (0.03–0.05 mg/kg body weight, i.m.) + butorphanol (0.2–0.3 mg/kg body weight, i.m.) + propofol (3–4 mg/kg body weight, i.v.); acepromazine (0.03–0.05 mg/kg body weight, i.m.) + morphine (0.5 mg/kg body weight, i.m.) + propofol (1–2 mg/kg body weight, i.v.); and medetomidine (0.04 mg/kg body weight, i.m.) + propofol (1–1.5 mg/kg body weight, i.v.).

**Inhalation anesthesia:** Used for maintenance of anesthesia induced with intravenous agents.

*Halothane*: Anesthesia can be maintained with 0.8–2% concentration. The MAC is about 0.85%. It causes dose-dependent depression of the cardiac output and arterial blood pressure due to decreased plasma catecholamines. Dose-dependent reduction in rate and depth of respiration is also recorded. It also causes bradycardia due to activity in the vagus nerve. Halothane induces only moderate muscle relaxation and is a poor analgesic agent. Addition of opioid analgesic is advantageous. The incidence of hepatotoxicity is very low.

*Isoflurane*: It is a potent anesthetic agent, and therefore, the vaporizer must be precisely calibrated. Concentration required for maintenance is 1.5–2.5%. MAC in dogs is 1.28%. Other drugs used for inhalation anesthesia in dogs include enflurane, desflurane, and sevoflurane.

### 1.9.6 Anesthesia in Cat

**Injectable agents**: Cats object to being restrained, and therefore, injection of intravenous agent is difficult in conscious or un-premedicated cats.

*Ketamine*: Ketamine can be administered through i.v., i.m., or s.c. route. A dose of 10 mg/kg body weight i.v. or 20 mg/kg body weight i.m. can make the cat recumbent for 30 min. Ketamine initiates a state of catalepsy. It abolishes superficial painful stimuli but abdominal pain may still persist. Cats administered with ketamine exhibit marked muscle tone, and spontaneous movement unrelated to the stimulation may occur. Salivation is often profuse and premedication with atropine 0.03–0.05 mg/kg body weight is recommended. The effects of ketamine on the heart and respiration are minimal. A wide range of preanesthetics has been used to reduce emergence excitement and increased muscle tone: acepromazine 0.01–0.03 mg/kg body weight + ketamine 10 mg/kg body weight i.v. or 20 mg/kg body weight i.m.; xylazine 1.0 mg/kg body weight + ketamine 5 mg/kg body weight; diazepam 1 mg/kg body weight or midazolam 0.2 mg/kg body weight + ketamine 10 mg/kg body weight i.m.; and medetomidine 0.08 mg/kg body weight i.m. + ketamine 5–7 mg/kg body weight i.m.

*Propofol*: It has been a quite extensively used intravenous anesthetic in cats. Dose is 6–7 mg/kg body weight.

**Inhalation agents**: All inhalation anesthetics used in dogs may be used in cats in similar way.

### 1.9.7 Management of Pain

The International Association for the Treatment of Pain defined pain in human as 'An unpleasant sensory and emotional experience associated with actual or potential tissue damage or described in terms of such damage'. Like human beings, fracture of a bone leads to severe pain and discomfort in animals as well. Prevention and treatment of pain and suffering of animals during the fracture, fracture fixation, and the postfixation period should be an important goal of veterinary orthopedic surgeons.

Pain in fracture cases is generally acute in nature, which can vary from mild to severe, and is induced by the trauma causing the fracture or fracture repair, especially surgical fixation. Based on the severity of tissue injury, pain may persist for a few days to weeks. Following a trauma, the magnitude of acute pain is highest during the initial 24–72 h, which normally responds well to analgesics. Early and stable fixation of fracture will reduce the intensity of pain. However, pain may be chronic lasting for months to years depending on the level of fracture repair and bone healing.

The various species of animals react differently to a trauma or a bone fracture. They may reveal different clinical signs suggesting (but not very characteristic to) pain and may respond differently to treatment. The individual response to trauma and the analgesic requirement may also vary greatly among the animals of a particular species. Nevertheless, it is essential to assess and control pain at the earliest as it can lead to early functional recovery and regaining of production.

The need to treat postoperative pain in animals is more compelling now than before. Nowadays, many veterinary practitioners use anesthetic drugs such as propofol, diazepam-ketamine, and isoflurane, which provide quick recovery from anesthesia. However, speedy anesthetic recovery is usually accompanied with profound pain after a surgery, except when analgesic drugs like opioids, alpha-2 adrenergic agonists, local anesthetics, or NSAIDs are used with these anesthetics. Further, the development of safe anesthetic techniques has allowed many veterinary surgeons to undertake more invasive procedures causing higher tissue damage and pain, necessitating the administration of drugs to mitigate pain.

It is difficult to estimate the intensity of pain experienced by an animal with a fracture; however, it is easy to predict and prevent/minimize the pain by knowing the extent of fracture and soft tissue trauma, the anatomical site, and the type of fixation technique used or to be used. Orthopedic procedures such as fracture fixation are always painful due to manipulation and trauma to the bone and surrounding soft tissues. Amputation can cause severe pain, especially on the high limb. Surgical procedures of the vertebrae can cause severe pain, especially of the cervical region (relatively less pain in the thoracic and lumbar regions).

Pain in animals may be recognized by deviations from normal behavior and appearance; however, they are not very consistent in all species of animals, and all the changes may not be seen in a particular animal. Pain may be recognized by the sudden changes in the behavior and temperament (e.g. a docile animal may suddenly become aggressive or an agile animal may become silent); abnormal vocalization (especially upon palpation of the injured site or if it is compelled to move); licking, scratching, or biting the aching area, sometime leading to self-mutilation;

guarding or protecting the affected area; changes in normal sleeping pattern; changes in posture or ambulation (lameness and limb disuse); changes in the activity (may become restless and repeatedly lie down and get up sometimes may become recumbent and lethargic or reluctant to move); inappetence (leading to cachexia); variation in facial expression (fatigue eyes, dilated pupils, drowsy, photophobia, etc.); extreme sweating and salivation (sweating is more frequent in horses than cattle); oculonasal discharge; grinding of the teeth (common in ruminants); and diarrhea or difficulty in defecation and urination.

Clinical signs associated with pain comprise of increase in heart rate, respiratory rate, body temperature, and blood pressure; peripheral vasoconstriction; cardiac arrhythmias; sweating and hyperventilation; reduction in peristalsis; elevated blood glucose, corticosteroid, and catecholamine concentrations; excessive shaking of heads, rubbing or scratching at the painful area, and vocalization during recovery from anesthesia; and kicking at their abdomen or rolling on their backs, seen especially in horses. However, it is often difficult to diagnose pain in animals based on any single clinical or laboratory finding. Rather, pain in animals can be perceived on the basis of a combination of one's skill to recognize the signs of pain and discomfort, understanding of animal behavior, and knowledge of the intensity of pain inherent with a specific surgery.

#### 1.9.7.1 Treatment of Pain

Although pain in animals may not be treated consistently or appropriately, the main objective of treatment is to minimize the pain and suffering of the animal, thereby hastening a return to normal function. Therefore, pain treatment can be considered successful if the animal can cope with the pain and perform its normal regular activities like eating, sleeping, and moving around.

Disruption of any tissue leads to pain, and trauma to the bone can cause severe pain. Hence, pain alleviation should be the priority in all cases of fractures soon after the trauma. Similarly, the patients should be given analgesics before recovery from anesthesia. The use of proper analgesics in the anesthetic protocol reduces the dose of general anesthetic required and thus reduces the extent of cardiovascular depression. Studies have demonstrated that administering analgesics before the induction of nociceptive stimulus (say surgical fixation of a fracture) can limit the excitation of the dorsal horn neurons in the spinal cord, thereby reducing the postoperative pain. It suggests that if analgesics are administered before the surgical fixation of a fracture (instead of after), postoperative pain can be minimized. As a general rule, pain management protocol should start before the surgery and should be continued during surgery and postoperative period. Administration of analgesics should be continued till the pain is reduced to a tolerable level. After a major surgery, it is advised to administer potent analgesics like narcotics during the initial 48–72 h; subsequently, relatively less potent NSAIDs may be sufficient.

Pain can be modified by intervening at various points along the pain transmission pathway. Nociceptive stimulation can be restricted by minimizing tissue trauma and/or by administering NSAIDs (like ketoprofen or carprofen), which diminish the production of prostaglandins and other substances (by inhibiting cyclooxygenase) that sensitize the nociceptors. Peripheral nerve transmission can be interrupted by the use of local anesthetic drugs for infiltration at the surgical site, blocking nerve roots, and intravenous administration for regional analgesia. Nociceptive transmission at the spinal cord level can be inhibited by systemic and epidural/subarachnoid administration of opioids or alpha-2 adrenergic agonists or epidural/subarachnoid administration of local anesthetics. The brain pathways can be modulated by systemic administration of opioids or alpha-2 adrenergic agonists. The use of balanced or multimodal analgesia may act at different levels to maximize pain control with minimal drug doses and clinical side effects. Further, by ensuring that the animal is comfortable, normothermic, and free from environmental disturbances during recovery and postoperative period, pain can be controlled (as anxiety and fear may magnify the hypothalamic response to pain).

Selecting a particular drug or dosage of a drug used for pain relief in animals depends on several factors. Treatment of pain must be aimed at individual patient, based on the species, breed, age of the animal, surgical procedure, degree of tissue trauma, etc. A drug with known analgesic property, such as opioids, alpha-2 adrenergic agonists, local anesthetics, or NSAIDs, should be used. Sedatives can be used to reduce anxiety, but they generally have poor analgesic properties. The effects of therapy should be carefully monitored with respect to the dose and frequency of administration, which may be modified based on the particular animal's needs. Administration of analgesic drugs should be started before the start of surgery to reduce postoperative pain and hyperalgesia. Despite all analgesic drugs having some harmful effects, proper selection of drugs and dosages customized for the individual patient can minimize the detrimental effects. Further, the use of a combination of drugs from different pharmacological classes (multimodal analgesia) may provide more effective analgesia with reduced dosages of individual drugs and their side effects.

### Analgesic Drugs

Doses and routes of administration of analgesics in different species of animals are listed in Tables 1.8, 1.9, 1.10, and 1.11.

## 1.10 Methods of Fracture Reduction

The basic principles of fracture treatment are reduction of fracture segments and their stabilization till the healing of the bone and restoration of function [23, 79]. Reduction refers to bringing the fracture segments to near normal anatomical alignment. In incomplete fractures with the bone segments in place, fracture reduction is not required. Similarly, in certain type of complete fractures with little or no overriding of bone segments, fracture reduction may not be required. If bone segments can be aligned properly, imperfect apposition of the segments is acceptable in clinical situations as long as normal function and appearance are restored. When reduction of bone segments is necessary, it must be carried out under deep sedation or general anesthesia as the reduction of fracture segments is very painful. Further, sedation/anesthesia also brings about muscle relaxation, which facilitates reduction.

The fracture reduction can be achieved either by *closed*, *open*, or *semi-open* method. Reduction of fracture without incising the skin or exposing the bone, through external manipulation, is called *closed* reduction. The technique involves holding the major bone segments over the skin, separating the impacted broken ends by traction if needed and then aligning them to the near normal anatomical position. Normally, after a closed reduction, fracture is immobilized with an external fixation technique, although in certain internal fixation, reduction can be achieved externally as in fresh cases of incomplete/greenstick fractures of femur in young animals without bone displacement. Closed reduction is generally indicated in fresh lower limb fractures, comprising only two bone pieces with little or no overriding of the bone segments. Closed reduction is done only when the bone segments are easily palpable with less muscular coverage. It reduces the risk of soft tissue trauma from the surgical incision and also the cost of initial treatment.

Under sedation/anesthesia, the animal is secured in lateral recumbency. Fractures of the metacarpus, metatarsus, and radius-ulna, which have least soft tissue covering and are oriented along the long axis of the limb, can be reduced by applying traction along the limb. Holding the limb in an upright position helps in muscle relaxation and hence facilitates fracture reduction, in addition to allowing optimal surgical preparation of the suspended limb. A rope or bandage is tied to the toe/hoof of the affected limb and traction is applied along the axis of the limb. The traction, counter-traction, and manipulation bring about reduction in fresh cases with little overriding of bone segments. In large animals, the rope can be secured to the dorsal, lateral, or palmar/plantar aspects of the pastern to alter the direction of pull and to facilitate fracture reduction. If it fails, as in cases with severe overriding of bone segments, toggling/angulation/tenting method can be used. In this method, the limb is carefully bent at the fracture site until the two bone segments are met to form an angle with each

**Table 1.8** Doses of analgesics for use in dogs

| Drug | Dose (mg/kg body weight) | Route | Frequency/duration |
|---|---|---|---|
| *Opioid agonists* | | | |
| Fentanyl[a] | 0.001– 0.002 | i.v. | 0.25–0.5 h |
| | 0.001–0.006[b]/h | CRI | Duration of infusion |
| | | | +~0.5 h |
| | 0.01–0.04[c]/h | CRI | Duration of infusion |
| | | | +0.5 to 1.0 h |
| Hydromorphone | 0.02–0.1 | i.v., i.m., s.c. | 1–4 h |
| Methadone | 0.1–1.0 | i.v., i.m., s.c. | 1–4 h |
| Oxymorphone | 0.02–0.1 | i.v., i.m., s.c. | 1–4 h |
| Morphine[a] | 0.05–1.0 | i.v., i.m., s.c. | 1–4 h |
| | 0.1–0.3/h | CRI | Duration of infusion |
| | | | +0.5–1.0 h |
| Preservative-free morphine | 0.1–0.2 | Epidural | 6–24 h |
| *Partial opioid agonist* | | | |
| Buprenorphine | 0.005–0.02 | i.v., i.m. | 4–8 h |
| *Opioid agonist-antagonist* | | | |
| Butorphanol | 0.1–0.5 | i.v., i.m., s.c. | 0.25–2.0 h |
| *Alpha-2 agonists*[e] | | | |
| Medetomidine | 0.01–0.04 | i.m. | 0.5–2.0 h |
| (Postop, low dose) | 0.001–0.002 | i.v. | 0.5–1.0 h |
| Xylazine | 0.1–0.5 | i.m., s.c. | 0.5–2.0 h |
| (Postop, low dose) | 0.1–0.2 | i.v. | 0.5–1.0 h |
| *Local anesthetics* | | | |
| Bupivacaine | 1.5–3.0 | Local blocks | 2–6 h |
| | | Intrapleural | |
| | 1.0–1.5 | Epidural | 4–6 h |
| | 0.1–0.5[f] | Epidural | 4–6 h |
| Lidocaine | 1–2 | Local blocks | 1–2 h |
| | | Prior to bupivacaine | |
| *NMDA receptor antagonist* | | | |
| Ketamine | 0.25–0.5 | i.v. | Loading dose |
| | 0.01–0.02/h | CRI | Duration unknown |
| *NSAIDs*[g] | | | |
| Carprofen | 2.2 | s.c., i.m., p.o. | 12 h |
| | 4.4 | s.c., i.m., p.o. | 24 h |
| Deracoxib | 3–4 | p.o. (max. 7 days) | 24 h |
| | 1–2 | p.o. | 24 h |
| Firocoxib | 5 | p.o. | 24 h |
| Ketoprofen | 1–2 | s.c. | 24 h |
| Meloxicam | 0.2 | i.v., s.c., p.o. (once) | 24 h |
| | 0.1 | i.v., s.c., p.o. | 24 h |

Adapted from Hellyer, P.W., Robertson, S.A., and Fails, A.D. 2007. Pain and its management, *In:* Lumb & Jones' Veterinary Anesthesia and Analgesia, Edn 4, *Edited by* William J. Tranquilli, John C. Thurmon, Kurt A. Grimm, Blackwell Publishing, Oxford OX4 2DQ, UK, pp. 49–50 [84]

*BID*, twice a day; CRI, constant-rate infusion; i.m., intramuscularly; i.v., intravenously; NMDA, N-methyl-D-aspartate; NSAIDs, non-steroidal anti-inflammatory drugs; p.o., per os (orally); s.c., subcutaneously; s.i.d., once a day

[a]Fentanyl doses may be increased incrementally above the recommended dose, provided the patient is monitored for respiratory depression and bradycardia

[b]High doses of fentanyl are associated with bradycardia and hypoventilation and usually decrease anesthetic gas requirements

[c]Must be administered slowly to avoid side effects, such as hypotension and excitement

[d]These doses have been compiled from many sources and reflect doses used by the authors. The wide variability of recommended doses appears related to the variety and severity of stimuli used to establish the individual drug's analgesic activity in a given species. Doses are intended as guidelines only. Clinical judgment must be exercised to provide effective analgesia in a given situation

[e]Postsurgical doses and duration of effect have not been clearly established. Use cautiously to avoid profound cardiac depressant effects. [f]Bupivacaine dose when combined with preservative-free morphine at 0.1 mg/kg

[g]Do not use in the presence of hypovolemia, hypotension, renal disease, gastrointestinal bleeding, or coagulopathies

**Table 1.9** Doses of analgesics for use in cats

| Drug | Dose (mg/kg body weight) | Route | Comments |
|---|---|---|---|
| *Opioids* | | | |
| Butorphanol | 0.1–0.4 | i.v., i.m. | Short acting (less than 90 min);<br>increasing the dose does not provide more intense or longer periods of analgesia |
| Buprenorphine | 0.01–0.02 | i.v., i.m., transmucosal | |
| Fentanyl | 0.005–0.01 | i.v. | May take up to 12 h to reach effective plasma concentration |
| | 25 μg/h patch | Transdermal | Uptake affected by body temperature |
| Hydromorphone | 0.05–0.1 | i.v., i.m. | SC route associated with vomiting.<br>Doses of 0.1 mg/kg and higher can produce hyperthermia |
| Meperidine | 5–10 | i.m. | Must not be given IV |
| Morphine | 0.2–0.5 | i.v., i.m. | May be less effective in cats compared with other species because of a lack of active metabolites |
| Oxymorphone | 0.05–0.01 | i.v., i.m. | |
| **NSAIDs** | | | Do not use in hypertensive or hypovolemic patients |
| Carprofen | 1–4 | s.c. | Not licensed for cats in the USA.<br>Should not be repeated |
| Ketoprofen | 1–2 | s.c. | Not licensed for cats in the USA.<br>Can be repeated with care (1–5 days at 1 mg/kg) |
| Meloxicam[a] | 0.2 or 0.1 | s.c., i.v., p.o. | One dose. Dose depends on degree of pain |
| | 0.1 | | Repeat once daily for 3 days |
| | 0.025 (0.1 mg/cat, lean weight) | | Alternate day or twice weekly |
| Local anesthetics | | | |
| Lidocaine | 2–4 | Local anesthetic blocks | Duration of action 1–2 h.<br>Constant-rate infusions not recommended in cats because of cardiovascular depression |
| Bupivacaine | 2 | Local anesthetic blocks | Duration of action 4–5 h |
| **Alpha-2 agonists** | | | Use with care in cats with cardiovascular disease |
| Medetomidine | 0.005–0.02<br>0.01 | i.v., i.m., s.c.<br>Epidural | Low doses combined with an opioid offer good sedation and analgesia |
| Others | | | |
| Ketamine | 2 | i.v. | No published data about cats on the efficacy of low-dose constant-rate infusions |

Adapted from Hellyer, P.W., Robertson, S.A., and Fails, A.D. 2007. Pain and its management, *In:* Lumb & Jones' Veterinary Anesthesia and Analgesia, Edn 4, *Edited by* William J. Tranquilli, John C. Thurmon, Kurt A. Grimm, Blackwell Publishing, Oxford OX4 2DQ, UK, p 51 [84]

*i.m.*, intramuscularly; *i.v.*, intravenously; *p.o.*, per os (orally); *s.c.*, subcutaneously

[a]The only licensed NSAID for cats in the USA. The oral formulation is off-label; however, this has been used in cats with careful attention to dose delivered

other (Fig. 1.30). Then, the apex of the angle is gently pushed away by slowly straightening the limb to impinge the fractured bone to bring about reduction. While doing so, care should be taken to prevent damage to the surrounding soft tissues by carrying out angulation in the direction of least resistance. Toggling technique is generally useful in transverse or near transverse fractures (dentated edges) in places with little soft tissue covering like the distal radius-ulna and tibia, metacarpal, and metatarsal bones. However, it should not be attempted in long oblique or

**Table 1.10** Doses of analgesics for use in horses

| Drug | Dose (mg/kg body weight) | Route | Frequency/ duration |
|---|---|---|---|
| **NSAIDs** | | | |
| Phenylbutazone | 2.2–4.4 | i.v., p.o. | SID-BID |
| Flunixin | 1.1 | i.v., i.m., p.o. | SID-BID |
| Ketoprofen | 2.2 | i.v., i.m. | SID-BID |
| Carprofen | 0.7 | i.v., p.o. | SID-BID |
| Opioids | | | |
| Butorphanol | 0.01–0.02 | i.v. | q 2 to 4 h |
| Morphine | 0.02–0.1 | i.v. | q 2 to 4 h |
| | 0.1–0.2 | Epidural | q 12 to 24 h |
| Preservative-free morphine (1 mg/mL) | 5–10 mL | Intra-articular | |
| Fentanyl | 0.001–0.002 | i.v. | |
| | 0.001 mg/kg/h | CRI | |
| Fentanyl transdermal patch | 1–3 patches per horse (10 mg or 100 μg/h patches) | 72 h | |
| Local anesthetics | | | |
| Lidocaine | 1 to 2 | Infiltration | 1–2 h |
| Lidocaine CRI | 2 | i.v. (loading dose administered over 20 min) | |
| | 30–50 μg/kg/min | CRI | |
| Bupivacaine | 1– 2 | Infiltration | 6–8 h |
| Alpha-2 agonists | | | |
| Xylazine | 1.0–2.2 | i.m. | 0.5–2 h |
| | 0.3–1.0 | i.v. | 0.5 h |
| | 25 mg total dose | Epidural, added to morphine | |
| Detomidine | 0.005–0.01 | i.v. | 1–2 h |
| | 0.01–0.02 | i.v., i.m. | 1–2 h |
| | 0.03–0.06 | Epidural | 2–3 h |
| | 0.01 | Epidural, added to morphine | |

Adapted from Hellyer, P.W., Robertson, S.A., and Fails, A.D. 2007. Pain and its management, *In:* Lumb & Jones' Veterinary Anesthesia and Analgesia, Edn 4, *Edited by* William J. Tranquilli, John C. Thurmon, Kurt A. Grimm, Blackwell Publishing, Oxford OX4 2DQ, UK, p 52 [84]

*BID* twice a day, *CRI* constant-rate infusion, *i.m.* intramuscularly, *i.v.* intravenously, *p.o.* per os (orally), *SID* once a day

comminuted fractures and also old fractures with overriding segments. Toggling may also aggravate longitudinal fissures leading to comminution of fractures. In fractures of the proximal bones with heavy soft tissue covering (such as the humerus, femur, and tibia), it is difficult to reduce bone segments by traction, which may often lead to overriding of the fracture segments. However, pulling the rope in cranial or caudal direction may facilitate fracture reduction. Alternate methods which can be used to aid fracture reduction are the local anesthetics, general anesthetics, muscle relaxants, and fragment distractors. The main disadvantage of closed reduction is decreased ability to achieve anatomical realignment at the fracture site, especially in proximal bones.

Open reduction is achieved under general anesthesia by directly exposing the fracture segments through a skin incision. Open reduction is done primarily along with internal fixation, although at times it is done with external fixation or external skeletal fixation, commonly indicated in fractures with severe comminution and/or overriding of bone segments. As the fracture segments are directly visualized, manipulation is easy in early cases. With severe overriding of

**Table 1.11** Doses of analgesics for use in ruminants and swine

| Drug | Dose (mg/kg body weight) | Route | Frequency | Species |
|---|---|---|---|---|
| NSAIDs | | | | |
| Aspirin | 50–100 | p.o. | q 12 h | Cattle |
| | 50–100 | p.o. | q 12 h | Sheep/goat |
| | 10 | p.o. | q 4 h | Swine |
| Phenylbutazone | Not recommended | | | Cattle |
| | 5 | i.v., p.o. | Daily | Sheep, llama |
| | 4 | i.v., p.o. | Daily | Swine |
| Flunixin | 1.1 | i.v. | q 12 h | Cattle, llama |
| | 2.2 | i.v. | q 12 h | Sheep |
| Ketoprofen | 1–3.3 | i.v., i.m. | Daily | Ruminants/llama |
| Opioids | | | | |
| Butorphanol | 0.044–0.07 | i.v. | q 4 h | Cattle |
| | 0.05–0.2 | i.v., i.m. | q 4 h | Camelid |
| | 0.1–0.5 | i.v., i.m., s.c. | q 4 h | Sheep |
| | 0.1–0.2 | i.v., i.m., s.c. | q 4 h | Goats |
| Buprenorphine | 0.005–0.01 | i.v., i.m., s.c. | q 12 h | Sheep, goats |
| Morphine | 0.05–0.5 | i.v., i.m., s.c. | q 4 to 6 h | Ruminants/camelids |
| | 0.1 | Epidural | q 12 h | Ruminants/camelids |
| | 0.2 | i.v., i.m. | q 4 to 6 h | Swine |
| Fentanyl patch | 0.002–0.004 | i.v. | q 0.25 to 0.5 h | Ruminants |
| | 0.002 (equivalent to 15 mg/70 kg sheep) | Transdermal | q 72 h | Sheep |
| Local anesthetics | | | | |
| Lidocaine | Do not exceed 10 mL (2% lidocaine) | | | Adult sheep/goats |
| | Do not exceed 1 mL (2% lidocaine) | | | Dehorning young kids |
| | 4–5 mL (2%) | Epidural | | Cattle |
| | 1–2 mL (2%) | Epidural | | Sheep |
| Bupivacaine | 1–2 mg/kg | Infiltrations | | Ruminants/camelids |
| Alpha-2 agonists | | | | |
| Xylazine | 0.1 | i.m. | As needed | Cattle |
| | 0.05–0.1 | i.m. | As needed | Sheep |
| | 1 | i.m. | As needed | Swine |
| Detomidine | 0.01 | i.v. | As needed | Cattle |

Adapted from Hellyer, P.W., Robertson, S.A., and Fails, A.D. 2007. Pain and its management, *In:* Lumb & Jones' Veterinary Anesthesia and Analgesia, Edn 4, *Edited by* William J. Tranquilli, John C. Thurmon, Kurt A. Grimm, Blackwell Publishing, Oxford OX4 2DQ, UK, p 53 [84]
*i.m* intramuscularly, *i.v.* intravenously, *PO* per os (orally), *s.c.* subcutaneously

bone segments and in old cases with fibrous adhesions, manual reduction of bone segments is difficult. In such cases, careful dissection/separation of soft tissues around the fractured bone should be done to exteriorize the bone segments, and reduction can be achieved with the help of bone clamps by traction or toggling method. In open reduction, perfect bone alignment can be achieved without soft tissue interposition between the bone segments.

## 1.11 Timing and Selection of Fracture Fixation Technique

Immobilization of broken bone segments is an important aspect of fracture treatment. Some fractures may not require immobilization to ensure union, whereas some fractures may be immobilized using simple external fixation techniques such as splints and bandages to achieve satisfactory bone union, and excessive immobilization may be actually harmful in some

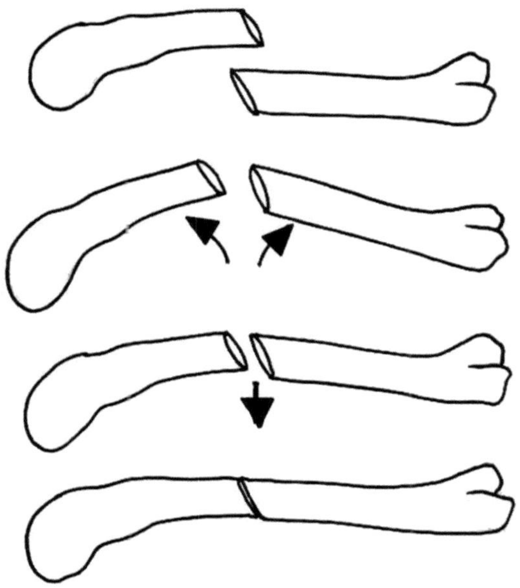

**Fig. 1.30** Toggling method of bone reduction

cases. However, some other fractures require rigid immobilization using either external skeletal fixation or internal fixation of the bone. There are mainly three reasons for immobilizing a fracture: (i) to relieve pain associated with broken bone, (ii) to prevent dislodgement or angulation of the bone segments, and (iii) to avert any movement between the bone ends that might hamper healing at the fracture site. In general, if reduction is required to align bone segments, immobilization is also needed to avoid their further displacement. In human patients, if the broken bone segments are not displaced much at the time of the original injury (if the original position is acceptable), it may not be necessary to immobilize the fracture, whereas in animal patients, if the fractured bone segments are not immobilized, they are more likely to get displaced subsequently, and more often, a simple closed fracture may get open and contaminated. Hence, fractured limb should be immobilized immediately through temporarily using the available external fixation techniques such as splints and bandages or cast application, before deciding on the definitive (operative) fixation.

During fracture stabilization, emphasis should be given on soft tissue preservation and minimal tissue damage while providing stable bone fixation to achieve desirable bone healing in optimal time duration [80]. It is therefore a balance between carpentry and gardening. This balance is important especially in complex trauma patients with severe soft tissue injury [81]. More emphasis to biological fixation may often lead to insufficient stabilization and vice versa; hence, inherent biological and mechanical needs of specific patient should be taken into consideration.

### 1.11.1 Timing of Definitive Fixation

Timing of operative fracture fixation is not only important with respect to outcome of fracture but also for financial considerations. By optimizing the time of fracture management, the morbidity, mortality, and hospital stay related to fracture care can be minimized, and also, long-term outcomes may be improved.

Haemodynamic stability of the patient is an important factor that should be taken into account while deciding the timing of fixation. In multiple trauma patients, delaying or limiting early orthopedic intervention is beneficial. In patients with blunt trauma having thoracic and soft tissue damage, early definitive fixation of the long bones (particularly intramedullary nailing) may result in complications such as respiratory distress and multiple organ failure. Hence, timing of fracture care is dependent on adequate resuscitation, and it is ensured that vital physiological parameters such as heart rate, blood pressure, and urine output are normal before surgical fixation of fracture. Reversal of coagulopathy and correction of core body temperature are also important to favorable outcome. In a human study, 100% mortality was reported when core body temperature was not restored before surgical treatment. Management of lung injury should also take precedence over definitive bony stabilization. Inflammation remains elevated during the initial 2–4 days after injury, indicating sustained inflammatory response and ongoing fluid imbalance; surgical procedure should be avoided during this phase to reduce the rate of complications.

Another major concern pertaining to the timing of surgical fixation is the extent of soft tissue injury and open wound associated with fractures [82]. The status of the soft tissues even in closed fractures is often the principal decisive factor of delayed fracture fixation. Open fractures need urgent attention but delay the definitive fracture fixation. The timing of wound closure in open fracture is also an important issue. In clean wounds, it is possible to close the wounds after the initial irrigation and debridement. But when the condition of the tissue is doubtful, skin closure may be done by only keeping adequate drainage, or delayed closure may be preferred. Closure of wounds should generally be undertaken between the fourth and seventh day or may be allowed to heal by second intention if the wound bed is not clean and ready. When the wound bed is clean and fracture fixation is stable, flap coverage can be undertaken within 72 h.

High-energy gunshot wounds are always treated as open fractures [83]. Therefore, the decision on fracture fixation, whether temporary external fixation or definitive fixation, should be made based on the degree of soft tissue damage, viability, and contamination. Delaying the definitive fixation not necessarily increases the hazard of infection, but early antibiotic administration (such as cephalosporin) is essential to control infection.

The timing of surgical fixation in veterinary orthopedics is often complicated with many issues unrelated to the fracture; it is also sometimes dictated by the availability of expertise and implants for fracture fixation and economic considerations, especially in ruminants. Nevertheless, once the animal is otherwise healthy and haemodynamically stable, definitive fracture immobilization should be undertaken as early as possible, which will not only help reduce complications but also achieve early functional recovery.

### 1.11.2 Selection of Fixation Technique

Many factors should be considered while selecting a technique for fracture management, namely, the species of the animal, the fracture type and location, the extent of soft tissue injury, the presence or absence of open wound, the behavioral nature of the animal, the facilities available, and the experience of the veterinary orthopedic surgeon. The following questions should be answered before attempting any treatment: (i) Can the fracture be optimally reduced by closed method or open reduction needed?; (ii) Can the fracture be adequately stabilized using any of the external fixation techniques?; (iii) Is the surgical treatment really required?; (iv) Which is the ideal technique of fixation?; (v) What is the type and utility of animal – whether it is a pet?, a food animal?, or a production animal?; (vi) What is the potential economic or genetic value of the animal?; (vii) Can the animal owner afford the treatment and take care of his animal after bone fixation?; and (viii) What is the other best option if the 'ideal treatment' is not possible?

In general, fractures in dogs, cats, sheep, and goats can be treated more easily than in large animals, mostly due to relatively less body weight. Almost all the advanced fracture fixation techniques and implants available for use in human patients can be employed in small animals. Sheep and goats are more docile than dogs and cats and hence are easier to manage during fracture repair. Fractures in large animals are not as easy to treat as in small animals, due to heavy weight, non-availability of proper fixation implants, and difficulty in postoperative care and management. Nevertheless, cattle and buffaloes are better orthopedic patients as they are more sensible in handling a fractured limb, spend majority of time lying down, less likely to develop contra-lateral limb breakdown and stress laminitis, do not resist having orthopedic devices on their limbs, and have remarkable bone healing capacity and lesser susceptibility to infection than horses.

Age of the injured animal should also be taken into account while selecting a fracture fixation technique. Young animals make better orthopedic patients, as they are easy to manage during postoperative period (due to less body weight and easy to handle) and have tremendous bone healing potential due to increased metabolic rate and faster skeletal growth. Hence, most of the distal limb fractures can be managed using external fixation techniques, whereas fractures in the proximal bones (e.g. femur) can be treated using simple IM fixation technique. In young animals, damage to the growth plate should also be taken into account. As most of the long bone fractures in young animals are located at the metaphyseal/epiphyseal region, any technique used to stabilize the bone segments should not damage the growth plate; reaming of the medullary cavity and bone plate fixation should be avoided (e.g. distal growth plate of the femur is responsible for 70–80% of long bone growth). In very old geriatric patients also, internal fixation of fracture should be avoided.

The type and location of fracture is another important factor determining the selection of fracture fixation technique. Fractures of the axial skeleton (including skull and vertebral column) are usually managed by only providing confinement and rest, especially in large animals, because external or internal fixation is not practical. In general, fracture in proximal limb bones such as the femur and humerus may not be amenable to external fixation techniques, and fractures below the stifle or elbow joint are better treated using external fixation techniques. Similarly, forelimb fractures can be better managed using external fixation techniques such as cast application, as it is relatively straighter than hindlimbs, and tibial fractures are difficult to treat using external fixation techniques as it is difficult to stabilize the stifle joint (due to conical shape of the limb with more soft tissues). Diaphyseal fractures can be relatively easy to treat using any of the internal fixation techniques than metaphyseal or epiphyseal fractures, as fracture reduction is easy and there is greater purchase of implants. Further, fractures near or involving a joint need more rigid fixation, often using transarticular fixation, to achieve early bone healing with minimal callus formation. Simple transverse or oblique fractures of the diaphysis can be treated using IM pin fixation, whereas a comminuted fracture needs to be immobilized using a more rigid bone plate or interlocking nail.

The degree of soft tissue trauma is also an important factor determining the selection of a fracture fixation technique. Animals with open fractures are more difficult to treat. In principle, a fixation technique used in open fractures should not only provide rigid bone fixation but also allow soft tissue drainage and regular dressing of the open wound. Hence, a suitable external skeletal fixation technique is preferred; and cast application should not be done; if unavoidable, a window should be opened in the cast at the wound site. Similarly, internal fixation technique should also be avoided, as a buried implant may harbor infection.

The cost of treatment and utility of the animal are other important determinants of fracture fixation in animal patients, except may be in small animal practice. While many of the dog owners may be ready to bear the treatment expenses, in small and large ruminants, the value of the animal and economics of fracture treatment must be kept in mind. If the animal owner is unable to bear the cost and still insists on a treatment, simple procedures such as stall rest and application of splints and bandages or plaster cast should be considered wherever possible rather than to attempt an ideal treatment option which may be complicated and more expensive. The utility of the animal should also be considered before attempting a fracture repair, especially in production and working animals. A lactating cow or a buffalo may not lose productivity even if some degree of fracture malunion occurs. However, a working bullock or a horse following a fracture will require restoration of near normal function of the affected limb.

Proper case selection is also important for successful outcome of a fracture repair. Recumbent animal with multiple fractures/injuries is a poor subject for surgery. Usually, it is futile to attempt repair of a long bone fracture in adult cattle or buffaloes which are recumbent for a period longer than 48–72 h. If the animal owner is willing, euthanasia is always a practical proposition in such cases. The success of fracture treatment depends to a great extent on the experience and insight of the surgeon and cooperation of the animal owner and the patient. If the owner is not cooperative in following instructions or is negligent with the aftercare of his animal, even the best technique applied with a high degree of precision and skill will fail to produce satisfactory results. Similarly, there are greater chances of failure if the animal is vicious and uncooperative, which is, however, not in the hands of a surgeon. The use of a more common technique by a relatively inexperienced surgeon may yield better results than a newer and technically superior technique followed by an otherwise experienced surgeon. There are many treatment methods available for the stabilization of fractures; the choice of the fixation method must be based on which method best accomplishes functional restoration with least complications and patient risk. Hence, the surgeon should use his wisdom while selecting a suitable fracture fixation technique based on his experience and the facilities available at hand.

## Chapter 1: Sample Questions

**Q. No. 1: Mark the correct answer**

1. The bone cells responsible for the formation of the matrix
   (a) osteocytes (b) osteoblasts (c) osteoclasts (d) mesenchymal cells
2. The nutrient artery supplies to
   (a) outer 1/3 of the bony cortex (b) inner 1/3 of the bony cortex (c) outer 2/3 of the bony cortex (d) inner 2/3 of the bony cortex
3. Primary bone healing cannot occur in the presence of
   (a) micromotion (b) fracture gap (c) rigid fixation (d) none of the above
4. The rate of fracture healing can increase in the presence of
   (a) infection (b) bone loss (c) soft tissue trauma (d) controlled exercise
5. Long, spiral fracture is generally caused by
   (a) compression force (b) shearing force (c) torsional force (d) bending force
6. Which of the following vitamins is important for bone formation?
   (a) Vitamin B (b) Vitamin C (c) Vitamin D (d) Vitamin E
7. During early stages of fracture healing, the external callus is mainly supplied by
   (a) nutrient artery (b) periosteal arteries (c) metaphyseal arteries (d) medullary artery
8. A fracture with at least three bone fragments which are interconnected to each other is known as
   (a) compound fracture (b) complex fracture (c) comminuted fracture (d) multiple fracture
9. Bone mineral is mostly composed of
   (a) calcium sulfate (b) calcium carbonate (c) calcium phosphate (d) calcium hydroxide
10. Increase in bone length is brought about by
   (a) osteochondral growth (b) enchondral growth (c) appositional growth (d) endochondral growth

**Q. No. 2: State true or false**

1. Periosteum has an outer cambium layer containing osteoprogenitor cells and an inner fibrous layer.
2. Callus formation may take place independent of haematoma formation.
3. Bone healing cannot occur without the formation of periosteal callus.
4. Osteoclasts may appear in the early stage of fracture healing.
5. During bending of the bone, electronegativity exists in the convex side and electropositivity in the concave side.
6. Healing of the cortical bone is faster than the cancellous bone.
7. Cartilagenous callus forms from vascular periosteum, while bony callus forms from avascular periosteum during fracture healing.
8. Healing of the bone will never occur in the presence of infection.
9. Corticosteroid administration may delay the fracture healing.
10. The cartilagenous model of bones is formed only during embryonic life.

11. The calcification of intercellular substance of the cartilage is known as endochondral ossification.
12. Vitamin C has antioxidant and anti-inflammatory properties and is necessary for bone collagen synthesis.
13. Electronegativity favors osteoclastic activity, whereas electropositivity is associated with osteoblastic activity.
14. Metaphyseal fractures usually heal faster than diaphyseal fractures.
15. Periosteal callus formation is useful to provide fracture stability in early stages of fracture healing.
16. Gunshot injury usually leads to comminuted fracture.
17. Articular cartilage has no blood supply but richly supplied with nerve endings.
18. Parathyroid hormone is released from the parathyroid gland in response to lowered blood calcium ion concentration.
19. Analgesics should be administered before the surgical fixation of a fracture to minimize the postoperative pain.
20. Titanium is an ideal material for implantation due to its high strength, low weight, excellent corrosion resistance, and total biocompatibility.
21. Mg alloys are biodegradable metals best suited for development of orthopedic implants due to their biocompatibility, biodegradability, and acceptable mechanical properties.

**Q. No. 3: Fill in the blanks**

1. Osteocytes surrounded by mineralized matrix are interconnected by ________________ _______ through the __________________ _______ system.
2. Osteoclasts help in dissolution and removal of the minerals and matrix by production of ____________________________ and _____ ____________________________.
3. Organic matrix of the bone predominantly consists of ________________________ and ___________________________, whereas the inorganic mineral comprises of ______________________________________ ___________.
4. The basic structural unit of lamellae concentrically arranged about the Haversian canal is called________________________.
5. The complete outer surface of the bone is covered by __________________________ _, except at the ends (joints), which is covered with ____________________________ ______.
6. The principal blood vessel supplying a long bone with blood is ____________________ _________, which penetrates the cortex through the _____________________________ _ and enters the medullary cavity.
7. In endochondral ossification, the bone is formed from ___________________________ _______, whereas in intramembranous ossification, the bone is directly formed from ____________________________________.
8. When two apposing forces approach one another on the same plane, it is called as _______________________, whereas when two opposing forces act through one plane, it is called ___________________________.
9. Different phases of secondary bone healing are ____________________________, ______ ____________________, and ______________ ______________ phase.
10. _________________________________ alloys are most widely used for manufacturing orthopedic implants worldwide.

**Q. No. 4: Write short note on the following:**

1. Endochondral ossification
2. Composition of the bone
3. Circulation of the bone
4. Secondary bone healing
5. Fracture forces
6. Instruments for bone plating
7. Non-biodegradable polymer implants
8. Pain management in orthopedic patients

## References


1. Clarke, B. 2008. Normal bone anatomy and physiology. *Clinical Journal of the American Society of Nephrology* 3 (Suppl. 3): S131–S139.
2. Florencio-Silva, R., G.R. da Silva Sasso, E. Sasso-Cerri, M.J. Simões, and P.S. Cerri. 2015. Biology of bone tissue: structure, function, and factors that influence bone cells. *BioMed Research International* 2015: 17. https://doi.org/10.1155/2015/421746. Artcle ID: 421746.
3. Buckwalter, J.A., M.J. Glimcher, R.R. Cooper, and R. Recker. 1996. Bone biology. I: structure, blood supply, cells, matrix, and mineralization. *Instructional Course Lectures* 45: 371–386.
4. Capulli, M., R. Paone, and N. Rucci. 2014. Osteoblast and osteocyte: games without frontiers. *Archives of Biochemistry and Biophysics* 561: 3–12.
5. Boivin, G., and P.J. Meunier. 2002. The degree of mineralization of bone tissue measured by computerized quantitative contact microradiography. *Calcified Tissue International* 70 (6): 503–511.
6. Franz-Odendaal, T.A., B.K. Hall, and P.E. Witten. 2006. Buried alive: how osteoblasts become osteocytes. *Developmental Dynamics* 235 (1): 176–190.
7. Civitelli, R., F. Lecanda, N.R. Jørgensen, and T.H. Steinberg. 2002. Intercellular junctions and cell-cell communication in bone. In *Principles of bone biology*, ed. J.P. Bilezikan, L. Raisz, and G.A. Rodan, 287–302. San Diego, CA: Academic Press.
8. Yavropoulou, M.P., and J.G. Yovos. 2008. Osteoclastogenesis—current knowledge and future perspectives. *Journal of Musculoskeletal & Neuronal Interactions* 8 (3): 204–216.
9. Buckwalter, J.A., and R.R. Cooper. 1987. Bone structure and function. *Instructional Course Lectures* 36: 27–48.
10. Fetter, A.W. 1985. Normal bone anatomy, section one: structure and function of bone. In *Textbook of small animal Orthopaedics*, ed. C.D. Newton and D.M. Nunamaker, 9–20. Philadelphia: J.B. Lippincott.
11. Rhinelander, F.W. 1972. Chapter 1: Circulation in bone. In *The biochemistry and physiology of bone*, ed. G. Bourne, vol. 2. New York: Academic Press.
12. Rhinelander, F.W. 1974. Tibial blood supply in relation to fracture healing. *Clinical Orthopaedics* 105: 34–81.
13. Rhinelander, F.W. 1968. The normal circulation of diaphyseal cortex and its response to fracture. *Journal of Bone and Joint Surgery* A50 (4): 784–800.
14. Cashman, K.D., and F. Ginty. 2003. *Bone*, 1106–1112. New York: Elsevier.
15. Vanputte, C.L., J.L. Regan, and A.F. Russo. 2013. Skeletal system: bones and joints. In *Seeley's essentials of anatomy and physiology*, 8th ed., 110–149. New York: Mc Graw Hill.
16. Wojnar, R. 2010. *Bone and cartilage–its structure and physical properties*. Weinheim: Wiley-VCH Verlag GmbH & Co.
17. Calvi, L.M., N.A. Sims, J.L. Hunzelman, M.C. Knight, A. Giovannetti, J.M. Saxton, H.M. Kronenberg, R. Baron, and E. Schipani. 2001. Activated parathyroid hormone/ parathyroid hormone-related protein receptor in osteoblastic cells differentially affects cortical and trabecular bone. *The Journal of Clinical Investigation* 107 (3): 277–286.
18. Miao, D., and A. Scutt. 2002. Recruitment, augmentation and apoptosis of rat osteoclasts in 1,25-(OH)2D3 response to short-term treatment with 1,25-dihydroxyvitamin D3 in vivo. *BMC Musculoskeletal Disorders* 7: 3–16.
19. Raisz, L.G., and G.A. Rodan. 1998. Embryology and cellular biology of bone. In *Metabolic bone disease and clinically related disorders*, ed. L.V. Avioli and S.M. Krane, 3rd ed., 1–22. New York: Academic Press.
20. Zafalon, R.V.A., B. Ruberti, M.F. Rentas, A.R. Amaral, T.H.A. Vendramini, F.C. Chacar, M.M. Kogika, and M.A. Brunetto. 2020. The role of vitamin D in small animal bone metabolism. *Meta* 10 (12): 496. https://doi.org/10.3390/metabo10120496.
21. Boudrieau, R.J. 1991. Foreword, fracture management: 1. *Seminars in Veterinary Medicine and Surgery (Small Animal)* 6 (1): 1–2.
22. Schwarz, P.D. 1991. Biomechanics of fracture and fracture fixation. *Seminars in Veterinary Medicine and Surgery (Small Animal)* 6 (1): 3–15.
23. Smith, G.K. 1985. Biomechanics pertinent to fracture etiology, reduction and fixation. In *Textbook of small animal Orthopaedics*, ed. C.D. Newton and D.M. Nunamaker, 195–230. Philadelphia: J.B. Lippincott Co.
24. Muller, M.E., S. Nazarian, P. Koch, and J. Schatzker. 1990. *The Comprehensice classification of fractures of long bones*. Berlin: Springer-Verlag.
25. Meinberg, E.G., J. Agel, M.D. Karam, C.S. Roberts, and J.F. Kellam. 2018. Fracture and dislocation classification compendium - 2018. *Journal of Orthopaedic Trauma* 32 (Suppl 1): S1.
26. Aithal, H.P., and G.R. Singh. 1999. A survey of bone fractures in cattle, sheep and goats. *The Indian Veterinary Journal* 76: 636–639.
27. Aithal, H.P., G.R. Singh, and G.S. Bisht. 1999. Fractures in dogs: a survey of 402 cases. *Indian Journal of Veterinary Surgery* 20: 15–21.
28. Aithal, H.P., and G.R. Singh. 1999. Pattern of bone fractures caused by road traffic accidents and falls in dogs: a retrospective study. *The Indian Journal of Animal Sciences* 69: 960–961.
29. Kumar, P., H.P. Aithal, P. Kinjavdekar, Amarpal, A.M. Pawde, K. Pratap, and G.S. Bisht. 2013. The occurrence and pattern of simple and compound fractures in limb bones in different domestic animals:

a retrospective study of 989 cases. *Indian Journal of Veterinary Surgery* 34: 35–40.
30. McKibbin, B. 1978. The biology of fracture healing in long bones. *Journal of Bone and Joint Surgery* 60-B: 150–162.
31. Kaderly, R.E. 1991. Primary bone healing. *Seminars in Veterinary Medicine and Surgery (Small Animal)* 6 (1): 21–25.
32. Schelling, S.H. 1991. Secondary (classical) bone healing. *Seminars in Veterinary Medicine and Surgery (Small Animal)* 6 (1): 16–20.
33. Cruess, R.L., and J. Dumont. 1985. Healing of bone. Section Four: Conditions influencing fracture healing. In *Textbook of small animal orthopaedics*, ed. C.D. Newton and D.M. Nunamaker, 58–61. Philadelphia: J.B. Lippincott Co.
34. Cashman, K.D. 2007. Diet, nutrition and bone health. *The Journal of Nutrition* 137: 2507S–2512S.
35. Karpouzos, A., Diamantis, E., Farmaki, P., Savvanis, S. And Troupis, T. 2017. Nutritional aspects of bone health and fracture healing. Journal of Osteoporosis 2017; 2017:4218472. doi: https://doi.org/10.1155/2017/4218472
36. Heaney, R.P. 2002. Protein and calcium: antagonists or synergists? *The American Journal of Clinical Nutrition* 75: 609–610.
37. Wengreen, H.J., R.G. Munger, N.A. West, D.R. Cutler, C.D. Corcoran, J. Zhang, and N.E. Sassano. 2004. Dietary protein intake and risk of osteoporotic hip fracture in elderly residents of Utah. *Journal of Bone and Mineral Research* 19 (4): 537–545.
38. Fischer, V., M. Haffner-Luntzer, M. Amling, and A. Ignatius. 2018. Calcium and vitamin D in bone fracture healing and post-traumatic bone turnover. *European Cells & Materials* 35: 365–385.
39. Stockman, J., C. Villaverde, and R.J. Corbee. 2021. Calcium, phosphorus and vitamin D in dogs and cats. Beyond the bones. *Veterinary Clinics of North America: Small Animal Practice* 51 (3): P623–P634.
40. Morton, D.J., E.L. Barrett-Connor, and D.L. Schneider. 2001. Vitamin C supplement use and bone mineral density in postmenopausal women. *Journal of Bone and Mineral Research* 16 (1): 135–140.
41. Roman-Garcia, P., I. Quiros-Gonzalez, L. Mottram, L. Lieben, K. Sharan, A. Wangwiwatsin, J. Tubio, K. Lewis, D. Wilkinson, B. Santhanam, N. Sarper, S. Clare, G.S. Vassiliou, V.R. Velagapudi, G. Dougan, and V.K. Yadav. 2014. Vitamin B12-dependent taurine synthesis regulates growth and bone mass. *The Journal of Clinical Investigation* 124 (7): 2988–3002.
42. Sandukji, A., H. Al-Sawaf, A. Mohamadin, Y. Alrashidi, and S.A. Sheweita. 2010. Oxidative stress and bone markers in plasma of patients with long-bone fixative surgery: role of antioxidants. *Human & Experimental Toxicology* 30 (6): 435–442.
43. Aerssens, J., R. Van Audekercke, P. Geusens, L.P.C. Schot, A.A. Osman, and J. Dequeker. 1993. Mechanical properties, bone mineral content, and bone composition (collagen, osteocalcin, IGF-I) of the rat femur: influence of ovariectomy and nandrolon decanoate (anabolic steroid) treatment. *Calcified Tissue International* 53 (4): 269–277.
44. Ahmad, F., S.M. Yunus, A. Asghar, and N.A. Faruqi. 2013. Influence of anabolic steroid on tibial fracture healing in rabbits – a study on experimental model. *Journal of Clinical and Diagnostic Research* 7 (1): 93–96.
45. Maiti, S.K., M. Hoque, H.P. Aithal, and G.R. Singh. 1999. Repair of experimental fracture under influence of anabolic steriod: Clinico radiological study. *Intas Polivet* 2: 29–31.
46. Deka, D.K., L.C. Lahon, J. Saikia, and A. Mukit. 1994. Effect of clssus quadrangular/s in accelerating healing process of experimentally fractured radius-ulna of dog: a preliminary study. *Indian Journal of Pharmacology* 26: 44–45.
47. Hoque, M., S.K. Maiti, N. Hoque, G.R. Singh, H.P. Aithal, N. Kumar, and Kalicharan. 2004. Evaluation of alcoholic extract of bamboo (*Bambusa arundinacea*) buds on fracture healing in rabbits. *The Indian Journal of Animal Sciences* 74: 915–919.
48. Russo, C.R. 2009. The effects of exercise on bone. Basic concepts and implications for the prevention of fractures. *Clinical Cases in Mineral and Bone Metabolism* 6 (3): 223–228.
49. Heckman, J., J. Ryaby, J. McCabe, J.J. Frey, and R.F. Kilcoyne. 1994. Acceleration of tibial fracture-healing by non-invasive, low-intensity pulsed ultrasound. *The Journal of Bone and Joint Surgery A* 76: 26–34.
50. Kristiansen, T.K. 1990. The effect of low power specifically programmed ultrasound on the healing time of fresh fractures using a Colles' model. *Journal of Orthopaedic Trauma* 4: 227–228.
51. Hoque, M., S.K. Maiti, H.P. Aithal, G.R. Singh, N. Kumar, P. Singh, and K. Charan. 2003. Effect of static magnetic field in fracture healing in goats: an experimental study. *The Indian Journal of Animal Sciences* 73: 275–277.
52. Mollon, B., V. da Silva, J.W. Busse, T.A. Einhorn, and M. Bhandari. 2008. Electrical stimulation for long-bone fracture-healing: a meta-analysis of randomized controlled trials. *The Journal of Bone and Joint Surgery A* 90: 2322–2330.
53. Scott, G., and J.B. King. 1994. A prospective, double-blind trial of electrical capacitive coupling in the treatment of non-union of long bones. *Journal of Bone and Joint Surgery* A76: 820–826.
54. Shakya, G., M.M.S. Zama, H.P. Aithal, R. John, and M. Baghel. 2014. Biochemical changes following electro-acupuncture and static magnetic field therapy in rabbits for bone defect healing. *Veterinary World* 7: 83–86.
55. Peng, J., J. Zhao, Y. Long, Y. Xie, J. Nie, and L. Chen. 2019. Magnetic materials in promoting bone

regeneration. *Frontiers in Materials* 6. https://doi.org/10.3389/fmats.2019.00268.
56. Smith, G.K. 1985. Orthopaedic biomaterials. In *Textbook of small animal Orthopaedics*, ed. C.D. Newton and D.M. Nunamaker, 231–241. Philadelphia: J.B. Lippincott Co.
57. Suryavanshi, A.V., V. Borse, V. Pawar, K.R. Sindhu, and R. Srivastava. 2016. Material advancements in bone-soft tissue fixation devices. *Science Advances Today* 2 (2016): 25236.
58. Black, J. 1980. Biomaterials for internal fixation. In *Fracture treatment and healing*, ed. B. Heppenstall, 113. Philadelphia: WB Saunders.
59. Navarro, M., A. Michiardi, O. Castano, and J.A. Planell. 2008. Biomaterials in orthopaedics. *Journal of The Royal Society Interface* 5: 1137. https://doi.org/10.1098/rsif.2008.0151.
60. Ma, R., and T. Tang. 2014. Current strategies to improve the bioactivity of PEEK. *International Journal of Molecular Sciences* 15: 5426–5445.
61. Richard WG Jr., Matthew J, Thompson (2018). Carbon fiber implants aid fixation of extremity fractures in oncology cases. Orthopedics Today, October 2018.
62. James, J.P. 2016. Recent advancements in magnesium implants for orthopedic application and associated infections. *Clinical Trials in Orthopedic Disorders* 1: 138–144.
63. Liu, C., Z. Ren, Y. Xu, S. Pang, X. Zhao, and Y. Zhao. 2018. Biodegradable magnesium alloys developed as bone repair materials: a review. https://www.hindawi.com/journals/scanning/2018/9216314/. Article ID 9216314.
64. Prakasam, M., J. Locs, K. Salma-Ancane, D. Loca, A. Largeteau, and L. Berzina-Cimdina. 2017. Biodegradable materials and metallic implants-A review. *Journal of Functional Biomaterials* 8: 44. https://doi.org/10.3390/jfb8040044.
65. Shuai, C., S. Li, S. Peng, P. Feng, Y. Lai, and C. Gao. 2019. Biodegradable metallic bone implants. *Materials Chemistry Frontiers* 3: 544–562.
66. Mukherjee, D.P., and W.S. Pietrzak. 2011. Bioabsorbable fixation: scientific, technical, and clinical concepts. *The Journal of Craniofacial Surgery* 22: 679–689.
67. Boccaccini, A.R., M. Erol, W.J. Stark, D. Mohn, Z. Hong, and J.F. Mano. 2010. Polymer/bioactive glass nanocomposites for biomedical applications. A review. *Composites Science and Technology* 70: 1764. https://doi.org/10.1016/j.compscitech.2010.06.002ff.
68. Newton, C.D. 1985. Examination of the orthopaedic patient. Section one: evaluation of the nonemergency patient. In *Textbook of small animal orthopaedics*, ed. C.D. Newton and D.M. Nunamaker, 125–128. JB Lippincott: Philadelphia.
69. Adams, S.B. 1985. The role of external fixation and emergency fracture management in bovine orthopedics. *The Veterinary Clinics of North America. Food Animal Practice* 1: 109–129.
70. Anson, L.W. 1993. Emergency management of fractures. In *Textbook of small animal surgery*, ed. D. Slatter, 2nd ed., 1603–1610. Philadelphia: W.B. Saunders Company.
71. Aithal, H.P. 2015. Management of fractures. In *Handbook on field veterinary surgery*, ed. M.M.S. Zama, H.P. Aithal, and A.M. Pawde, 145–154. New Delhi: Daya Publishing House, Astral International Pvt. Ltd.
72. Aithal HP, Singh GR (Amarpal), Mogha IV, Gupta OP, Kumar N, Hoque M (1997) Epidural ketamine and xylazine for hind quarter surgery in ruminants: a study on 35 clinical cases. The Indian Veterinary Journal 74: 625–626
73. Amarpal, P. Kinjavdekar, H.P. Aithal, and A.M. Pawde. 2013. *Anaesthesia and Analgesia for Veterinary graduates*. New Delhi: Satish Serial Publishing House.
74. Kinjavdekar, P., H.P. Amarpal Aithal, M. Hoque, S.K. Maiti, and G.R. Singh. 2006. Comparison of systemic and epidural xylazine and ketamine anaesthesia for external skeletal fixation in cattle. *The Indian Journal of Animal Sciences* 76: 998–1000.
75. Sharma, D., H.P. Aithal, Amarpal, P. Kinjavdekar, A.S. Mudasir, S. Sahu, and Priya Singh. 2021. Effect of medetomidine-ketofol-isoflurane anaesthesia on the clinicao-physiological and haemodynamic stability in canine orthopaedic patients. *Indian Journal of Veterinary Surgery* 42: 56–60.
76. Sharma, D., H.P. Aithal, Amarpal, P. Kinjavdekar, M.A. Shah, M.A. Rashmi, and M.A. Rafee. 2017. Analgesic and haematobiochemical effects of dexmedetomidine-ketofol-isoflurane anaesthesia in canine orthopaedic patients. *Indian Journal of Veterinary Surgery* 38: 100–103.
77. Surbhi P, Kinjavdekar, H.P. Amarpal Aithal, A.M. Pawde, and V. Malik. 2010. Comparison of analgesic effects of meloxicam and ketoprofen using university of Melbourne pain score in clinical canine orthopaedic patients. *Journal of Applied Animal Research* 38: 261–264.
78. Surbhi, P. Kinjavdekar, Amarpal, H.P. Aithal, A.M. Pawde, M.C. Pathak, B.M. Borena, and V. Malik. 2010. Physiological and biochemical effects of medetomidine-butorphanol-propofol anaesthesia in dogs undergoing orthopaedic surgery. *Indian Journal of Veterinary Surgery* 31: 101–104.
79. Singh, A.P., G.R. Singh, H.P. Aithal, and P. Singh. 2020. The musculoskeletal system; section D: fractures. In *Ruminant surgery: a textbook of the surgical diseases of cattle, buffaloes, camels, sheep and goats*, ed. J. Singh, S. Singh, and R.P.S. Tyagi, 2nd ed., 465–527. Chennai: CBS Publishers & Distributors Pvt Ltd.
80. Palmer, R.H. 2011. Preoperative planning in fracture treatment. In *Small animal orthopedic surgery*, ed. R.H. Palmer, 28–33. http://1filedownload.com.
81. Aron, D.N., R.H. Palmer, and A.L. Johnson. 1995. Biologic strategies and a balanced concept for repair of highly comminuted long bone fractures.

*Compendium on Continuing Education for the Practising Veterinarian* 7: 35–49.
82. Johnson, A.L. 1999. Management of open fractures in dogs and cats. *Waltham Focus* 9 (4): 11–17.
83. Doherty, M.A., and M.M. Smith. 1995. Contamination and infection of fractures resulting from gunshot trauma in dogs: 20 cases (1987-1992). *Journal of the American Veterinary Medical Association* 206: 203–205.
84. Hellyer, P.W., S.A. Robertson, and A.D. Fails. 2007. Pain and its management. In *Lumb & Jones' veterinary anesthesia and analgesia*, ed. W.J. Tranquilli, J.C. Thurmon, and K.A. Grimm, 4th ed. Oxford: Blackwell Publishing.

# Principles of Fracture Fixation Techniques

# 2

**Learning Objectives**

You will be able to understand the following after reading this chapter:

- Principles and application of different external techniques of fracture fixation such as bandages, splints, slings, casts, and modified Thomas splint
- Basic principles and techniques of internal fixation such as intramedullary pins/nails, bone plate, and screws, minimally invasive percutaneous osteosynthesis, and ancillary fixation devices such as orthopedic wires and screws
- Indications, biomechanics, and different types of external skeletal fixation systems, linear ESF systems for small animals, transfixation pinning and casting, bilateral linear ESF system for large animals, circular ESF, epoxy-pin fixation, and complications of ESF

**Summary**

- Splint and bandage, the most economical orthopedic application, can be used as a first aid to stabilize fractures temporarily, to prevent preoperative or postoperative swelling or as a primary fixation method in closed fractures of the distal limb bones especially in lightweight animals.
- Velpeau sling is used to hold the shoulder joint in flexion, while Ehmer sling is used to stabilize the hip joint.
- Fiberglass cast, a synthetic alternative to the plaster of Paris cast, is preferred for both small and large animal applications as it has greater strength and durability, is lightweight, sets quickly, and allows immediate weight-bearing on the limb.
- Intramedullary (IM) Steinmann pin is the most widely used internal fixation device in veterinary practice as it can resist bending forces well and maintain bone alignment due to its central position in the medullary cavity. Cross IM pinning can provide stable fixation of small segment fractures, such as supracondylar femoral fractures, with minimal damage to the growth plate.
- Interlocking nail system is useful to repair comminuted long bone fractures, as the nail is secured to the bone cortex using fixation bolts that provides rotational stability and prevents collapse of fracture segments. Locking plate with threaded screw holes is biomechanically

(continued)


H. P. Aithal et al., *Textbook of Veterinary Orthopaedic Surgery*,
https://doi.org/10.1007/978-981-99-2575-9_2

superior to conventional dynamic compression plate.
- In minimally invasive plate osteosynthesis technique, a bone plate is applied in a bridging fashion through small incisions without exposing the fracture site.
- External skeletal fixation (ESF) is a versatile and minimally invasive orthopedic procedure with excellent mechanical properties allowing early return to function of the affected limb.
- The circular and hybrid ESF systems can provide stable fixation of long bone fractures and are effective to treat fractures in angularly placed bones such as the tibia and transarticular stabilization of fractures with small bone segments near the joint.
- The epoxy-pin fixation technique, wherein the bent fixation pins are incorporated within the epoxy mold to construct the connecting side bars, can be easily applied with minimal facilities and can provide stable fixation of fractures in different species of animals weighing up to about 100 kg.

Fracture fixation techniques can be broadly classified as external fixation techniques, internal fixation techniques, and external skeletal fixation techniques. The basic principle of any technique is to provide stable bone fixation by immobilizing the fractured bone segments to enable early bone healing and functional recovery of the injured limb. The way and the extent to which it is achieved, however, differ among the techniques, apart from the fracture configuration and location.

## 2.1 External Fixation Techniques

External fixation or external coaptation, often called as conservative fracture management, refers to immobilization of fractures and other skeletal abnormalities with devices applied externally, without the use of any invasive technique. External coaptation has been the most widely used technique for fracture management in man and animals for centuries. Although materials may have changed, techniques largely remain the same with few modifications. Among the external fixation techniques practiced today, bandage and splints, plaster/synthetic cast, modified Thomas splints, and splint-cast combinations are widely used in both small and large animal practices [1–6]. As external coaptation techniques are relatively inexpensive and non-invasive, they are frequently applied even in situations where they are not ideal or where there is a high probability of complications (where probably surgical fixation is recommended), mostly due to financial or other constraints. Nevertheless, external coaptation is an integral part of every form of orthopedic therapy, be it to prevent swelling, as a first aid to treat fractures temporarily, as a primary means of fixation in specific fractures, or as an additional support in various conditions such as internal fixation of comminuted unstable fractures, arthrodesis, tendon suturing, etc. Proper case and technique selection is essential for successful outcomes.

### 2.1.1 Bandages

Application of bandage and splint is the simplest and probably the most economical orthopedic application (Fig. 2.1). It does not need any special materials or instruments and can be easily applied. It looks quite easy to apply bandage and splints, but it may get loosened when not tight enough or may cause serious complications when too tight.

Application of bandages may help to cover the wounds and prevent preoperative or postoperative swelling and as a first aid stabilize fractures temporarily. For bandaging, the animal is properly restrained in lateral recumbency, and the affected limb is held upwards. In forelimb applications, the elbow joint is held in fully extended position, whereas in the hindlimbs, the stifle joint is held partially extended. Help can be taken from an assistant to keep the limb in extended position using an anchor tape/adhesive tape applied along the limb extremity or a cotton bandage tied around and above the toes. Cotton stripes are put between the toes, and adequate

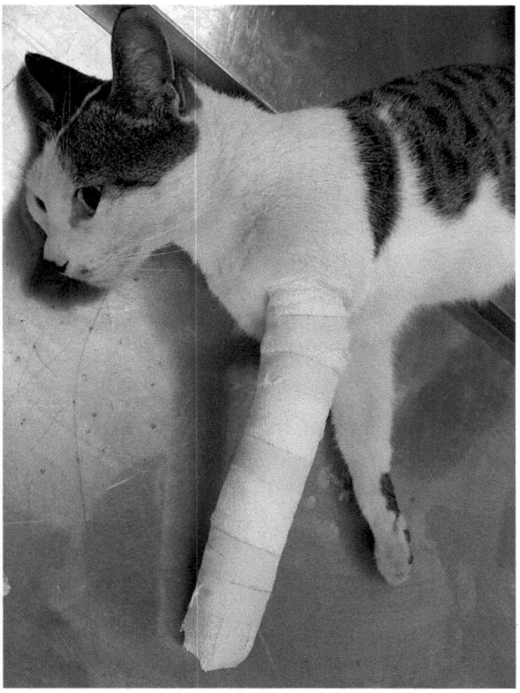

**Fig. 2.1** Application of bandage to stabilize the forelimb in a cat

padding of the limb is done by wrapping an even layer of cotton roll around the limb, starting from the distal end, including the fractured bone, and up to above the joint proximally. Cotton gauze is then firmly applied by twisting over the cotton padding from the distal to the proximal end, so as to leave 1–2 cm of cotton strip out of the bandage proximally. The cotton gauze is then quickly twisted back from the proximal to the distal end, with each new twist covering 1/2–2/3 of the previous. This 'to and fro' covering of cotton gauze is done for 3–4 times. The distal end of the limb may be covered using additional gauze flaps placed from the dorsal to the plantar aspect and then secured with twisting the bandage roll around the limb. Finally, after making sure that the bandage is uniform and firm, if needed, additional coverings are reinforced. An adhesive tape is then wrapped around the limb in a circular fashion intermittently to secure the bandage. The bandage so applied should be changed every 3–4 days depending on the case situation, especially in cases with open wounds/fractures.

Elastic bandage can be used to protect from postoperative oedema and swelling. Normally, the bandage is directly applied over the skin, and if there is a need to keep the bandage for more than 3–4 days, it may be applied over the first layer of the cotton padding. While applying the bandage over the limb, it is important to make sure that the pressure is adequate with same level of elasticity. The end of the bandage is secured with an adhesive tape to prevent loosening, and the proximal edge of the bandage is stuck to the skin.

*Robert-Jones bandage* is used to prevent soft tissue inflammation and to temporarily immobilize the stable limb fractures below the elbow or stifle joint [7]. In this technique, 3–4 thick layers of cotton padding are done around the leg (as described above), which is then tightly and uniformly compressed by covering with cotton gauze roll. Thick cotton padding around the limb prevents any chance of vascular compromise while tightening the gauze roll. If the outer covering is not tightened firmly, there is possibility of slipping of bandage. This can be prevented by applying adhesive tape along the lateral and medial side of the leg from proximal to distal (with a long tail projecting at the tip of the toe) before the cotton is applied and turning it backwards (180°) to stack it to the bandage before completion. This 'massive' bandage often causes inconvenience to the animal. Hence, the *modified Robert-Jones bandage* having much less cotton padding is commonly used in small animals and small ruminants (Fig. 2.2). The bandage can incorporate splints or casts to increase its rigidity. Two to four wooden or aluminum stripes can be sandwiched between the layers of the bandage equally around the leg or a half-leg; molded thermoplastic cast (caudal half for the front leg, cranial half for the hind leg) can be used to make the bandage stiff and strong. The tips of the toes may be excluded while bandaging, which may allow for daily inspection, but too much exposure and constriction around the toe should be avoided not to obstruct the venous blood flow causing swelling. The Robert-Jones bandage is effective for short-term applications only. The elastic

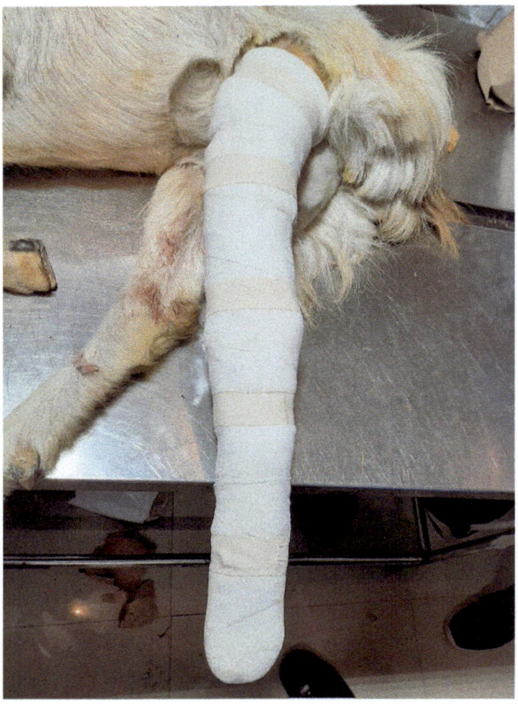

**Fig. 2.2** Modified Robert-Jones bandage application to stabilize tibial fracture in a goat

bandage provides the compression to the surface of the limb for very short duration, lasting for not more than 24–48 h; hence, it is inappropriate for any use beyond 1–2 days.

### 2.1.2 Splints

Splints cover only a part of the limb surface, unlike casts which encircle the entire limb. They are indicated in stable closed fractures distal to the proximal 1/3 of the radius or tibia (mostly with intact ulna or fibula). Open fractures with wounds and unstable comminuted fractures are contraindications for its use. Splints can be either prefabricated (mostly made of plastics or aluminum) or custom-made (plaster/fiberglass cast or thermoplastics). Preformed splints are more convenient but they often do not fit adequately. The disadvantage with wooden or plastic sticks is that they do not adapt to the leg (the leg is adapted to the splint), whereas the cast splint can adapt to the contours of the leg. Hence, wooden sticks or plastics can only be used for first aid and for temporary stabilization of fractures and not preferred for definitive treatment (Fig. 2.3). Thermoplastic material is also not used as definitive fixation device as it also does not adapt to the contours of the leg and hence may not provide stable fixation of fracture segments. Molding several layers of casting tape to the limb produces better fracture stability and a more comfortable fit for animal applications. Plaster of Paris can be easily molded along the contours of the leg and is quite resistant against bending load; however, it is not resistant against humidity and may lose its strength upon wetting. Newer synthetic cast materials such as fiberglass cast are strong and can mold to the shape of the limb, but it is costly and more expensive.

Splints should be applied along the length of a fractured leg, distally from the point of the toes/hoof and proximally up to the joint above the fracture site. It should include the carpal joint in metacarpal fractures and the tarsal joint in case of metatarsal fractures, whereas in fractures distal to

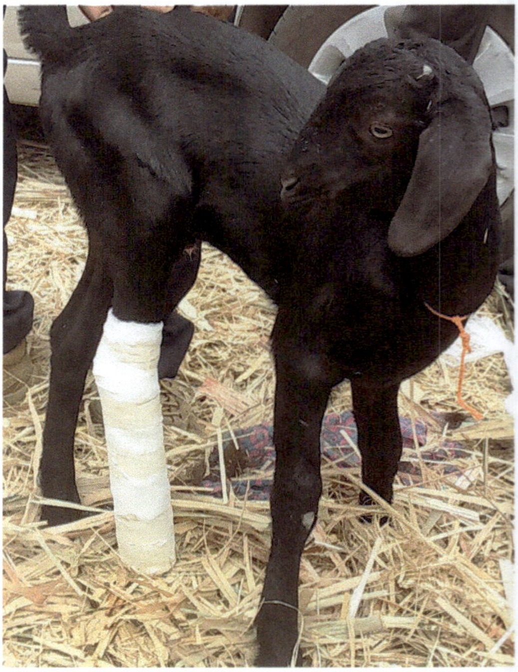

**Fig. 2.3** Application of splint and bandage to stabilize metatarsal fracture in a kid

the elbow (distal 2/3 of radius-ulna) or stifle (distal 2/3 of tibia-fibula) joints, the splint should extend up to the olecranon and tibial tuberosity, respectively (Fig. 2.4). Half/hemi-splint, covering half of the leg surface is generally ideal, as it provides support to the broken bone, allows for swelling, and is easily removed. In forelimbs, the splint is applied along the caudal surface of the antebrachium, as the ulna is longer and courses more superficially than the radius. In hindlimbs, the splint is applied along the cranial surface of the crus as the tibia is located at the cranial aspect and the presence of the Achilles tendon caudally may not allow its proper placement.

For application of splint, under deep sedation, the animal is restrained with the fractured limb downwards but slightly tilted on its back. Fracture segments are reduced and the limb is held extended. The whole leg is then padded with a thin cotton layer, covering the areas of bony prominences, followed by a layer of cotton gauze bandage. A 6–8-layer plaster strip is immersed in warm water (till the air bubbles stop coming), squeezed to remove excessive water, compressed uniformly, and applied at the right place. When still wet, the plaster is contoured to the surface of the limb and allowed to harden. The splint edges are then smoothened by trimming with a pair of scissors (POP) or a saw (fiberglass), and the splint is properly placed. The uncovered part of the leg is padded with the cotton to fill the gap. The plaster splint along with the cotton is then secured around the limb by applying cotton gauze roll from the distal to the proximal end.

In large animals, splint and bandage is often used for temporary stabilization of fractures in straight long bones such as the metatarsus, metacarpus, and radius-ulna (Fig. 2.5). It can also be used as a primary fixation method, especially in lightweight animals. Under sedation, the animal is restrained in lateral recumbency with the fractured leg held uppermost. A long length of cotton gauze/rope is loosely tied around and just above the hoof, to help reduce the fracture by applying traction and counter-traction and to keep the limb in extended position with the help of an assistant. After sprinkling talcum powder over the limb, 'adequate' padding of the limb is done by wrapping an even layer of cotton around the limb. A roll of cotton gauze is then firmly wrapped around the limb starting from the distal extremity of the limb and moving upwards, leaving about 1–2 cm cotton strip out of the bandage at the proximal end. After a layer of bandaging, two wooden/metal splints of appropriate length

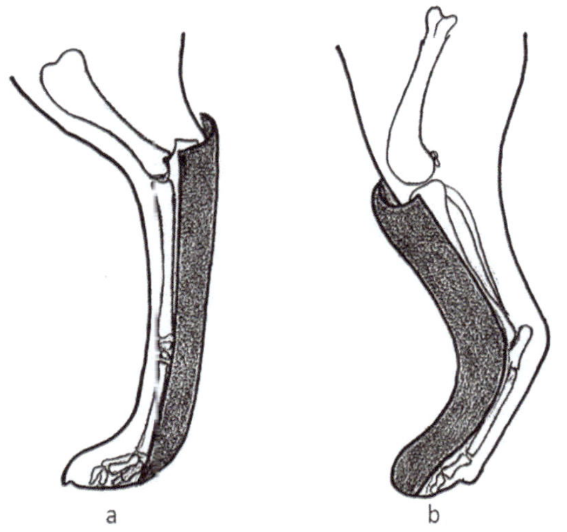


**Fig. 2.4** Application of splint in the forelimb (**a**) and hindlimb (**b**)

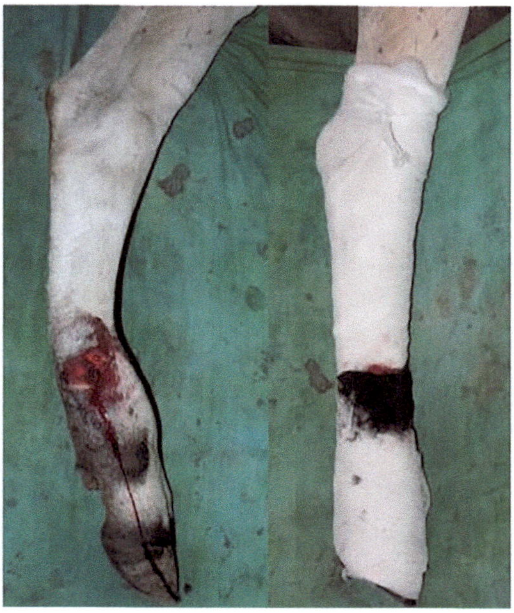

**Fig. 2.5** Application of splint and bandage to stabilize open fracture of the metatarsus in a calf

are placed at 90° to each other (one on the medial/lateral aspect and another on the caudal/cranial aspect). In heavy animals, 3–4 splints may be used and are secured by tying cotton gauze roll/ropes around. The width and thickness of the splint may vary as per the animal's size, but it should not be very light (may break during weight-bearing) or very heavy (may interfere with normal weight-bearing). The length of the splint should span from the hoof up to the joint above the fracture site. The cotton gauze roll is then wrapped over and above the splints by incorporating them within. Depending on the case, several layers of wrapping are done. Extra turns of gauze roll are taken at the distal and proximal ends to secure the splints properly, and at the level of the joints, extra layers of wrapping are done in figure of '8' fashion to provide additional support against bending stress. Before applying the final layers of the bandage, the anchor tapes/ropes are released by loosening/cutting, and the extra length of cotton sticking out is reflected back and included in the bandage. The splint and bandage is then secured by applying adhesive tape rolls around at places, especially at the distal extremity, proximal end, and at the level of joints.

### 2.1.3 Slings

Slings are infrequently used for external coaptation in animals [7]. Velpeau sling is used to hold the forelimb joints (carpus, elbow, and shoulder) in flexion by bandaging the limb against the body, thus preventing weight-bearing on the affected limb (Fig. 2.6). It is indicated in stabilization of minor fractures of the scapula and humerus or reduced shoulder luxation. The sling can be applied in standing awake animals or in recumbent animals under general anesthesia. The paw and carpus are held in a slightly flexed position, and cotton padding is done followed by wrapping of the elastic bandage roll. By placing the padded portion in the axillary region, the wrap is continued to cover the elbow and shoulder, holding the limb to the side of the torso and encircling the body. Padding is ideally wrapped behind and in front of the opposite limb alternatively to prevent its slippage. While bandaging, a small window may be left at the distal end of the limb to visualize the toes.

Ehmer sling, which is more popular in veterinary practice, prevents the patient from weight-bearing on the bandaged hindlimb (Fig. 2.7). It is indicated to provide stability following reduction of a cranio-dorsal luxation of the hip joint. The sling if applied properly helps to abduct and internally rotate the femur and thus keep the femur head within the acetabular cavity. This is not indicated in ventral dislocation of the hip, as abduction of the limb may lead to re-luxation. The technique includes soft padding of the hind paw and metatarsal region followed by elastic gauze application starting from the lateral surface of the paw. The gauze roll is then progressed upwards on the medial side and over the quadriceps. By flexing the leg, the bandage roll is continued laterally over the thigh and medial to the hock joint to take it around the paw. This process is repeated 2–3 times and then the gauze bandage is wrapped around the body by keeping the limb close to the body in a flexed position. At the end, the gauze bandage is fixed using one or two pieces of adhesive tape to prevent loosening of the bandage. The sling is kept in place for about 10–15 days to achieve full stability of the joint, constantly observed, and if get wet or loosened, it is reapplied.

### 2.1.4 Plaster Cast

Plaster cast is the most widely practiced external fixation technique in both small and large animals [2, 6–8]. Plaster bandage consists of a cotton bandage impregnated with plaster of Paris that hardens upon wetting. Plaster of Paris is anhydrous calcium sulfate that has been heated. In the presence of water, the soluble form of calcium sulfate becomes insoluble (hardening) with production of heat (exothermic reaction):

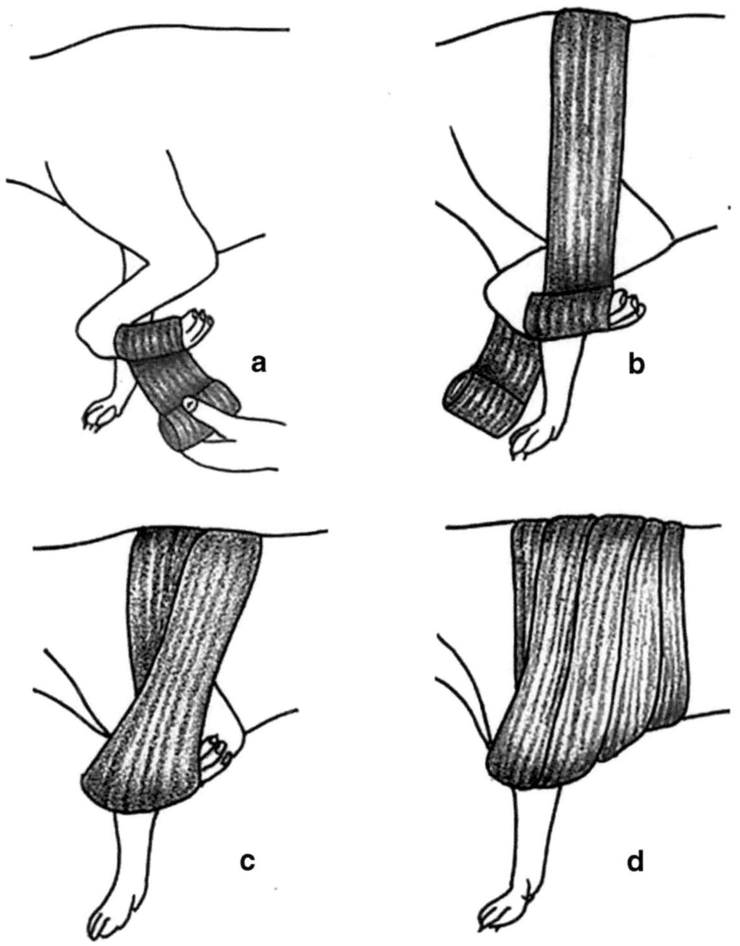


**Fig. 2.6** Velpeau sling: (**a**) the paw of the affected limb is loosely wrapped around (lateral to medial) using a gauze bandage; (**b**) by keeping the carpus, elbow, and shoulder joints in flexed position, the gauze bandage is taken over the lateral aspect of the limb and chest and brought behind the opposite axilla; (**c**) several such layers of gauze are applied taking around the flexed carpus; (**d**) gauze bandaging is completed by taking several layers of wrap around the chest and secured

$$2\,(CaSO_4 \cdot H_2O) + 3\,H_2O \rightarrow 2\,(CaSO_4 \cdot 2H_2O) + \text{Heat}$$

#### 2.1.4.1 Indications and Contraindications

It is indicated in fractures below the mid-diaphysis of the radius or tibia (below the elbow or stifle joint) and is most suitable for straight limb applications like fractures of the metacarpus, radius-ulna, and metatarsus. Plaster should be used in only those fractures which can be closely reduced and maintained with at least 50% of the bone ends in contact. Further, fractures that are expected to heal relatively rapidly are chosen for cast application to reduce the chances of cast-related complications. Plaster cast is contraindicated in proximal bones such as the femur and humerus, as the joints above (hip and shoulder joints) cannot be stabilized adequately by a cast. Generally, it is not indicated in open fractures with soft tissue injury.

Plaster should be applied in fresh cases with no or little soft tissue swelling or when the inflammatory swelling has subsided (after 3–4 days of initial injury), to prevent cast loosening and slippage. Until then, the limb may be immobilized using temporary splinting and bandaging.

#### 2.1.4.2 Biomechanics

Full cylindrical cast of adequate thickness, which conforms to the limb and immobilizes the joints above and below the fracture site, can effectively neutralize bending and rotational forces; however, it is generally unable to resist compressive, shear, and tensile forces. A cast applied straight is

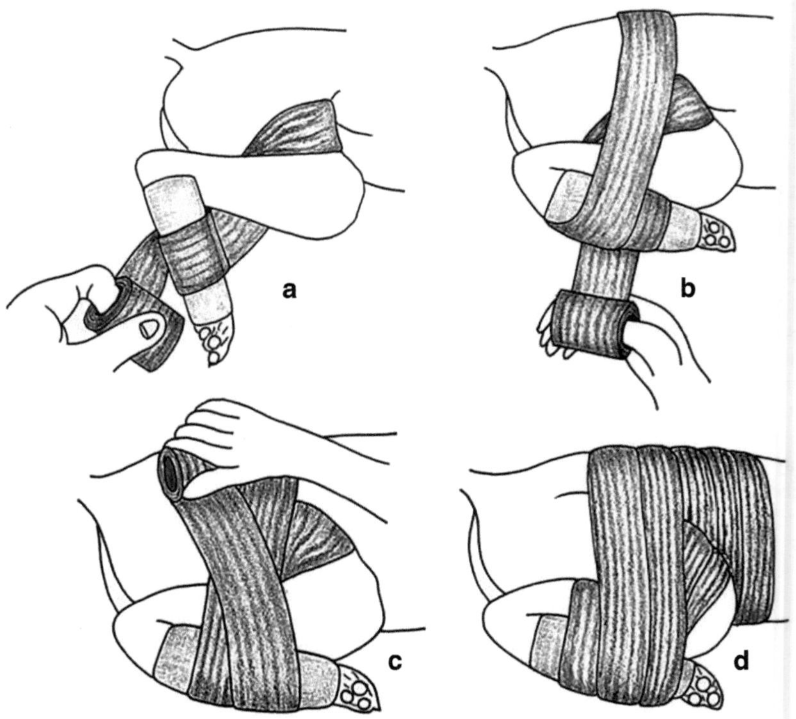


**Fig. 2.7** Application of Ehmer sling: (**a**) the hind paw and metatarsal region are soft padded and the elastic gauze is applied starting from the lateral surface of the paw and is then progressed upwards on the medial side and over the quadriceps; (**b**) by flexing the leg, the bandage roll is continued laterally over the thigh and medial to the hock joint to take it around the paw; (**c**) rolling of bandage is repeated 2–3 times; and (**d**) the gauze bandage is wrapped around the body by keeping the limb close to the body in flexed position and secured using clips or adhesive bandage application

better able to resist fracture forces than that applied angularly. As the cast is applied around the limb (bone surrounded by soft tissues), there exists a certain distance between the cast and the bone; therefore, the level of fixation stability achieved is much less than internal fixation and also external skeletal fixation, where the bone segments are directly immobilized using fixation implants. Hence, the bones having least coverage of soft tissues, such as radius-ulna, metacarpus, and metatarsus, are better suited for cast application.

Fracture immobilized by a cast heals by secondary healing, i.e. through external callus formation (suggesting adequate stability to allow revascularization and callus formation), but stability is insufficient to allow primary bone union (micro-movement at the fracture site persists).

#### 2.1.4.3 Technique

Usually, the animal is restrained in lateral recumbency with the fractured limb positioned upwards, under deep sedation or general anesthesia. An assistant can help to maintain proper alignment of bone segments and ensure the correct positioning of the limb. In small animals, adhesive tapes (anchor tape) may be placed along the medial and lateral sides of the foot extending about 10 cm beyond the toes, to hold the limb in an extended position. A cotton bandage may also be tied around the toes to hold the limb and apply tension. In large animals, rope restraint may be used; in heavy animals, the limb can be pulled by applying traction using the wires placed through the holes drilled in the hoof wall.

In general, the limb is placed in a comfortable position, with the normal standing angle preferred during casting. The limb should be dry before cast application. The talcum powder may be sprinkled over the limb (shaving is not needed), and an even layer of cotton is applied around the leg in order to protect bony prominences. The cotton padding is extended 1–2 cm beyond the cast to prevent direct contact with the skin. Over-padding should be avoided to prevent cast loosening; further, it may impair immobilization by allowing movement of fracture segments within the cast. A tube of stockinette firmly fitting the limb may be slipped along the length of the limb (Fig. 2.8). If not, a roll of cotton bandage may be used to wrap

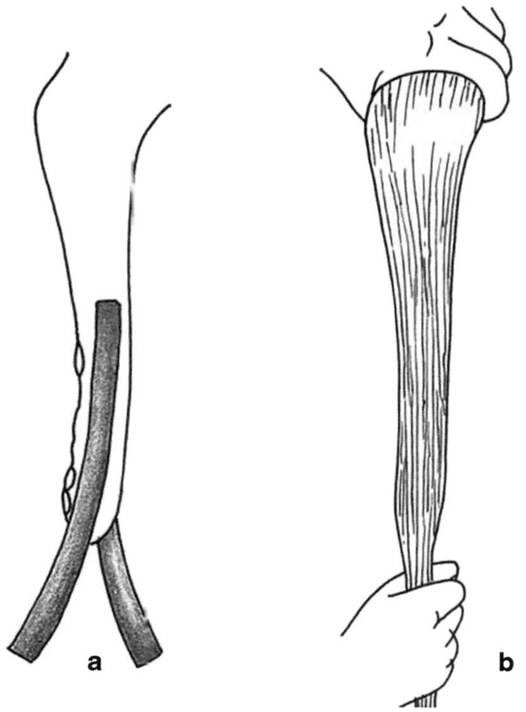


**Fig. 2.8** Application of plaster cast: (**a**) adhesive tapes applied along the medial and lateral sides of the foot extending beyond the toes to hold the limb in extended position; (**b**) a stockinette is slipped along the length of the limb (adopted from Leighton, R.L. 1991. Principles of conservative fracture management: splints and casts. Semin Vet Med Surg. 6 (1): 39–51.)

the limb in spiral fashion. An assistant (may be two are required in large animals) can hold the limb in traction by grasping the stockinette/cotton bandage above and the anchor tape/rope below the area to be covered by the cast.

Plaster of Paris bandage is soaked in warm water for a few seconds until air bubbles cease to appear. It is then removed from the water, squeezed, and wrapped over the limb, starting at the fracture site from the distal to the proximal (Fig. 2.9). Subsequently, remaining POP bandages are applied one by one along the entire limb except for the toe pads in dogs and hooves in large animals. A strip of a few (6–8) layers of plaster can be made wet and applied firmly along the caudal surface of the limb to provide greater strength to fixation (Fig. 2.10). During cast application, formation of folds or indentations should be prevented as they may cause injury and necrosis of the underlying skin. Overstretching and tightening of the plaster cast around the limb should also be avoided.

The strength of the cast can be increased and weight reduced by incorporating the splints within the cast, especially in large animals. Two wooden/metal rods can be placed $90^0$ to each other. In large animal applications, a 'U'-shaped walking bar (metal strip) may be placed under the hoof and incorporated into the cast (Fig. 2.11). This can reduce the loading forces on the distal limb and thus help protect the fracture site.

The plaster is molded by rubbing with wet hand after each layer before hardening. And before applying the final layers of cast, the tapes and the stockinette are reflected back onto the cast at both ends. If a rope is used, one should not forget to untie the knot (if applied) before allowing the cast to set. At the end, a wet polythene sheet may be pressed over the wet cast to smoothen the surface.

The plaster cast should generally extend from the toe/hoof up to above the level of the joint proximal to the fracture site. In heavy animals, the full-limb cast extending up to the elbow or stifle joint should be applied even if the fracture is in the metacarpus or metatarsus, especially if it is at the proximal end of the bone near the carpal/tarsal joint. The thickness of the cast may vary depending on the case. In small animal applications, 4–5-layer thick cast is usually adequate; in calves weighing up to 150 kg, 6–8-layer thick cast may be required; and in adult large animals, 12–16-layer thick casts may be needed. The cast should be thicker at the level of the joints (applied in figure of 8 fashion), especially at the hock joint (hindlimb) to resist the stress concentration due to the angulation and movement of the joints.

The plaster is then allowed to become dry and hard before letting the animal bear weight on the limb. This may take about 30–45 min in small animals and about 1–2 h in large animals. However, complete drying and hardening of the cast

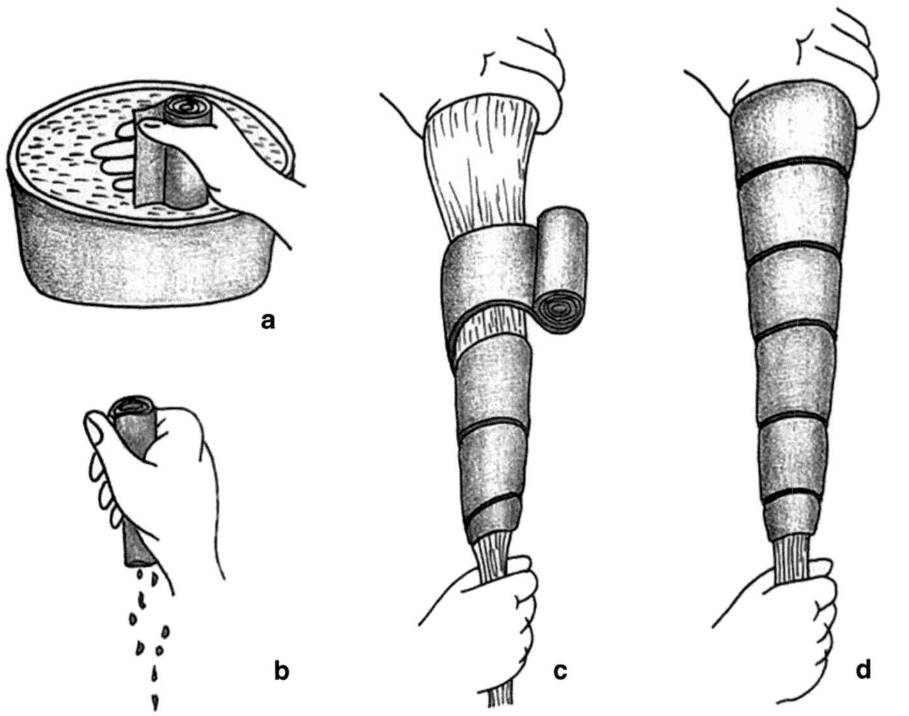


**Fig. 2.9** Application of plaster cast: (**a**) POP bandage is soaked in warm water for a few seconds until air bubbles cease to appear; (**b**) POP bandage is removed from the water and squeezed; (**c, d**) POP bandage is then wrapped around the limb, starting at the fracture site from the distal to proximal (adopted from Leighton, R.L. 1991. Principles of conservative fracture management: splints and casts. Semin Vet Med Surg. 6 (1): 39–51.)

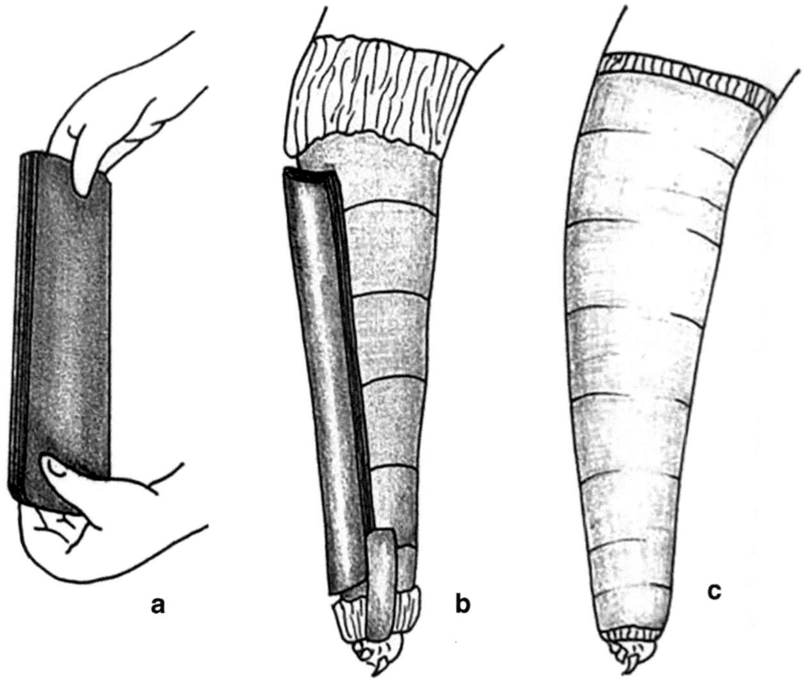


**Fig. 2.10** Application of plaster cast: (**a**) a strip of a few layers of plaster (6–8) is made wet, (**b**) it is then applied firmly along the caudal surface, and the tapes and the stockinette are reflected back onto the cast at both ends, and (**c**) the final layers of cast are applied, molded by rubbing the layers of cast using a wet hand; a wet plastic sheet may be used to smoothen the surface, and it is then allowed to dry (adopted from Leighton, R.L. 1991. Principles of conservative fracture management: splints and casts. Semin Vet Med Surg. 6 (1): 39–51.)

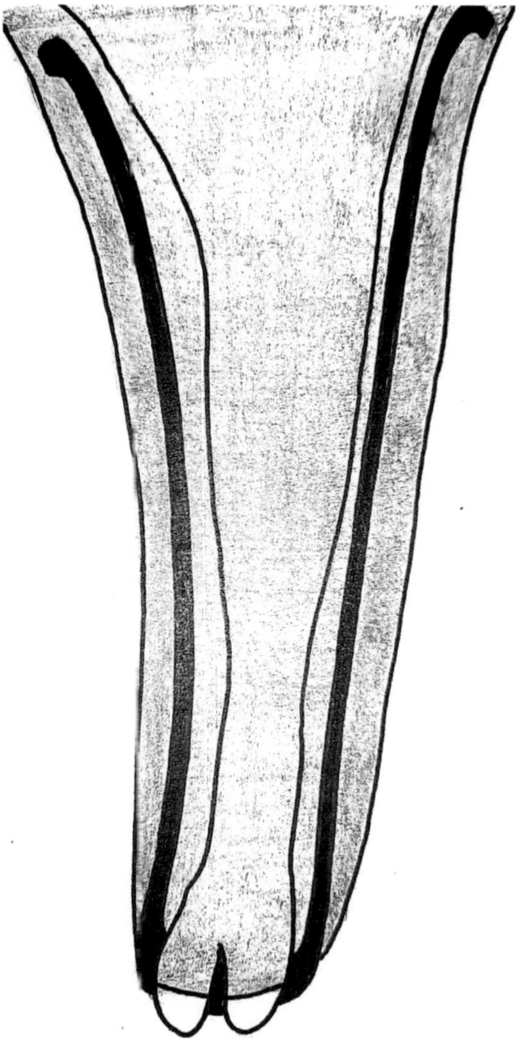

**Fig. 2.11** Placement of U-shaped bar under the hoof will help reduce the load on the distal limb

(attaining full strength) may take 24–72 h depending on the thickness.

'Bi-halving' can be done after applying the cast, allowing it to set, and then making it into two halves by cutting longitudinally along the medial and lateral aspects of the cast. After placing back the halved cast on the limb, it is then wrapped with an elastic bandage to hold it firmly. Bi-halving a cast allows examination of the underlying soft tissues if need arises and allows easy removal of the cast if swelling develops, and it can be reapplied. This technique is often used in small animals and rarely practiced in large animals, as bi-halving reduces the fixation strength of the cast considerably.

#### 2.1.4.4 Post-application Care and Management

In open fractures, for drainage and daily dressing of the skin wound, an opening (window) is made in the cast at the level of the wound. The window at the wound site can also be left at the time of cast application. One should remember that creating a 'window' in the cast will reduce its strength considerably and make the window site prone for breakage, especially when it is at the level of joints.

Complications can occur with application of cast both in small and large animals [2, 9–11]. The toes/hooves are inspected several times during the first 48 h for any swelling, coldness, or constriction. If the toe/hoof gets swollen or gets cold, pressure at the end of the cast should be relieved by removing the cast, and the cast may be reapplied after swelling subsides. Similarly, if the cast gets loosened and slips (due to subsiding of inflammatory swelling present earlier), the cast should be reapplied.

The plastered animal should be kept in a dry place (to prevent the cast from getting wet) with soft bedding (to prevent slippage). Wetting is more common in hindlimbs due to urination; it weakens the cast and may lead to its breakage. Plastic (polythene) sheets may be wrapped around the cast to prevent wetting.

Cast may be retained for up to 3–4 weeks in young dogs, sheep, and goats and 4–6 weeks in adult dogs, sheep/goats, and calves. In adult large animals, clinical union of fracture (development of bridging callus with adequate fracture stability) may normally take place by 8–10 weeks, but often, it may require 12–16 weeks or more. Plaster is removed using a saw after radiographic fracture union (complete bony union with obliteration of fracture line), which generally takes a few weeks to months after the clinical union. After removal of the cast, the affected limb is massaged to promote circulation. Movement is restricted till the limb regains its normal function.

### 2.1.5 Fiberglass Cast

Fiberglass cast, unlike traditional plaster cast, is strong, lightweight, and radiolucent. Due to its desirable qualities, fiberglass cast has become the preferred type of casting both in human and veterinary orthopedics [12–16].

#### 2.1.5.1 Advantages over Plaster Cast

Fiberglass cast is made of water-activated polyurethane resin combined with bandaging materials, so it offers greater strength and durability. It weighs less and hence more comfortable to the patient. The setting time is very quick and therefore needs less care and restraint during application, and the animal can be allowed to use the limb almost immediately. Fiberglass cast is radiolucent and hence allows better radiographic evaluation of fracture repair. It is also water impermeable (waterproof); therefore, the inside padding does not get wet. If the cast gets wet, it quickly becomes dry.

#### 2.1.5.2 Drawbacks

Fiberglass cast is costlier than traditional plaster cast; hence, it may be a constraint in veterinary practice. As fiberglass cast hardens quickly, there is less time to apply. The synthetic materials leave less room for swelling; if more tightly applied, it may lead to vascular compromise. Knitted fiberglass and resin bandages are less moldable than a traditional plaster, so sometimes a less comfortable fit is achieved. Fiberglass bandage is less smooth and more likely to snag clothing or to cause skin bite injuries.

#### 2.1.5.3 Technique

Technique of application of fiberglass cast is almost similar to that of plaster cast. The fractured limb is first padded with cotton or any other waterproof padding material. Then, the knitted fiberglass bandage is wrapped around the limb in several layers (Fig. 2.12). The use of stockinettes and/or cast padding is essential to avoid direct contact between the cast and the skin. Wearing of protective gloves is a must during its application to prevent sticking of the cast material (once get stick, it is difficult to remove).

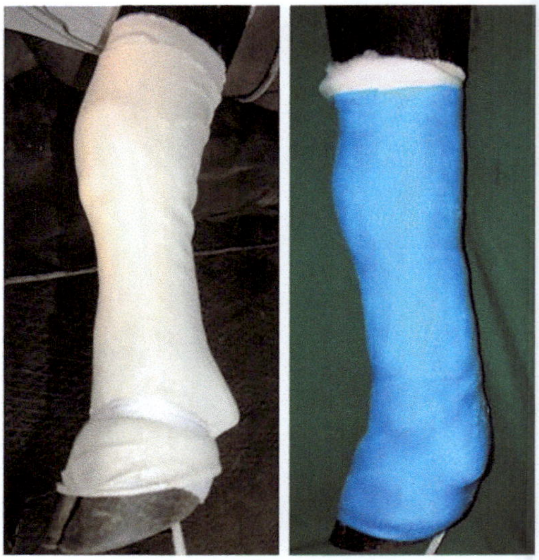

**Fig. 2.12** Application of fiberglass case in metacarpal fracture in a buffalo

When the cast material is immersed in water, it should be squeezed firmly before applying. Cast should be applied quickly, to prevent premature hardening. Application of 3–4 layers of the cast is enough in small animals and 6–8 layers in large animals. Further, application of additional support strip or splints is not needed (stronger than plaster cast). The cast may be smoothed with a smoothing gel or lubricating gel.

#### 2.1.5.4 Post-application Care and Management

A fiberglass cast requires less care and maintenance than a plaster cast, and weight-bearing can be allowed as early as 15–20 min post-application. The limb immobilized with a fiberglass cast should be watched carefully in the first 24–48 h after the application for any swelling, coldness, or bad odor, as there is less room for swelling. Complications are more in equine patients (skin is more sensitive) than bovines. In case of any doubt, the cast should be removed and reapplied after the swelling subsides. For removal of the cast, an electric/power saw is needed, as it is difficult to cut the cast using a hand saw. While cutting the cast, it is taken care to prevent any possible injury to the skin.

### 2.1.6 Modified Thomas Splints

Modified Thomas splint (Schroeder-Thomas splint) is a whole limb traction splint, wherein the fracture ends are brought together and held in alignment by application of traction in specific directions using traction tapes/ropes/bandages, which are anchored to the supporting side rods [6, 7, 17]. This technique is not widely used in practice nowadays due to the advent of better internal and external skeletal fixation techniques; however, if properly used, it can give satisfactory results in many types of fractures, especially in small lightweight animals. Modified Thomas splint and cast combination has been used successfully for treatment of different long bone fractures in large ruminants too.

#### 2.1.6.1 Indications and Contraindications

Modified Thomas splints are generally indicated for treatment of fractures at the distal femur and humerus, tibia-fibula, and radius-ulna in dogs, cats, sheep, goats, and young calves. Splint-cast combination is indicated in heavy animals. It is either used as a sole method of fracture fixation or as an ancillary method along with internal fixation techniques such as intramedullary pins.

Modified Thomas splint is not indicated in long oblique and comminuted fractures, where it is difficult to reduce the fracture segments by close method and prevent overriding of bone ends. Further, fractures near the joints, unless properly reduced, may lead to malunion and degenerative joint disease.

#### 2.1.6.2 Materials Required

Aluminum rods (for dogs, cats, sheep/goats) or steel rods (for calves/foals) of varied diameter (5–7 mm is adequate in most cases; in adult large animals, 8–12 mm rods may be needed depending on the size of the animal), rod bender, pin cutter, cotton roll, gauze bandage, and adhesive tape are needed.

#### 2.1.6.3 Technique of Application

Under deep sedation/tranquilization (general anesthesia may be preferred where severe overriding of fracture segments is present), the animal is restrained in lateral recumbency with the fractured leg held upwards. The splint is customized to the individual case, so as to fit well to the front limb or hindlimb of the patient.

Firstly, the aluminum rod is bent to make a ring (1½ circle, taking the help of a splint mold or any cylindrical object of appropriate size) to properly fit in the patient's groin or axilla and secured using adhesive tapes (Figs. 2.13 and 2.14). The size of the ring should be kept adequate to accommodate wrapping of the ring with cotton roll and bandages. For hindlimb splint, the ring diameter should be the distance from the tuber ischii to the tuber coxae. For the forelimb, the distance from the axilla to the midpoint on the scapula should be the diameter of the ring. The ring is bent inwardly (toward medial side) at 45° angle from the vertical rods. The ring is then wrapped with a thin strip of cotton roll and secured with gauze bandage and adhesive tape. Sufficient padding is done at the bottom of the ring to protect the groin/axilla region when the splint is applied with the limb under traction.

The limb is temporarily inserted into the rings to determine the length of side rods. The length of the splint should be slightly longer than the extended limb. If the length is too long, it will hinder locomotion; and if it is short, proper tension cannot be applied. The total length of the rod is calculated as $2(3D + 1) + 2L + 20$, where $D$ = diameter of the ring and $L$ = length of the splint bar. For the forelimb, the diameter (D) is the length from axilla to midpoint of the scapula, and the length of bar (L) is the distance from axilla to the tip of the toe in an extended leg, whereas for the hindlimb, the diameter (D) is the length from tuber ischii to tuber coxae, and the length of bar (L) is the distance from the thigh to the tip of the toe in an extended leg.

For forelimb splint, both splint rods (cranial and caudal) are bent slightly at the level of the elbow to conform to the standing angle, whereas for the hindlimb, the caudal as well as the cranial

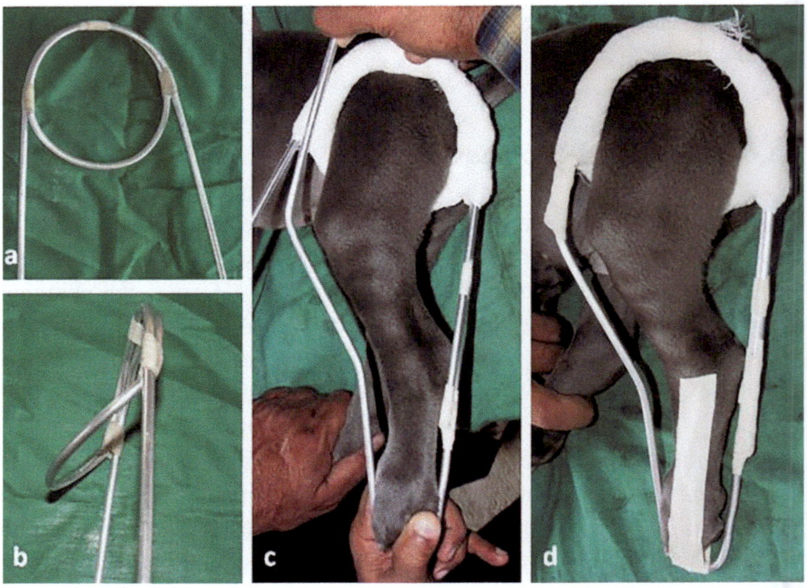


**Fig. 2.13** Application of Modified Thomas splint: (**a**) an aluminum rod is bent to make a ring (1½ circle) and secured using an adhesive tape; (**b**) the ring is bent at 450 angle from the vertical rods; (**c**) the limb is temporarily inserted into the rings to determine the length of side rods, and the side bar is bent at the level of the stifle and hock; (**d**) the extra length of the rod is cut and joined to give the final shape

rods can be bent to conform to the standing angles of stifle and hock joints, or the caudal rod can be kept straight without any bend and the cranial rod may be bent at stifle and hock (Fig. 2.15). The distal end of side rods is bent inwards and secured together using adhesive tape.

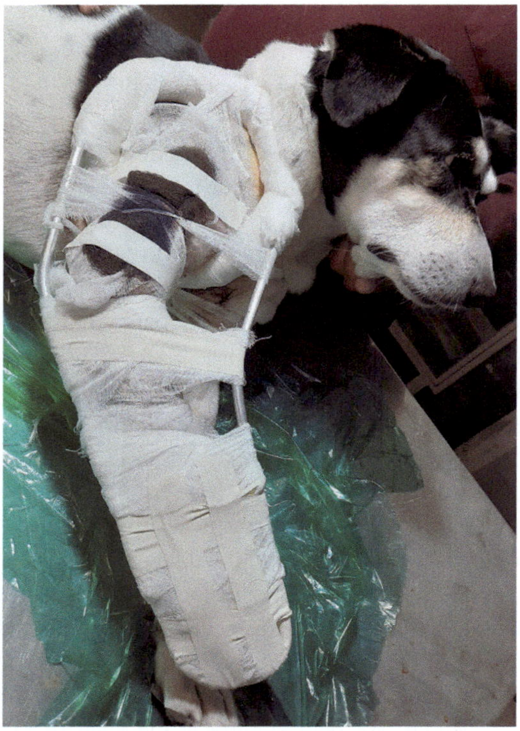

**Fig. 2.14** Modified Thomas splint application in the forelimb: note bending of both side bars at the level of the elbow

In bovine calves, iron/steel rods may be used in place of aluminum rods to construct the splint to provide greater strength to fixation (Fig. 2.16). Rings have to be secured by welding (rather than by adhesive tape), and an oval-shaped iron sheet of the size of hoof is welded at the distal end of side rods to provide a suitable anchorage for the hoof. The side rods of the splint are generally kept straight without any angulation/bending. The whole length of side rods may be tightly wrapped with gauze bandage, which is then anchored with adhesive tapes at different places.

At the distal extremity of the limb, adhesive tape strips are attached, one on the dorsal and another on the palmar/plantar surface, and the extended portions of the adhesive tapes are stuck together below the toes (dogs/cats) or hooves (sheep/goats) (Fig. 2.17). A thin layer of cotton roll is wrapped around the limb over the tape strips (from toe up to the knee/hock joint), which is then covered with a firm wrap of gauze bandage and anchored at places using circular wrap of adhesive tape to ensure that the tape strips applied on the limb do not slip while applying traction. In large animals, cotton rope may be anchored above the fetlock using a loose slip

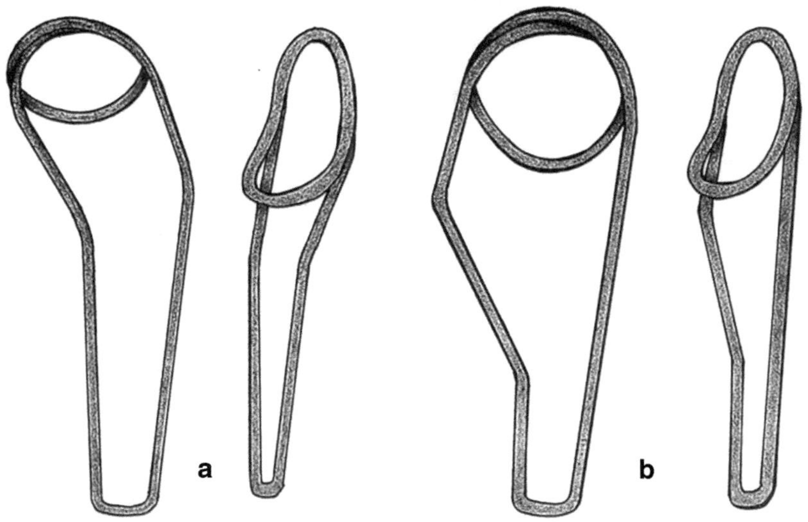


**Fig. 2.15** Modified Thomas splint: (**a**) for forelimb and (**a**) for hindlimb

knot in place of adhesive tape strips to enable traction with greater force.

The limb is inserted into the ring (bend should be held toward the inner/medial side of the limb) and ensured that the ring is properly and firmly fit in the region of the groin/axilla. Traction is applied at the extremity of the limb by tensioning the tapes/ropes and the tape strip/rope is secured to the 'U' portion of the splint under tension, in such a way that the leg is slightly rotated inwardly. Then, as per the fracture location and displacement of bone segments, the traction is applied at different levels, and the bones are fixed to the frame using cotton strips or bandages.

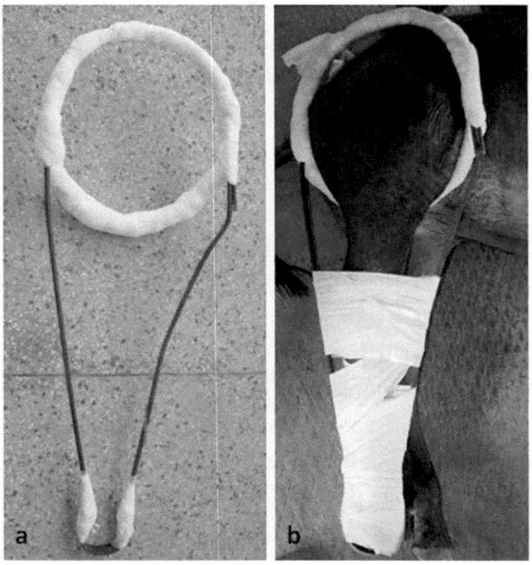


**Fig. 2.16** Construction of MTS ring using iron rod for calves: (**a**) the cut ends of rod are joined by welding; a flat iron sheet is welded at the distal end to seat the hoof; (**b**) the limb is then inserted in the MTS ring, and the limb is anchored

#### 2.1.6.4 Application of Traction

The fracture site is supported and secured to the side rods with the help of cotton strips/bandages for applying traction at least at two locations (one above and one below the fracture site) around the non-fractured bones of the limb.

To apply traction, the cotton strip/bandage is secured to the side bar toward the direction at which the traction is desired (say, cranial). It is then wrapped around the portion of the limb by taking it through the medial, caudal, and lateral sides and bringing it back to the original side bar with firm traction, to allow pulling of that portion of the limb toward the side bar (cranial). Few more layers of similar wrappings may be done to provide additional support. The cotton bandage is then encircled around the limb including both side rods 2–3 times and secured using an adhesive tape.

In middle or distal diaphyseal fractures of humerus, the side rods are bent at a more acute angle at the elbow, and both the foot and the radius-ulna are drawn caudally by using traction

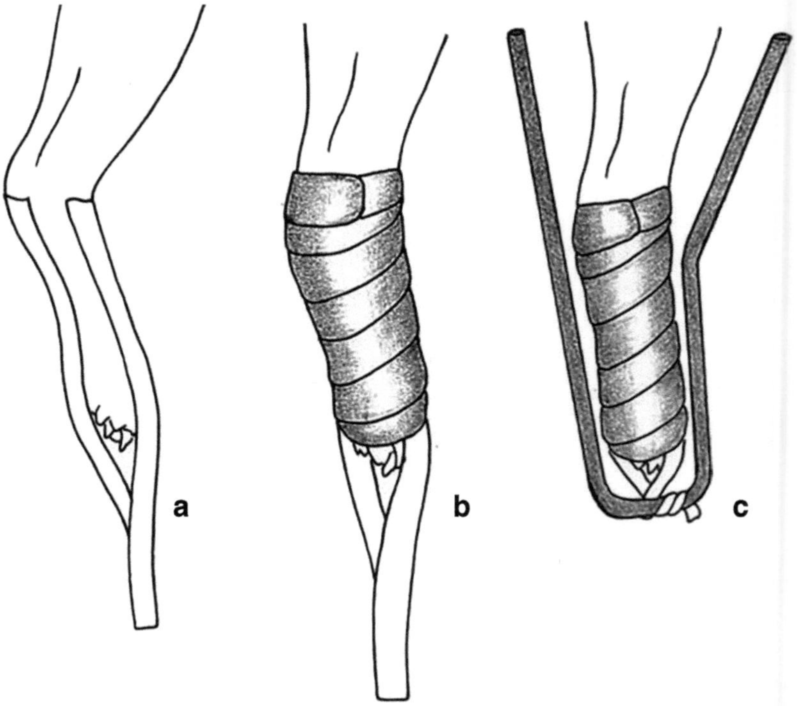


**Fig. 2.17** Anchoring the limb in MTS: (**a**) adhesive tape strips are applied on the dorsal and palmar/plantar aspect, and the extended portions of the adhesive tapes are stuck together below the toes; (**b**) wrapped around the limb using cotton roll and gauze bandage; and (**c**) securing the tape strip to the 'U' bottom of the splint under tension

bandages (Fig. 2.18). In middle or proximal diaphyseal fractures of the radius-ulna, the side rods are only slightly angled at the elbow to provide an almost straight pull on the limb; the traction is applied caudally at the lower limb as well as at the humerus.

In fractures of the femur or tibia, the lower limb cotton strip/bandage should secure the foot in caudal position. The proximal strip should pull the tibia and stifle (in femoral fractures) or the femur (in tibial fractures) toward the cranial side (Fig. 2.19).

In fractures of carpals/metacarpals, the side bars of the splint are more acutely bent at the hock corresponding to the normal standing angle of the joint. The distal bandage strip should hold the foot caudally and the proximal strip should draw the femur cranially.

Once the splint is properly secured and traction applied appropriately, the entire splint may be covered with a stockinette or cotton bandage rolls and secured using adhesive tapes at desired places, before allowing the weight-bearing on the limb.

#### 2.1.6.5 Postoperative Care

The animal must be checked frequently for any injury at the groin or axilla that may have been caused due to rubbing of the ring. The splint is kept in place for 3–6 weeks as per the fracture type and location or till the radiographic healing occurs. All skin wounds created by rubbing of splint, if any, may be treated with antibiotic ointment/powder.

### 2.1.7 Thomas Splint-Cast Combination

#### 2.1.7.1 Indication

Modified Thomas splint-cast combination is indicated for treating closed radius-ulna and tibial fractures in heavy large animals, in which full-limb cast alone does not provide adequate immobilization [2, 18–20]. Generally, it is not recommended in very young animals and also in cases of severe comminuted fractures and in fractures near the joint (metaphyseal or epiphyseal fractures).

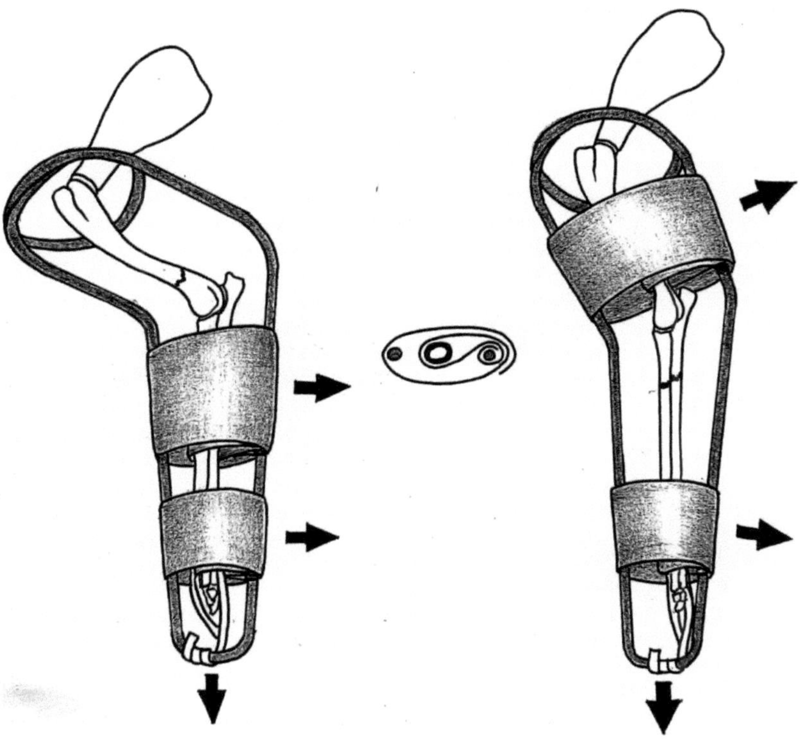

**Fig. 2.18** Application of traction using modified Thomas splint in forelimb fractures

#### 2.1.7.2 Biomechanics

The fractured limb is spared from weight-bearing stresses, which are taken by the splint rods, preventing collapse of the fracture segments. Adequate immobilization of fracture segments allows healing of the bone by external callus formation.

#### 2.1.7.3 Technique

Under sedation or general anesthesia, the animal is positioned in lateral recumbency with the affected limb held upwards. The limb is held in extended position using a tape strip/traction rope tied above the pastern. Alternatively, holes can be drilled in the hoof wall of both distal phalanges, and a suitable size wire threaded through these holes can be used to apply traction and subsequently secure the limb with the splint rod.

An appropriate size steel rod (10–12 mm) is bent from the middle of the rod (using a template) to make a ring (1½ circle), with the extended part of the rod to make the legs (side rods) of the splint (Fig. 2.20). The splint ring should be large enough to properly fit into the axilla or groin region without causing any harm to the bony prominences. Care is also needed to avoid exerting pressure on the scrotum in bulls and udder in dairy cows. The ring is bent at its middle to about 30–40° toward the inner/medial side, and the rod extending from the ring is cut to the limb length. The contralateral normal limb may be used to measure the normal length of the limb.

A second piece of the rod is bent to a U-shaped bar, cut to the length of limb, and fixed to the extended bars of the ring and to the ring itself using adhesive tapes or welded in case of iron/steel rods to provide adequate strength to the splint. The distal end of the splint may be welded to a steel plate, conforming to the hoof. The side rods are not generally bent but kept straight.

The ring is padded using cotton roll and bandages and secured using adhesive tape. The inner portion of the ring must be adequately padded to avoid pressure sores. The side bars of the

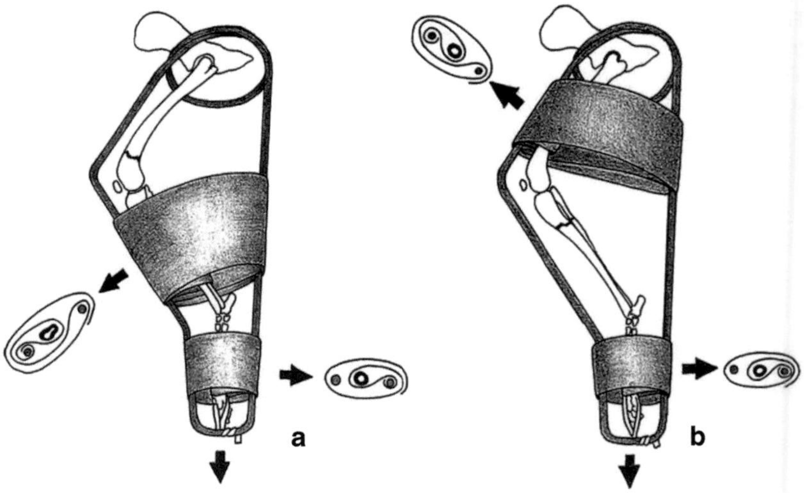


**Fig. 2.19** Application of traction using modified Thomas splint in hindlimb fractures

splint may be padded with foam rubber pipe/ cotton roll and bandages for insulation.

The limb is inserted into the ring and the distal end of splint (U-bar) is attached to the foot using the wires threaded through the hoof wall. The splint is firmly anchored in the axillary or groin region so that maximum load can be transferred. However, the limb is fixed to the splint with minimum traction (traction applied should only be sufficient to keep the limb extended and hold the bone segments in alignment) to avoid pressure sores at the contact points of the splint in the axillary or inguinal area and to prevent interference in venous drainage and locomotion.

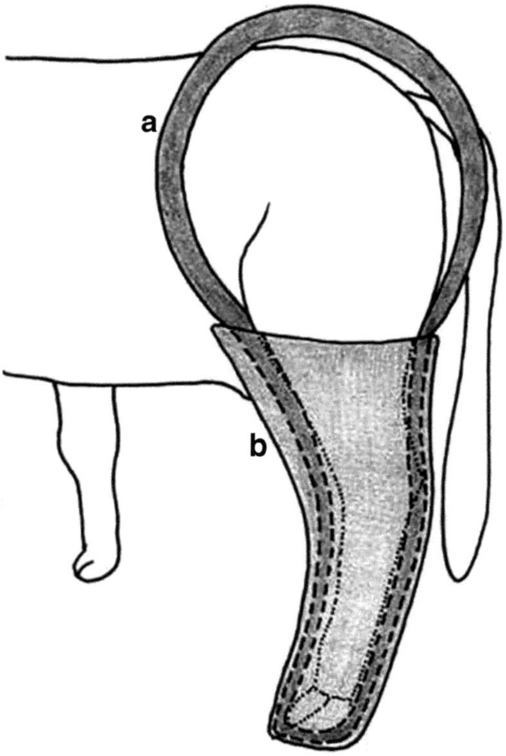


**Fig. 2.20** Modified Thomas splint-cast combination: (**a**) MTS ring, (**b**) cast applied around the side bars

The cast (preferably fiberglass/POP) is applied first directly over the fractured limb constructing a lightweight cast. Care is taken to prevent medial bowing of the limb by supporting the carpus or hock joint with a sling of plaster bandage. The cast is fixed to the splint using a casting tape, and the splint is then incorporated within the cast to make a splint-cast unit, which would help to prevent limb movement and rotation during locomotion.

In the forelimbs, the limb is attached to both side rods of the splint throughout the length, whereas in the hindlimbs, the thigh is attached to the cranial rod, the hock is attached to both side rods, and the limb below the hock is attached to the caudal side bar of the splint using a casting tape. Generally, the total cast material required is less (about 1/3 to ½ less) than the full-limb cast alone. It is better to extend the cast proximally up to the medial aspect of the ring to strengthen the splint and also to prevent the opposite limb from getting entrapped and to prevent urine and manure accumulation between the skin and the cast.

#### 2.1.7.4 Postoperative Care, Management, and Complications

The animal must be assisted while getting up during the first few days until it learns to rise on its own without help, especially a heavy animal [13]. The animal must be watched frequently to make sure that it is not lying on the splint side. The animal must be inspected for any loosening of the cast around the fracture site leading to slipping of the splint, which can occur after the initial soft tissue swelling subsides. Refracture may be seen in some cases of slipped splint. Hence, in such cases, the splint-cast should be replaced. The animal must also be checked frequently for any injury or decubital ulcers in the flank and inguinal area under the ring; decubital ulcers may also occur due to prolonged recumbency and struggling to rise. They should be checked and treated properly. Splint-cast is kept in place for 6–8 weeks depending on the type and location of fracture and animal's age and weight.

Laxity in the immobilized limb immediately after removal of the cast is common, which can be reversed gradually by regular exercise. Poor alignment and lateral deviation/outward rotation of the limb are common complications; however, it generally does not adversely affect the fracture healing and functional recovery of the limb.

## 2.2 Internal Fixation Techniques

Internal fixation of fractures by open reduction provides good alignment and rigid fixation of the bone segments. In small animal practice, internal fixation is the preferred method for fixation of long bone fractures, especially of the femur, humerus, and tibia. It can be achieved either by intramedullary fixation techniques like pinning/nailing or by extramedullary techniques like bone plating. Screws, wires, and staples are generally used as ancillary fixation devices along with plates and nails.

### 2.2.1 Intramedullary Pin/Nail

Intramedullary (IM) Steinmann pins are most commonly and widely used for fracture fixation in veterinary practice [21–23]. Nail/IM pin can be used either alone or along with other ancillary techniques like cerclage wiring. Due to their central position within the medullary cavity, IM pins can resist bending forces well and maintain alignment. Single IM pin cannot, however, resist compression and rotational forces. The technique of IM pinning is simple and needs minimum instruments, such as variable size Steinmann pins, Jacobs chuck with handle and key, and pin cutter in addition to the general surgical instruments. There are different types of IM pinning techniques.

#### 2.2.1.1 Single IM Pin

It is indicated in simple transverse or slight oblique diaphyseal fractures of long bones (mostly the femur, humerus, and tibia). The pin can be introduced either by normograde technique (through one end of the bone) or by retrograde technique (through the fracture site) [21] (Fig. 2.21). In retrograde pinning, after exposing the fracture site through standard surgical incision, the fracture segments are identified and reduced either manually or using forceps. While separating and exteriorizing the bone segments, the bone ends are protected by covering with finger tips, so that the sharp bone ends do not damage the surrounding soft tissues and especially the vessels and nerves. At the exposed distal end of the proximal bone segment, a Steinmann pin of adequate diameter is inserted into the medullary cavity using a chuck until the pin exits the proximal bone cortex (Fig. 2.22). Subsequently, the chuck is reversed and the pin is withdrawn from the proximal end up to the level of fracture site. The bone segments are then aligned and the pin is driven into the medullary cavity of the distal bone segment until it reaches the distal metaphysis or epiphysis, where a resistance to pin insertion is felt. At this time, the chuck is removed, and the extra length of the pin is cut short at the proximal end using a

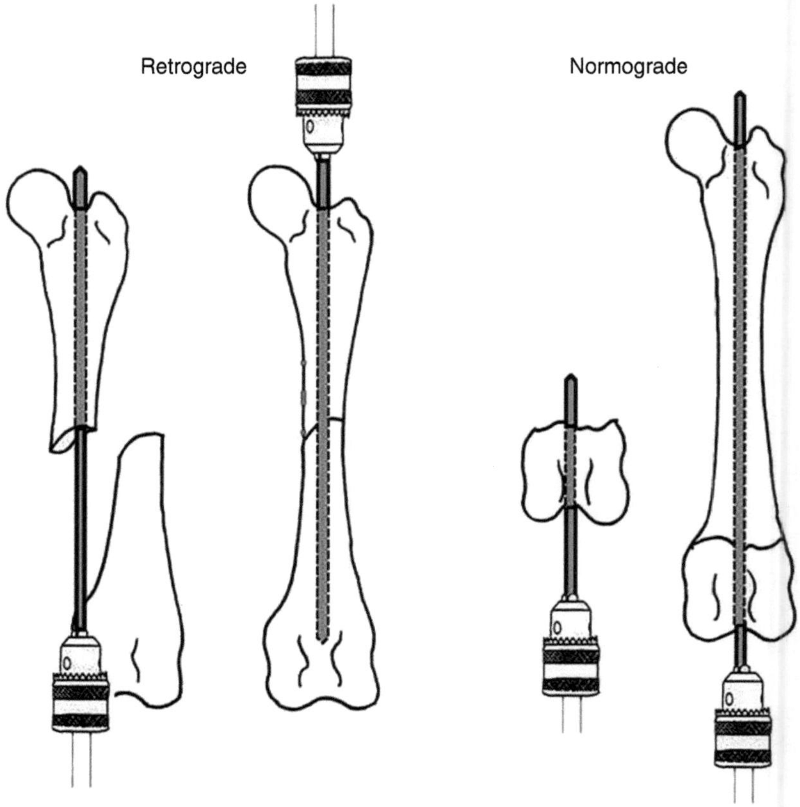


**Fig. 2.21** Retrograde and normograde technique of IM pin fixation

pin cutter. The cut end of the pin is then pushed into the metaphysis/epiphysis by gently hitting the cut end of the pin using the T-handle. Rotating the pin at the point of final seatment should be avoided as it may loosen the pin and predispose to pin migration. Subsequently, the skin is drawn over the cut end of the pin and an interrupted suture may be applied.

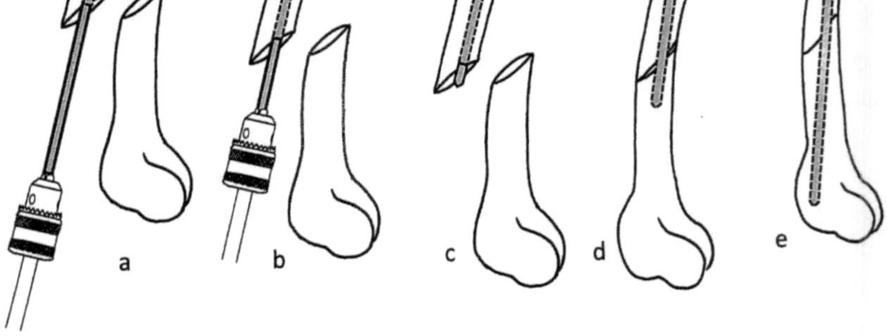


**Fig. 2.22** Retrograde technique of IM pin fixation in the femur: (**a**) insertion of IM pin through the distal end of proximal fragment using a chuck; (**b**) the pin inserted through the proximal cortex; (**c**) the pin is withdrawn from the proximal end up to the level of fracture site; (**d**) the bone fragments are aligned and the pin is then driven into the distal bone fragment; and (**e**) the pin is seated in the distal metaphysis/ epiphysis

In normograde technique of pinning, the Steinmann pin is inserted from one end of the bone. Normograde pinning is often done by closed/blind method in recent incomplete or simple transverse and sort oblique fractures with minimal displacement of bone segments after closed reduction [24, 25]. In long oblique/spiral and comminuted fractures, open reduction and fixation are always done. Once the pin reaches at the fracture site, the bone segments are reduced and the pin is then inserted into the medullary cavity of the opposite bone segment. The pin is driven up to the level of metaphysis and ensured that it is properly seated, and then, the extra length of the pin is cut close to the skin level.

There are some basic principles of IM pinning [23, 26]. One should not use pin fixation for non-reconstructable and unstable fracture configurations (comminuted fractures) and where uncontrolled loading is predicted. One should have a pack of large number of pins of different diameter and always select two pins of the same length, one pin for insertion and one pin to be used as a 'measuring pin' to estimate the depth of pin insertion in the medullary cavity. It is always better to select a smaller-diameter pin first, because we can easily remove and replace it with a larger pin, if needed. But if we use larger diameter pin first, it cannot be replaced by a smaller pin, and it may lead to pin loosening and migration. Assessment of pin seating can be done by (i) feeling resistance to further insertion, (ii) a measuring pin, or by (iii) radiographic examination. One should not cut and countersink a pin unless we are absolutely certain of its proper position, which can be confirmed by radiography or by image intensifier.

The retrograde pinning has the advantage of simpler passage of pin and easier selection of pin diameter, whereas normograde pinning has the advantage of accurate placement of pins and better purchase at the smaller bone segment (mostly used in metaphyseal/epiphyseal fractures). The diameter of the pin should be near to that of the medullary cavity, i.e. 70–90% of medullary cavity diameter (Fig. 2.23). The pin should run the whole length of the bone and then anchored at the distal metaphysis or epiphysis. The main

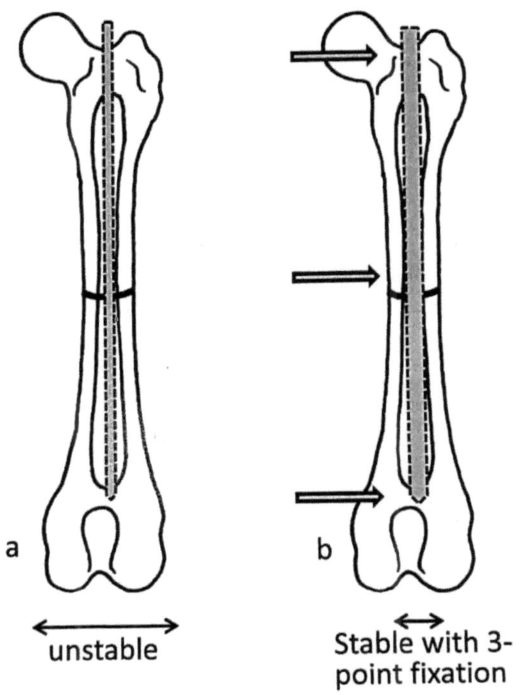


**Fig. 2.23** Improper (**a**) and proper (**b**) fixation of IM pin in the medullary cavity

limitation of single IM pin fixation is its inability to resist rotational forces and inability to hold the bone fragments in comminuted fractures. The use of full-cerclage or hemi-cerclage wires along with single IM pin provides greater stability against the rotational forces, especially in long oblique/spiral fractures.

#### 2.2.1.2 Stack Pins

The use of more than one pin (of relatively small diameter) is indicated in transverse or slight oblique fractures of long bones to provide more stable fixation [27]. It is also indicated in long bones with relatively large medullary cavity, where a single pin cannot fill the medullary cavity adequately (calves and foals in particular). The use of more number of pins can snugly fit the medullary cavity and thus provide enhanced stability against shear and rotational forces [21]. Each pin is inserted through a separate proximal hole into the medullary cavity, preferably allowing the opposite ends of the pins to diverse within the opposite metaphysis

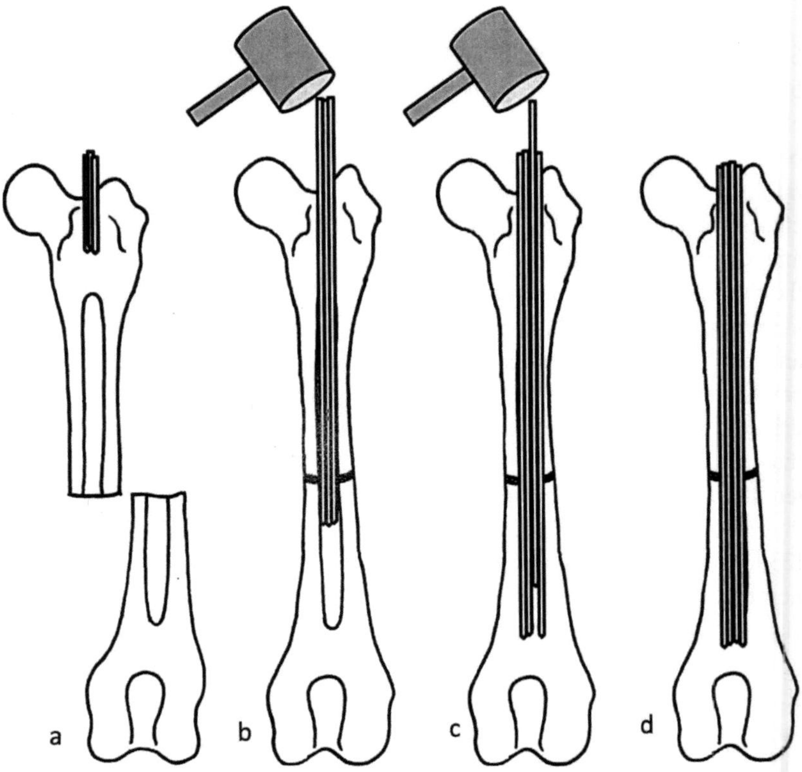


**Fig. 2.24** Technique of stack pinning: (**a**) more than one pins (3–4) are inserted through the proximal fragment through separate holes in the cortex; (**b**) bone fragments are reduced and the pins are driven across the fracture line into the distal fragment; (**c**) if needed, one or two more pins are inserted between the multiple stack pins to snugly fit in the medullary cavity; and (**d**) all the pins are then seated in the distal metaphysis, and the extra length of the pins is cut short at the proximal end

(Fig. 2.24). This technique also cannot completely resist the rotational forces and sometimes may lead to pin loosening and migration.

#### 2.2.1.3 Rush Pins

Rush pins, described by Dr. Leslie Rush, are solid curved cylindrical pins [22, 28]. Rush pin has a hooked end, which helps to drive and seat the pin in the bone, and another end is tapered that helps to bounce off the opposite inner cortex of the bone and thus prevent penetration of the bone cortex. Rush pins are indicated for the stabilization of metaphyseal/epiphyseal fractures of long bones, especially at the distal femur and proximal humerus or tibia. Two pins are passed from opposite sides (normally medial and lateral) of the cortex in the smaller bone segment (Fig. 2.25). The pins are inserted at about 30° angle to the long axis of the bone so that they cross each other above the fracture site and then glance off the endosteal surface of the diaphyseal bone to provide spring loaded tension. Bending the pins into a slight curve prior to insertion (prestressing) is useful to prevent penetration of the opposite cortex. Paired Rush pins held in spring loaded tension are expected to provide rotational stability. Rush pinning is contraindicated in very young animals, where the soft bony cortex (with relatively large medullary cavity) may get easily penetrated by the pin. Rush pinning may damage the growth plate leading to its rapid closure and shortening of the bone. Rush pins are also contraindicated in cases where there is longitudinal crack in the bone segment.

#### 2.2.1.4 Cross IM Pins

Cross intramedullary pins (two small diameter Steinmann pins/K-wires) can also be used instead of Rush pins, and they are allowed to exit from the opposite end of the bone to facilitate pin removal in the later stage. This dynamic cross IM pinning using small diameter pins provides stable fixation of small fracture segments (mostly supracondylar femoral fracture or proximal tibial fracture) with minimal injury to the physeal plate [29, 30]. The technique of pin insertion and

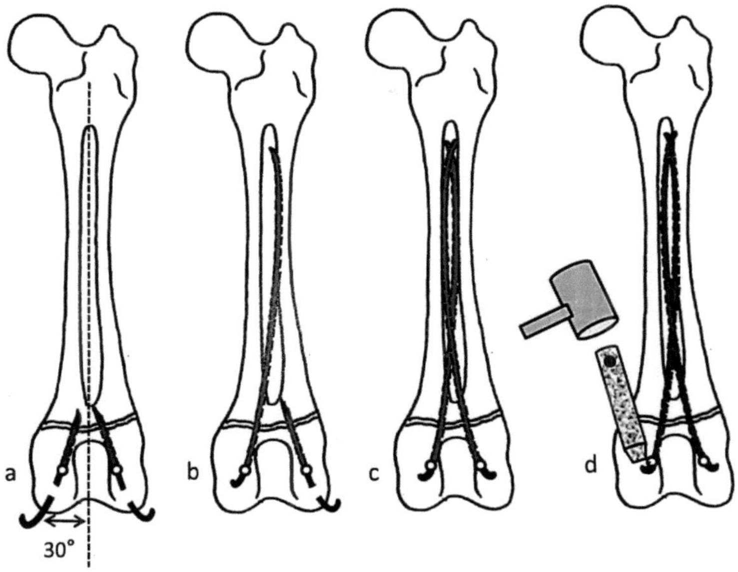


**Fig. 2.25** Technique of Rush pinning: (**a**) two proper size Rush pins are inserted on opposite sides of the small distal fragment, alternatively, at an acute angle ($30^0$) to the long axis of the bone to exit at the fracture site; (**b**) bone fragments are held in reduction and the pins are alternatively driven into large proximal fragment; (**c**) once the pins are driven completely, they glance off the opposite cortex and are held in spring loaded tension; and (**d**) the pin can be removed using Rush pin driver/extractor and a mallet

removal is easier than Rush pinning (Fig. 2.26). As the pins are inserted from the outer surfaces of the condyles, there is generally no interference with the extension and flexion of the joint. Further, the pins are crossed and remain in spring loaded tension; hence, fracture fixation is more stable with rotational stability, and pin migration is also rare.

### 2.2.1.5 Kuntscher Nail

'Clover leaf' of 'V'-shaped Kuntscher nails are hollow IM nails with an 'eye' at either ends [31]. They have the advantage of lightweight and can provide three-point fixation. They are indicated in transverse or short oblique fractures of the long bones, especially the femur, humerus, and tibia, where the cortex is good with no longitudinal cracks [22]. The technique is preferred in calves, foals, small ruminants, and large dogs, where medullary cavity diameter is large. The medullary cavity is first reamed using a reamer, and then using a guide wire, a proper diameter K-nail is introduced through one end of the bone (normograde technique, through the trochanteric fossa in femur), driven across the fracture site (after reducing the bone segments using bone clamps) and placed in the distal metaphysis (Fig. 2.27). It is important to cut the nail at one end (lower) to the desired length before insertion by measuring the length of the medullary canal (using preoperative radiograph or using a guide wire during surgery) so that the other end of the nail with the 'eye' will be left on the upper side to facilitate removal of the nail after fracture repair. K-nail is removed by a K-nail extractor, which is attached to the nail through the 'eye'. K-nail extractor is a must during insertion of K-nail as well as for its removal.

### 2.2.1.6 Interlocking Nail

Interlocking intramedullary nail is a relatively new and an advanced device used mostly in human and small animal practice [32–37]; however, in recent years, it is becoming popular in large animal applications too [38–43]. The first interlocking nail (ILN) was described by the German surgeon Gerhard Küntscher in 1939. Johnson and Huckstep in 1986 first reported the use of ILN fixation in experimental dogs with comminuted femoral diaphyseal fracture, which required fluoroscopic guidance. Dueland and his colleagues from the USA in 1993 first reported the use of veterinary ILN system with an alignment guide (jig) for insertion of transverse locking screws. Since then, it is being used more frequently in small animal fracture fixation.

Interlocking nail is basically a cylindrical intramedullary (IM) nail with transverse

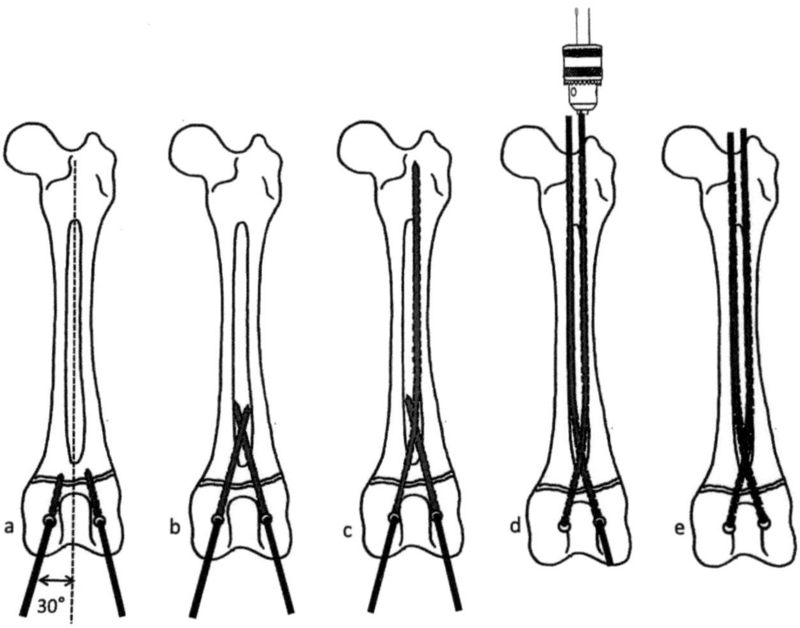


**Fig. 2.26** Cross IM pinning of supracondylar femur fracture: (**a**) two relatively small diameter pins are inserted from opposite cortices of the small distal fragment, alternatively, at an acute angle ($30^0$) to the bone axis to exit at the fracture site; (**b**) bone fragments are held in reduction and the pins are alternatively driven into the proximal fragment so that the pins are crossed in the medullary cavity above the fracture site; (**c**) the pins are further progressed into the proximal fragment to glance off the opposite cortex and exit from the proximal end; and (**d**) the pins are withdrawn from the proximal end so as to seat into the distal end just below the articular surface; and (**e**) the extra length of the pins is cut from the proximal end

cannulations secured (locked) in position by proximal and distal transfixing screws/bolts, which secure the nail to the bone cortex, thereby effectively neutralizing bending, rotational, and axial forces. It is performed using an image intensifier or a jig system.

Unlike a bone plate, the ILN allows biological osteosynthesis with minimal soft tissue trauma and vascular injury. Interlocking nail system is useful to repair simple and comminuted fractures of different long bones such as the humerus, femur, and tibia. Due to its mechanical advantages, the ILN provides rigid and stable bone fixation by neutralizing all the forces at the fracture site. As the implant is placed in the middle of the medullary cavity along the bone's biomechanical axis (like IM Steinmann pin), it effectively counteracts bending force. As the nail is secured to the cortex using fixation bolts, it provides rotational stability (resists axial and rotational forces unlike IM Steinmann pins) and prevents collapse and overriding of bone segments at the fracture site. Intramedullary position of ILN, unlike eccentric placement of bone plates, makes it more resistant to compressive, torsional, and bending forces. By increasing the number of fixation bolts in each bone segment and the locking mechanism in the nail, the strength of fixation can be increased, which is particularly important in large animal fracture fixations. The ILN also allows dynamization at the fracture site in delayed or non-healing cases.

Different systems of interlocking nails are available today, such as regular interlocking nails (Dueland), angle-stable interlocking nails (Dejardin), inverse interlocking nails (Unger and Brückner, Germany), etc. However, the Dueland ILN system is the basic and first ILN system

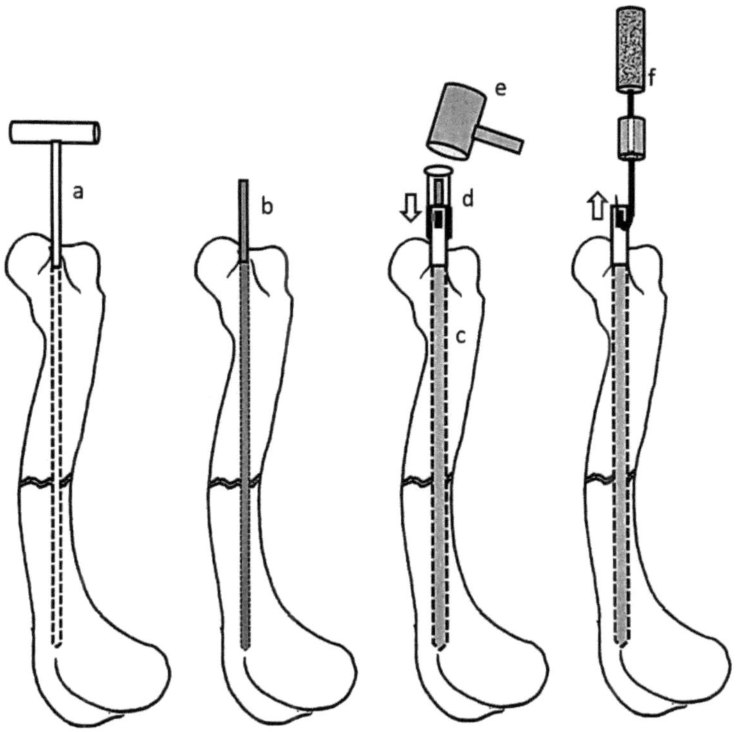


**Fig. 2.27** Technique of K-nailing: the medullary cavity is reamed using a reamer (**a**); a guide wire (**b**) is introduced into the medullary cavity (which will help measure the length of the bone and also guide the insertion of the nail); a proper diameter and length K-nail (**c**) is inserted along the guide wire (normograde) using the K-nail driver (**d**) and mallet (**e**) and seated in the distal metaphysis; K-nail extractor (**f**) attached to the nail through the 'eye' facilitates extraction of the nail

exclusively commercialized for use in veterinary practice and currently available commercially in India (Fig. 2.28).

The ILN is a solid steel rod with transverse openings usually at both ends. The one end of the nail has a trocar point to help in insertion and proper anchoring of the nail. The other end has negative threading (on the inner side), which helps to fix the alignment guide through the extension rod. The diameter of the nail generally ranges from 4 mm to 10 mm (Table 2.1), and any diameter nail can be custom-made. The lengths of 6–10 mm diameter nails vary from 120–230 mm, and 4 and 4.7 mm diameter nails vary from 68 to 134 mm. The number of holes in the nail vary from 3 (2 at one end and 1 at other end) to 4 (2 holes at both ends). The hole diameter varies from 2 to 4.5 mm. The holes are placed 22 mm apart in model 22 series (normally used for repair of diaphyseal fractures) and are placed 11 mm apart in 11 series (mostly used for repair of metaphyseal fractures). 4.0/4.7 mm nails are available only in the model 11 series.

Jig is an aiming device, which is fixed to the ILN using nail extension to facilitate correct placement of locking bolts/screws along the transverse openings of the nail without the need for image intensifier. The jig is attached to the nail with an extension so as to position it parallel to the nail with the jig holes corresponding to the nail holes. The nail extension, available as short or long extension, is temporarily attached to the nail to facilitate deep placement of the proximal nail end so that it does not protrude out of the bone once implanted. Locking screws (threaded)/bolts (smooth) are fixed in the *cis*- and *trans*-cortex of the bone through the hole in the nail, so that the nail is locked with the bony cortex and the bone and nail can act as a single unit.

Interlocking nails are commonly placed in different long bones, namely, femur, humerus, and tibia. The surgical approach for placement of ILN is same as IM pin fixation. The nail is introduced into the medullary cavity of long bones in normograde technique, either by closed or open approach (Fig. 2.29). Using a bone

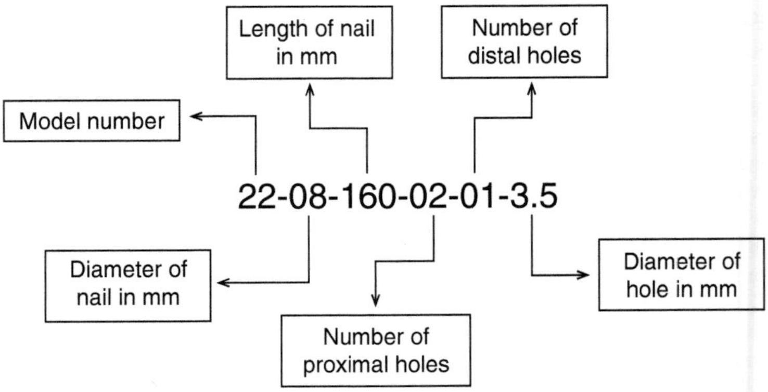


**Fig. 2.28** The inscription on an ILN

awl/Steinmann pin, a hole is created in the proximal bone cortex, which is enlarged with successively larger diameter reamers to a size that allows passage of the nail into the bone. The proper diameter nail with adequate length that can fit into the medullary cavity is chosen. A guide wire is passed in the proximal bone segment from the fracture site, so that it exits through the bone cortex and the skin at the proximal end. The nail attached to the jig is driven into the bone along the guide wire so that it is well seated in the proximal bone segment. Subsequently, the fracture segments are reduced, and the nail is further driven into the distal bone segment up to the level of metaphysis (till there is resistance to insertion). The holes for fixation screws/bolts are then drilled through predetermined sites by giving small stab incisions in the soft tissue and are directed through the bone and through the holes in the nail by utilizing the jig that aligns the drilling site with the holes in the nail.

If the screws/bolts are fixed in both proximal and distal bone segments, the fixation is called static (load-bearing mode), which is commonly used in small animals, especially in comminuted fractures with instability. Two screws/bolts fixed on both bone segments provide stable fixation. When the screw/bolt is fixed in only one bone segment, either proximal or distal, it is called dynamic fixation (load-sharing mode) allowing micromotion at the fracture site. Dynamic fixation does not neutralize rotational and axial forces and weight-bearing results in axial compression promoting bone healing. In large animal fixations, as many fixation bolts as possible should be used in proximal and distal bone segments to provide greater stability. In fractures of the distal metaphysis/epiphysis of the femur, the nail can be introduced through the intercondylar fossa to achieve greater purchase in the smaller distal segment. In canine femur, 4–8 mm nails are generally adequate. In bovine femur and humerus, 14–18 mm diameter straight nails are optimum, whereas in the tibia, 12–14 mm angular nails are adequate.

General guidelines for ILN fixation include selection of proper nail (appropriate diameter, length, and model) based on preoperative radiographs of the fractured bone and the contralateral intact bone. A Steinmann pin is used to create a hole in the bone cortex, and it is then passed in a retrograde (in femur/humerus) or normograde (tibia) fashion to establish an intramedullary channel in the proximal bone segment. Intramedullary reaming is not generally required and may be avoided to reduce endosteal injury and cortical ischaemia. ILN should be tightly fit with the jig for proper alignment of holes in the jig and nail, and the holes in the jig through which fixation bolts (proximal and distal)

**Table 2.1** Sizes of bone tap and drill bit in different diameter nails

| ILN diameter (mm) | 4 | 4.7 | 6 | 8 | 10 |
|---|---|---|---|---|---|
| Hole/screw/bone tap size (mm) | 2 | 2 | 2.7 | 3.5 | 4.5 |
| Drill bit size (mm) | 1.5 | 1.5 | 2 | 2.5 | 3.2 |

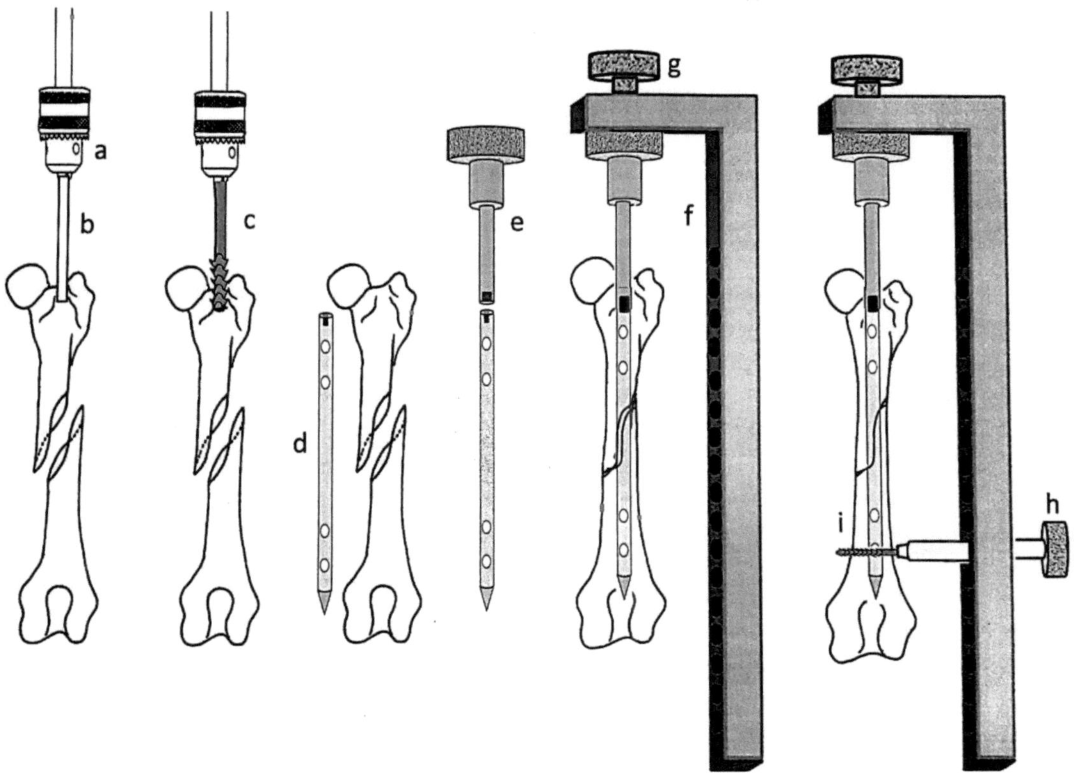


**Fig. 2.29** Technique of interlocking nail fixation: using a chuck (**a**) fixed with Steinmann pin (**b**), a hole is drilled in the proximal cortex; the intramedullary cavity is reamed with a corresponding size reamer (**c**); a guide wire is introduced into the medullary cavity in normograde manner, and a proper length nail (**d**) is selected; before insertion of the nail, holes along the jig arm corresponding to the holes in the selected nail should be noted; the nail attached to the extension (**e**) insertion tool (**g**) and firmly anchored to the jig (**f**) is inserted into the medullary cavity along the guide wire; the jig-nail unit is rotated to align in medio-lateral plane (desired for screw/bolt placement); then, interlocking screws/bolts are fixed first by drilling holes by placing guide sleeve/drill guide (**h**) and drill bit (**i**) in the corresponding hole in the jig; the most distal bolt is placed first, followed by other bolts in proximal and distal fragments as per the situation. At the end of fixation, the jig along with extension-insertion tool is detached from the nail by unscrewing, so that the nail will remain within the bone

need to be fixed should be ascertained based on the fracture location and configuration. The holes should not be drilled very close to the fracture site and should be at least 1 cm away. Undue pressure on the arm of the jig should be avoided while driving the nail (as it may lead to mal-alignment between the jig and nail) and ensure that the nail is properly seated in the distal metaphysis. Before drilling for transfixation bolts, if needed, the jig may be rotated to orient transfixation holes in the medio-lateral plane. The guide sleeve should always be used before inserting the drill/tap guides, and the holes are drilled using long drill bits without putting any pressure on the jig arm to ensure accurate drilling. A transfixation hole may be drilled in the proximal bone segment first, and the drill bit is left in situ to temporarily stabilize the jig to ensure accurate drilling in the distal bone segment. Before drilling any transfixation holes in the distal segment, it is ensured that the distal bone segment is rotationally aligned with proximal segment. After drilling at the most distal hole and inserting the drill bit in the distal bone segment, rotate the distal segment to ascertain that the distal drill bit has engaged the nail; if engaged, the nail will not rotate with the distal segment, and if not, the nail will freely rotate. Care should be taken while placing the distal-most screw as there is every chance for getting misplaced. It is better to fix two fixation bolts on both bone segments, but in distal metaphyseal fractures, at least one bolt/screw should be placed in the small distal bone segment. It is also advised not to leave an empty hole at the fracture site.

Interlocking nail can be placed in semi-closed manner; hence, soft tissue morbidity and vascular interference are lesser leading to biological osteosynthesis as compared to plating. It also permits early weight-bearing and return of limb function. The nail can be removed after bone healing, but it is not necessary to remove it if there are no complications.

The common complications with ILN include malpositioning of the nail in the medullary cavity leading to mal-alignment of the nail and jig and damage to the threaded proximal end of the nail. Misplacement of locking bolts/screws in the distal hole of the nail is also common. Other complications may include bending and breakage of screws and angular deformation of the nail. Complications of bone healing such as delayed union, non-union, and osteomyelitis can also be seen at times.

Hybrid ILN-ESF systems have been developed to improve the bending and torsional stiffness and overcome slack and interfragmentary movements. Type I ESF can be connected to ILN by tie-in configuration using an ILN extension or extended locking bolts. ILN can also be combined with epoxy-pin fixation using extended locking bolts. These hybrid fixators have the advantage of achieving dynamization at the fracture site by controlled destabilization. Further, it also facilitates easy removal of ILN after bone union. However, complications such as difficulty in postoperative care, poor patient tolerance, loosening of external pins, pin-tract infections, and additional soft tissue trauma offset the mechanical advantages of hybrid constructs. Attempts have also been made to combine ILN with bone plates (plate-ILN construct) to achieve maximum mechanical advantages of both implants in a single system so that all the forces acting at the fracture site can be more effectively neutralized.

The angle-stable ILNs have been developed to enhance the construct stability of the standard ILN by improving the torsional and bending deformation and by reducing slack and interfragmentary motion. The basic design of an angle-stable ILN is almost similar to standard ILN, with some modifications. The locking bolt has a threaded conical central part that matches with the shape and threads of the nail holes to create an angle-stable rigid fixation between the bolt and nail. The solid triangular end of the bolt is designed to engage the *cis*-cortex and is driven into the nail, and the thinner cylindrical end is designed to engage the *trans*-cortex. The locking bolts are available in different diameters, and they can be cut to appropriate length as per the requirement. The AS-ILN has been designed in an hourglass shape, which reduces damage to medullary circulation and increases overall construct stability. The core diameter of the nail is relatively less; hence, it is easy to insert without reaming the medullary cavity. The bullet-shaped distal tip of the nail minimizes tissue trauma, especially injury to the joint. AS-ILN is currently available in 6 mm, 7 mm, and 8 mm diameters, ranging in lengths from 122 to 203 mm.

Even though interlocking nail systems from different manufacturers are available for use in small animals, ILN systems for use in large animal fracture repair are not freely available commercially. Mostly, the implants developed for use in human applications are being used in large animals, but they are not strong enough due to their tubular designs, which compromise the fixation strength. However, a prototype of equine interlocking nail (manufactured by IMEX Veterinary, Longview, TX, USA) [44, 45] and bovine interlocking nails (Nebula Surgical Pvt. Ltd., Rajkot, India) [39, 41] for use in the humerus, femur, and tibia of young horses and bovines has been developed.

#### 2.2.1.7 Interlocking Nails for Bovine

The ICAR-Indian Veterinary Research Institute has developed interlocking nails for fixation of fractures in bovine tibia and femur. The tibial ILN developed using 316L stainless steel has a diameter of 12 mm and length of 250 mm (Fig. 2.30). The nails are solid and have 9 holes, either all holes threaded or non-threaded (smooth), along

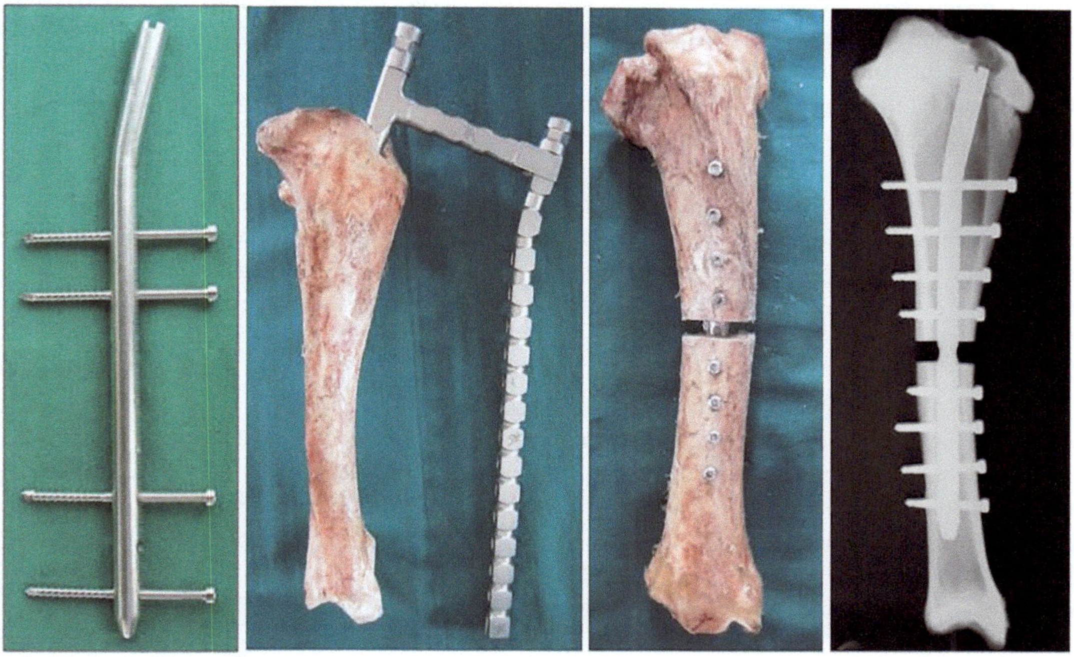


**Fig. 2.30** Angular interlocking nail developed for bovine tibia; ILN with locking bolts (**a**), placement of ILN using the jig in a cadaver tibia (**b**), ILN-tibia bone construct (**c**), and lateral radiograph of ILN-tibia construct (**d**)

its length to facilitate application to a variety of diaphyseal fracture configurations. The direction of holes is cranio-caudal. The nails are given a cranial angular bend of 10° at the proximal one-fifth of length to facilitate easy insertion and alignment with the medullary cavity of the tibia. Locking bolts are of 4.9 mm diameter (self-cutting trocar tip, self-tapping) and are either standard bolts (high pitch) for nails with non-threaded holes or a modified locking bolts (with low pitch), having two types of threads, the proximal part with threads complementary to hole threads to snugly fix the bolt with the nail in locking fashion (in nails with threaded holes) and the distal part with threading as of standard locking bolt (Fig. 2.31).

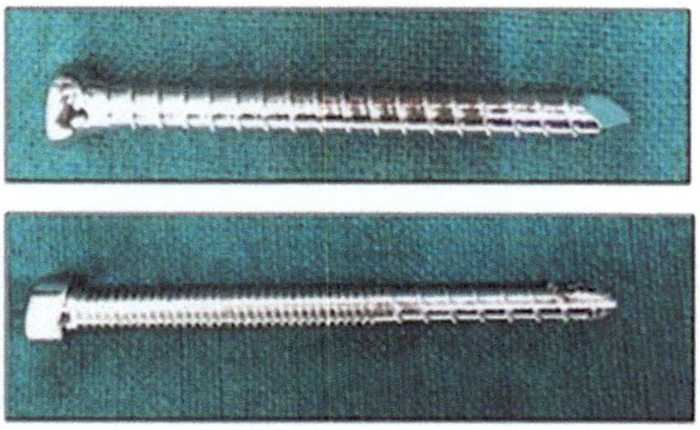


**Fig. 2.31** Locking bolts used in bovine ILN for the tibia; standard locking bolt (**a**) and modified locking bolt (**b**)

The nail-bone (buffalo tibia) constructs (with 10 mm mid-diaphyseal transverse ostectomy) developed using 4 or 8 standard locking bolts and 8 modified locking bolts were subjected to axial compression and 3-point cranio-caudal bending and torsion tests using a universal testing machine. ILN-bone constructs with 8 bolts were significantly stronger than the constructs with 4 bolts under compression, bending, and torsion loads [39]. The constructs with 8 modified bolts showed highest mechanical values. The compressive stiffness was 1.852 ± 0.04 MPa, yield load 18.475 ± 0.40 kN, and ultimate failure load 21.6 ± 0.39 kN. Bending moment was 419.03 ± 10.61 Nm, stiffness 0.583 ± 0.01 MPa, yield load 6.15 ± 0.17 kN, and ultimate failure load 6.33 ± 0.16 kN. Yield loads under compression and bending in constructs with modified bolts were significantly higher than in constructs with standard bolts. Under torsion, the constructs with 8 modified locking bolts showed ultimate failure load of 265.53 ± 10.23 Nm and ultimate failure displacement of 31.79 ± 0.82°. Both in vitro mechanical tests and clinical studies have shown that ILN developed for bovine tibia was sufficiently strong to stabilize diaphyseal fractures in young adult cattle and buffaloes weighing up to about 250–350 kg.

The ILNs developed for bovine femur (with solid or tubular shaft) measured 16 mm in diameter and 240 mm in length. The tubular nail has an inner diameter of 10 mm. The nails had 8 threaded holes (4 each in the proximal and distal part), for fixation of 6 mm locking bolts (Fig. 2.32). The nails were subjected to in vitro mechanical tests and clinical application.

For mechanical testing, nail-bone constructs were prepared using cadaver buffalo femur bones. The constructs developed using either solid or tubular ILNs (with eight 6-mm diameter, self-cutting trocar tip modified locking bolts, 40–75 mm length) with 5-mm mid-diaphyseal osteotomy were subjected to compression and cranio-caudal bending and torsion tests [41]. The compressive stiffness (MPa), yield load (kN), and ultimate failure load (kN) recorded for solid and tubular nails were 5.77 ± 0.23 and 5.35 ± 0.12, 46.89 ± 0.66 and 45.22 ± 0.86, and 51.39 ± 0.52 and 49.98 ± 0.51, respectively, with no significant difference between the solid or tubular nail constructs. The bending stiffness (MPa), bending moment (Nm), yield load (kN), and ultimate failure load (kN) for solid and tubular nail-bone constructs were 1.07 ± 0.05 and 0.86 ± 0.09, 680.55 ± 10.83 and 622.59 ± 23.13, 8.32 ± 0.25 and 7.36 ± 0.31, and 9.49 ± 0.28 and 8.18 ± 0.35, respectively (bending moment and failure load significantly different between the nail constructs). Under torsion testing, ultimate failure load (kN) and failure displacement (°) recorded for solid and tubular nail-bone constructs were 331.56 ± 4.87 and 312.48 ± 2.71 and 20.27 ± 0.39 and 18.33 ± 0.37, respectively (failure load significantly different between the nail constructs). These results suggested that solid nails were mechanically more stronger than tubular nails, but both solid and tubular nails were sufficiently strong to immobilize femur fractures in young adult cattle and buffaloes weighing at least 250–350 kg.

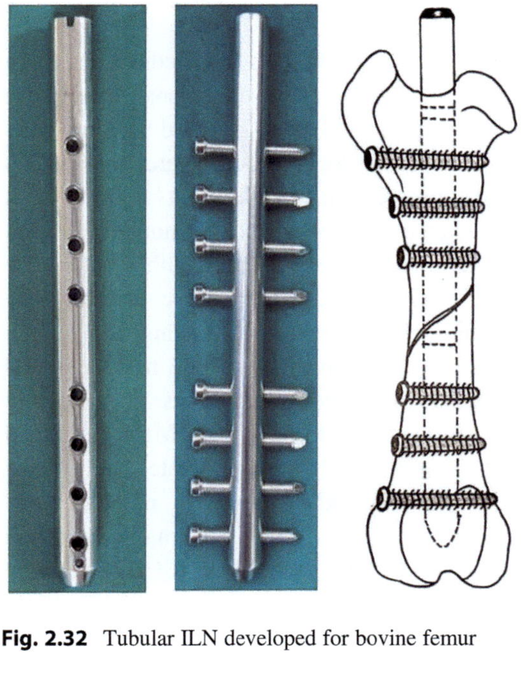

**Fig. 2.32** Tubular ILN developed for bovine femur

The interlocking nail provides rigid fixation of the bone allowing early weight-bearing and functional recovery of the limb. Additionally, the soft tissue morbidity is also minimal. The nail can be removed after bone healing, but it is not necessary to remove it if there are no complications. Non-availability of proper size and shape of the nail and the cost of the instruments, however, limit their routine use in large animal applications.

## 2.2.2 Bone Plate and Screw Fixation

Bone plate and screw fixation provides rigid and stable internal fixation, especially in unstable comminuted fractures [22, 46–49]. It also facilitates early mobilization of the joints leading to quick functional recovery of the affected limbs. Plates can be used to function in different ways (Fig. 2.33):

**Fig. 2.33** Functions of plate: Neutralization, transmits the force from one end of the bone to another via the plate; compression, plate fixed in tension side of the bone or fixed in principles of DCP brings compression between the bone ends favoring bone healing; buttress plate, bridges the diaphyseal bone defect and thus prevents collapse and shortening at the fracture site; and bridge plate, the plate is attached to the main fragments spanning the fracture site and restores the bone length and alignment

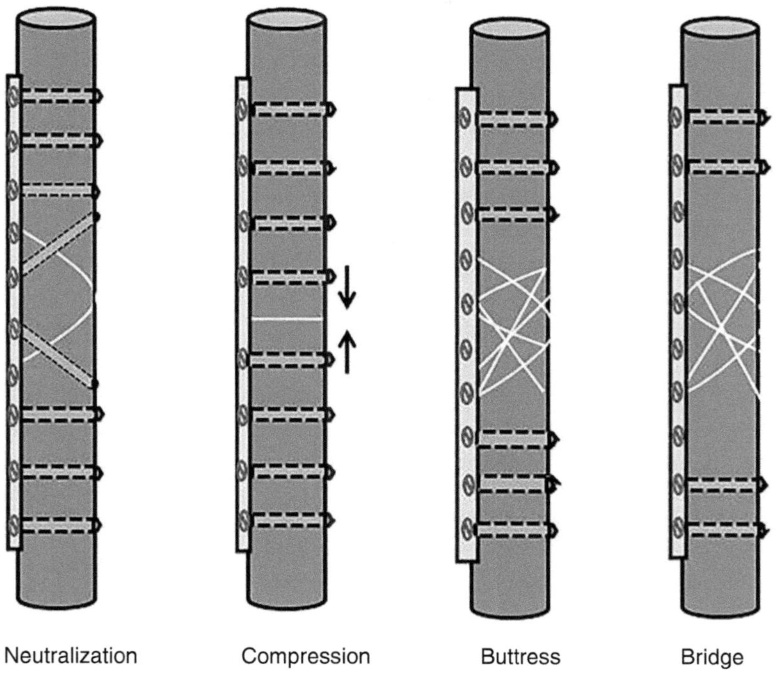


(i) *Neutralization plate*: Here, the plate acts as a bridge to protect a comminuted area that has been constructed with lag screws. It transmits the force from one end of the bone to another via the plate, bypassing the area of fracture, and thus acts as a mechanical link between the main bone segments above and below the fracture site. It does not produce compression between the bone segments.

(ii) (ii) *Tension band plate/compression plate*: Compression of the main segments of a fracture can result in absolute stability, with complete abolition of interfragmentary movement. By fixing the plate on the tension side of the bone (such as the lateral side of the femur, the craniolateral aspect of the tibia, the anterior aspect of the humerus, the anterolateral aspect of the radius, and the caudal aspect of the proximal ulna) (Fig. 2.34) and by the use of dynamic compression plate principle, compression can be achieved at the fracture site.

(iii) (iii) *Buttress plate*: The plate is used to bridge a diaphyseal defect with a comminuted fracture or a gap filled with a

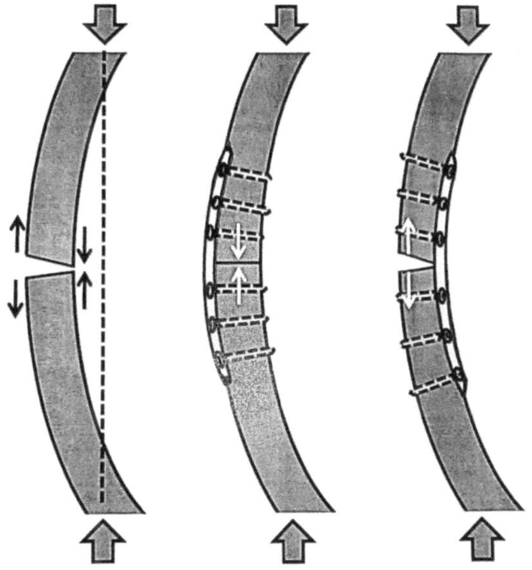

**Fig. 2.34** Why should the plate be applied on the tension side of the bone? Normally, a long bone is subjected to bending stress (tension on one side and tension on the opposite side). If the plate is fixed on the tension side, compression occurs between the bone ends on opposite side favoring bone formation. If plate is fixed in compression side, gapping occurs on the tension side leading to fixation failure

bone graft or a substitute. Its function is to prevent the fracture from collapsing until the new bone fills the diaphyseal bone defect. The buttress plate is never applied under tension.

(iv) (iv) *Bridge plate*: In comminuted diaphyseal fractures with severe soft tissue injury, a plate is often attached to the main bone segments spanning the fracture site. It is used to restore the bone length and alignment, even though fixation stability is less. This technique allows biological healing with external callus. Bridge plating is often performed by minimally invasive surgery.

There are four basic types of plates: (i) straight rigid plates for diaphysis, (ii) flexible/cuttable plates which can be easily contoured to the bone surface/cut to the desired length, such as reconstruction plates and veterinary cuttable plates, (iii) special plates like mini plate, 'T'/'L' plate for the epiphysis and metaphysis of long bones, and (iv) special plates for specific applications like angled/hooked plates for the proximal and distal end of long bones like the femur, acetabular plate, tibial plateau leveling osteotomy (TPLO) plate, pancarpal and pantarsal arthrodesis plates, etc. Straight plates are most widely used for repair of long bone fractures in veterinary practice. Special T/L plates offer greater purchase in small segment fractures, as 2–3 screws can be easily fixed. Reconstruction plates are more often preferred in fractures of irregular bones such as the mandible and pelvis as these plates can be more readily contoured to the irregular bone surfaces.

The selection of bone plate is made carefully based on animal's size and age, the bone involved, and the type and location of fracture (Table 2.2). Commonly, 2.7 mm and 3.5 mm plates are used in small animals; however, 1.5 mm and 2.0 mm plates are often used, especially in cats. In large animal applications, generally, 4.5 and 5.5 mm broad plates are utilized. Plates selected should be large enough to neutralize the forces acting at the fracture site but not too thick or heavy for the bone they cover. Before application, the plate should be contoured to the shape and curvature of the bone. Plates should be fixed using at least four cortices or two screws on both sides of the fracture site. There should be no gap between the bone and the plate and between the plate and screw head.

For application of plate, the fracture site is approached as per the standard procedure, and the soft tissue is then retracted along the whole length of the affected bone. Fracture segments are then reduced in their original position. After selecting a proper size plate, it is contoured to the bone accurately using a plate bender. The contoured plate is placed on the bone centered over the fracture and aligned along the axis of the bone and secured using bone-holding forceps. To ensure proper alignment of the plate along the axis of the bone, screws can be first fixed at either ends of the plate. Then, the fracture alignment can be re-checked before remaining screw holes are drilled and screws fixed. On the other hand, if plate-bone alignment can be easily ensured, the screws can be first fixed in the screw holes close to the fracture site on both sides of the fracture. The screws in the remaining holes of the plate are then fixed alternatively in both bone segments. Once all the screws are inserted, the correct alignment of the fracture segments is ascertained, and the screws are tightened one by one.

Screw holes in the bone are predrilled using a proper size drill bit, which is one size smaller than the screw size (Table 2.3). After drilling the hole in one of the screw holes, the screw length is measured by considering the plate thickness, and the proper length screw is chosen. If self-tapping screws are used, they can be directly inserted into the hole. If non-self-tapping screws are chosen, then the drill holes need to be tapped using a threaded tap (of same size as screw). Threads carved in the tap are sharper than the screw threads, and tapping helps to clear the bone debris and facilitate screw insertion. Tapping also reduces the heat generation during the screw insertion.

#### 2.2.2.1 Dynamic Compression Plate

Dynamic compression plate (DCP), first introduced in 1969, is an improvised plate having special oval holes unlike traditional plates with round holes. The DCP allows achieving axial

**Table 2.2** Choice of plate size in different long bones in relation to animal's body weight

| Body weight | | | | | | |
|---|---|---|---|---|---|---|
| Type of long bone | Type of bone plate | ≤10 kg | 10–20 kg | 20–30 kg | 30–40 kg | >40 kg |
| Humerus/femur/tibia | DCP/LC-DCP/LCP | 2.0 | 2.7/3.5 | 3.5 | 3.5/4.5 | 4.5 |
| | VCP | 1.5/2.0 | 2.7 | | | |
| Radius-ulna | DCP/LC-DCP/LCP | 2.0 | 2.7 | 3.5 | 3.5 | 4.5 |
| | VCP | 1.5/2.0 | 2.0/2.7 | | | |

*DCP* dynamic compression plate, *LC-DCP* limited contact dynamic compression plate, *LCP* locking compression plate, *VCP* veterinary cuttable plate

compression at the fracture site (without a tension device) by eccentric placement of screws. When a screw is tightened along the sloping design of the oval screw hole, the plate moves away from the fracture resulting in compression of the bone segments [50–55].

A DCP is applied by drilling a hole in one of the bone segments (say, proximal segment) close to the fracture site (about 1 cm away) using a neutral guide, and the plate is then secured by inserting a screw. Another screw hole is then drilled eccentrically in the opposite bone segment (say, distal segment) close to the fracture with the aid of a loaded (eccentric) drill guide (Fig. 2.35). Insertion of screw through the eccentrically drilled hole and tightening against the slope of the screw hole result in self-compression of fracture by displacing the plate. The remaining screws are then inserted alternatively in the proximal and distal bone segments using the neutral drill guide. It is also possible to use more than one eccentrically placed screw on either side of the fracture. Before the second compression screw is tightened, the first screw has to be loosened to allow the plate to slide and achieve compression at the fracture site; the first compression screw is then tightened.

Bone plating requires complete exposure of the fractured bone, sometimes leading to disruption of soft tissue attachments and hence vascular compromise at the fracture site. When the plate is rigidly fixed, it may protect the underlying bone from loading stresses. This 'stress protection' along with vascular compromise may lead to weakening of the bone (osteoporotic). In recent years, limited contact dynamic compression plates (LC-DCPs) have been developed [52, 54, 56]. These plates are designed to reduce the contact between the plate and the bone with the presence of undercuts beneath and between the screw holes. This in turn reduces the stress protection and vascular compromise and thus allows periosteal callus formation at the fracture site. In LC-DCP, the holes are symmetrical, which allows eccentric placement of a screw in either direction. It helps to achieve compression at any level along the plate and thus facilitate treatment of a segmental fracture. LC-DCP also allows relatively more inclining of screws (40°) along the longitudinal direction than a DCP (25°). LC-DCPs are now being used more frequently in clinical practice than before.

The DCPs are available for small animal use in a variety of sizes like, 2.0, 2.7, 3.5, and 4.5, which are used with 2 mm, 2.7 mm, 3.5 mm, and 4.5 mm cortex screws, respectively. 4 mm cancellous screw can be used with DCP 3.5, and 6.5 mm cancellous screw can be used along with DCP 4.5. Whereas in large animal applications, 4.5 or 5.5 broad DCPs are used, broad DCPs are wider and thicker than standard DCPs (4.5 mm broad DCP has a width of 16 mm and thickness of 4.8 mm as against 13.5 mm width and 4.2 mm thickness of standard narrow DCP) and have

**Table 2.3** The sizes of drill bit and tap for different sizes of screw

| | | | | | | | | | | |
|---|---|---|---|---|---|---|---|---|---|---|
| Screw size (mm) | 1.0 | 1.3 | 1.5 | 2.0 | 2.4 | 2.7 | 3.5 | 4.0 | 4.5 | 5.5 |
| Drill bit size (mm) | 0.8 | 1.0 | 1.1 | 1.5 | 1.8 | 2.0 | 2.5 | 2.5 | 3.2 | 4.0 |
| Tap size (mm) | 1.0 | 1.3 | 1.5 | 2.0 | 2.4 | 2.7 | 3.5 | 4.0 | 4.5 | 5.5 |

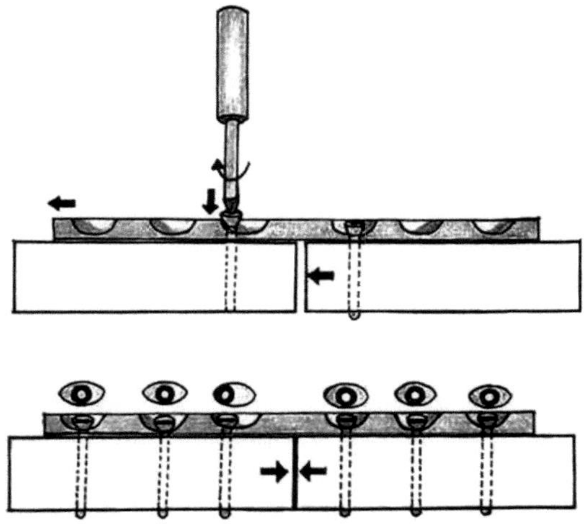

**Fig. 2.35** In dynamic compression plating, a hole is drilled in the center of the screw hole close to the fracture site in the proximal bone fragment using a neutral guide, and the plate is then secured by inserting a screw. An eccentric hole is drilled in the screw hole in the distal bone fragment close to the fracture site with the help of an eccentric drill guide. As the screw is inserted and tightened through the eccentrically drilled hole, the fracture is self-compressed by displacing the plate. The remaining screws are then inserted alternatively using the neutral drill guide

staggered screw holes. In heavy large animals, double plates are recommended for fixation of fractures in load-bearing bones. Though plates have been developed specifically for use in large animal orthopedics, they are not readily available. Compression can also be obtained with any of the straight plates by using a compression device (Fig. 2.36). Here, a suitable length plate is used across the fracture site and is fixed to one (proximal) fracture segment using one or more screws. At the opposite (distal) end of bone segment, the compression device is fixed using a small cortical screw and is anchored with the last screw hole. As the screw in the device is tightened, the plate is pulled toward the device achieving compression between the fracture segments. Subsequently, the screws are fixed in the remaining holes of the plate, and then, the compression device is removed by loosening the small screw fixing the device.

*Plate luting*: Fixation stability with a bone plate is achieved from friction between the plate and the bone, and therefore, it is directly proportional to the extent of plate contact with the bone cortex. The technique of 'plate luting' has been developed to obtain maximum plate-bone contact, through interfacing a layer of bone cement between the plate and the bone. Plate luting is mostly used in large animal fixations to achieve greater fixation strength [57, 58]. The technique involves placement of all screws in the plate first, and then, the screws are loosened to lift the plate off the bone. PMMA dough (incorporated with a broad-spectrum antibiotic) is filled between the bone and the plate, and all the screws are soon tightened, and the excess spilled cement is removed. Hardened PMMA cement, filled between the plate and screws and in the screw holes around the screw heads, provides stable plate-bone fixation. While applying PMMA dough, care should be taken to prevent penetration of bone cement into the fracture line, which may hamper bone healing. Further, as hardening of PMMA (polymerization) is an exothermic reaction with releasing of heat, the bone and the implants have to be cooled using cold saline solution during the process.

#### 2.2.2.2 Veterinary Cuttable Plate (VCP) and Reconstruction Plates

Veterinary cuttable plates are special plates that can be customized for use in bones of varied length by cutting them to desired length [59, 60]. VCP is not a compression plate. They are available in two sizes: small plates can accommodate 1.5 mm and 2.0 mm screws, and larger plates can accommodate 2.0 mm and 2.7 mm screws. The length of plate is 30 cm having 50 round holes. As these plates are relatively weak, they can be used only in small animals with simple fractures.

Reconstruction plates are flexible plates, which can be contoured in two planes [61]. The presence of deep notches between the screw holes makes them relatively flexible but much weaker than standard bone plates. The different sizes of plates available are 2.7, 3.5, and 4.5. The plates have oval holes, which allow for compression between the bone segments. Reconstruction plates are particularly useful for fixation in pelvic

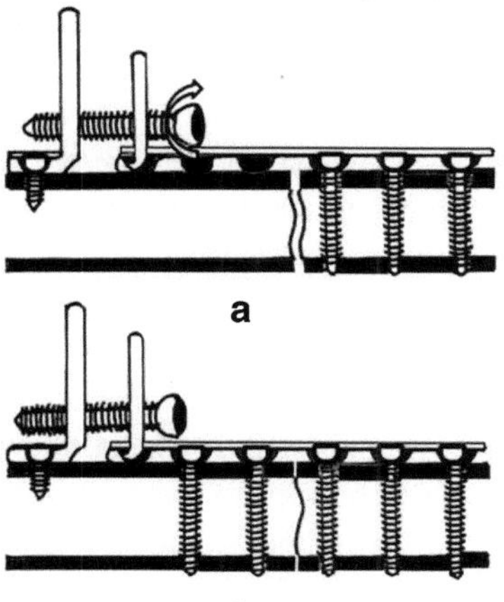


**Fig. 2.36** The use of a compression device to achieve compression between fracture fragments: (**a**) a plate is applied across the fracture site and is attached to the proximal fragment with 2–3 screws, and at the opposite end of fracture fragment, the compression device is fixed with a small cortical screw and is attached to the last screw hole; (**b**) the compression device is tightened to bring the two bone fragments closer; (**c**) with the fragments in the proper position, the screws are fixed in the distal aspect of the plate; (**d**) the device is then detached by removing the small screw

fractures, mandibular fractures, and distal humeral or femoral fractures.

#### 2.2.2.3 Special and Mini Plates

Special T- and L-plates are available in variable sizes (2.0, 2.7, and 3.5) for veterinary applications. Other special plates include acetabular plates (2.0 and 2.7) [62, 63], hook plate for proximal femoral fracture, tibial plateau leveling osteotomy plate, pantarsal and pancarpal arthrodesis plates, and tubular plates for bones with minimal soft tissue coverage and osteoporotic bones, etc. Small fragment mini plates are also available in variable sizes (1.0, 1.3, 1.5, and 2.0), shapes, and lengths as T-plate, L-plate, round-hole plate, cuttable plate, and DCP [64]. Generally, self-tapping screws are used. Mini plates are commonly used for fractures of the mandible, maxilla, metacarpals, and metatarsals in small breed dogs and cats.

#### 2.2.2.4 Locking Plate-Screw Systems

Locking plate-screw system, a more recent concept, is a bone plate having threaded screw holes that allow locking head screws to snugly fix into the plate. This combination of plate and screw functions as a fixed-angle device [65–72]. Locking plate systems have several advantages over other conventional plating systems. The locking plate is biomechanically superior to traditional DCP [73, 74]. In the DCP, friction at the bone-plate interface brings about compression of the plate to the bone; as the axial load is increased, the screws may start toggling and loosening, leading to fracture instability and implant failure. Thus, it is difficult to attain and maintain adequate screw-plate stability, especially in unstable comminuted fractures and in metaphyseal and osteoporotic bones. The conventional plate fixation may also compromise the periosteal circulation and vascularity at the fracture site. The locking plate need not be in close contact with the underlying bone; hence, perfect contouring of the plate is not essential. Thus, reduced contact between the plate and the bone can help preserve the periosteal circulation and reduce osteoporosis underneath the plate. The locking plates do not cause friction between the plate and the screws, and the angularly stable screw-plate interfaces provide stable fixation. In other words, the locking plates act as external fixators positioned under the skin with little distance between the bone and plate, providing more stable fixation. Further, the screws need not be fixed through both bone cortices (can only be fixed in the near cortex); it allows locking plates to be used in a variety of applications like in mandibular and acetabular fractures and in double plate fixations.

### Locking Compression Plate

Innovation of locking compression plate (LCP) is the presence of combi holes to allow fixation of either locking head screws or conventional non-locking screws (Fig. 2.37). The locking compression plates with combi holes are available in standard DCP/LC-DCP sizes of 3.5, 4.5, and 5.5. Combi hole has one part similar to standard compression plate that allows fixation of conventional screw allowing compression or an angled lag screw [65]. The other part of the hole is threaded, which allows fixation of locking head screw exactly at perpendicular to the plate, providing angular stability. Special threaded drill guide, which can fix to the hole threads, facilitates precise drilling for fixation of locking screws. Depending on the situation and function, the plate can be used as a compression plate or a fixed angle internal fixator. Locking head screws are available in two forms, either only self-tapping screws (for fixation in unstable fracture conditions) or self-drilling and self-tapping screws (for unicortical fixations). Locking screws have smaller threads (as there is no need to achieve compression between the plate and the bone) and have a larger core diameter (ensures greater bending and shear strength). Locking screws are designed with new Stardrive head, which can withstand 65% greater insertion torque than conventional hexagonal head, and it is also self-retaining (screw stays on the screwdriver).

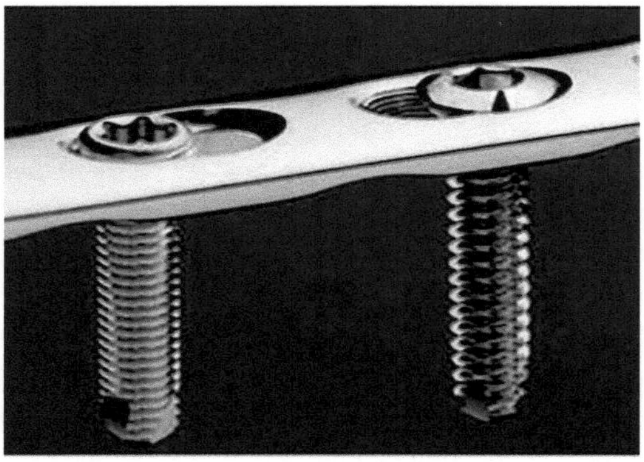

**Fig. 2.37** Locking plate with combi holes fixed with locking and non-locking screws

Locking compression plates can be used to treat most of the fractures where plating is indicated, especially in unstable conditions. In small animals and in sheep and goats, 2.7/3.5 plates can be used to immobilize the fractures of different long bones such as the femur, humerus, tibia, and radius-ulna, apart from the mandibular, pelvic, and spinal fractures. In large animals (horses, cattle, and buffaloes), diaphyseal fractures of the tibia and radius are more amenable to plate fixation, although they can also be used to treat certain fractures of the femur, humerus, metacarpus, and metatarsus using 4.5/5.5 broad locking compression plates.

### Locking Plate (UniLock)

The UniLock locking plate has round holes with locking mechanism for fixation of locking head screws [75]. This is available in two systems, 2.0 (allow 2.0 mm locking screws) and 2.4 (allow 2.4 and 3.0 mm locking screws), which allow fixation of self-tapping locking screws. Locking screws are fixed perpendicular to the plate using special threaded drill guide. The UniLock plates can be particularly useful in mandibular and pelvic fractures and small bones of dogs and cats.

### String of Pearls (SOP) Plate

SOP plate with locking mechanism is a unique fixation system; mechanically, it acts as an internal external fixator [70]. Its design allows the use of cortical screws as locking screws and allows contouring in six degrees of freedom (mediolateral bending, cranio-caudal bending, and torsion) with high bending strength. The SOP plate is narrower but has greater moment of inertia than DCP, LC-DCP, or LCP of similar size. Mechanically, the bending strength of SOP is 30–50% greater than conventional plates.

Basically, the plate has two components, cylindrical and spherical, arranged alternatively. The cylindrical component (internode) is designed to contour the plate by bending or twisting. The spherical component (node) is designed to accept the head of a standard screw; as the screw head is tightened, the screw threads get locked along the threads carved within its deeper part to provide rigid fixation. Both bicortical and monocortical screws can be fixed in SOP plates.

SOP plates are available in two sizes, 2.7 and 3.5. As it can be bent and twisted to contour to the shape of the bone, it has a variety of clinical applications like long bone fractures, pelvic and acetabular fractures, and spinal fractures. Bending and twisting, however, reduce the plate strength (twisting should not be more than 20° per internode). SOP plate cannot be used to achieve compression but can be used as a buttress or neutralization plate.

#### Clamp-Rod Internal Fixator (CRIF)

The CRIF is another versatile system, which consists of a rod, clamps, and standard screws. It can be readily contoured to the bone surface and easily applied with minimal instrumentation, and it is relatively economical [43, 76–78]. CRIF system favors vascularization at the fracture site as only the clamps placed along the rod touch the bone. Clamps can be arranged on either side of the rod contouring to the outer surface of the bone to provide rigid fixation. Tightening of screws allows firm fixation of the clamps to the rods. The available CRIF systems can utilize 2.0, 2.7, 3.5, and 4.5 mm screws, for use in different long bones of small animals and young large animals.

### 2.2.2.5 Contoured Locking Plates for Bovines

The novel locking plates specifically contoured to different long bones such as the radius, femur, and tibia (designer plates) have been developed by the Indian Veterinary Research Institute, using 316L stainless-steel alloy for use in large bovines [41, 79, 80]. The plates are contoured to the cranial surface of the radius, craniolateral surface of the femur, and craniomedial surface of the tibia. The screw holes are placed in two rows and are directed in different planes to facilitate proper placement and fixation of screws in the bone cortex and also to provide greater fixation stability.

The contoured plate developed for the radius has a length of 180 mm, thickness 4.5 mm, and width 32 mm (Fig. 2.38). The plate has 7 combi holes on medial and lateral border each, and the distance between the two screw holes (longitudinal) is 15 mm. Curvature of the plate (arc) is 45° (1/8th of circle). The plate has two additional locking holes at both ends between the two rows of combi holes. Both rows are angled at each other at about 40° to prevent penetration of medial and lateral radial surfaces during screw fixation.

The locking plate developed for the femur has a length of 180 mm, thickness 4 mm, and width (straight) 35 mm at proximal and distal portions and 32 mm at the central portion (Fig. 2.39). The number of combi holes on medial and lateral border is 8 each, and the distance between the two screw holes is 25 mm, whereas the distance between the screw holes on the same border (longitudinal) is 10 mm. The medial border of the plate is straight, whereas the curvature of the plate on the lateral border (arc) is 45° (1/8th of circle), which is nearly flattened at the distal end. The plate has two additional locking holes, one at either ends, between the two rows of screw holes. The holes on both rows are placed alternatively and angled at each other at about 40° to prevent collision and proper purchase of screws in both bone cortices (cis- and trans-cortices) during screw fixation.

The locking plate developed for the tibia has a length of 240 mm, thickness 5 mm, and maximum and minimum width of 55 mm and 24 mm (Fig. 2.40). The number of holes on the cranial and caudal border is 8 and 7, respectively. The distance between two screw holes (longitudinal) is 15 mm. The tibial plate has three additional combi holes in between the two rows of screws. The first five screws in the craniomedial row are at an acute angle to the screws of caudal row to allow the craniomedial screws to enter the far cortex without penetrating through the lateral surface of the bone.

The threaded component of combi holes in all the plates can accept 5.0 mm locking screws with a core diameter of 4.4 mm and a thread pitch of

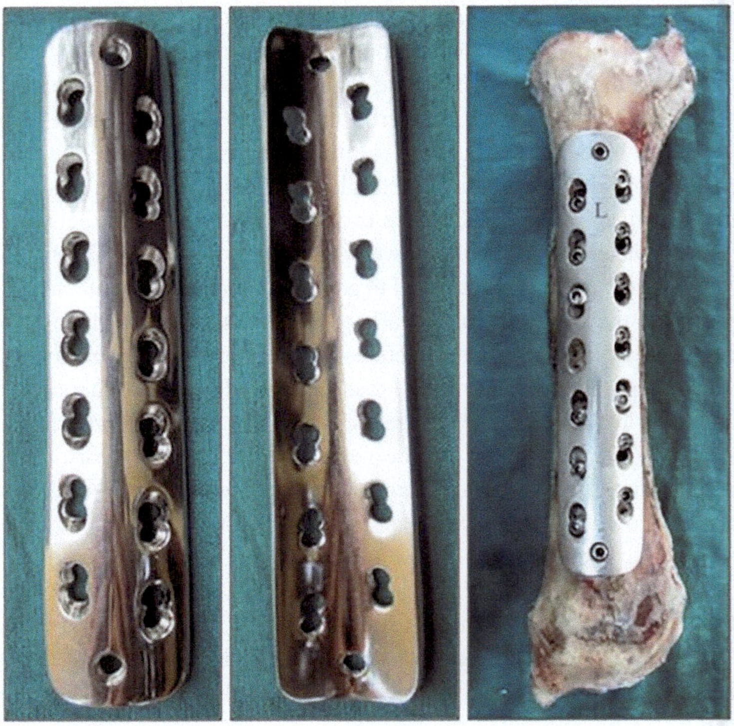


**Fig. 2.38** Contoured locking compression plate developed for bovine radius

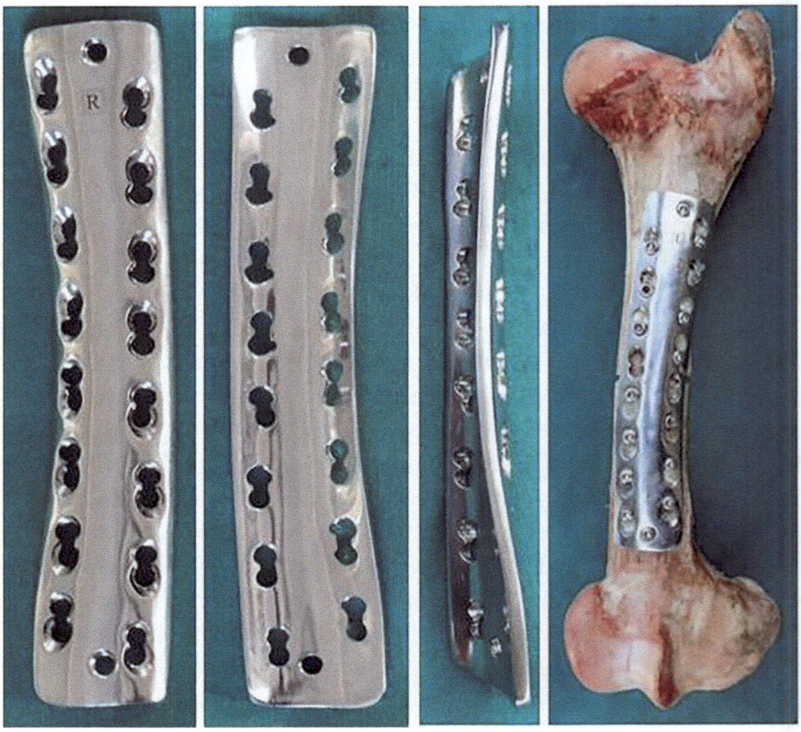


**Fig. 2.39** Contoured locking compression plate developed for bovine femur

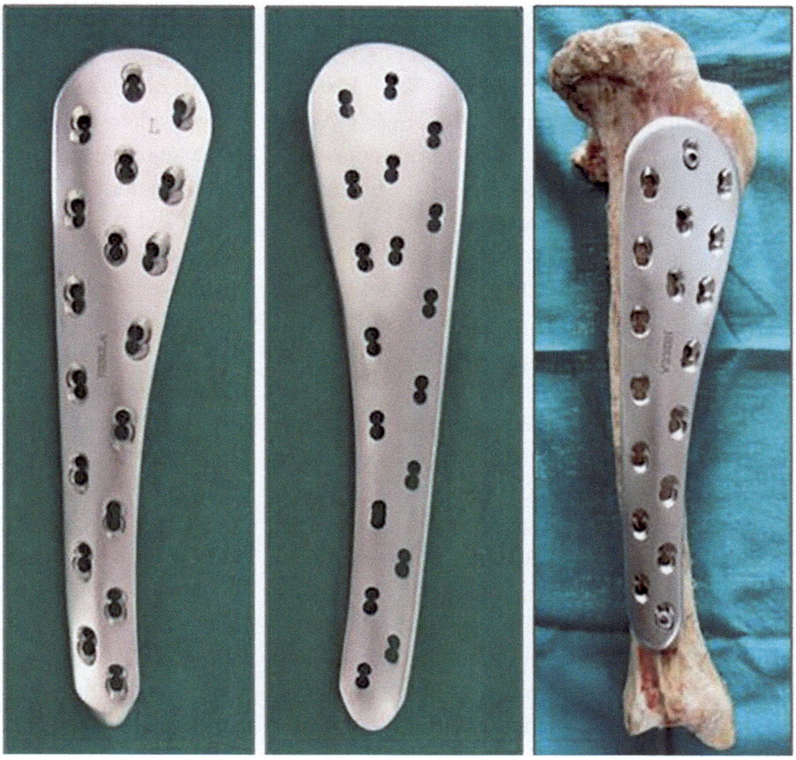

**Fig. 2.40** Contoured locking compression plate developed for bovine tibia

1 mm. The oval component can accept 4.5 mm cortical screws with a core diameter of 3.0 mm, thread pitch of 1.75 mm, and head diameter of 8 mm.

The novel locking plates developed for different bones were subjected to in vitro mechanical tests using plate-bone constructs developed using buffalo cadaver bones. In the radius, mid-diaphyseal transverse osteotomy model was used; in the tibia, a long oblique osteotomy was used; and in the femur, a transverse ostectomy with a 5 mm gap was used to develop bone-plate constructs. Different locking plate-bone constructs were subjected to axial compression and cranio-caudal 3-point bending and torsion (only femur constructs) tests and compared with different plate-bone constructs such as non-locking plate-bone, single locking plate-bone, and double locking plate-bone constructs using a universal testing machine. For compression testing, specimens were loaded in compression at a constant actuator displacement rate of 10 mm/sec until failure; for bending, the central load support contacted the cranial aspect at the center of the specimen, and load was applied at 10 kN per second until failure. For torsion testing (0–2000 Nm TTM), with the longitudinal axis of the femur aligned along the axis of rotation, each bone or construct was externally rotated, so that the cranial aspect of the femur moved medially relative to the mid-shaft, at 5°/sec until failure occurred.

The novel locking plate-radius constructs under compression showed mean (±SE) stiffness of 3.59 ± 0.47 MPa, yield load of 22.65 ± 2.03 kN, and ultimate failure load of 22.65 ± 1.91kN. Under the bending test, the mean (±SE) bending moment was 514.07 ± 55.06 Nm, stiffness 0.61 ± 0.09 MPa, yield load 8.73 ± 0.95 kN, and ultimate failure load 10.82 ± 1.16 kN.

The novel locking plate-femur bone constructs showed 5.19 ± 0.15 MPa stiffness, 45.13 ± 0.76 kN yield load, and 49.31 ± 0.57 kN ultimate failure load under compression. Under bending, mean (±SE) stiffness was 0.93 ± 0.08 MPa, bending moment 620.00 ± 24.56 Nm, yield load

7.09 ± 0.50 kN, and ultimare failure load 8.51 ± 0.45 kN. Under torsion, mean (±SE) ultimate failure load was 245.64 ± 4.47 kN and ultimate failure displacement was 21.66 ± 0.48°.

The novel locking plate-tibia constructs exhibited mean (±SE) compressive stiffness of 4.0 ± 1.04 MPa, yield load of 24.07 ± 3.45 kN, and ultimate failure load of 25.85 ± 4.32 kN. The mean (±SE) bending moment was 565.37 ± 79.3 Nm, stiffness 0.58 ± 0.11 MPa, yield load 7.9 ± 1.14 kN, and ultimate failure load 9.83 ± 1.38 kN.

The novel locking plates designed and developed for fixation of different long bones of a bovine were well contoured and could fit well on the respective bone surfaces. Fixation of the bone with contoured locking plate was mechanically stronger than the standard single locking compression plate fixation and was almost as strong as double plate fixation. These contoured locking plates look promising to treat long bone diaphyseal fractures in adult cattle and buffaloes, which are otherwise difficult to treat by conventional plate fixation. However, they need to be tested in more number of cases in a variety of clinical settings.

Locking plates have certain limitations. Fracture has to be properly reduced before fixing the plate, as the bone segments cannot be manipulated once a locking screw is fixed through the plate. The cost of locking plates is also more than conventional plates, which may limit their use in routine veterinary practice.

#### 2.2.2.6 Minimally Invasive Percutaneous Plate Osteosynthesis (MIPO)

In recent years, more focus in fracture repair has been given on minimally invasive fixation techniques. After the advancements in the development of rigid fixation systems such as LCP, a new technique of fracture fixation, i.e. less invasive stabilization system (LISS) or minimally invasive percutaneous osteosynthesis (MIPO), is gaining popularity [81–84].

In MIPO, a bone plate is fixed through two small incisions made away from the fracture site and hence referred as percutaneous plating (Fig. 2.41). As the fracture site is not directly exposed and minimally disturbed, this technique allows biological bone healing. In this technique, a bone plate is fixed in the proximal and distal bone segments in a bridging fashion across the fracture site. The bone segments are first reduced by closed or indirect methods. Two small skin incisions are made one on either end of the fractured bone, and using a blunt instrument such as artery forceps, a subcutaneous tunnel is created between the soft tissues and the periosteum connecting the two incisions. The plate is then inserted through one of the incisions along this tunnel, sliding across the fracture site on the periosteal surface of the bone, toward the opposite incision. The plate is aligned along the bone and screws are fixed at both ends of the plate through the insertion incisions, and if needed, additional stab incisions are made to fix more screws. Usually, only 2–3 screws are fixed at both ends of the plate leaving the screw holes at the center blank (bridge plating).

MIPO has the advantage of reduced operative time once familiar with the procedure. It lowers the risk for bacterial infection due to decreased duration of surgery, limited soft tissue trauma, and reduced fracture site contamination. It preserves the haematoma formed at the fracture site contributing to early callus formation and bone healing. MIPO also causes minimal damage to the periosteal vascular supply in comparison to conventional plating, which in turn may hasten fracture healing. With MIPO, the postoperative pain is relatively lesser, and the fracture healing is more rapid than traditional plating due to minimal skin incision and manipulation of bone segments. Even though MIPO has similar advantage as external skeletal fixation in terms of fracture healing, postoperative care of patient is less with MIPO.

The main disadvantage with MIPO is that the technique is difficult and challenging to learn and apply. Further, it may not be suitable for fractures requiring more rigid and stable fixation, especially in small segment fractures, and in articular fractures which require precise anatomic reduction and interfragmentary compression. With MIPO, fracture site cannot be directly visualized,

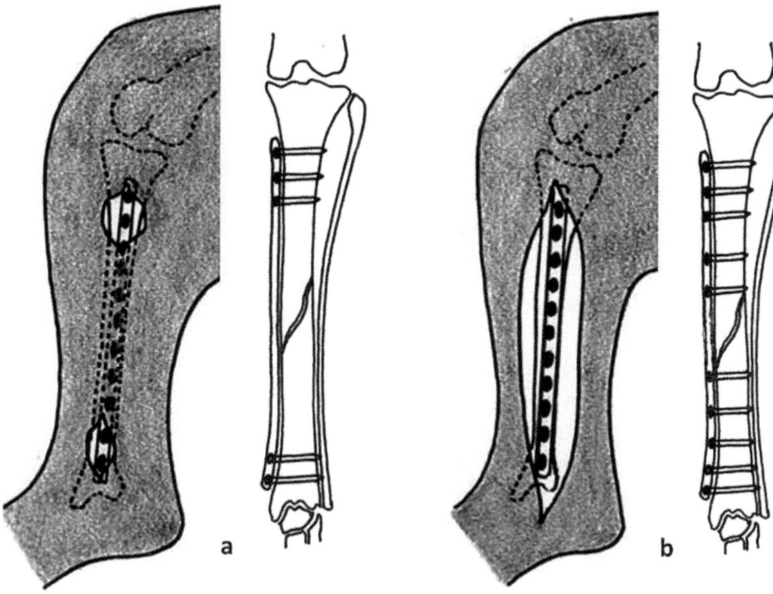


**Fig. 2.41** Minimally invasive plate osteosynthesis (MIPO) (**a**) vs. standard bone plate fixation (SBPF) (**b**). MIPO is less traumatic, less rigid, but more biological. SBPF is more traumatic, less biological, but more rigid

and therefore, there is a need for intraoperative fluoroscopy or radiography, which may increase the risk of radiation exposure for both the patient and the surgical team.

## 2.2.3 Ancillary Fixation Devices

### 2.2.3.1 Screws

Screws have been used in many ways in orthopedic applications [7, 46, 47, 49, 54] (Fig. 2.42). Generally, screws are not used as sole fixation devices as they cannot resist bending, rotation, or axial loads. They are used as ancillary fixation devices along with primary fixation devices such intramedullary pins/nails or bone plates, where screws can stabilize the fracture and keep the bone fragments in anatomic alignment. The screw is often used to provide compression between the bone segments, so that the fractured bone can heal faster. Any screw used to bring interfragmentary compression is called as a lag screw, which not only reduces the gap between the fracture segments but also decreases the stress on the primary fixation implant. Usually, half-threaded screw is used as lag screw, wherein the near cortex is over-drilled automatically leading to compression of bone segments while tightening the screw. If fully threaded screw is used as lag screw, the near cortex must be over-drilled to achieve compression (Fig. 2.43). If the compression is achieved by the fixation device alone, it is called *static* compression, and if the body weight or muscle force is utilized to achieve additional compression, it is called *dynamic* compression.

Screw can be either cortex or cancellous type. Cortex screws, which are designed to anchor in the cortical bone, have fine threads (with relatively larger core diameter and smaller pitch) along their shaft. Cortex screws are commonly available in sizes varying from 1.5–5.5 mm (1.5, 2.0, 2.5, 3.5, 4.5, and 5.5 mm) in diameter with varied lengths. Most frequently used 3.5 mm cortex screw has a 6 mm head with a 3.5 mm hexagonal recess, the outer thread diameter is 3.5 mm, and the core diameter is 2.4 mm, whereas cancellous screws having coarse threads (with lesser core diameter and larger pitch) are designed to anchor in softer cancellous bone. A 3.5 mm cancellous screw has an outer thread diameter of 3.5 mm and core diameter of 1.9 mm. Cancellous screws can be fully threaded or half-threaded having a smooth unthreaded portion, which is normally used as a lag screw. Locking head screws, used along with locking plates, have

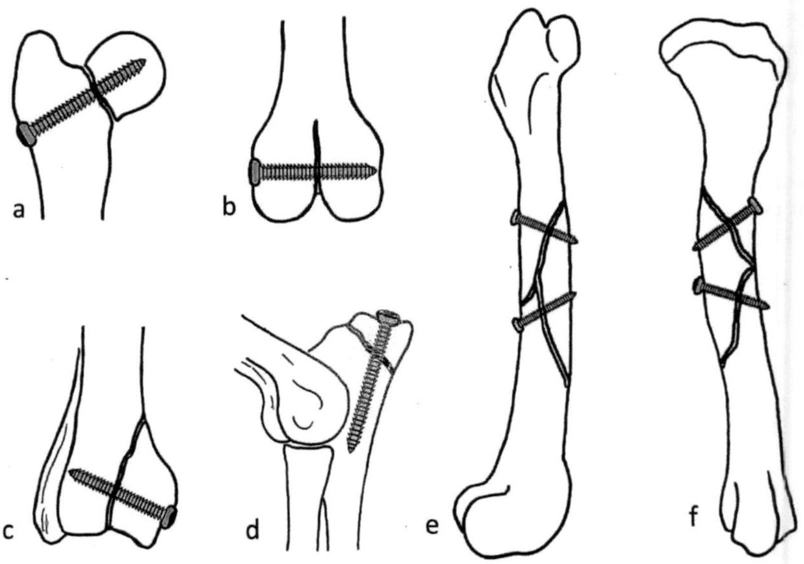


**Fig. 2.42** Fixation of screws in different fractures/bones: (**a**) femur neck fracture, (**b**) intercondylar fracture of the femur, (**c**) distal epiphyseal fracture of the radius, (**d**) olecranon fracture of the ulna, (**e**) comminuted fracture of the femoral diaphysis, and (**f**) comminuted fracture of the tibial diaphysis

core diameter larger with smaller threads than standard bone screws; the pitch of the screws is also smaller, and it matches with the pitch of the threads on the screw head. A 3.5 mm locking screw typically has thread diameter of 3.5 mm and core diameter of 2.9 mm with 1.24 mm thread pitch.

Screws can be self-tapping or non-self-tapping. Self-tapping screws are designed to directly insert into a predrilled hole in the bone, without tapping (creating threads in the bone). Self-tapping screw can allow withdrawal and reinsertion through the predrilled hole without losing its grip; but if misdirected, it can damage the previously cut threads. Hence, it is inappropriate to use self-tapping screw as a lag screw, whereas non-self-tapping screws require cutting threads in the predrilled hole in the bone using a tap having sharp threads corresponding to the profile of screw threads, before their insertion. These screws can be withdrawn and reinserted without fear of accidentally cutting a new track, as it is unable to cut threads in a dense bone. Self-drilling self-tapping screw can cut through the bony cortex and is designed for use in locking plate systems for unicortical fixation.

Generally, solid screws are used; however, cannulated screws with a hollow shaft are often

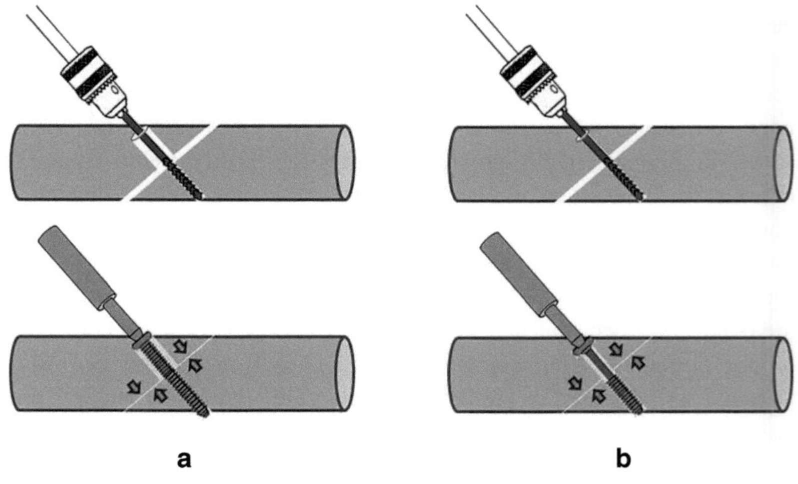


**Fig. 2.43** Application of lag screw: in fully threaded cortical screw (**a**), the near cortex must be over-drilled to achieve interfragmentary compression, whereas in half-threaded cancellous screw (**b**), the near cortex is automatically over-drilled while tightening the screw which brings about compression between the fragments

used in specific applications. Cannulated bone screws are available in sizes 3.5 mm and 6.5 mm. The cannulated screw can be placed at exact location using Kirschner-wire as a guide. A small K-wire is first drilled across the fracture line, usually under C-arm fluoroscopic visualization, and the cannulated screw is then slid along the wire down into the bone using a special driver. Care should be taken not to penetrate the articular surface while placing the screw in the subchondral bone near the joint. The K-wire is then withdrawn to complete the procedure. Cannulated bone screws can be used as lag screws particularly in the metaphyseal or epiphyseal fractures of the distal humerus and distal or proximal femur.

#### 2.2.3.2 Wires

*Kirschner- or 'K'-wires* are handy orthopedic devices used in many different ways for reduction and temporary or final stabilization of fractures. They are also used as guide wires during the application of cannulated screws or nails. The difference between a pin and a wire is their diameter. Pins are between 1.5 mm and 6.5 mm in diameter, whereas Kirschner-wires are between 0.9 mm and 1.5 mm in diameter. K-wire is used to reduce comminuted bone segments before the placement of primary fixation device, to stabilize small bone segments or as a primary intramedullary device to immobilize a long bone fracture [85]. K-wires can also be used in a crossed fashion (cross pinning or cross IM pinning) to help stabilize fractures at the epiphyseal/metaphyseal region of long bones, as in cases of supracondylar femoral and humerus fractures or in proximal tibial fractures in young animals. The main advantage with a K-wire is that as it is very small, the fixation is minimally invasive and non-traumatic. Hence, it can be placed safely through an articular surface or across an open physeal (growth) plate without causing significant injury. K-wires are also widely used in external skeletal fixation systems, especially in circular fixators, which use relatively small diameter pins.

*Orthopedic wire* is available on a spool or in individual preformed loops (eyelet wires). It is used most widely as an adjunct to IM pinning or bone plating to provide rotational stability [7, 21]. Generally, 0.6–1.2 mm (18–24 G) thick wires are used in small animals and 1.2 to 2.0 mm (14–18 G) wires in large animal fixations. It can be used either as full-cerclage wire or hemi-cerclage wire [26, 86, 87].

The full-cerclage wire is placed around the circumference of the bone, generally to hold small fracture fragments together in a comminuted fracture or to achieve compression between long oblique/spiral fracture segments (Fig. 2.44). Spool wire is cut to the desired length and the cut ends are secured by twisting with pliers, needle holders, or special twisting instruments. While passing the wire around the bone, care should be taken not to entrap any soft tissue. A needle holder or a wire passer can help in safe passage of the wire. The wire should be firm, and even tension should be applied along the two ends during twisting to ensure proper intertwining of the two cut ends, instead of twisting one wire end around the circumference of the other (Fig. 2.45). The wire is usually cut at the third or fourth twist. It is advised to bend the twist knot down along the bone surface to prevent possible injury from the protruding wire to any surrounding neurovascular structures (Fig. 2.45b). However, one should remember that bending causes a 30% loss of wire tension.

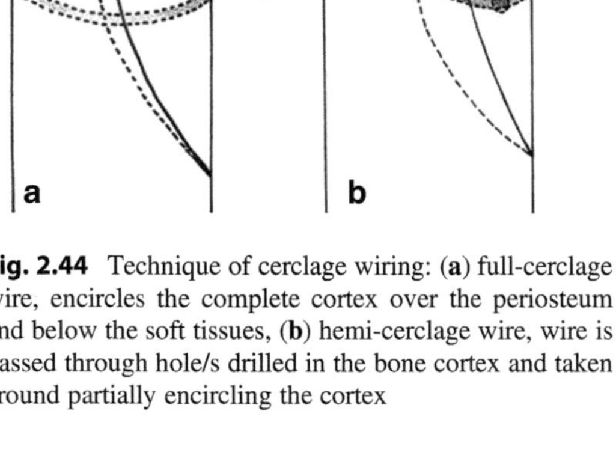


**Fig. 2.44** Technique of cerclage wiring: (**a**) full-cerclage wire, encircles the complete cortex over the periosteum and below the soft tissues, (**b**) hemi-cerclage wire, wire is passed through hole/s drilled in the bone cortex and taken around partially encircling the cortex

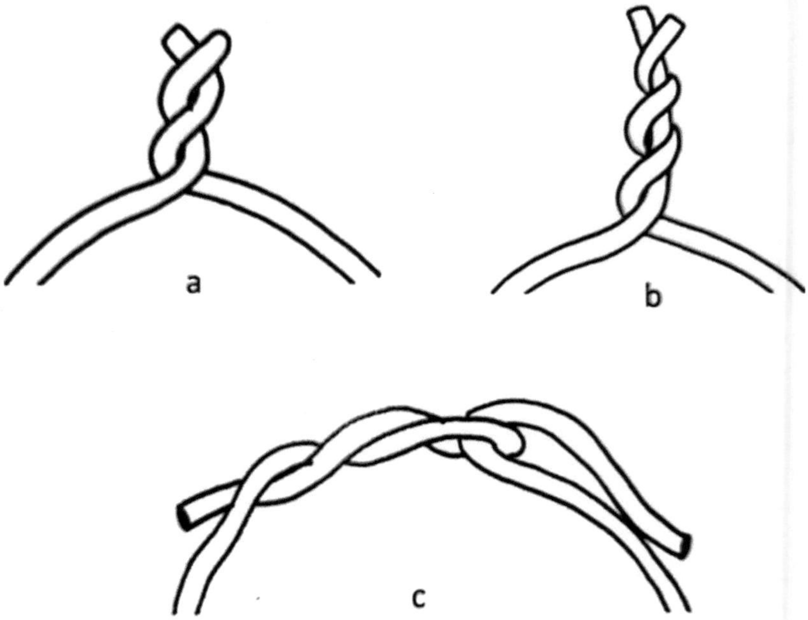


**Fig. 2.45** Technique of orthopedic wire tightening: (**a**) symmetric twist knot (correct), (**b**) asymmetric twist (incorrect), and (**c**) eyelet loop knot. (**d**) Full-cerclage wires used to secure the bone fragments in a comminuted fracture of the femur immobilized with interlocking nail

On the other hand, loop knots have been shown to produce a greater wire tension than twist knots. In this technique, the preformed (eyelet) loop wire is placed around the bone, and by taking through the eye loop, it is tightened using a special tightening instrument. After achieving the desired tension, it is bent over the loop along the bone surface and cut about 2–3 cm from the eye loop. Twist-knotted wires provide greater resistance to knot failure than single-loop knotted eyelet wires, but final wire tension (thus compression) on the bone is greater with loop-knotted wire. A double-loop knotted wire provides greater final wire tension and resistance to knot failure.

Cerclage wires should be used to stabilize only reconstructable fractures (long oblique or spiral fractures or single large butterfly fragment). Wires should not be used if the bone is not cylindrical in shape. Monofilament wire with sufficient strength should be used, and braided wire should never be used. A minimum of two cerclage wires should be applied and are placed at least 0.5 cm (or half the bone diameter) away from the fracture line and spaced approximately 1 cm (or bone diameter) apart. The wire is always placed perpendicular to the bone's axis directly on the periosteum without interposition of the soft tissues. All wires are placed and tightened before closure. To prevent slip of wire and subsequent loosening, the wire may be passed and secured through a hole drilled in the bone cortex or secured by notching the cortex or placing a small K-wire.

Properly tightened and applied cerclage wires do not interfere with the blood supply to the underlying cortical bone. Likewise, cerclage wires can also be placed around immature bone without disrupting bone growth. However, loose wires shift back and forth along the cortical bone and disrupt the blood supply by damaging the periosteal vessels and compromising blood flow through the bony cortex and predispose to infection.

Hemi-cerclage wires are used to counter the rotational or shear forces in transverse and short oblique fractures. The orthopedic wire is passed through a hole drilled in the bone so that it only partially encircles the bone. The wire is placed before the fracture is reduced and tightened after fracture reduction. Tightening of hemi-cerclage

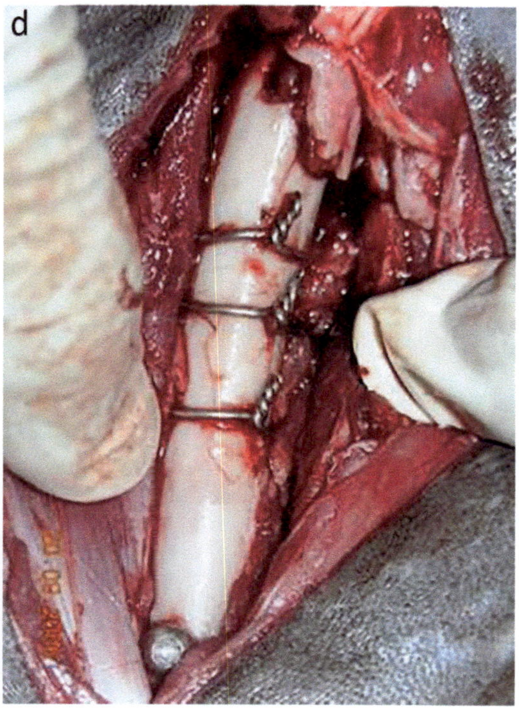

**Fig. 2.45** (continued)

wire should be just enough; excessive tightening may distract the fracture on the opposite cortex. If distraction is suspected, another hemi-cerclage wire can be used on the opposite side. Hemi-cerclage or full-cerclage wires can also be used to reduce the fracture and keep the bone segments in alignment during primary bone fixation with IM nail/plate and screws, especially in severely displaced/comminuted fractures of long bones such as the tibia.

Orthopedic wire can also be used for stabilization of avulsion fractures (especially of os-calcis and olecranon) to counteract tension force (Fig. 2.46). Here, two holes are drilled at the center of the bone in the proximal and distal bone segments, medio-laterally almost equidistant from the fracture line. Two wire pieces (long enough to approximate and twist the opposite ends) are then passed, one each through the proximal and distal holes. Subsequently, they are tightened uniformly on both sides in the form of figure eight wire or as a mattress suture. This type of fixation is particularly useful in fractures with small bone segments, especially in young lightweight animals. However, one should be careful not to put undue tension on the wires, which may cut through the soft bone of young animals.

*Tension band wire*: It is indicated for the treatment of avulsion fractures, wherein the avulsed bone segment is constantly subjected to distraction/tensile force through the attached muscle, tendon, or ligament. Tension band wires not only counteract the tensile force acting on the avulsed bone segment but also bring about compression between the fracture segments. Common fractures that are amenable to tension band wiring are that of thw olecranon, greater trochanter, patella, tibial tuberosity, and os-calcis [88, 89].

Tension band fixation consists of dual K-wires that fix the avulsed bone fragment back to the shaft and orthopedic wire that passes through a hole in the distal bone segment and behind the cut ends of K-wires twisted in a figure of '8' form (Fig. 2.47). Twists are placed on each side of figure of 8 wire and loops are tightened simultaneously [90] (Fig. 2.47b). The purpose of K-wires is to maintain fracture alignment and provide rotational stability; the figure of 8 cerclage counteracts the tensile forces of the tension attachment on the avulsed bone and converts these forces into vectored forces that compress the fracture as the animal bears weight. Tension band wires should be avoided in places where it involves active growth plate as it may cause premature closure of the growth plate (if used, it should be removed within 4 weeks).

#### 2.2.3.3 Postoperative Care and Management with Internal Fixation

Postoperatively, broad-spectrum antibiotics and non-steroidal anti-inflammatory/analgesic drugs should be given for 3–5 days. The antibiotic coverage may be extended if inflammation persists or infection develops. Prolonged use of anti-inflammatory drugs should be avoided as they may hinder bone healing.

Post-surgery, the animals should be restricted to cages/stalls, for the initial 2–3 weeks. Only minimum weight-bearing should be allowed on the operated limb, to prevent any complications.

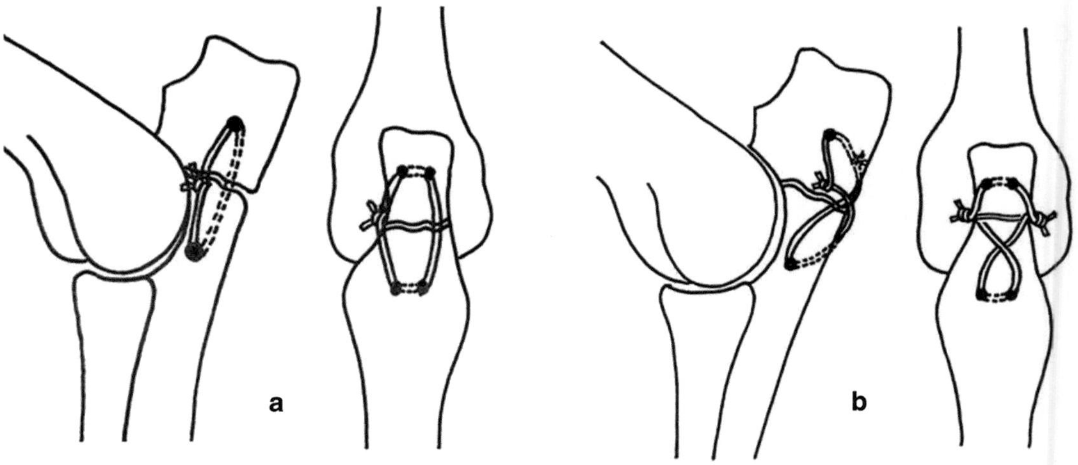


**Fig. 2.46** Orthopedic wire fixation for avulsion fracture: (**a**) as a Mattress suture, (**b**) as figure of 8

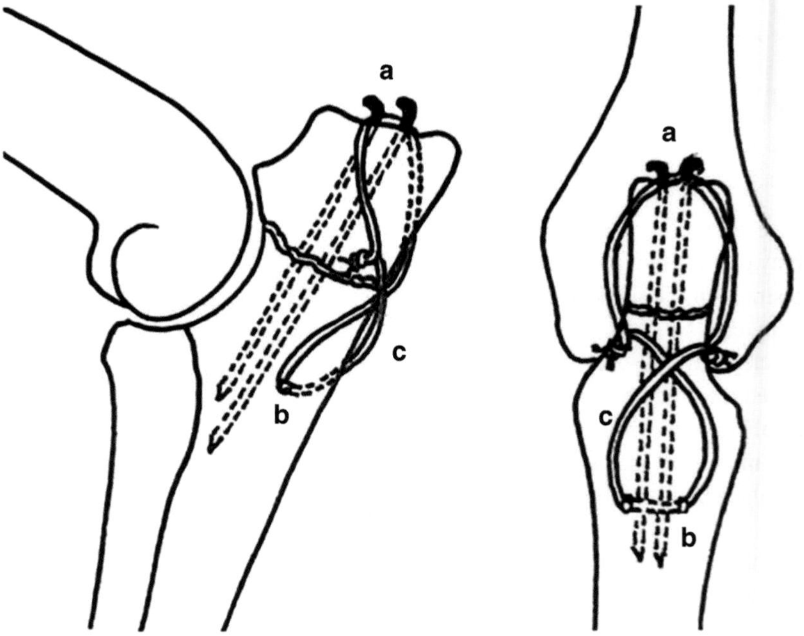


**Fig. 2.47** Tension band wiring for fixation of avulsion fracture: (**a**) K-wires, (**b**) hole drilled in the bone, (**c**) orthopedic wire. (**d**) Tension band wiring in a dog with olecranon fracture

In cases of small animals, generally, the internal fixation provides rigid and stable bone fixation, and chances of implant/fixation failure are rare. Weight-bearing can be gradually increased as the fracture site consolidates. Early weight-bearing should be encouraged (as far as possible), as it will help to hasten bone healing. In large animals, special care is needed during the period of anesthetic recovery and in the immediate post-fixation period. During the period, complications such as implant failure and refracture are more common, especially in horses. However, internal fixation of fractures is associated with considerable risk both in horses and cattle. Contralateral limb laminitis is more common in horses, but in cattle, it is less common as cattle prefer to lie

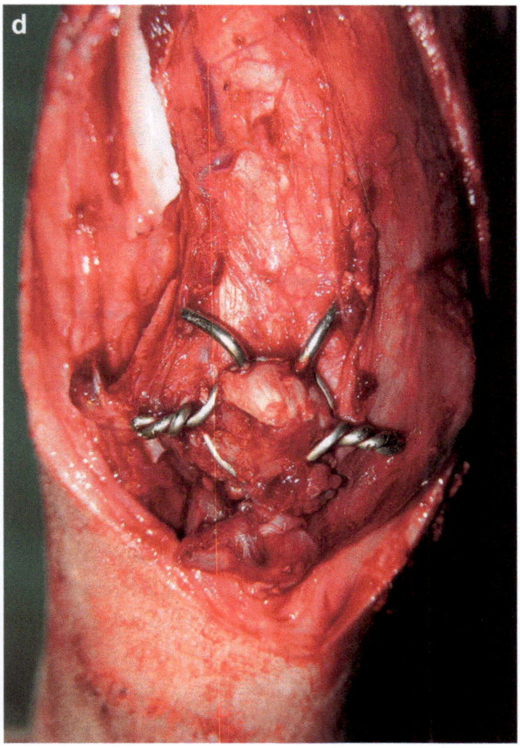


**Fig. 2.47** (continued)

down more often than horses. Bending of the contralateral limb is more often seen in young animals. In cases where the animal is unable to get up or struggle while getting up, decubital ulcers may develop. Hence, soft padding should be provided at the stalls/sheds.

Implant removal after bone healing is not always necessary. Generally, if the fracture heals without any complications, there is no need to remove the implants. If complications arise, such as implant failure or infection, the implants should be removed. It is generally easy to remove an intramedullary pin in small animals with a small skin incision under sedation and local analgesia, whereas bone plates and screws and interlocking nails are not often removed both in small and large animals, as they require extensive surgery for removal. However, if nails and plates are kept in situ for a prolonged period, they may get trapped within the bone or bony callus and may cause stress protection resulting in refracture in later dates. If and when an internal fixation device is removed, the affected limb should be temporarily immobilized using splints and bandages for a few days to avoid chances of refracture.

## 2.3 External Skeletal Fixation

External skeletal fixation (ESF) indicates immobilization of a debilitating musculoskeletal injury (normally bone fractures, but often joint dislocations, tendon/ligament injuries, etc.) utilizing multiple percutaneous fixation pins (transfixation pins/transcortical pins), which are connected to make a rigid external frame or scaffold, spanning the region of instability. Parkhill devised the concept of ESF in 1897 to stabilize open fractures and malunions of the extremities. In the first half of the last century, veterinarians such as Ehmer, Leighton, Schroeder, and Stader developed various designs of external skeletal fixators. ESF has been used in both human and veterinary orthopedic applications for more than 100 years, but it has only recently (during the last 20–30 years) enjoyed resurgence of popularity among veterinarians [91–99]. Renewed interest in the use of ESF has occurred for several reasons: an increasing occurrence of severe bone injuries related to vehicular and firearm accidents; advances in biomechanical studies of ESF and fracture healing that have reduced the incidence of fixator related complications; and the versatility of fixators for use in treatment of a variety of conditions such as fractures, delayed and non-unions, arthrodesis and limb deformities, etc. Even though ESF has been widely used in small animals to treat various fractures, arthrodesis, and limb-lengthening procedures, it has not got widespread acceptance in large animal practice due to lack of appropriate fixation implants that can endure heavy weight of the animals that can be applied in angularly placed bones and due to postoperative management problems. The cost of treatment is also a hindering factor for use of ESF in large animals. Although open fracture repair and stabilization using pins and wires or plates and screws have remained viable treatment modalities, more attention has been given recently to minimal surgical invasion and external

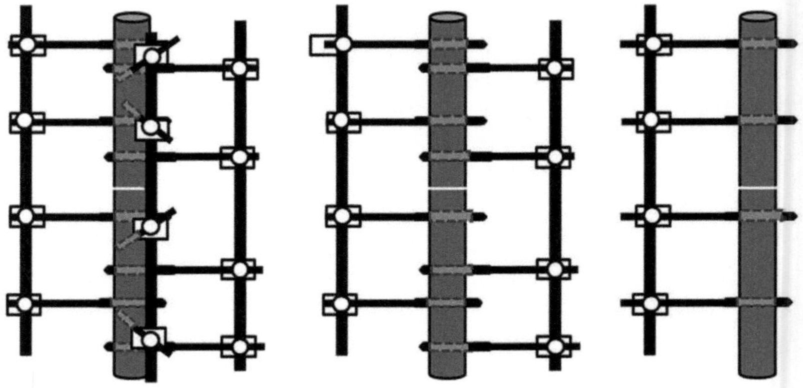

**Fig. 2.48** Dynamization, more rigid to less rigid fixation, by gradual destabilization of fixator components

fracture stabilization, and ESF is being used more frequently in both pets and livestock. It has allowed repair of some fractures that are unmanageable by use of conventional techniques.

### 2.3.1 Indications

ESF has been recommended for the treatment of long bone fractures below the stifle or elbow joints, where cast immobilization is not suitable or provides satisfactory level of fixation (above the mid-diaphysis of the radius/ulna or tibia). Fractures with open wounds and soft tissue injuries can also be better managed using an ESF, as they cannot be suitably treated using casts, splints, or their combinations [100]. It is useful especially in open, comminuted, and infected long bone fractures, where internal fixation in not advised and also suitable for transarticular application [101] for arthrodesis or temporary immobilization during healing of the soft tissues (ligament/tendon injuries) [102] or bone fractures of the extremities (metaphyseal/epiphyseal fractures).

### 2.3.2 Advantages of ESF

External skeletal fixation offers several advantages, such as quick functional recovery of the injured limb with excellent mechanical properties, allowing correction of rotational or angular deformities by adjusting the external frames even after fixation of the bone; avoidance of surgical trauma to the injured or normal tissues and hence protecting the circulation at the fracture site; and avoidance of infection associated with the buried implants. It also preserves the fracture haematoma and bone stimulatory proteins released during the fracture, allowing natural or biological healing to occur with a periosteal or endosteal callus [92, 94, 103–105].

Diversity in design and versatility of the ESF techniques allow their application to numerous types of fractures and are useful to treat short-segment fractures also. Fixation is useful in reserving the bone length and alignment, and removal of the implant after fracture union is easy. ESF is also useful for transarticular application in cases with severe soft tissue injury or comminution of the bone at the end of long bones. It preserves the joint range of motion and allows multiple applications with reusability of components. ESF also allows providing dynamization at the fracture site to hasten bone healing [106] (Fig. 2.48). Dynamization, however, is insubstantial in large animal applications, as providing rigid and stable fixation is most important and less rigid fixation leading to fixation failure is one of the major concerns. In the treatment of fractures, the use of closed reduction and stabilization via external skeletal fixation better preserves the periosteal circulation than bone plate fixation with open method.

### 2.3.3 Disadvantages of ESF

Though ESF offers several advantages, it has certain limitations. Penetration of fixation pins through the soft tissues may injure the vessels, nerves, and tendons, impairing the neuromuscular functions. The open skin-pin interfaces may allow the entry of bacterial infection. Eccentric placement of the ESF connecting elements (far from the central axis of the bony column) may often put ESF devices at a mechanical disadvantage when compared to intramedullary nails and bone plates. Postoperative care and management are difficult due to the presence of fixator components exposed externally.

### 2.3.4 Fixator Configurations and Types

According to the shape/configuration of the external frame connecting the transfixation pins, ESF is classified as either linear fixator, circular fixator, or hybrid fixator [96, 103, 107–109]. Based on the number of skin surfaces penetrated by the pins, ESF can be unilateral (pins enter the skin from one surface and penetrate only till it exits the opposite cortex) or bilateral (pins enter from one surface and exit from the opposite surface). As per the number of planes involved in the fixator, an ESF can be uniplanar, biplanar, or multiplanar.

In small animal practice, unilateral or bilateral linear fixation systems are often used, and in large animals, mostly bilateral systems are used. Unilateral fixator is mostly used in an upper extremity (humerus or femur, usually along with IM nails) or mandible, etc., because the anatomical structure precludes placement of a connecting bar on the medial side, whereas bilateral fixators are commonly used in distal limb bones such as the radius, tibia, metatarsals, and metacarpals, where medial and lateral limb surfaces are easily accessible. Circular fixators are also used in both small and large animal fracture fixation. They can be used in any bone where bilateral multiplanar fixators can be applied but are particularly useful for trans-tarsal applications in the hindlimb (fractures of the tibia and proximal metatarsus, luxation of tarsal joints, etc.).

### 2.3.5 Biomechanics of ESF

External skeletal fixation involves fixation of fractured bone using pins transfixed through bone segments, which are then externally connected to form a rigid frame. Fracture stability is achieved by transfer of loads between the major bone segments through the fixator components spanning the fracture site. Therefore, mechanical stability of a fracture immobilized by ESF is determined by (1) the material characteristics of the bone and fracture configuration, (2) the material properties of the ESF components, and (3) the design of the ESF [95, 104, 110–114].

#### 2.3.5.1 The Material Characteristic of the Bone and Fracture Configuration

The diaphysis of a long bone has more dense cortical (lamellar) bone than the metaphysis or epiphysis having less dense cancellous (spongy) bone. Further, the diaphysis is more cylindrical in shape than the metaphysis or epiphysis, which are more irregular. Therefore, implant holding power of the diaphyseal bone is more than the metaphyseal or epiphyseal bone.

Fracture configuration also influences the mechanical stability of a reconstructed bone (Fig. 2.49). When an ESF is applied for fracture stabilization, a varying proportion of load is shared by the fixator and the reconstructed bone. In a transverse fracture with compression between the bone segments, much of the ground reaction force is transmitted axially along the bone segments across the fracture line; hence, the loading of the fixator components and the pin-bone interfaces is the least (ideal load-sharing fixation). In an oblique or comminuted fracture having a large butterfly fragment that is anatomically reconstructed with full-cerclage wires or lag screws (stabilized with interfragmentary compression), the ESF takes most of the ground reaction load as compared to the reconstructed bone (a partial load-sharing fixation), whereas in a highly comminuted fracture that cannot be

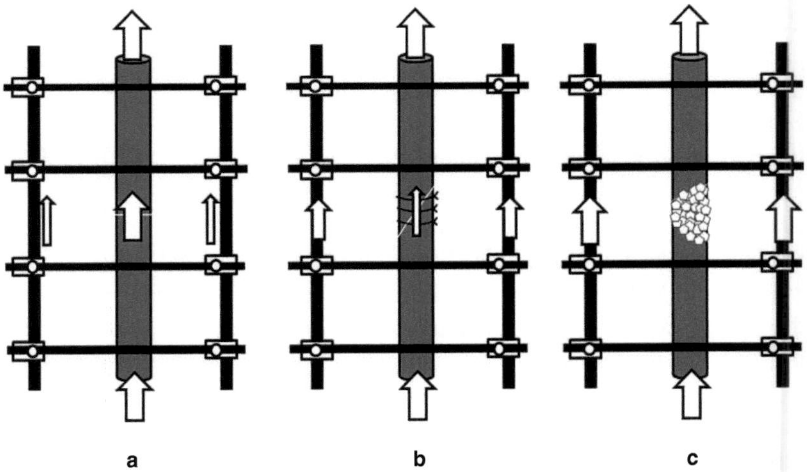


**Fig. 2.49** Load sharing by the fixator under different fracture conditions: (**a**) transverse fracture, (**b**) oblique fracture with cerclage wiring, (**c**) comminuted fracture

anatomically reconstructed, none of the ground reaction force is transmitted through the bone column; instead, all of the load is transmitted from the distal bone segment to the proximal bone segment through the pin-bone interfaces and fixator components (buttress or non-load-sharing fixation).

#### 2.3.5.2 The Material Properties of the ESF Components

Traditionally, ESF components have been fabricated from stainless steel. The connecting bars/rings made of mild steel, aluminum, or carbon composites have also been used. Stainless steel is a sufficiently strong material than aluminum and mild steel. Mild steel is stronger than aluminum and economical. Stainless steel is also generally more rigid and stronger than carbon fiber, but it may undergo plastic deformation with progressive loss of strength at higher loads. Carbon fiber frames are stronger than aluminum frames but costlier than aluminum or stainless-steel frames. Further, carbon fiber frames can delaminate when clamps are tightened on it, which limits their use for multiple applications. As aluminum and carbon fiber are lightweight and less rigid, their frames should be thicker than that of stainless-steel frames to maintain comparable rigidity.

The methyl methacrylate used to construct a connecting bar in free-form fixation systems has certain advantages such as lightweight and more economical than standard steel connecting bars and clamps. But to achieve comparable mechanical strength, acrylic connecting bars should be about four times larger in diameter than stainless-steel connecting bars (20 mm diameter acrylic column is almost similar to 5 mm diameter stainless-steel rod). Once hardened during frame construction, acrylic connecting bars cannot be adjusted. Acrylic is also more brittle and hence can develop cracks. Further, during hardening (polymerization-exothermic reaction) of acrylic, heat is generated (>55 °C); hence, there is a possibility of thermal injury to the tissues. However, this can be minimized by wetting/rinsing the transfixation pins with cold saline during the period and also by keeping a safe gap of about 10 mm between the skin and the acrylic column. The use of epoxy putty for construction of external frame has also shown promising results in terms of mechanical strength of the fixator, which is as good as methyl methacrylate. With epoxy putty, construction of connecting bars is technically easy, and heat generation is also less (because polymerization reaction is slower in epoxy than acrylic).

#### 2.3.5.3 The Design of the ESF

The strength and stiffness of an ESF construct are also determined to a large extent by the implant design of different ESF components.

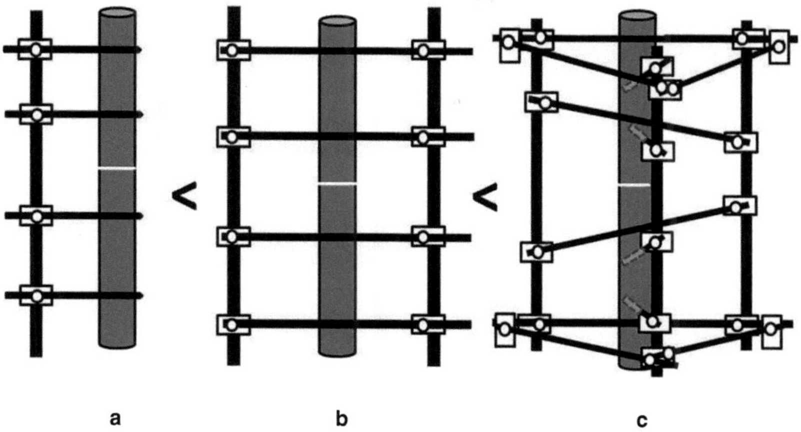


**Fig. 2.50** Mechanical strength increases as the complexity of the design increases

*Frame configuration:* The unilateral uniplanar fixation systems are mechanically the weakest (Fig. 2.50). In unilateral fixation systems, the axial extraction force for transcortical pins is greater when the pins engage to both cortices than that engages to only one cortex. Divergent pins increase the torsional stability and yield higher resistance at the fracture site as compared to parallel pins.

Bilateral linear fixator designs provide superior biomechanical stability than that of unilateral designs, irrespective of the pin size and number. Multiplanar fixators having four connecting bars (quadrilateral) placed equidistantly from one another are mechanically superior to bilateral fixators. The number of connecting bars (more number, greater stability) and the size of the connecting bars (increased size, greater stability) used also affect the fixation stability.

Regardless of the fixator design, the clamps joining the fixation pins to the connecting bars are the weak link in the fixator assembly. If not applied properly, it may cause movement and instability at the pin-bone interfaces leading to loosening of the pin and fracture instability. Hence, in large animal applications, fixation bolts are preferred over clamps, to provide more stable fixation between the pin and connecting bar.

Circular external fixation (CEF) allows axial micromotion at the fracture site without affecting the fixation stability [113]. With CEF systems, the distribution of bending and torsional loads is more uniform across the fractured bone with transfer of greater axial load along the fracture. The CEFs are less rigid but are more resilient (load-bearing capacity) than linear fixation systems.

In CEF, relatively small diameter pins are used under tension. Tensioning of pins increases the axial stiffness. It has been seen that a properly tensioned 1.6 mm pin can be as stiff as a 4 mm non-tensioned pin. However, pin should not be tensioned more than 50% of its yield strength (i.e. 105 kg for 1.5 mm pin and 150 kg for 1.8 mm pin) to avoid deformation and breakage of pin. Further, the effect of tensioning is more in small diameter pins, and as the pin diameter increases (large animal applications), tensioning effect reduces.

The angle between the opposing (cross) pins in a ring also impacts the fixation stability; to maximize stability, this angle must be close to 90°. Eccentric position of the bone within the ring reduces the axial and torsional stiffness. The use of beaded pins (olive wires) minimizes the translation of bone segments along the axis of the pin and thus significantly enhances bending stiffness and fixation stability.

*Number of pins in each bone segment:* The more the number of fixation pins in each bone segment, the larger the surface area for stress distribution and, hence, the greater the fixation stiffness (Fig. 2.51). The use of two or more

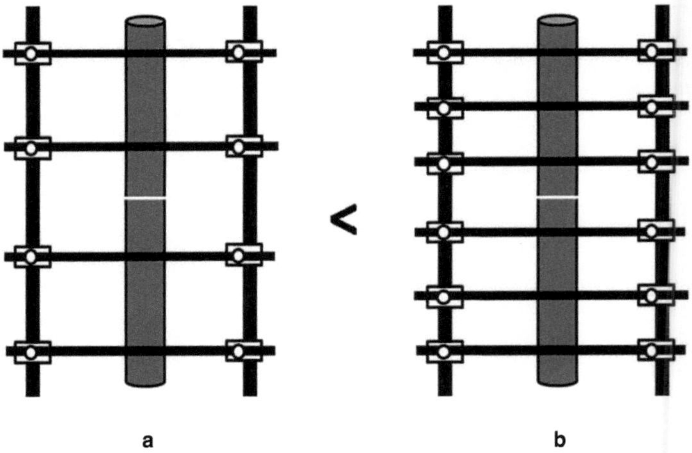


**Fig. 2.51** Mechanical strength increases by increasing the number of pins

pins (in linear systems)/rings (in circular systems) in each bone segment significantly increases fixation stability as compared to single pin/ring fixation. However, adding more than four pins per bone segment does not increase fixation stiffness but may increase the potential for pin-tract infection.

*Pin design:* Smooth (non-threaded) pins have least axial extraction strength and have the tendency for premature loosening and fixation failure and hence should be avoided in linear ESF systems. Among the threaded pins, the axial extraction force is greater in positive-profile pins than negative-profile pins. Among the different pin tip styles, trocar points are better penetrable than chisel or diamond points, but they cause higher temperature along the pin tract. Experimental results have shown that the use of wire ropes (braided steel wires) instead of monofilament pins of the same diameter can provide greater stiffness with respect to transverse loads, indicating that a wire rope may be a viable alternative to a monofilament pin as the transosseous component, especially in large animal circular fixation systems; however, it has not resulted in clinical applications, may be due to technical difficulties.

*Pin diameter:* Pin diameter also influences the fixation rigidity both in linear and circular fixation systems, as it has a direct effect on stability at pin-bone junctions. The larger pins bend less and hence produce less movement between the pin and bone. Pin stiffness is directly proportional to its radius (fourth power); hence, larger pins provide more rigid fixation (Fig. 2.52). But pin diameter should not exceed 20–25% of the bone diameter to avoid the risks of iatrogenic fracture through the pin tract and catastrophic failure of fixation.

*Pin length:* The strength and stiffness of fixation are inversely proportional to pin length, which also implies to the position of the

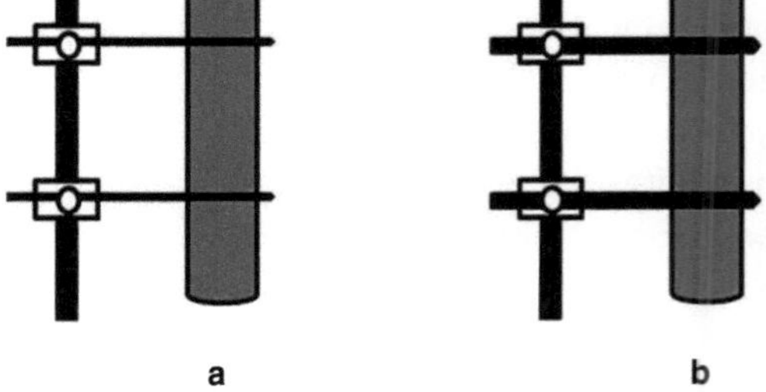


**Fig. 2.52** Mechanical strength increases by increasing the diameter of pins

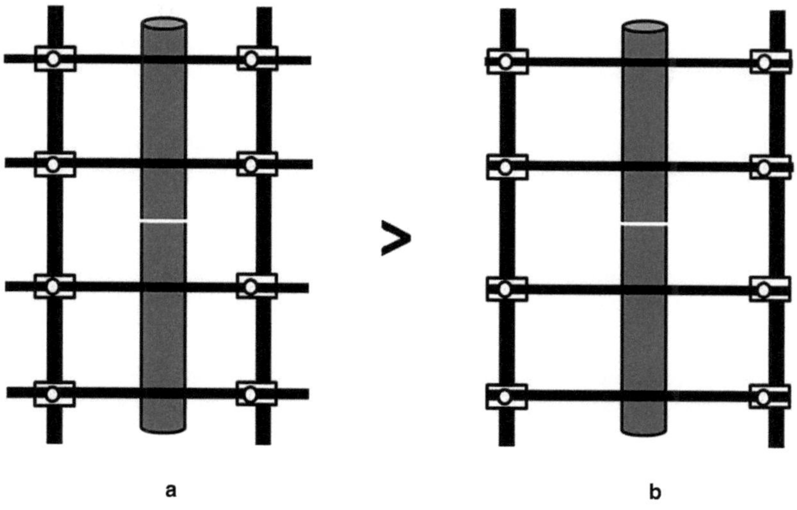


**Fig. 2.53** Mechanical strength decreases as the distance from the bone to the connecting rod increases

connecting bar/ring on the fixation pins. Irrespective of fixator configuration, by minimizing the distance from the bone to the connecting bar, the fixation rigidity can be increased (Fig. 2.53); doubling this distance has been shown to reduce the resistance against compressive load by about 25%. If the distance between the bone and connecting bar/ring is less, the working length of the pin will be shorter. Hence, the pin will be less flexible causing less movement at the pin-bone interfaces. Clinically, it has been recommended placing the clamps about 1–2 cm from the skin surface.

*Pin placement:* Proper placement of the pins relative to the bone is critical to augment the strength and stiffness of the fixator construct. The pin must be placed at the center of the medullary cavity of the bone, so as to penetrate both bone cortices, to maximize stability and prevent iatrogenic fracture. Increasing the distance between the pins increases the working length of the connecting bar bridging the fracture zone and thereby increases its deflection (and fracture gap deformation) with weight-bearing. It is also advised to distribute the pins throughout the length of the bone segments (by using more pins) to disperse the load evenly. Pins close to the fracture are placed about 1–2 cm from the fracture line.

In bilateral linear and circular ESF systems, pins are always placed parallel to each other and perpendicular to the long axis of the bone; angling of pins does not offer any significant mechanical advantage. However, in unilateral systems, divergent pins are used to increase the yield strength; pins close to the fracture are angled to shorten the working length of the connecting bar.

### 2.3.6 Linear External Skeletal Fixation Systems for Small Animals

External skeletal fixation (ESF) is an ever-evolving system. In the 1940s, Emerson Anton Ehmer working with the Kirschner Manufacturing Co., Washington, developed the Kirschner-Ehmer splint, popularly called as KE device. The KE device became synonymous with the external skeletal fixator for several generations of veterinarians and has been widely used in small animal applications [105]. However, due to several disadvantages of KE device, such as mechanical weakness, poor understanding of the system, and high patient morbidity, the popularity of ESF system is reduced by the early 1980s. Subsequently, better understanding of the ESF system led to improved design of fixation pins and KE clamp and a trend toward more rigid fracture fixation. Further improvements in ESF devices were directed to simplify some of the complex frame geometries with the KE device, which led to improved ESF systems such as IMEX™, SecurOS™, Innovative Animal Products™, and Synthes ESF system. These ESF devices have significant improvements in ESF design that improved technical ease of application; increased fixation rigidity, with simplified frame configurations; and decreased patient morbidity.

The standard ESF systems developed for small animal applications have often tried for large animal fixations. However, the mechanical limitations of most of these ESF devices markedly limit their application in large animals. The major limitation is the inability of conventional ESF systems to sustain the heavy weight-bearing loads, leading to fixation failure, especially at the clamps used to connect the fixation pins to the connecting rods. Implant failure in large animals is mostly attributed to loosening of pin-bone interfaces. Heavy weight-bearing loads placed on transfixation pins may cause deflection of pins and thus significant strain at the pin-bone interfaces leading to bone resorption. Resorption of the bone along the pin-bone tracts can further increase pin movement, thus setting in vicious cycle of pin motion and bone resorption, resulting in reduced fixator stiffness and fixation failure. Although various ESF devices developed for humans and small animals have been used in experimental and clinical studies in large animals, the results with type II configurations were satisfactory in lightweight calves and foals weighing less than 150 kg, and type I (half-pin) designs were successful only to a limited extent.

A typical ESF device is made up of (1) fixation pins, (2) linkage devices (fixation clamps, pin grippers), and (3) connectors (connecting rods/connecting bars/sidebars). Connectors and linkage devices together form ESF frame.

#### 2.3.6.1 Frame Configurations

ESF systems for small animal applications are available in different frame configurations: unilateral or bilateral (based on the side) and uniplanar, biplanar, or multiplanar (based on the plane) [90, 109] (Fig. 2.54). Taking both the side and plane into consideration, ESF frames can be further classified as detailed below:

- *Unilateral-uniplanar (type Ia)*: Fixator frame projects from only one side (mostly lateral) of the limb and occupy just one plane. The frames are constructed entirely of half-pins.
- *Unilateral-biplanar (type Ib)*: It is a combination of two distinct type Ia frames. Type Ib frames also protrude from only one distinct side of the limb, but the frame occupies two planes. Many modifications of the type Ib frame have been described.
- *Bilateral-uniplanar (type II)*: The frame projects from two sides of the limb (usually medial and lateral) but occupy only one plane. These frames are made of either entirely full-pins or a combination of full- and half-pins. Accordingly, type II frames are sub-classified as either 'maximal' or 'minimal'. A maximal type II frame has full-pins in all locations, whereas a minimal type II frame has at least one full-pin each in the proximal and distal bone segments and half-pins in the remaining locations.
- *Bilateral-biplanar (type III)*: It is a combination of type I and type II frames. It can be constructed in many different ways.

#### 2.3.6.2 Fixation Pins

Fixation pins are of different types. Based on their placement, pins can be called as either half-pins or full-pins. A half-pin penetrates one surface of the skin and both bone cortices. A full-pin (through and through) enters through a skin surface (near), penetrates both bone cortices, and exits through the opposite (far) skin surface.

According to their design, pins can be classified as non-threaded (smooth) or threaded. Historically, smooth pins were used in ESF systems. The placement of pins at divergent angles is recommended to increase the fixation stability,

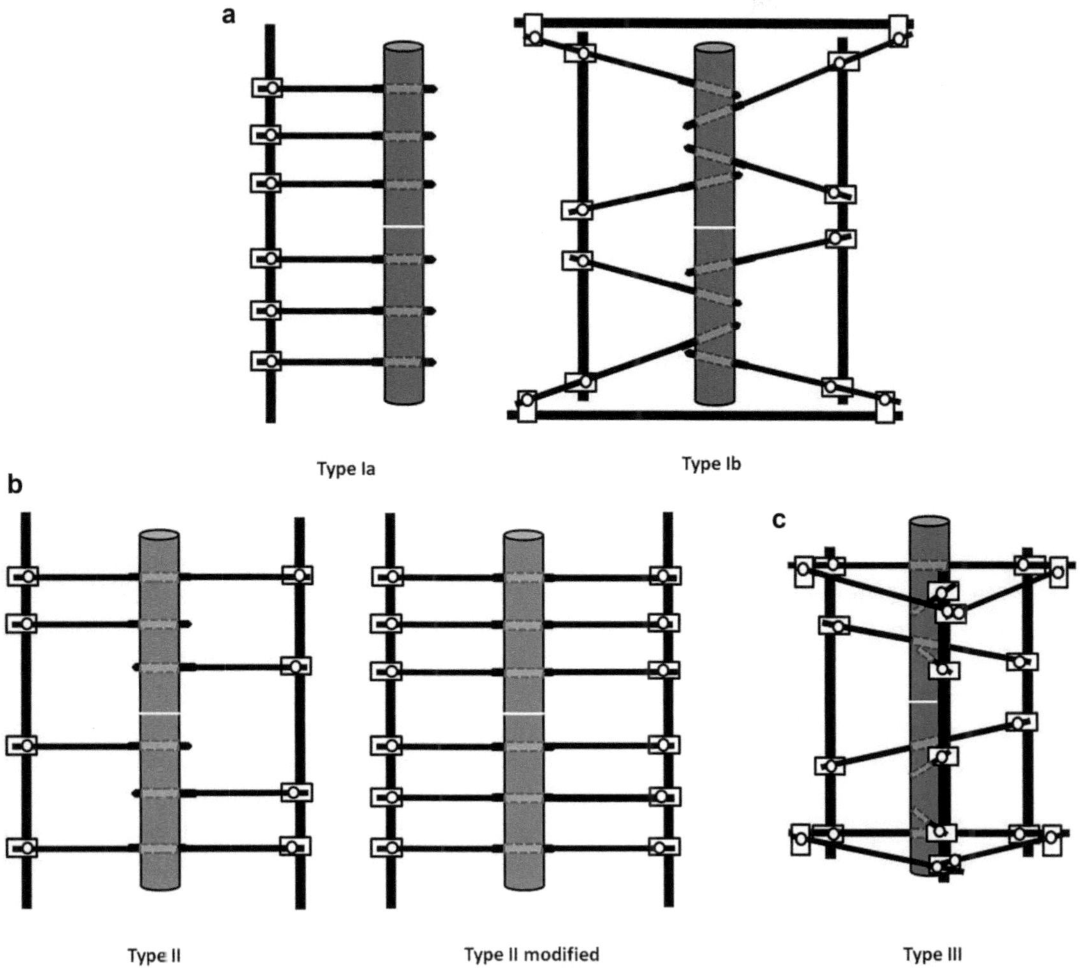


**Fig. 2.54** Classification of ESF frames based on the side and plane: (**a**) unilateral-uniplanar (type Ia), unilateral-biplanar (type Ib), (**b**) bilateral-uniplanar (type II and type II modified), and (**c**) bilateral-biplanar (type III)

but it does not prevent pin loosening and associated morbidity. Threaded pins allow an interlock between the pin and the bone such that this pin-bone interface is much more stable when compared to use of non-threaded pins. Hence, currently most often, threaded pins are used in ESF designs.

Threaded pins can be sub-classified according to the thread profile (negative vs. positive), location of the thread (centrally threaded vs. end-threaded), or recommended use (cancellous vs. cortical).

Threaded pins manufactured by cutting threads into the core of the pin are called negative-profile pins. In partially threaded negative-profile pin, the junction of the threaded and non-threaded portion is the weak point due to the concentration of bending stress leading to cracks. In early ESF devices (such as IMEX and KE), these negative-profile pins were mostly used to provide some pin-bone interface stability when compared with smooth non-threaded pins. Modern ESF devices are designed in such a way that the positive-profile pins can be used at any position within a fixator due to improved clamp configurations such as the Secur-U™ clamp (SecurOS) and the IMEX-SK™ clamp (IMEX). Due to the improvements in these fixation systems and the advantages of positive-profile pins, the use of negative-profile pins is declining. In positive-profile pins, the threads are built above the pin core; hence, they have good holding power when implanted in the bone and are quite resistant to fatigue failure [115]. These pins are available from IMEX™, SecurOS™, and Innovative Animal Products™ in end-threaded and centrally threaded designs.

Fixation pins can also be classified based on their thread form as cortical or cancellous. Cortical pins have large number of fine threads per unit length, which is ideal for hard lamellar bone as it has greater surface area of contact through thread-bone interfaces. Cancellous pins have more coarse thread pattern with fewer threads per unit length, designed particularly for use in sites where the bone is very soft such as the metaphyses or epiphyses of long bones.

#### 2.3.6.3 Linkage Devices (Fixation Clamps/Pin Grippers)

Connecting rods and linkage devices (clamps) are the essential frame components of an ESF. Linkage devices are specific to the manufacturers. Some of the commonly available systems are described below, but there are many other systems marketed around the world that may differ in a variety of ways but not necessarily inferior.

*KE clamp*: Three different sizes (small, medium, and large) of KE clamps are available. The KE single clamp has a bolt portion holding a U-shaped body. The clamp is primarily used to join the fixation pin to the connecting bar. Pin is attached through a small gripping channel present in the bolt, while a large gripping channel at one end of the U-shaped body is used to fix the connecting rod (Fig. 2.55). The clamp can also be used to make articulations in biplanar configurations and in tie-in configurations wherein an intramedullary pin is connected to an external fixation frame. The KE double clamp has two large rod-gripping channels, which is designed for attaching one connecting rod to another and is also useful for connecting an IM pin to a fixation frame. The limitation of KE clamps is that when adequately tightened to achieve firm fixation between the connecting bar and the clamp, the U-shaped body of the clamp may get deformed, which has to be restored to its original shape prior the reuse. This can be done by springing open the U-shaped body with a pin cutter applied to the open end of the 'U'. Due to mechanical inferiority of the clamps and the technical limitations of their use, KE device is currently not commonly used as compared to more modern/advanced ESF devices.

*Secur-U ™ clamp*: The Secur-U clamps are available in small and medium sizes. The clamp has three parts: a U-shaped body, a round head, and bolt that attaches the head to the body and tightens the clamp. The U-shaped body has an opening for the connecting bar, and the head portion has two holes each accommodating different diameter pins. The SecurOS™ fixator overcomes the problems with the KE splint, as positive-profile pins can be placed in any clamp position by using an aiming device. Tightening of the clamp may cause only slight deformation of the head portion against the connecting rod; hence, when used for the second time, the head should be rotated 180° so that there will be a different contact area. The clamp can be ideally tightened to 7.34 Nm of torque by using the precision torque wrench. Another clamp, the *Augmentation Clamps*™ made by SecurOS, is used to attach an augmentation plate to build a stiffer, more compact frame.

*IMEX-SK™ clamp*: The IMEX-SK™ fixator also overcomes many of the limitations of KE splint. SK clamps are also available in three different sizes (mini, small, and large). The clamps have three different components: a two-piece body, a long pin-gripping bolt, and another short secondary bolt. The two-piece body made of black anodized aluminum has the rod-gripping channel at the center, and the pin-gripping bolt with a slotted washer and nut goes through the bottom portion of the body and the secondary bolt through the top portion. Clamps can be fixed at the desired position along the connecting rod. The washer in the pin-gripping bolt permits effective gripping of different diameter pins. The presence of large hole in the pin-gripping bolt allows predrilling and fixation of positive-profile pins

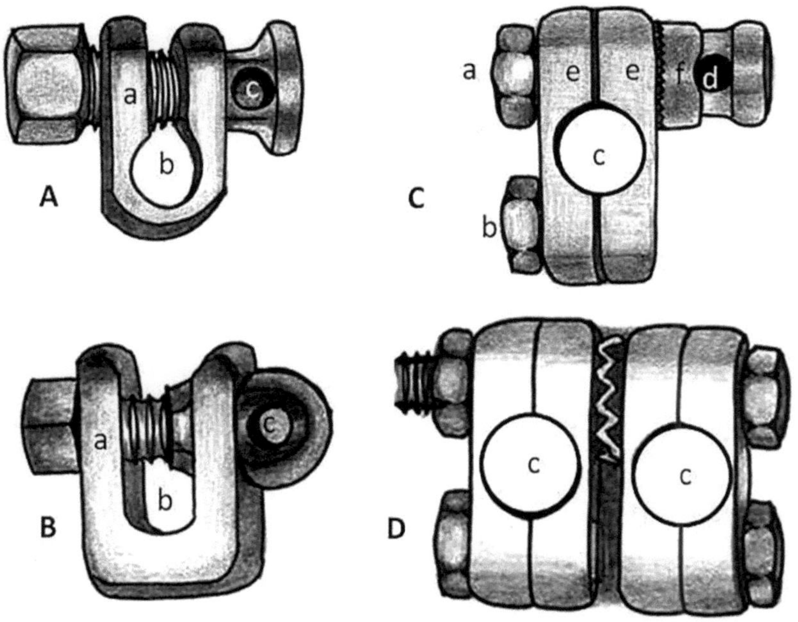


**Fig. 2.55** Different types of fixator clamps: (A) KE clamp with U-shaped clamp body (**a**), rod-gripping channel (**b**) and pin-gripping channel (**c**); (B) Secur-U ™ clamp showing U-shaped clamp body (**a**), opening for connecting bar (**b**) and opening for fixation pin (**c**); and (C and D) IMEX-SK™ clamps with bolt for fixation pin (**a**), bolt for connecting bar (**b**), opening for connecting bars (**c**), opening for fixation pin (**d**), halves of clamp body (**e**) and slotted washer (**f**)

directly through the clamp. The secondary bolt which is unique to the SK clamp design helps to properly secure the connecting rod with additional grip and also allows the use of clamp as a drill guide as well as a targeting device. The secondary bolt is loosely tightened to hold the clamp in the desired location on the connecting rod and to maintain the position of the clamp while predrilling and placing a fixation pin. The connecting rods in SK splint are made from carbon fiber composite, titanium, or aluminum (instead of stainless steel), which permit the use of increased rod diameter and strength without excess weight.

#### 2.3.6.4 General Principles of ESF Application

Many of the principles of ESF application are the same regardless of the specific device used [98, 103, 116, 117]. The use of the more modern ESF devices available today can improve the clinical outcomes because of enhanced technical simplicity of application and mechanical superiority of the devices themselves.

*Anesthesia and restraint*: The patient is anesthetized, the hair is clipped, and skin is prepared with scrubbing as for any orthopedic procedure. The surgical field must include a joint above and below the fracture, and it is properly draped. The animal is restrained in dorsal recumbency and the limb is suspended in a hanging limb position throughout the surgical procedure, especially for fixation of radius-ulna or tibia-fibula fractures, whereas in humerus or femur fractures (where typically unilateral fixators are used), the animal may be positioned in lateral recumbency with the affected limb facing upwards.

*ESF frame construction*: The planned frame configuration including pin selection should be sketched prior to surgery and placed near the radiographic viewer, which will act as a guide during fracture fixation. With the KE device, it is important to anticipate the desired number of fixation pins so that an appropriate number of clamps can be positioned on the connecting bar in the beginning since it is very difficult to add or remove clamps later during the repair, whereas SecurOS™ or IMEX-SK™ clamps can be added to the connecting rods at any point during the procedure. The distal-most and proximal-most pins are usually placed first (Fig. 2.56). These pins are then fixed to a connecting rod through the clamps to construct the frame. Fracture

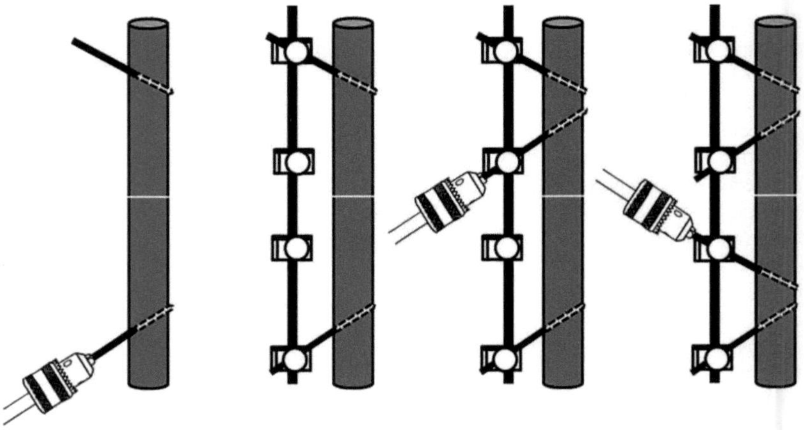

**Fig. 2.56** Technique of ESF application: the proximal-most and distal-most pins are usually placed first; subsequently, remaining pins are inserted using the clamp as guide

reduction and alignment are fine-tuned at this time prior to placing pins in the middle-clamp positions. Subsequently, predrilling and pin placement are done through the clamps (KE and IMEX-SK™ devices) or with the aid of an aiming device (SecurAim ™) to ensure placement of the pin in an appropriate position relative to the connecting bar. Pins should be positioned about 1–2 cm off the fracture line. In multiplanar frames (type Ib and type III), two uniplanar frames are interconnected. As metallic multiplanar frames tend to obstruct the radiographic visualization of the fracture, the two frames can be articulated after postoperative radiographs are made.

*Pin selection*: The selection of appropriate size pin depends on the bone diameter. Larger diameter pins are much stiffer; however, the penetration of the bone by excessively large pins will weaken the bone. By and large, the pin diameter should not be more than 20–25% of the bone diameter. Threaded pins are preferable to non-threaded pins because of their superior holding power in the bone. Positive-profile threaded pins offer the additional advantage of resistance to breakage. Negative-profile threaded pins may be preferred where the bone diameter is small to minimize risk of iatrogenic fracture through the pin tract. With modern ESF devices which allow the use of different pin sizes, smaller-size positive-profile threaded pins may be preferred instead of negative-profile pins. Cancellous fixation pins may be used in the metaphyseal regions of different long bones; however, placement of cancellous pins in other locations risks iatrogenic fracture through the pin tract.

*Pin placement and insertion*: Fixation pins are placed through 'safe' corridors to reduce the risks of musculotendinous or neurovascular injury. As a general rule, medio-lateral or latero-medial pin placement is safe than cranio-caudal placement. About 1–2 cm-long release incision is made (proximal to distal) in the skin at the proposed site of pin placement. A haemostat is used to bluntly dissect down and make a small 'grid' along the soft tissues down to the underlying bone. It is advised to make a slightly larger soft tissue corridor than the pin size because any tension of soft tissues on the fixation pin may cause irritation and inflammation. Soft tissues are retracted away from the pin during pin placement by use of a haemostat spread at the tips or use of a drill sleeve. It is always preferred to predrill the pin tract with a drill bit measuring about 10–15% smaller in diameter than the pin, before the pin placement. Ensure that the pin tract is made at the center of the bony cortex. Half-pin is then advanced through the soft tissue corridor and inserted along the predrilled hole in the bony cortex (using a power drill) so as to penetrate the far cortex. The entire trocar point should exit with 1–2 threads coming out of the far cortex to maximize stability. In case of a full-pin, it is advanced through the soft tissue corridor and both cortical surfaces to exit the far skin surface. At the exit point, a small skin incision is made, and using a haemostat, the soft tissues are retracted to create a corridor around the pin.

For drilling, a slow-speed power drill is used; a hand chuck or high-speed drill (>400 rpm) is not recommended. Hand chuck insertion creates an excessively large pin tract due to chuck wobbling, whereas high-speed drill insertion generates excessive frictional heat causing necrosis of the bone around the pin tract. Both methods risk premature pin loosening and associated pain, poor-limb use, and loss of fracture reduction.

It is also important to drill in small pulses (with 30 s between the pulses) to allow for dissipation of heat generated. If stuck, the pin should be retracted and reinserted after a while. While drilling, cold isotonic solution is dropped continuously at the pin site to minimize thermal injury to the tissues. To achieve stable fixation, at least two pins are fixed in each bone segment. The distance between the skin and connecting rod should be minimum; however, at least 1–2 cm gap should be kept between the skin and the connecting rod to allow soft tissue swelling and regular dressing of pin-skin interfaces. Except in unilateral linear fixation systems, pins are always placed parallel to each other and perpendicular to the bone axis.

ESF is often used along with intramedullary pin, as in 'tie-in' configuration (Fig. 2.57). In this case, the fracture is first reduced by inserting a relatively small diameter Steinmann pin into the medullary cavity. Unilateral ESF is then fixed on the lateral surface of the limb by inserting two end-threaded bicortical half-pins, one at each end. After ascertaining adequate bone reduction, additional half-pins may be reinforced as per the need. The protruding end of the IM pin is then anchored (tied-in) with proximal end of the ESF using a clamp.

Post-fixation radiographs are made to assess proper placement of fixation pins in the bone. After reviewing the radiographs, if needed, it is preferable to advance a pin that was not placed deeply enough into the bone, rather than retracting a deeply seated pin (retraction of the pin disrupts the pin-bone interface and hence increases the risk of premature pin loosening). Final adjustments are then made and all the clamps are tightened.

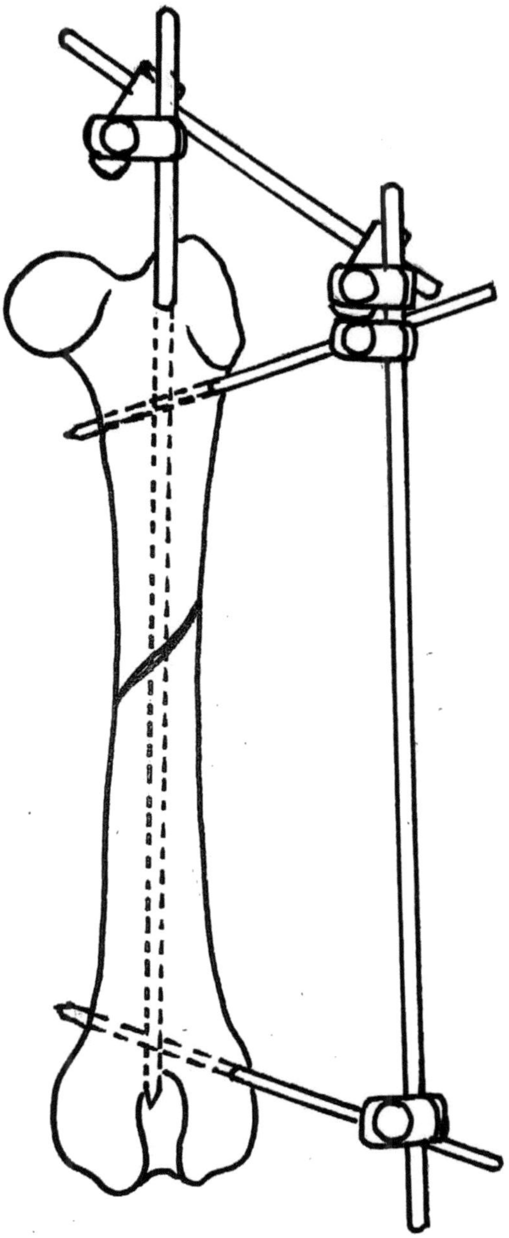

**Fig. 2.57** Tie-in ESF fixation

#### 2.3.6.5 Postoperative Care and Management

Immediately after the surgical fixation, the external fixator components and the surgical area should be cleansed of debris and blood clots and allowed to dry. Cut ends of fixation pins are flushed, and protective caps may be applied to prevent injury to the animal as well as the handler while dressing. The skin-pin interfaces are cleaned with an antiseptic solution (0.05% chlorhexidine or 1% povidone iodine), an antibiotic ointment is applied, and then a sterile non-adherent dressing is done around the surgical area to cover the open wound or skin incision and the skin-pin interfaces. It is also advised to apply a compressive bandage on the operated limb, similar to a Robert-Jones bandage, which would help absorb exudates from the pin-skin interfaces and decrease postoperative swelling [107]. A course of broad-spectrum antibiotic is given for a period of 3–5 days, especially in open fractures to prevent bacterial infection. If bandaging is done, it should be replaced after 1–2 days. Daily cleaning and dressing of the surgical site may continue till the release incisions/wounds are healed.

The animal's activity should be restricted in the postoperative period to prevent any complications and allow for bone healing. The patient may be confined to a cage/limited area to prevent running, jumping, or playing and allowed only leash walking. This movement restriction should continue until the radiographic confirmation of bone union. It is important to inform the animal owner about the importance of movement restriction and daily cleaning and dressing of pin-skin interfaces for successful outcome of fixation and bone healing.

The patient should be subjected to follow-up examinations at regular intervals. Although the interval of examinations may differ from case to case, it is advisable to inspect more frequently in the initial stages, especially the fixator components, and if needed, corrections (tightening the loose components) may be done. Subsequently, clinical and radiographic examinations may be carried out at 15-day intervals till radiographic bone healing. If delayed healing is suspected, staged destabilization of the fixator construct can be done (starting from sixth week) by removing certain part/s of the frame. This 'dynamization' reduces fixator stiffness and increases micro-movement at the fracture site leading to accelerated bone healing. The fixator is removed after the radiographic evidence of bone healing (bridging callus). For removal of fixator, the animal may be sedated and fixation pins are cut using a pin cutter, and the cut pins are pulled using a plier or hand chuck. The pin tracts are flushed with sterile saline or antiseptic solution, and the limb is temporarily bandaged for 2–3 days. The pin tracts are not sutured but allowed second intention healing to occur.

## 2.3.7 Transfixation Pinning and Casting in Large Animals

Transfixation pinning and casting (TCP) is the most commonly used external skeletal fixation technique in large animal practice. It can be applied as a 'hanging limb pin cast' or as an 'external skeletal fixator'.

### 2.3.7.1 Hanging Limb Pin Cast

In hanging limb pin cast, one or two transfixation pins are placed medio-laterally in the proximal bone segment of a fracture, and a full-limb cast is applied by anchoring the cast with the pin/s (Fig. 2.58). In this scenario, the load (body weight) is taken by the pin/s and transferred to the cast, sparing the fracture site. The distal part of the limb is 'free' and it 'hangs' inside the cast [13, 118].

#### Principle of Hanging Limb Pin Cast

During cast application, fracture site stability is achieved by immobilizing the joints above and below the fracture. However, inclusion of both joints in the cast is not always possible because of anatomical disposition of some bones. Fractures of the proximal tibia (and often the radius) in heavy large animals cannot be adequately stabilized using a plaster cast because the stifle or elbow joint cannot be appropriately secured in the cast. In hanging limb pin cast, the pin(s) used in the proximal bone segment helps secure the cast and prevent its downward slipping.

#### Technique

Under general anesthesia or deep sedation with regional nerve block, the animal is restrained in lateral recumbency with the injured limb

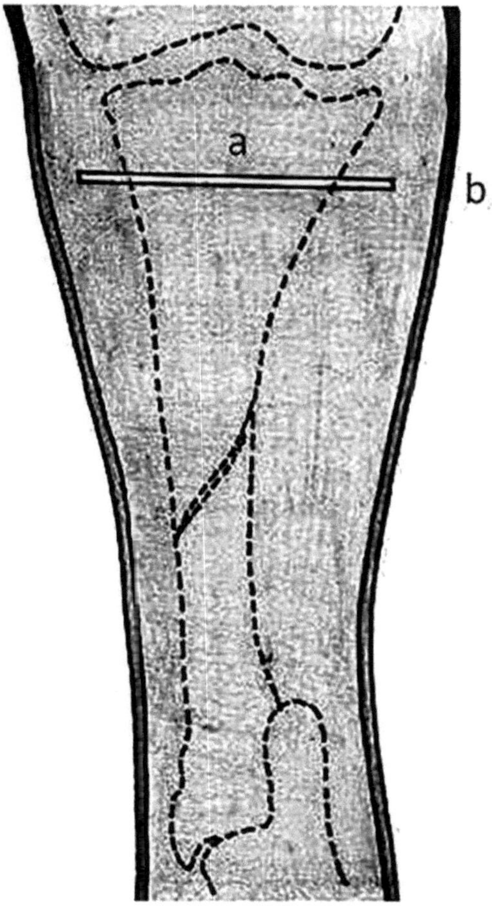


**Fig. 2.58** Hanging limb pin cast: (**a**) Steinmann pin, (**b**) cast

positioned upwards. The area proximal to the fracture site is shaved and prepared aseptically. The proposed site of pin insertion (usually one) is marked on the skin on the outer surface (usually lateral). A small release incision is given in the skin (proximal to distal orientation) at the proposed site of pin insertion in the proximal bone segment. A hole is predrilled through the center of the bone cortex (perpendicular to the bone axis) along the proposed line of pin insertion, using an electric drill and a drill bit (about 0.5 mm smaller than the pin diameter). A proper size pin (about 6–7 mm Steinmann pin) is then inserted through the predrilled tract, so as to exit it through the far cortex and the skin on the opposite surface (standard pin insertion technique as described before is followed while passing the transfixation pin). The extra length of the pin is cut and the pin-skin interfaces (on both skin surfaces) are dressed with sterile gauze and antiseptic solution. The fracture segments are aligned by closed reduction using traction and countertraction and held in extension using a rope tied at pastern region. The whole limb is padded using cotton, and a full-limb cast (plaster of Paris or fiberglass) is then applied in such a way that the cut ends of the pin are buried within the cast.

#### Postoperative Care and Management

Postoperatively, broad-spectrum antibiotic and analgesic-anti-inflammatory drug are administered for 3–5 days. The animal is closely observed for any soft tissue infection or necrosis around the pin exit points.

#### Limitations/Disadvantages

With handing limb pin cast, it is not possible to prevent overriding of bone segments in case of an oblique or spiral fracture, and it does not provide adequate fixation of a comminuted fracture. Placement of pin only in proximal bone segment does not prevent rotation of the distal bone/limb and hence cannot provide as stable fixation as transfixation pinning of both bone segments.

### 2.3.7.2 Transfixation Pinning and Casting (TCP) as an ESF

This technique includes placement of at least two fixation pins in both major bone segments (proximal and distal) and application of a full-limb cast to stabilize the fracture site [2, 13, 119, 120] (Fig. 2.59). The advantages of pin-cast ESF as compared to hanging limb pin cast is relatively more rigid fixation of fracture with limited movement of fracture segments within the pin-cast. Further, with pin-cast ESF, the cast need not span the adjacent joint (such as stifle); however, full-limb cast is always preferred, especially in heavy large animals.

#### Technique

Under general anesthesia (or deep sedation with regional nerve block), the animal is positioned in lateral recumbency. The affected leg is drawn out of the operation table and held in extended position. The whole length of the injured bone is aseptically prepared by shaving and scrubbing.

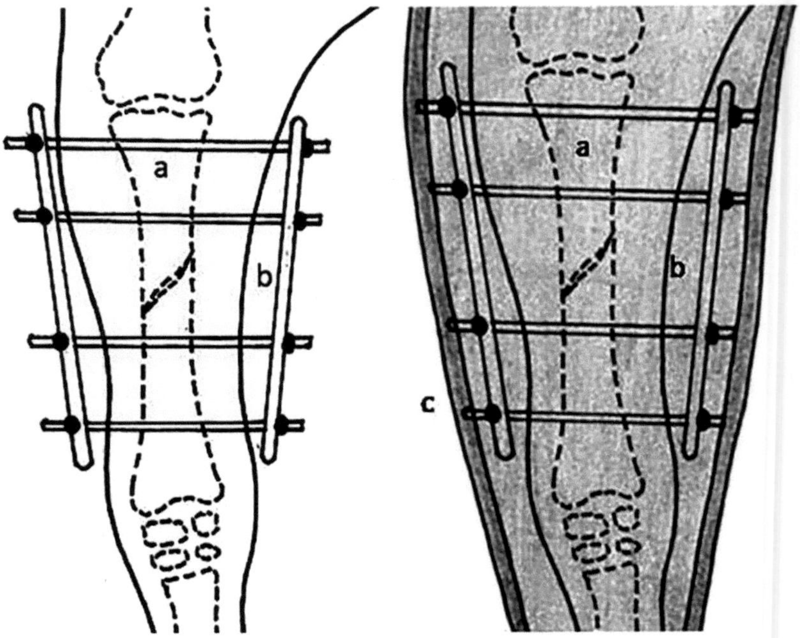


**Fig. 2.59** Transfixation pinning and casting: (**a**) Steinmann pin, (**b**) side bar, (**c**) cast

The bone segments are aligned by close reduction using traction and counter-traction and held in extension using a rope tied around the pastern. The proposed sites of pin insertion are marked on the skin along the bone (upper surface). Small release incisions are made in the skin at the proposed sites of pin insertion. Subsequently, optimum size pins (smooth or threaded pins, a least two each in the proximal and distal segment) are drilled through predrilled holes in the bone cortex, so as to exit from the opposite bone cortices and the skin (through release incisions made in the skin at the pin exit points). The size of the pins is selected based on the animal's body weight; usually, 6–7 mm pins are adequate in adult large animals.

The transfixation pins are inserted using a low-speed electric drill, following proper pin insertion principles. All the pins are passed parallel to each other and perpendicular to the bone's axis. The pins emerging from the skin surfaces on medial and lateral surfaces are then connected using connecting bars (metal/plastic/wooden) to give greater strength to fixation. The extra length of the pins is cut, and the pin sites are protected using sterile gauze with antiseptic solution. Subsequently, a full-limb cast is applied routinely so that the cut ends of the pins are buried within the cast. Plaster of Paris or fiberglass cast can be used, but fiberglass cast has distinct advantage of lightweight and greater strength.

In open fractures, a 'window' is kept at the level of skin wound to allow for drainage and daily dressing. Keeping a window, however, does not give satisfactory results always, and the patient may feel discomfort due to the development of swelling at the defect site. The cast is cut and transfixation assembly is removed once the clinical union of fracture is evident, usually after 10–12 weeks in adult large animals.

#### Advantages

The biomechanical advantage of TPC includes rigid bone fixation due to the least distance between the bone and the external frame. With TPC, fixation pins can be placed at desired locations (as per the fracture configuration), and it need not dictated by the typical ESF clamp or rod position. Further, the mechanical (weight-bearing) load is distributed by sharing with the cast.

**Disadvantages**

Complications such as soft tissue infection, bone necrosis, and periosteal reaction around the transfixation pins can often occur, which are difficult to assess and treat. It is not possible to adjust the fracture reduction and alignment after the cast application. There can be difficulty in managing wounds (with open fractures) and problems in assessing the development of cast sores.

### 2.3.8 Linear External Skeletal Fixation Systems for Large Animals

It is a great challenge to treat long bone fractures in large animals, especially open infected fractures. As most of the bone fractures are open in nature, the fixation device should not only provide rigid fixation and well tolerated by the animal but also allow drainage and daily dressing of the open wound. Further, any fixation technique developed for large animals should also be less cumbersome to apply by practicing veterinary surgeons at field level for its wide acceptance. ESF devices developed specifically for use in large animal applications [13, 121–125] are not commercially available.

A full-pin type II ESF device has been developed for equines by Nunamaker and Nash in 2008 [126–128]. The original design comprised of partially threaded self-tapping fixation pins with core diameter of 8.6 mm at threaded portion and 9.6 mm at non-threaded portion. The connecting bars are developed from composite polyurethane reinforced with stainless-steel rods. The device was designed specifically for distal limb fractures (metacarpals and metatarsals), wherein transfixation pins placed in the proximal bone segment are connected to the opposing connecting rods that are attached to a foot plate (which is rounded and angled 15–25° from the ground surface). The foot plate in turn is fixed to a customized bar shoe. Further modification of the design included an additional tapered sleeve over the smooth pins (7.94 mm), which can be compressed against the bone cortices by tightening the nuts along the inbuilt threads on the pin ends. This improved design has greater fixator stability especially at bone-pin interfaces. The fixator construct has been found to have adequate stiffness and strength to allow immediate full weight-bearing by adult animals. The modified design can support about ten times the animal's weight, as compared to the original version, which can support three times the body weight.

A novel bilateral external fixation device has been developed at the Indian Veterinary Research Institute, Izatnagar (UP), India, which comprises of a pair of threaded solid cylindrical connecting rods (sidebars), having a hexagonal flat inbuilt nut at the center and threads carved in opposite directions on both sides from the center (to allow distraction or compression of bone segments after bone fixation by turning the connecting rod in opposite directions) (Fig. 2.60) [13, 121–123]. Multiple fixation bolts help to secure the fixation pins at desired levels as per the fracture location. This fixator is unique in that it is simple and less cumbersome to apply, and fracture reduction and compression can be achieved even after bone fixation.

#### 2.3.8.1 Fixator Components

*Connecting rods (side bars)*: The stainless-steel connecting rods measure 14 mm in diameter with different lengths (22–45 cm). The center of the connecting rod has an inbuilt hexagonal nut (2 cm wide) to facilitate turning of connecting rod with a wrench. On either side, the threads are carved in opposite directions (pitch 2 mm), 'positive (right hand thread)' and 'negative (left hand thread)'.

*Fixation bolt*: The fixation bolts are in the form of rectangular blocks, having an eccentrically placed threaded hole to get secured along the connecting rods and on the other side an 8 mm smooth hole drilled perpendicular to the length of connecting rod to accept a 6–7 mm pin. The threads carved in the fixation bolts are either in 'positive (right hand)' or 'negative (left hand)' direction to secure along the corresponding side of the connecting rod. Variable number of fixation bolts can be fixed along the connecting rod at desired levels (to secure the pins exiting the bone segments).

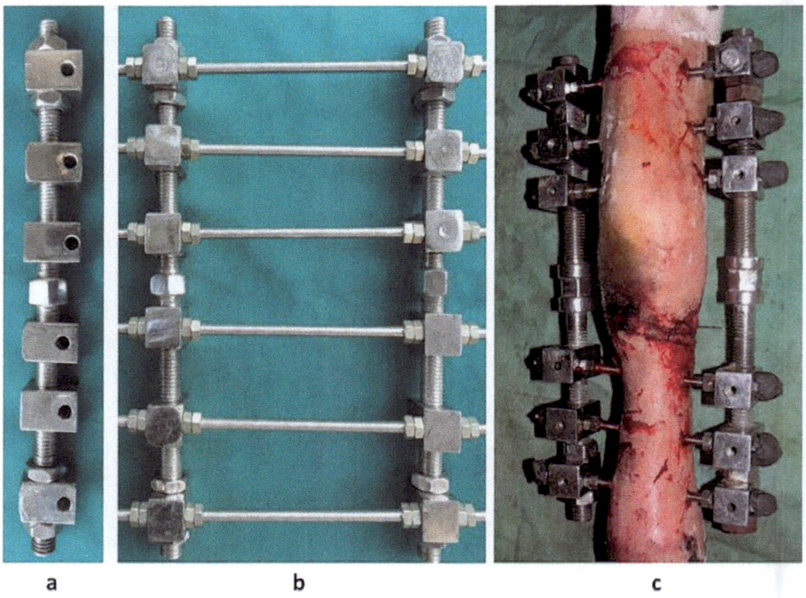

**Fig. 2.60** Different parts of novel bilateral linear fixation device: (**a**) connecting rod with clamps and check nuts fixed on either side of the outermost clamps; (**b**) ESF assembly with 6 fixation pins connected to connecting bars through clamps; and (**c**) fixator applied transarticularly to repair proximal metacarpal fracture in a cattle

*Check nuts*: Two small check nuts (for fixation along the threaded pins) are tightened on either side of the fixation bolts along the threaded pin to prevent loosening of the pin-bolt assembly. Two large nuts (for fixation along the connecting rods) are tightened on either side of outermost fixation bolts along the connecting rod to tightly secure the fixation bolts to prevent their rotation and thus achieve rigid fixation.

*Transfixation pins*: Fully threaded pins can be of negative profile or positive profile (positive-profile pins are preferred). Thread designs may be cortical or cancellous as per the location. 6–7 mm diameter pins are commonly used in adult large animals.

#### 2.3.8.2 Indications

It is indicated for the treatment of fractures in different straight long bones such as the radius-ulna, metacarpus, metatarsus, and phalanges in cattle, buffaloes, and horses. It is particularly useful to treat open infected fractures, where cast immobilization is not indicated and internal fixation (like bone plate or nail) is not desired and also suitable for transarticular application during arthrodesis or temporary immobilization of the joint to allow healing of soft tissues (ligament/tendon injuries) or fractures of bone extremities.

#### 2.3.8.3 Advantages

Novel bilateral ESF provides rigid fixation of fractures in straight long bones of large animals. Fractured bone segments can be reduced or compressed even after fixation of pins, by turning the hexagonal nut at the center of the connecting rods in opposite directions. The device is simple and less cumbersome to attach and assemble during bone fixation. The fixator design allows its usage in different straight long bones of varied length and in transarticular applications. Transfixation pins of different diameter can be fixed at desired locations. Wound dressing and care of the fixator assembly is easy during the convalescent period. As the device has minimal parts, the cost of manufacturing is less.

#### 2.3.8.4 Principles and Guidelines for Application

*Survey radiography:* Radiographs (orthogonal views) of the fractured bone are made to determine the fracture location and configuration and to plan for fixator application (to decide the size and number of fixation pins, location of pin insertion, etc.).

*Anesthesia and restraint*: Using general anesthesia, the animal is restrained either in dorsal recumbency with the limb suspended or in lateral recumbency with the fractured limb extended outside the operation table (which will facilitate through and through pin insertion) and the open wound facing the surgeon (to help reduce the bone segments and keep watch on bone alignment during fixator application). While general anesthesia is always preferred in small animals and horses, deep sedation with regional or spinal analgesia can be used in small and large ruminants, especially in hindlimb applications.

*Preparation of the surgical site*: The hair is clipped and skin is prepared with surgical scrubbing. The preparation of surgical field must include a joint above and below the fracture, and the area is properly draped. The fracture segments are reduced and held in alignment using traction and counter-traction. In case of a compound fracture, the open wound is cleaned and dressed using cotton bandage to prevent further contamination of the wound. In stable fractures, skin sutures may be applied (to cover the fracture site) leaving sufficient gap between the sutures for drainage. The proposed sites for placement of transfixation pins are chosen (using radiographic images) and marked considering the safe corridors (generally medio-lateral/latero-medial).

*Selection of pins and preparation of fixator assembly*: A proper diameter pin (not exceeding 20% of the bone diameter) is selected. In medium-sized animals weighing about 300–400 kg, 6 mm fully threaded positive-profile pins may be used; in heavy animals (>400 kg), 7 mm pins are indicated. It is important to anticipate and decide the desired number of fixation pins (based on the radiographic evaluation) before surgical fixation so that appropriate number of fixation bolts can be positioned along a pair of connecting rods. Two check nuts are placed on either side of the outermost fixation bolts along the connecting rods on both ends. The length of the connecting rods is decided as per the fracture location and configuration and the number of pins needed; in mid-diaphyseal fractures, normally four pins (two in both bone segments) are fixed, but in transarticular fixations (proximal or distal metacarpal or distal radial fractures), 5–6 pins may be needed; hence, relatively long connecting rods have to be selected so as to span the carpal/fetlock joint.

*Pin insertion technique*: Standard pin insertion technique (as described before) is followed while inserting the transfixation pins. All the pins are inserted one by one in a single plane (medio-lateral) and parallel to each other and perpendicular to the long axis of the bone (Fig. 2.61a). It is also ensured that all the pins are inserted up to the same level to facilitate fixing of the connecting rods.

*Fixation of pins with the connecting rods*: Once all the pins are passed, two small nuts are inserted through both ends of the threaded pins and are brought close to the skin (Fig. 2.61b). It is ensured that the clamps in the connecting rods are spaced as per the location of transfixation pins. The pins are then fixed to the connecting rod by inserting them into the fixation bolts (through the pin holes). It is advised to insert all the pins to the corresponding clamps at a time. Similarly, the pins that exit from the opposite skin surface are also connected to another connecting rod (Fig. 2.61c, d).

Once both connecting rods are fixed, they are brought close to the skin by gentle maneuvering (if needed central hexagonal nut may be slightly hammered down) and are fixed at the desired level, so that both connecting rods lay parallel to each other (Fig. 2.61e). The distance between the bone and the connecting rods should be kept minimum; however, at least 15–20 mm gap between the skin and connecting bars is needed to allow soft tissue swelling and regular dressing of pin-skin interfaces. Subsequently, two more nuts are inserted through both ends of the threaded pins (Fig. 2.61f). The pins are cleaned from any tissue debris before inserting the nuts for smooth passage. The nuts on either side of the fixation bolts, along the threaded pins, are tightened against the bolts to achieve stable pin-bolt junctions (Fig. 2.61g). The check nuts on either side of outermost fixation bolts along the connecting rod are then tightened to rigidly secure the fixator assembly (Fig. 2.61i). The extra length of pins is cut, and the cut ends may be sealed using epoxy putty to prevent possible injury to the contralateral limb and to the handler during routine wound dressing (Fig. 2.61k, l). The surgical/open wound is approximated by

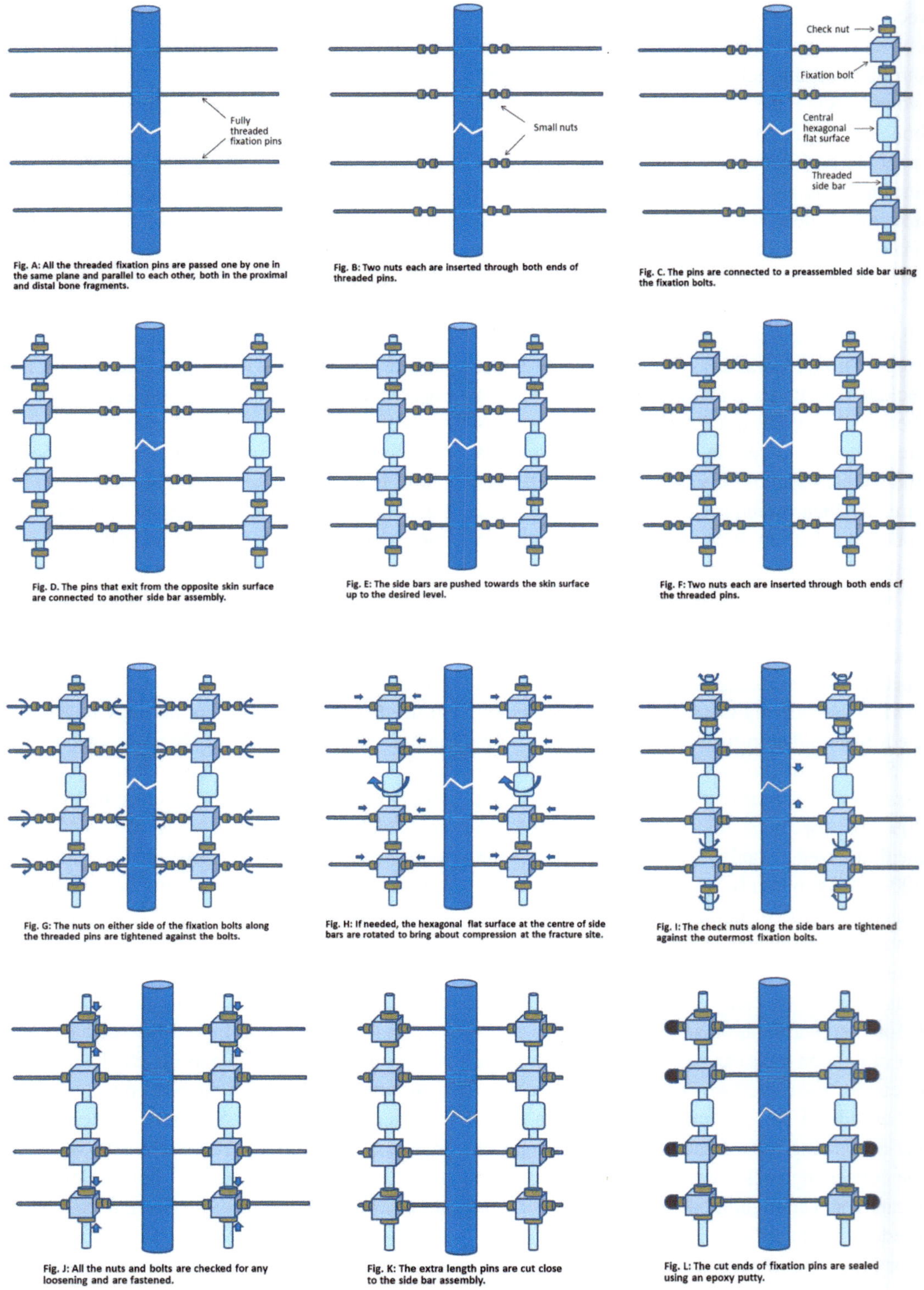


**Fig. 2.61** Technique of application of bilateral linear fixator

placing interrupted skin sutures when possible (if not done before).

#### 2.3.8.5 Postoperative Care and Management

Management of animals in the immediate postoperative period (48–72 h) is more critical as they may feel discomfort by the presence of the external frames. The animal may take some time to get accustomed to the fixator; hence, regular observation of the animal is required during the period. Broad-spectrum antibiotic and anti-inflammatory/analgesic drugs are given for 3–5 days. As an ESF is generally applied in an open infected fracture, prolonged antibiotic therapy may be needed. In such cases, it is always advised to change the antibiotic, as per the sensitivity test results.

Regular antiseptic dressing of the pin-skin interfaces and the skin wound (in case of open fractures) is done till the healing occurs. Pin site discharge is common with ESF; hence, prolonged dressing of the pin site is needed using an antiseptic solution like chlorhexidine or povidone iodine and an antibiotic solution. The ESF frame may be covered with a sleeve or bandage to prevent licking of the pin-skin interfaces. The movement of the animal should be avoided during the post-fixation period; however, walking should not be restricted for prolonged period, as it is an excellent form of physical therapy, which can help in early bone union.

#### 2.3.8.6 Removal of Fixator

After the radiological union of the fracture (generally 8–12 weeks), the pins are cut using a pin cutter and the ESF frame is removed. The cut pins are pulled out of the limb with pliers. After removal of pins, the pin tract is cleaned with an antiseptic solution. The limb may be temporarily splinted and the activity of the animal restricted for another week or so.

### 2.3.9 Circular External Skeletal Fixation

Circular external fixation (CEF) system was first described by a Russian scientist, Ilizarov, in the early 1960s. In CEF systems, relatively small diameter wires/pins are fixed under tension across a ring anchoring at both ends; such pins placed under tension provide good axial strength. Due to the mechanical advantage, Ilizarov model of CEF systems has been extensively used for treatment of a variety of musculoskeletal disorders like fractures, dislocations, arthrodesis, correction of angular deformities, and limb-lengthening procedures in human as well as small animal practice. Even though CEF systems were first introduced in the early 1990s for small animal applications, it has only recently attracted the attention of large animal orthopedic surgeons mostly for fracture fixation in large animals. The most commonly used CEF system in small animal applications is marketed by IMEX Veterinary Inc. However, there are many other systems available across the world. Nevertheless, CEF systems developed specifically for use in large animals are not commercially available.

#### 2.3.9.1 Fixator Components

Apart from fixation pins, the circular fixation system comprises of three basic components: rings, connecting rods, and fixation bolts [13, 91, 95, 103, 129] (Fig. 2.62).

*Circular rings* (half-rings): A typical CEF system consists of four full rings or eight half-rings (two rings blocks in each major bone segment). The number of rings required in a particular case may depend on the bone involved and the location of fracture. Transarticular fixations generally require more number of rings, and often to maintain the normal joint angle and movement, ¾ rings or ½ rings are used.

Circular rings made from different materials such as stainless steel, carbon fiber, and aluminum are available for use in small animals. The rings ranging in diameter from 50 to 150 mm are available; the ring size depends on the site of application and the size of animal, but it should be large enough to maintain a gap of about 2–3 cm between the skin and ring around the limb. The thickness of the rings varies with the material used; carbon fiber and aluminum rings are thicker than stainless-steel rings.

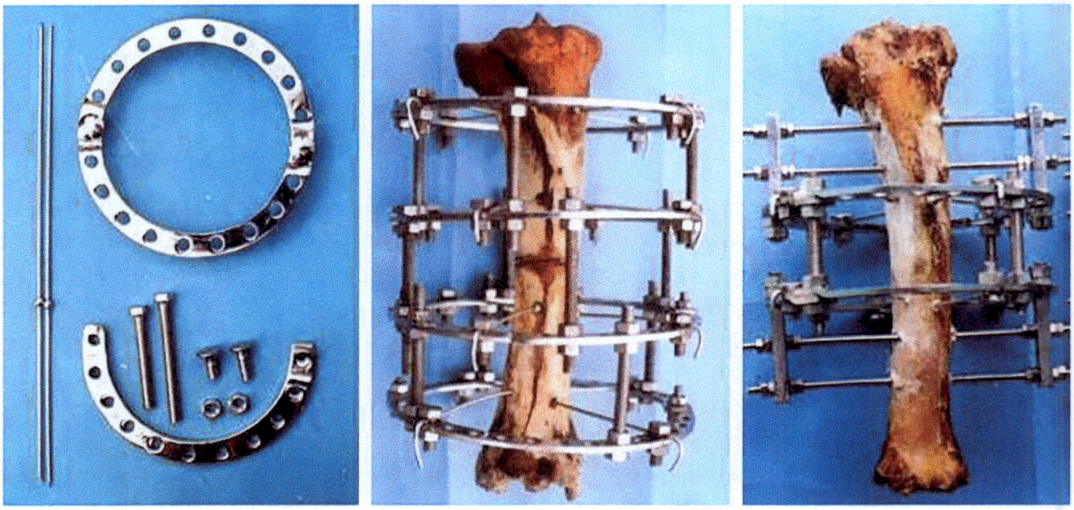

**Fig. 2.62** Components of CEF and hybrid fixation systems for large animals

For large animal applications, CEF rings made of stainless steel, aluminum, and mild steel have been developed. The steel rings measuring 5 mm thickness and 20 mm width having 18–28 equidistant holes (10 mm diameter) to accommodate connecting rods and fixation bolts (8 mm) are mechanically adequate in most adult large animals. Although ring diameter may vary as per the location of fracture (tibial fractures require relatively large diameter rings, while metacarpal/metatarsal fractures need only small diameter rings) and the animals' weight, about 150–220 mm inner diameter rings are generally required for large animals. The fixation systems developed using mild steel or aluminum are sufficiently rigid and are more economical for fixation in large animals.

*Fixation pins*: They can be smooth or beaded (olive wire). Beaded/olive wires are specialized wires with a larger diameter bead/ball at their midpoint, preventing movement of the bone (translation) in relation to the pin. They strengthen the fixation and allow translation of bone segments when traction is applied from the opposite end. 1.0–1.8 mm (1.0, 1.2, 1.4, 1.5, 1.6, and 1.8 mm) wires/pins are generally used in small animals based on the body weight and bone fracture location (1.0 mm in cats and toy breed dogs to 1.8 mm in giant breed dogs). 2.0–2.5 mm pins may be used in young large animals, calves and foals weighing <100 kg; in animals weighing about 100–200 kg, 3 mm pins; in animals weighing about 200–300 kg, 3.5 mm pins; and in heavy adult animals weighing >300 kg, 3.5–4.5 mm pins. A pair of pins (cross pins) is fixed to each ring under tension using fixation bolts.

*Fixation bolts/nuts*: Bolts are slotted or cannulated to fix the transfixation pins to the rings. Cannulated bolts have better pin holding strength and are preferred especially in large animal fixation systems [129]. The hole/slot present in the bolt should be optimum to accept the fixation pins intended for use.

*Connecting rods/nuts*: The number of connecting rods required between each ring block may vary based on the weight of the animal and required fixation rigidity. A minimum of 2–3 connecting rods are used in small animal applications, and at least four rods are fixed in large animals, between the rings by tightening nuts on either side of the rings. The distance between the rings can be adjusted by tightening or loosening the nuts to provide tension or compression between the fracture segments. Five to six millimeter diameter connecting rods are usually used in small animal fixation systems and 8–10 mm connecting rods in large animal fixation systems.

Hybrid external skeletal fixation (HESF) is becoming popular to treat fractures with short segment. Here, the small bone segment near the joint is stabilized using small diameter pins anchored to a ring, and primary large bone segment is stabilized with linear components and pins. As the hybrid frame combines both linear and circular ESF frames, it has the advantages of both the systems and superior mechanical properties [130, 131]. In large animal fracture fixations, hybrid fixation systems are useful to treat fractures of the middle to proximal diaphysis of the tibia and radius, where it is often difficult to fix a circular ring (due to large soft tissue covering and eccentric placement of the bone) [132, 133]. Further, by using linear fixator elements, relatively smaller-size rings can be used, which in turn increases fixator stiffness.

#### 2.3.9.2 Indications

In small animals, CEF is indicated for treatment of certain fractures which are otherwise difficult to treat (severely comminuted open fractures). Other indications are correction of angular deformities, treatment of non-unions, extremity lengthening, and arthrodeses, etc. [91, 98, 134]. In large animals, CEF is mostly used for treatment of long bone fractures, especially of the tibia, where cast application does not provide adequate level of fixation and linear fixation systems are not advised [13, 121, 129, 135–138]. As CEF is less traumatic with the use of relatively small diameter pins, it is also indicated in open fractures with severe soft tissue injuries to achieve more biological healing. CEF is also indicated in transarticular (particularly transtarsal) applications [139]. Fractures of extremities of long bones can also be better treated using a circular or hybrid ESF.

#### 2.3.9.3 Application of CEF

*Survey radiography*: Radiographs (orthogonal views) of the fractured bone are made before planning for surgical fixation, which will help determine the fracture configuration and location and plan for fixator application (to decide the size and number of fixation pins, location of pin insertion, etc.). Radiographs of the contralateral limb often help determine the normal length of the bone.

*Anesthesia and restraint:* Under general anesthesia, the patient is preferably restrained in dorsal recumbency with the affected limb under suspension. In large ruminants involving hindlimb surgeries, regional/epidural analgesia can be used along with deep sedation, and the animal can be restrained in lateral recumbency with the fractured limb extended outside the operation table and the open wound facing the surgeon, to facilitate fracture reduction and fixation.

*Preparation of the surgical site:* The hair is clipped and skin is prepared with surgical scrubbing as for any orthopedic procedure. The preparation of the surgical field must include a joint above and below the fracture, and the whole area is properly draped. Once the surgical site is properly prepared, the proposed sites for placing the transfixation pins are chosen (using radiographic images) and marked.

*Construction of fixator assembly*: Proper diameter pins, connecting rods, and rings are selected (as described before). The fixator frame can be preassembled based on radiographs and then modified slightly at the time of surgery (Fig. 2.63). The frames should have a minimum of two rings in each major bone segment. The rings are spread along the entire length of each bone segment to achieve maximum mechanical advantage. In case one of the fracture segments is too small, only one ring is positioned at the level of small bone segment, and two rings are positioned at the adjoining normal bone (for transarticular fixation). The rings are interconnected using four equidistantly placed connecting rods between each ring block using nuts. Once all the rings are properly positioned along the connecting rods, the connecting rod-ring interfaces are stabilized by tightening the nuts on either side of the rings.

The fractured limb is inserted into the preassembled CEF frame and held in such a way that the fractured bone is centered within the ring block and the rings are aligned with the chosen level of pin insertion sites.

*Fracture reduction*: Fracture can be reduced either by closed method or by open method.

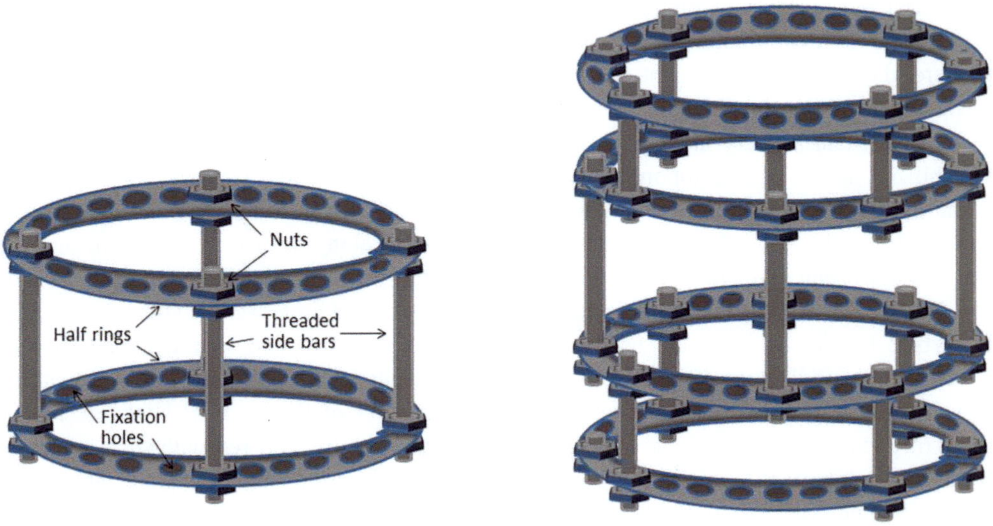


Fig. A: Two half rings are joined to form a full ring, two full rings are joined using 4 threaded side bars and nuts.

Fig. B: Additional rings are joined by using 4 threaded side bars between the rings to make at least a 4-ring fixator construct (the number of rings and the distance between the rings is determined by the type and location of fracture-radiographic examination).

**Fig. 2.63** Construction of CEF frame

Closed reduction is less traumatic and does not disturb the blood circulation at the fracture site and facilitate biological healing. Fracture healing and functional recovery are rapid with closed fracture reduction. Closed reduction can be more easily achieved in distal bones of the limb due to least soft tissue covering, especially in fresh cases. If required, semi-open method (by giving a small incision or by extending the wound margin) can be adopted to reduce the bone fragments. In cases with severe overriding of bone segments and adhesions (long-standing cases), open reduction is advised.

*Pin insertion technique:* Standard pin insertion technique is followed (as described before in detail). About 0.5–1.0 cm long skin incision is made (proximal to distal) at the chosen site of pin insertion, and a similar incision is made at the pin exit point in the opposite skin surface. Predrilling is generally not practiced while passing the pins during CEF fixation. The selected fixation pins are introduced along the dorsal/ventral side of the ring. If possible, one of the cross pins is positioned above the ring and another below the ring to avoid collision within the medullary cavity. The pin is carefully introduced by hand through the soft tissues up to the level of the bone cortex to gently push aside the vessels and nerves. The pin should not be inserted too close to the fracture line (at least 10 mm gap should be present between the fracture line and the pin). The pins are crossed (at 60°–90° angle to each other) from craniomedial to caudolateral and caudomedial to craniolateral direction or vice versa. As the angle between the pins decreases, the bone segment may slide (translate) from the center of the ring. This translation of bone segments can be minimized by using olive wires/beaded pins. Pins are introduced using low-speed (ideal is 150–400 rpm), high torque power drills to avoid wobbling (which could cause premature loosening) and help reduce thermal necrosis of the bone tissue. It is important to drill in small pulses (with 30 s between the pulses) to allow for dissipation of heat generated. While drilling, sterile cold solution is continuously dropped at the skin-pin interface to minimize thermal injury.

It is advisable to first pass one pin each at the level of farther rings (proximal-most and distal-most) and loosely fix the pins to the rings using fixation bolts and nuts (this will allow proper positioning of fixator assembly and fracture

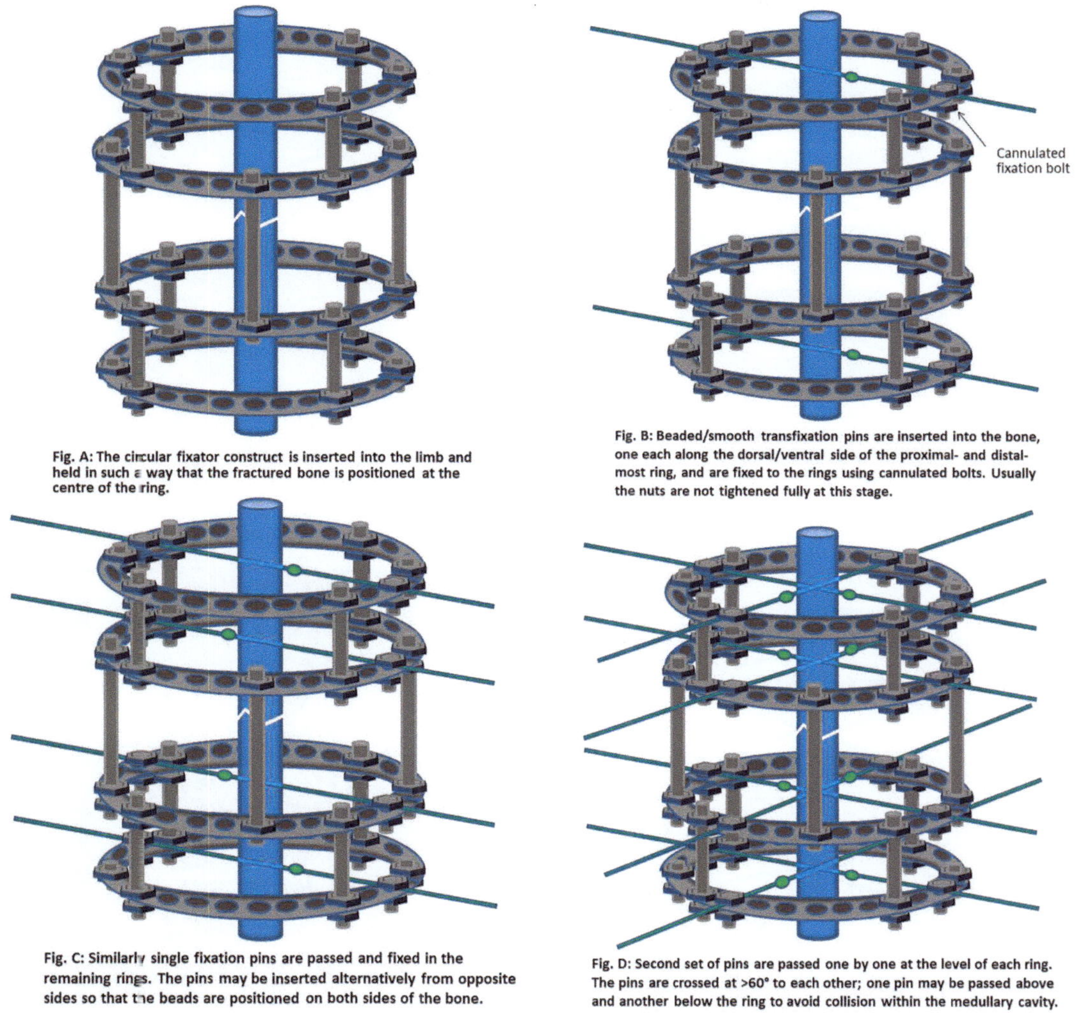


Fig. A: The circular fixator construct is inserted into the limb and held in such a way that the fractured bone is positioned at the centre of the ring.

Fig. B: Beaded/smooth transfixation pins are inserted into the bone, one each along the dorsal/ventral side of the proximal- and distal-most ring, and are fixed to the rings using cannulated bolts. Usually the nuts are not tightened fully at this stage.

Fig. C: Similarly single fixation pins are passed and fixed in the remaining rings. The pins may be inserted alternatively from opposite sides so that the beads are positioned on both sides of the bone.

Fig. D: Second set of pins are passed one by one at the level of each ring. The pins are crossed at >60° to each other; one pin may be passed above and another below the ring to avoid collision within the medullary cavity.

**Fig. 2.64** Technique of CEF application

reduction and alignment) (Fig. 2.64). Once it is ensured that the fixator frame is properly positioned along the fractured bone/limb and bone segments are adequately aligned, fixation pins are then passed at the level of remaining rings (closer to fracture site) alternatively and fixed to the rings. Once again, the alignment of the fixator and bone segments is re-checked, and if needed, the fixator frame can be slightly manoeuvered (by repositioning the fixation bolts along the ring) to correct. The second set of pins is then passed one by one at the level of each ring (either above or below the rings) and is fixed to the rings.

*Fixation of pins with the rings:* The transfixation pins are fixed to the rings using slotted or cannulated bolts. Slotted bolts are technically easier to adjust, but cannulated bolts provide greater stability to the fixation. The cannulated bolts are first inserted through both ends of the transfixation pin and slid along till they are at the level of the ring and then inserted into the fixation holes. Care should be taken not to bend the pin while approximating it to the ring. When required, fissured pin-nuts or washers can be used to achieve approximation. Fixation bolt is tightened to the ring using a nut at one end of the pin (beaded end of the pin in olive wires). The

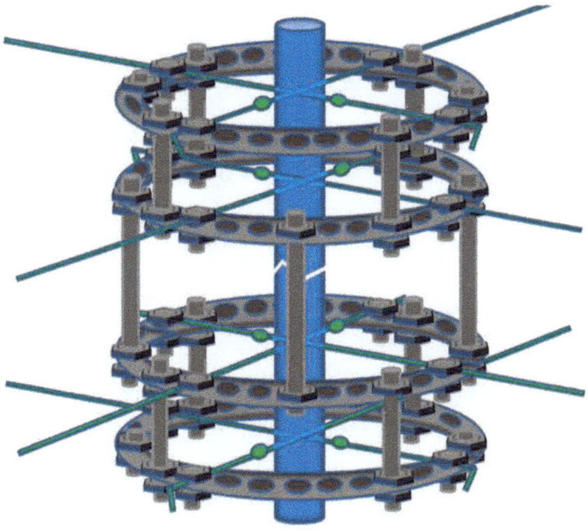

Fig. E: The fracture reduction is checked, and if needed the bone can be manipulated slightly to re-align the fragments. The pins are then fastened to the rings by tightening the nuts along the fixation bolts at the side of bead. The extra length of pin may be cut and bent towards the ring inwardly.

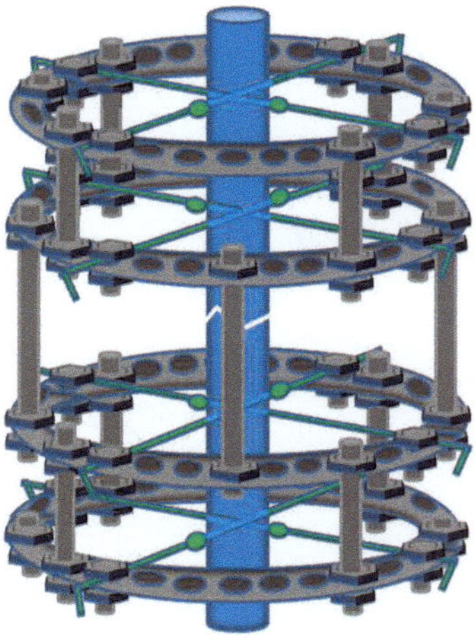

Fig. F: The pins are tensioned using a 'wire-tensioner' from the end opposite to the bead, and the fixation bolts are tightened to fix the pin to the respective ring before bending and cutting the extra length pins.

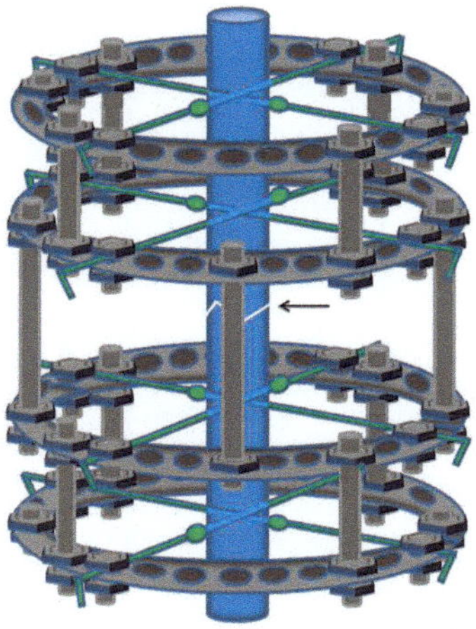

Fig. G: The bone fixation is re-checked, and compression can be achieved at the fracture site (arrow) by turning the nuts along the side bars between the central ring blocks. All the nuts are then checked and if needed tightened to secure the fixator assembly.

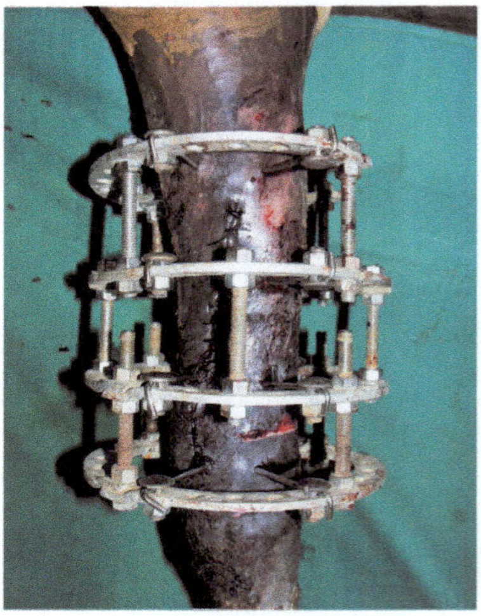

H. Clinical application of a four-ring CEF in a horse

**Fig. 2.64** (continued)

fixation pin is then tensioned from the other end, before fixing it with the ring to increase the fixation rigidity. As far as possible, all the pins are equally tensioned to share and distribute load equally. Generally, 20–30 kg force is adequate for animals weighing <10 kg (1 mm pin), 30–60 kg for animals weighing 10–20 kg (1.2 mm pin), and 60–90 kg for animals weighing >20 kg (1.5/1.6 mm pin). Tension should not be more than 30 kg in partial/incomplete rings. Similarly, each pin is snugly fixed to the ring one by one by tightening the nuts along the fixation bolts. Once the pins are fixed to the rings, the extra length of the pins is cut short (using a pin cutter), and the cut end is bent toward the ring and inwardly (with a plier) to avoid any damage to the patient and the handler from the cut end of the pins.

### 2.3.9.4 Postoperative Care and Management

Management of animals in the immediate post-fixation period is critical (especially large animals), as they may feel discomfort by the presence of the external fixator components. The animal may take some time to get accustomed; hence, regular observation of the animal is required during this period [129]. Regular antiseptic dressing of the pin-skin interfaces and the open wound (in case of open fractures) is done until the healing occurs. Pin site discharge is common; hence, prolonged dressing of the pin-skin interfaces is needed. A broad-spectrum antibiotic is administered for 5–7 days. If prolonged therapy is needed, the antibiotic may be changed as per the sensitivity test.

The fixator frame may be covered with a sleeve or wrapped with a bandage to prevent the animal from licking the pin-skin interfaces and biting the fixator components. However, it is not always required to wrap the fixator, and only the incision site/wound is dressed as the skin surface is generally protected from direct floor contact due to the presence of rings. The exercise is restricted in the immediate post-fixation period; however, walking in a closed enclosure should be allowed as early as possible, as it is an excellent form of physical therapy to accelerate bone healing and regain functional recovery.

#### 2.3.9.5 Removal of Fixator Assembly

After the radiological union of the fracture, the fixation pins are cut using a pin cutter. and the frame is removed. The pins are pulled out with pliers, making sure that the beaded pins are pulled from the side of the bead. After removal of pins, pin tract is cleaned with antiseptic solution, and the activity of the animal is restricted for another week. Generally, pin tracts heal quickly within a few days.

### 2.3.10 Acrylic- or Epoxy-Pin Fixation Systems

The connecting bars of an ESF frame can be constructed using acrylics, such as polymethyl methacrylate (PMMA) or epoxy materials, instead of steel rods to overcome some of the limitations of metallic fixator components. This type of 'free-form' fixation has the advantage that the pins can be passed at different directions regardless of the connecting bar/ring location, and any diameter pin can be used irrespective of the clamp size [140]. Such free-form fixation has been used since long to treat mandibular fractures in small animals and long bone fractures in birds with good success. The modified technique of epoxy-pin fixation described here is very versatile and mechanically strong [123, 141–145], and it can be used to treat various long bone fractures in different species of animals such as dogs, cats, sheep, goats, calves, foals, and birds [146–150]. Generally, all animals and birds weighing up to about 100 kg can be treated. It is economical and also easily applied by a practicing veterinarian with minimal facilities and expertise.

#### 2.3.10.1 Fixator Components

*Fixation pins*: In general, pins used in free-form fixation are slightly larger than typical CEF as pins cannot be tensioned to increase their strength. Smooth pins (Kirschner wires) of different diameter ranging from 1.2 mm to 2.0 mm are generally used in dogs and cats (based on body weight, 1.2–1.5 mm wires in the metacarpal and metatarsal bones, 1.5–2.0 mm pins in the radius-ulna and tibia), 1.5–2.0 mm pins in sheep and goats, and 2.0–3.0 mm pins in calves and foals. Pins over 3 mm cannot be used as they are difficult to bend.

*Acrylic/epoxy material*: For acrylic-pin fixation, any commercially available medical-grade acrylic material such as self-curing dental acrylic (Pyrax Polymars), which is easily available and economical, can be used. Along with this, polyvinyl chloride (PVC) pipes of desired diameter (20 mm diameter adequate in most applications) are needed to construct the connecting bars. For epoxy-pin fixation, any commercially available industrial-grade epoxy material can be used, such as M-seal (Pidilite Ltd). They are available as regular or fast curing; fast-curing epoxy can polymerize faster, leading to quick hardening once applied. About 200 g to 1 kg epoxy material may be required to construct a fixator frame as per the species and size of the animal and location of fracture.

#### 2.3.10.2 Indications

Indicated for fixation of long bone fractures (especially open infected fractures) below the elbow and stifle joints in dogs, cats, sheep, goats, calves, foals, and birds (weighing up to 100 kg). It is also indicated for immobilization of joints (below the elbow and stifle) by transarticular fixation (joint luxations, tendon and ligament injuries, and for arthrodesis, etc.) and correction of angular limb (antebrachial) deformities. Fractures of the mandible can also be treated effectively by epoxy-pin fixation.

#### 2.3.10.3 Advantages

Free-form fixation provides stable fixation of fractures in lightweight animals (<100 kg). The technique is very versatile, as the epoxy-pin connecting bars can be angled at the level of the joint without compromising the fixation stability and the connecting bars/rings of different diameters can be constructed. The technique is least cumbersome, does not require fixation clamps or any special instruments/materials, and is economical too. The device is lightweight; hence, small animals and birds can tolerate well. This is very easy to design and apply in clinical situations by practicing veterinarians in any remote corner with minimal facilities and expertise.

#### 2.3.10.4 Technique of Application

*Survey radiography*: Radiographs (orthogonal views) of the fractured bone help to determine the fracture type and location and plan for fixator application (to decide the size and number of fixation pins, fixator design, etc.).

*Anesthesia and restraint*: In dogs, cats, foals, and birds, general anesthesia is advised. In sheep, goats, and calves, fixation can be done with deep sedation under regional anesthesia; in hindlimb fractures, epidural analgesia can be used, and in forelimbs, nerve blocks can be used. General anesthesia may be needed in some cases, especially for forelimb fixations. The animal is positioned as for any ESF application. A cotton rope tied at the level of the digits/hoof can help to suspend the limb or may be used to pull the limb straight manually to help in fracture reduction and restraining of the animal during fixator application.

*Fracture reduction and alignment*: After preparing the fractured limb for aseptic surgery by hair clipping and scrubbing, the fracture segments are reduced and aligned by closed method using traction and counter-traction. Fracture reduction may be easily achieved in metacarpal and metatarsal bones in all species of animals and also in radius-ulna fractures in dogs, cats, sheep, and goats. In some cases, fracture is reduced by maneuvering through the open wound. If needed, the skin wound may be slightly extended to reduce the overriding bone segments. In most fractures of the straight bones, reduced bone segments can be maintained in apposition manually; if needed, bone-holding forceps may be used. In cases of severe overriding, especially in fractures of the tibia, hemi-cerclage wiring may be done to reduce and temporarily stabilize the bone segments. If the fracture reduction is stable, the skin wound may be sutured using simple interrupted sutures by keeping enough space between the sutures for drainage and dressing. Suturing may also be done after fixator application; however, it is slightly more difficult. It is not advised to completely close the skin wound, and in most cases, it may not be possible. Suturing the skin may help in bringing the soft tissue cover around the fracture site and also help secure the reduced bone segments in alignment until fixator application.

*Fixation of pins*: The proposed sites for transcortical passage of pins (based on radiographic evaluation) are marked on the skin as per the fracture type and fixator design, and small release incisions (4–5 mm) are made. In bilateral uniplanar designs, at least two pins are passed either medio-laterally or latero-medially in both proximal and distal fracture segments (Figs. 2.66, 2.67, 2.68, 2.69, 2.70, 2.71, and 2.72). In multiplanar linear and circular designs, the pins are passed in the same plane from craniomedial to caudolateral and caudomedial to craniolateral directions or vice versa; two pins are passed at one point at an angle of about 60° or more; at least two-point fixation is provided in both fracture segments. Increasing the number of pins increases the fixation rigidity, and it is desirable to use maximum number of transcortical pins spanning the whole length of the bone. When fracture is at one end of the bone (one of the fracture segments is very small), at least two pins are passed in the adjacent normal long bone, spanning the joint area (transarticular fixation). Using standard technique (as described before), the transfixation pins are inserted.

#### 2.3.10.5 Construction of ESF Frame Using Acrylic

After all the pins are inserted, the pins in the same plane are affixed to the PVC pipes (by piercing the pipe through and through the pin ends) to prepare a temporary scaffold of connecting bars (in uniplanar design, two connecting bars, and in multiplanar design, four connecting bars) (Figs. 2.65 and 2.66). The connecting bars (PVC pipes) are aligned close to the skin leaving a gap of about 2 cm from the skin. The connecting bars on both sides can also be joined at proximal and distal ends (by using a single long PVC pipe),

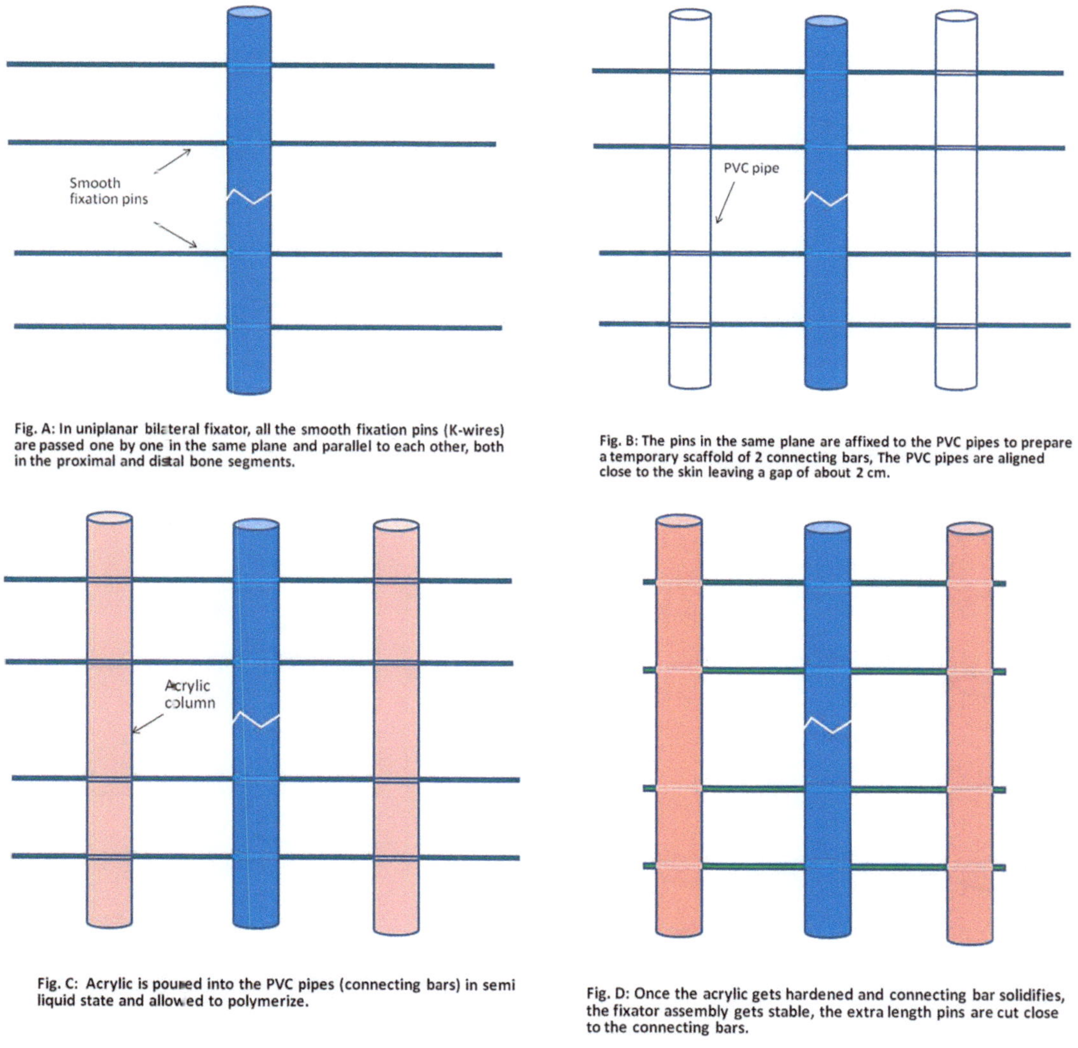


**Fig. 2.65** Acrylic-pin external skeletal fixation technique

which will help prevent movement of pins during the post-fixation period. The acrylic powder (polymer) and liquid hardener (monomer) are mixed in a pre-cooled glass beaker with the help of a spatula, immediately before application with continuous stirring, to maintain a flowing consistency. If it becomes hard due to delay in application, it should be discarded and a fresh mix prepared. Acrylic is poured into the PVC pipes in semi-liquid (dough) state with the hollow pipes sealed at the bottom using an adhesive tape. Care should be taken to prevent any leakage of the liquid acrylic from the points of pin insertion, by reinforcing the pin insertion points with an adhesive tape. The acrylic dough is allowed to flow down the pipe making sure that the complete PVC column is filled uniformly without leaving any air pockets. The acrylic is then allowed to polymerize and harden for 10–15 min. As polymerization is an exothermic reaction releasing heat, thermal injury to the tissues may occur, which can be prevented by using cold saline and ice packs around the skin. The fumes produced during polymerization are noxious and toxic; hence, one should wear mask while mixing acrylic powder with liquid, and adequate care is

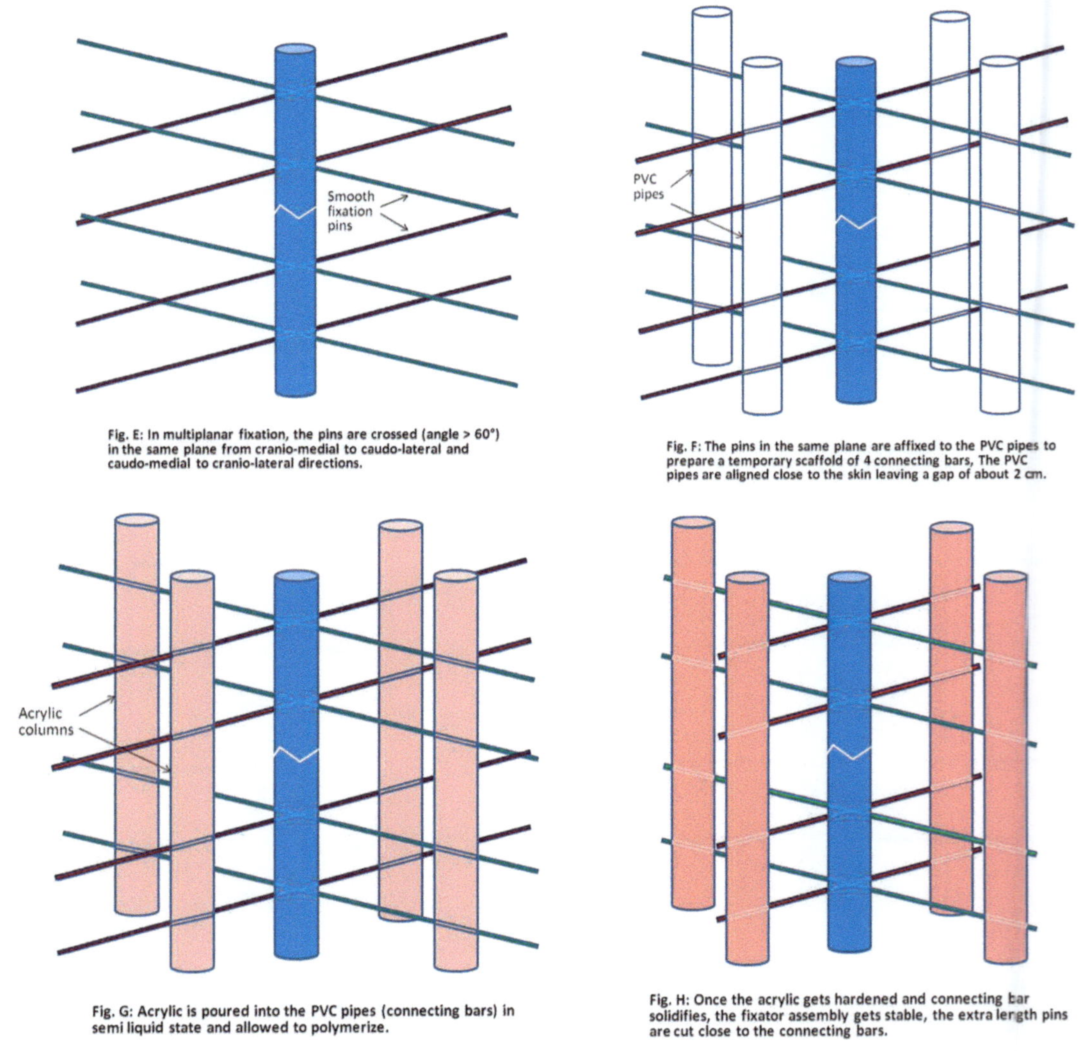


**Fig. 2.65** (continued)

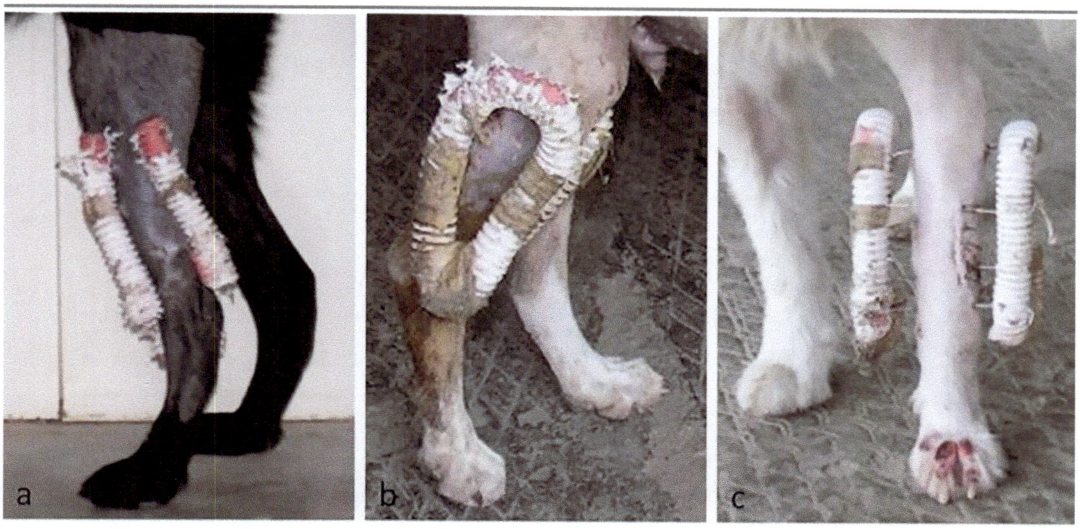


**Fig. 2.66** Acrylic-pin ESF (multiplanar type III) applied for treatment of tibial and radius-ulna fractures in dogs. (**a**) four independent connecting bars are constructed, (**b** and **c**) connecting bars on both sides are joined at the proximal and distal ends, which provide more stable fixation by preventing bone translation

taken to reduce the production of fumes by mixing acrylic part by part in a pre-cooled glass beaker.

#### 2.3.10.6 Construction of Pin Scaffold for Epoxy-Pin Fixation

Once all the transfixation pins are placed, the pins in the same plane are bent toward the fracture site (proximal pins are bent downwards; distal pins are bent upwards) using a pin bender (Figs. 2.67 and 2.68). The pins are bent as close to the bone as possible, by leaving a gap of at least 2 cm between the skin and the connecting bar to allow inflammatory swelling and dressing of the wounds. The bent pins are joined using an adhesive tape. If the fixation pins are long enough, they may connect each other after bending. If the bent pins do not connect, additional pieces of pins can be used to join them. In multiplanar design, after joining the bent fixation pins to make connecting bar scaffold, the two connecting bars on each side may be joined at the proximal and distal ends (using additional pieces of pins) to make a rectangular frame, which can strengthen the fixation stability (Figs. 2.69, 2.70, 2.71, and 2.72). If the connecting bars are very long (as in transarticular fixation), additional articulations may be fixed between the connecting bars at the center of the frame. Alternatively, all the four connecting bars may be joined using additional pieces of pins at desired locations (at least one each at proximal and distal ends) of the scaffold to construct a circular fixator frame. Variable size/length/shape connecting bars/rings can be constructed on the spot as per the case situation.

#### 2.3.10.7 Application of Epoxy Dough Along the Pin Scaffold

After making the scaffold of interconnecting pins, the fracture fixation is checked for the alignment of bone segments again, as it is possible to correct minor defects in angulation/alignment even at this stage. After ensuring proper reduction of fracture segments, the epoxy resin and hardener are thoroughly mixed to make uniform colored dough. The epoxy dough is then applied along the pin scaffold so as to incorporate the bent pins within the mold (Figs. 2.67d, 2.69f, and 2.71e). The connecting bars and the circular rings are thus constructed keeping the fracture segments in alignment. Care is taken to maintain the continuity of the epoxy dough without any break/crack while constructing the fixator frame.

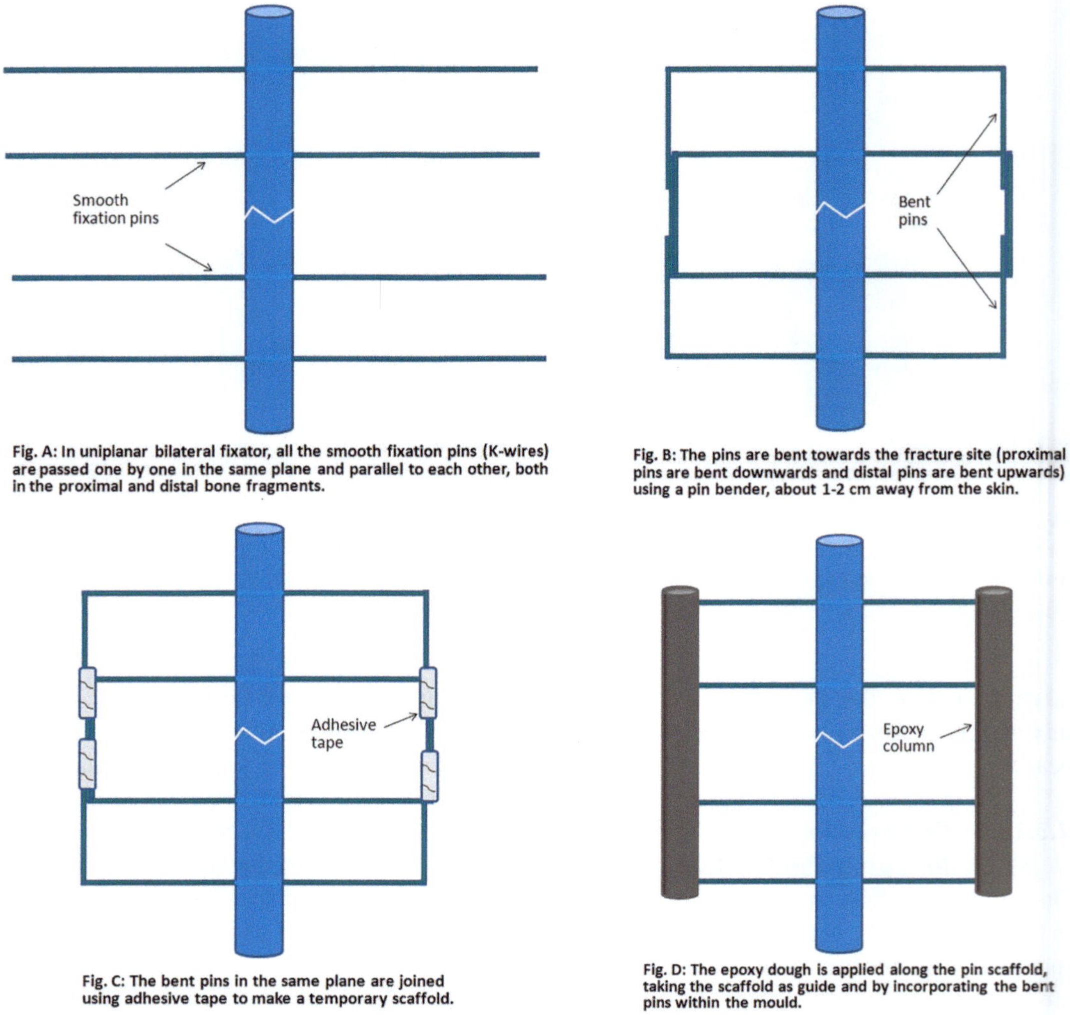


Fig. A: In uniplanar bilateral fixator, all the smooth fixation pins (K-wires) are passed one by one in the same plane and parallel to each other, both in the proximal and distal bone fragments.

Fig. B: The pins are bent towards the fracture site (proximal pins are bent downwards and distal pins are bent upwards) using a pin bender, about 1-2 cm away from the skin.

Fig. C: The bent pins in the same plane are joined using adhesive tape to make a temporary scaffold.

Fig. D: The epoxy dough is applied along the pin scaffold, taking the scaffold as guide and by incorporating the bent pins within the mould.

**Fig. 2.67** Bilateral uniplanar (type II) epoxy-pin fixation technique

The diameter of the connecting bars/rings may vary as per the fracture situation and weight of the animal. In small animals (dogs, cats, sheep, and goats), 10–20 mm diameter connecting bars, and in calves and foals, 20–25 mm diameter connecting bars may be needed. The surface of the connecting bars/rings is smoothened using oily/waxy surface. The epoxy-pin construct is then allowed to 'set (harden)' for about 30–60 min. During this time, the animal should be completely restrained to prevent any inadvertent movement of the fixator frame. Once hardened, the fixator frame becomes very strong, and the animal can be allowed to bear weight on the limb.

#### 2.3.10.8 Postoperative Care and Management

The animal should be allowed only limited weight-bearing soon after bone fixation. Weight-bearing can be gradually increased after about 1–2 weeks in stable fractures. In unstable fractures, prolonged immobilization may be needed to prevent any undue load at the fracture site. Regular antibiotic and anti-inflammatory drugs should be administered for 3–5 days, as

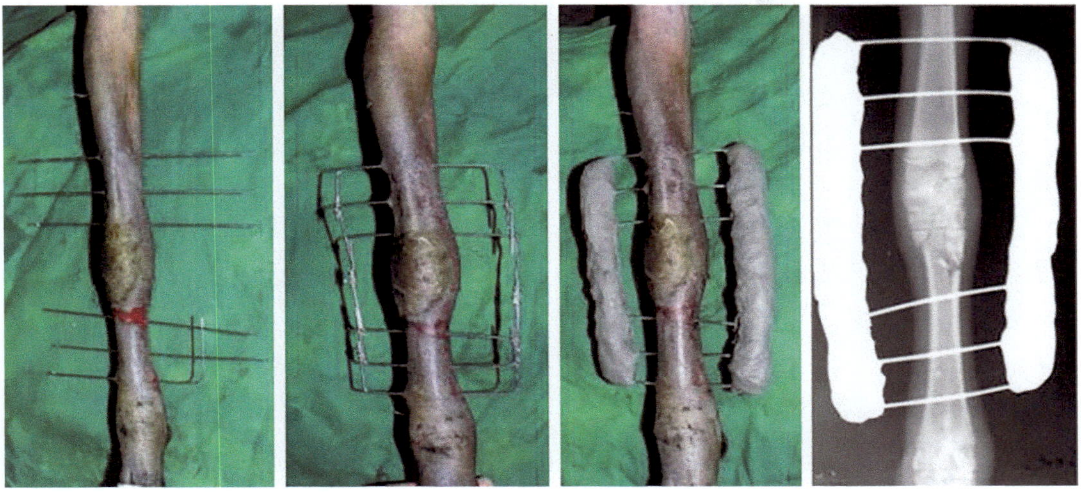

**Fig. 2.68** Bilateral uniplanar (type II) epoxy-pin fixation for fixation of proximal metacarpal fracture in a goat

per the case. If infection persists, prolonged antibiotic therapy is advised (as per the sensitivity test). The external fixator components are regularly watched for any change in the position and shape (bending/breakage) of fixator components. The pin-skin interfaces are regularly cleaned with antiseptic solution, so till complete healing of the open wound. Every 15 days, the animal is

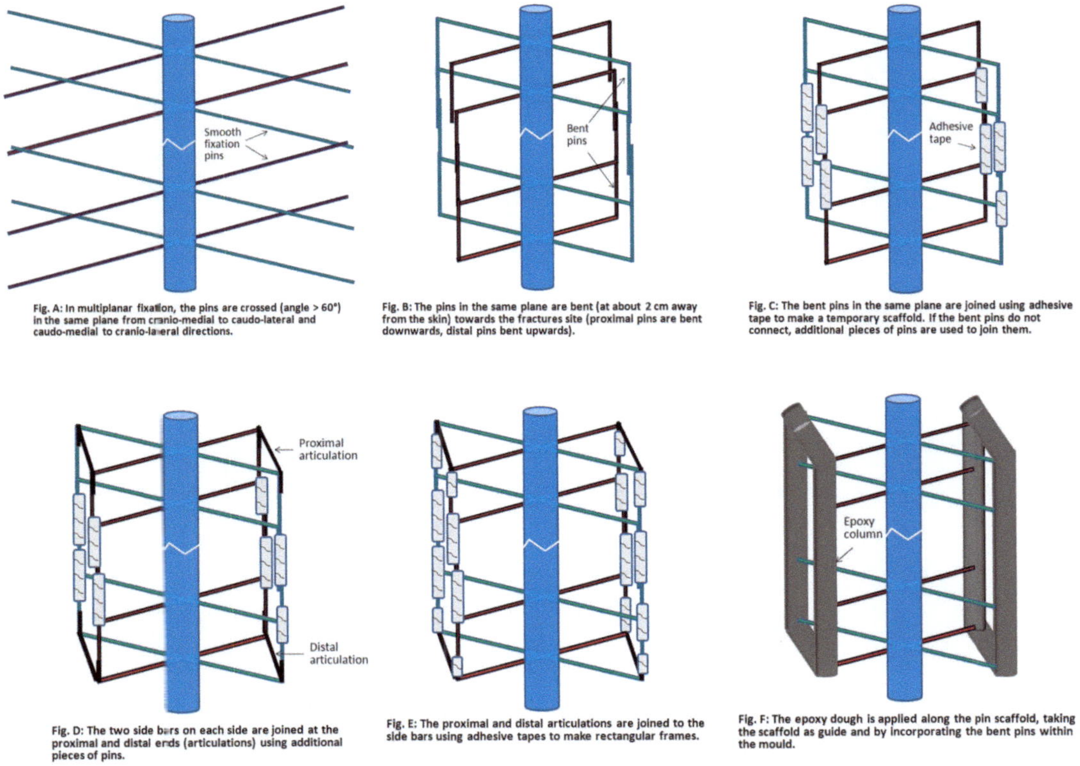


**Fig. 2.69** Bilateral multiplanar (type III) epoxy-pin fixation technique

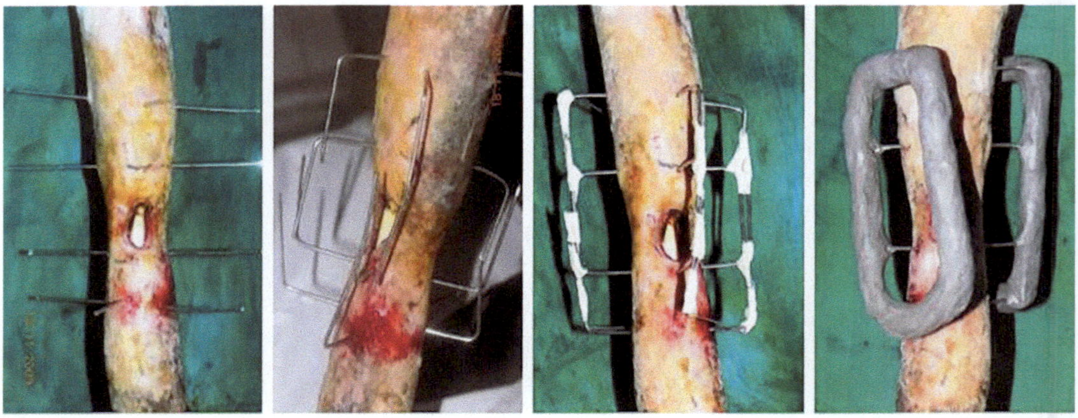

**Fig. 2.70** Bilateral multiplanar epoxy-pin fixation in the metacarpus of a calf

subjected to radiographic examination to observe for the status of fixation and bone healing.

#### 2.3.10.9 Removal of Fixator Assembly

Once the radiographic healing (bridging callus) is evident, the fixator assembly is removed by cutting the fixation pins (between the skin and connecting bars) on both sides using a pin cutter. The cut ends of the pins are pulled out using a plier, and the pin holes are flushed using an antiseptic solution such as povidone iodine. After the removal of the fixator, the limb may be provided

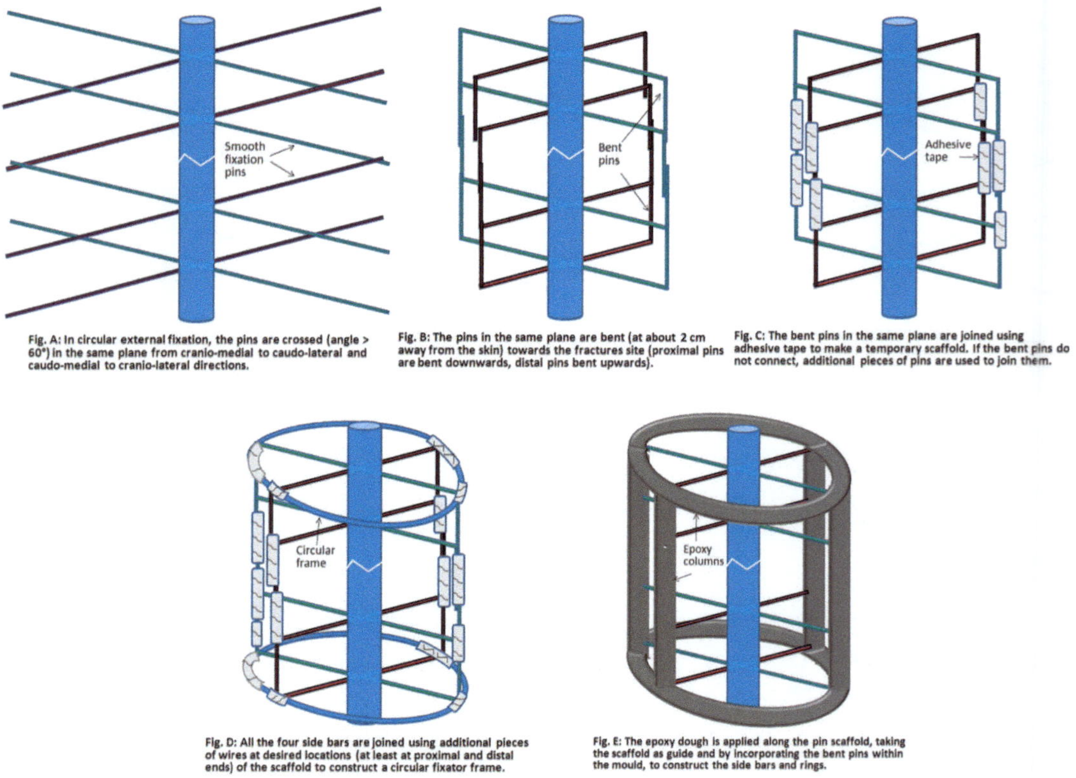


**Fig. 2.71** Circular epoxy-pin fixation technique

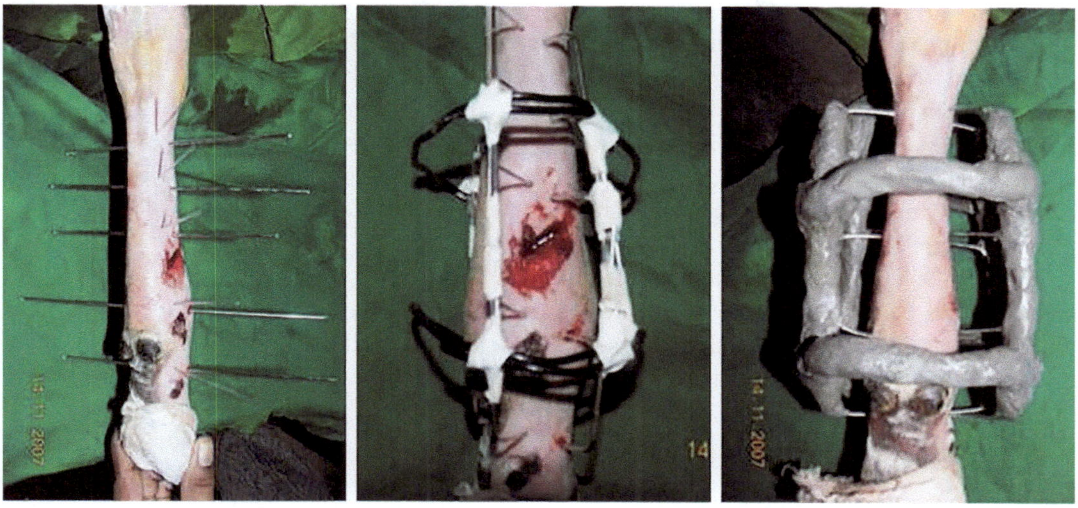


**Fig. 2.72**

with external support in the form of splint and bandages for 1–2 weeks.

### 2.3.11 Complications of ESF

After ESF application, certain complications can develop, which may include pin-tract sepsis and drainage, pin loosening and breakage, fracture instability, and pin-tract fractures. Most of these complications can be minimized by selecting appropriate fixation device, following proper technique of fixation along with good postoperative care and management.

The pin-tract infection and drainage are the most common complications reported with the use of an ESF both in pet and domestic animals. Slight pin-tract discharge is expected in the initial period of fixation. Pin-tract discharge is directly proportional to fixation rigidity; in most cases with rigid bone fixation, pin-tract discharge is the least, whereas instability at fracture site may increase the occurrence of pin-tract infection and drainage. Pin-tract drainage is generally more in proximal limb locations, where there is more soft tissue mass. Pin-tract drainage may be prevented or minimized by adopting proper fixation technique, including pin insertion (use of release incisions), and application of compressive bandage in the early post-fixation period.

Another complication commonly observed with ESF is loosening of fixation pins. Thermal necrosis of the bone around the pin tract during pin insertion can lead to resorption of the bone leading to widening of pin tracts and pin loosening. Predrilling the pin hole, drilling with low rpm power drill, use of cold saline solution at pin-skin interfaces while drilling, and drilling in small pulses by allowing 30 s between pulses can help reduce thermal necrosis along the pin tracts. High stress exerted at pin-skin interfaces (due to pin placement very close to the fracture), inadequate stiffness of ESF frame, excessive movement of soft tissues around the fixation pins (due to inadequate release of soft tissues during pin insertion), and development of infection along the pin tracts will also increase the chances of loosening of fixation pins. Loose pins can lead to continuous pain and may predispose to osteomyelitis, delayed union or non-union, and fracture disease. It is advised to remove the loose fixation pin, especially if the pin tract is infected, and make sure to increase the stability of ESF by using additional fixation pins if needed. In case of infection, the pin tract should be debrided and flushed with antiseptic solution along with administration of systemic antibiotics after antimicrobial sensitivity testing.

Fracture through pin tracts is another complication of ESF application but rarely reported. This normally results from improper surgical technique such as the use of large diameter pins (more than one third the bone diameter), placement of pins very close to fracture site or another pin, and inadequate movement restriction postoperatively. In such cases, it is advised to remove the broken pin and replace it with another pin placed in intact major bone segment to increase the fixator stability.

Laminitis of the contralateral limb is common in large animal ESF applications. Horses are more prone to contralateral limb laminitis than cattle. Prevention and management of this condition are detailed in Chapter 8.

## Chapter 2: Sample Questions

### Q. No. 1: Mark the most appropriate answer.

1. Intramedullary pinning is most resistant against
   (a) bending, (b) rotation, (c) tension, (d) torsion
2. Bone plating should be done at the following surface of a long bone.
   (a) compression side (b) tension side (c) lateral side (d) medial side
3. Technique of fracture fixation wherein multiple percutaneous, transcortical pins are passed in the proximal and distal bone segment and are connected to a rigid external frame is known as
   (a) external fixation (b) internal fixation (c) external skeletal fixation (d) none of the above
4. Which of the following is not true with respect to an ESF?
   (a) strength increases as complexity of design increases (b) increasing the number of pins increases fixator strength (c) the larger the pin diameter, the greater is the fixation stability (d) the more the distance from the bone to side bars increases, the more the fixation stiffness
5. Avulsion fracture of the olecranon can be better treated by
   (a) screw fixation (b) IM pinning (c) tension band wiring (d) cross pinning
6. Transfixation pinning and casting are a type of
   (a) external fixation (b) internal fixation (c) external skeletal fixation (d) none of these
7. The technique of choice for the fixation of a supracondylar femoral fracture is
   (a) retrograde technique of single pinning, (b) stack pinning, (c) cross intramedullary pinning, (d) K-nailing

### Q. No. 2: State true or false.

1. A plaster cast applied straight can neutralize bending and rotational forces but generally unable to resist compressive, shear, and tensile forces.
2. Creating an opening (window) in the cast will reduce its strength considerably and make the window site prone for breakage.
3. Modified Thomas splint is indicated in proximal femoral and humeral fractures.
4. IM nailing in a long bone fracture is contraindicated if periosteal system is already damaged.
5. In fractures with smaller bone segment, retrograde pinning is preferred due to accurate placement and better purchase of pin.
6. K-nails are not indicated if there are longitudinal cortical cracks in the fractured bone.
7. Plaster cast can be used for effective immobilization of fractures at the distal end of the femur.
8. Close pinning can only be used for recent stable fractures.
9. Internal fixation should be avoided in the presence of infection.
10. Periosteal stripping is preferred during plate fixation.
11. Cross IM pinning using small diameter pins can provide stable fixation of small fracture segments near the joint with minimal damage to the growth plate.
12. Interlocking nail is biomechanically superior to bone plate.
13. Limited contact DCPs with undercut can reduce the contact between the plate and the bone surface and in turn reduce the stress protection and vascular compromise.
14. Fully threaded cortical screw can be used as 'lag screw' by over-drilling the far cortex to achieve interfragmentary compression.

15. Positive-profile threaded pins are stronger than negative-profile threaded pins of similar size.
16. During ESF application, pins are introduced using high-speed, low torque power drills to avoid wobbling and reduce thermal necrosis of the bone.
17. A properly tensioned 1.6 mm K-wire provides stiffness equivalent to a 4 mm fixator pin.

**Q. No. 3: Fill in the blanks.**

1. ______________________ sling is used to hold the shoulder joint in flexion, while ____ ___________________ sling is indicated to hold the hip joint in flexed position.
2. Introduction of the pin for IM pinning through one end of the bone is called as __________ ______________ technique, and when it is introduced through the fracture site, it is termed as ______________________ technique.
3. The diameter of the intramedullary pin should be about ____________________ of medullary cavity diameter, to achieve adequate stability.
4. Interlocking nailing with fixation of either proximal or distal transfixation bolts is called as ______________________________, whereas fixation of both proximal and distal bolts is termed as ____________________ ________.
5. ________________________________ plates with threaded screw holes typically have combi holes to allow placement of either _________________________ or _____________________________ screws.
6. Minimally invasive plate osteosynthesis is ____ ____________ (less/more) traumatic, ______ _____________ (less/more) biological, and __________ (less/more) rigid than standard plate fixation.
7. An orthopedic wire placed around the circumference of the bone is called as ___________ ______________________, and a wire passed through a hole drilled in the bone to partially encircle the bone is __________________ _________.
8. The methods used to reduce thermal necrosis of tissues during ESF application include ____ _____________________, _____________ _________________, and ______________ _____________________.
9. Free-form fixation has the advantage of _____ _____________________________________-_______________, but the disadvantage is __ ____________________________________ ___.

**Q. No. 4: Write short note on the following.**

1. Principles of locking compression plate
2. Advantages of interlocking nailing
3. Minimally invasive plate osteosynthesis
4. Principles of external skeletal fixation
5. Plaster cast vs. fiberglass cast
6. Rush pinning vs. cross IM pinning
7. Dynamic self-compression plate vs. locking plate

## References


1. Adams, S.B., and J.F. Fessler. 1988. Fracture repair. In *Textbook of large animal surgery*, ed. F.W. Oehme, 2nd ed. Baltimore: Williams and Wilkins.
2. Anderson, D.E., and St. Jean, G. 2008. Management of fractures in field settings. *The Veterinary Clinics of North America. Food Animal Practice* 24: 567–582.
3. Charnley, J. 1963. 1963. The mechanics of conservative treatment. In *The closed treatment of common fractures*, ed. J. Charnley, 43–59. Philadelphia: Williams & Wilkins.
4. Dyce, J. 1998. Conservative management of fractures. In *BSAVA manual of small animal fracture repair and management*, ed. A.R. Coughlan and A. Miller. Cheltenham: British Small Animal Veterinary Association.
5. Harasen, G. 2012. Orthopedic therapy under wraps: the pros and cons of external coaptation. *The Canadian Veterinary Journal* 53: 679–680.
6. Leighton, R.L. 1991. Principles of conservative fracture management: splints and casts. In: fracture management. I, Boudrieau RJ (ed.). Semin Vet Med Surg Small Anim. 6: 39–51.
7. Nunamaker, D.M. 1985. Methods of closed fixation. In *Textbook of small animal orthopaedics*, ed. C.D. Newton and D.M. Nunamaker, 1st ed., 249–259. Philadelphia: JB Lippincott.

8. Hohn, R.B. 1975. Principles and application of plaster casts. *The Veterinary Clinics of North America. Small Animal Practice* 5: 291–303.
9. Levet, T., A. Martens, L. Devisscher, L. Duchateau, L. Bogaert, and L. Vlaminck. 2009. Distal limb cast sores in horses: risk factors and early detection using thermography. *Equine Veterinary Journal* 41: 18–23.
10. Meeson, R.L., C. Davidson, and G.I. Arthurs. 2011. Soft-tissue injuries associated with cast application for distal limb orthopedic conditions. A retrospective study of sixty dogs and cats. *Veterinary and Comparative Orthopaedics and Traumatology* 24: 126–131.
11. Tomlinson, J. 1991. Complications with fractures repaired with casts and splints. *The Veterinary Clinics of North America. Small Animal Practice* 21: 735–744.
12. Sangwan, V., G.P. Yadav, and A. Kumar. 2020. Aluminium splint incorporated fibreglass cast preserves limb function in bovines with olecranon fracture. *Veterinary and Comparative Orthopaedics and Traumatology* 33: 434–442.
13. Singh, A.P., G.R. Singh, H.P. Aithal, and P. Singh. 2020. Section D – fractures, chapter on the musculoskeletal system. In *Ruminant surgery: A textbook of the surgical diseases of cattle, buffaloes, camels, sheep and goats*, ed. J. Singh, S. Singh, and R.P.S. Tyagi, 2nd ed. New Delhi: CBS Publishers and Distributers.
14. Solanki, K.P., P.B. Patel, V.D. Dodia, J.V. Vadalia, R.J. Raval, H.M. Padheriya, and M.D. Khatariya. 2016. Comparative effectiveness of plaster of Paris and fibre glass casts in the management of long bone fractures in canines. *International Journal of Environmental Science and Technology* 5: 3512–3515.
15. Wilson, D.G., and R. Vanderby Jr. 1995. An evaluation of six synthetic casting materials. *Veterinary Surgery* 24: 55–59.
16. Wilson, D.G., and R. Vanderby Jr. 1995. An evaluation of fiberglass cast application techniques. *Veterinary Surgery* 24: 118–121.
17. Schroeder, E.F. 1933. The traction principle in treating fractures of the dog and cat. *The North American Veterinarian* 14: 32–36.
18. Adams, S.B., and J.F. Fessler. 1983. Treatment of radial, ulnar and tibial fractures in cattle, using a modified Thomas splint cast combination. *Journal of the American Veterinary Medical Association* 183: 430–433.
19. Baird, A.N., and S.B. Adams. 2014. Use of the Thomas splint and cast combination, walker splint, and spica bandage with an over the shoulder splint for the treatment of fractures of the upper limbs in cattle. *The Veterinary Clinics of North America. Food Animal Practice* 30: 77–90.
20. Ladefoged, S., S. Grulke, V. Busoni, D. Serteyn, A. Salciccia, and D. Verwilghen. 2017. Modified Thomas splint-cast combination for the management of limb fractures in small equids. *Veterinary Surgery* 46: 381–388.
21. Howard, P.E. 1991. Principles of intramedullary pin and wire fixation. In Fracture management. I, Boudrieau RJ (ed.). Semin Vet Med Surg Small Anim 6: 52–67.
22. Nunamaker, D.M. 1985. Methods of internal fixation. In *Textbook of small animal Orthopaedics*, ed. C.D. Newton and D.M. Nunamaker, 1st ed., 261–286. Philadelphia: JB Lippincott.
23. Rudy, R.L. 1975. Principles of intramedullary pinning. *The Veterinary Clinics of North America. Small Animal Practice* 5: 209–228.
24. Martin, R.A., J.L. Milton, P.K. Shires, et al. 1988. Closed reduction and blind pinning of selected fractures and luxations in dogs and cats. *Compendium on Continuing Education for the Practicing Veterinarian* 10: 784–799.
25. Newmann, M.E., and J.L. Milton. 1989. Closed reduction and blind pinning of 29 femoral and tibial fractures in 27 dogs and cats. *Journal of the American Animal Hospital Association* 25: 61–68.
26. De Young, D.J., and C.W. Probst. 1985. Methods of fracture fixation. In *Textbook of small animal surgery*, ed. D.H. Slatter, vol. 2, 1949–2014. Philadelphia: PA Saunders.
27. Chaffee, V.W. 1977. Multiple (stacked) intramedullary pin fixation of humeral and femoral fractures. *Journal of the American Animal Hospital Association* 13: 599–601.
28. Rush, L.V. 1959. Atlas of Rush pin technics. Berivon
29. Aithal, H.P., G.R. Singh, A.K. Sharma, and Amarpal. 1998. Modified technique of single pin fixation and cross intramedullary pin fixation technique for supracondylar femoral fracture in dogs: A comparative study. *Indian Journal of Veterinary Surgery* 19: 84–89.
30. Whitney, W.O., and S.C. Schrader. 1987. Dynamic intramedullary crosspinning technique for repair of distal femoral fractures in dogs and cats: 71 cases (1981-1985). *Journal of the American Veterinary Medical Association* 191: 1133–1138.
31. Jenny, J. 1950. Kuntscher's medullary mailing in femur fractures of the dog. *Journal of the American Veterinary Medical Association* 117: 381–387.
32. Déjardin, L.M., K.L. Perry, D.J.F. von Pfeil, and L.P. Guiot. 2020. Interlocking nails and minimally invasive osteosynthesis. *The Veterinary Clinics of North America. Small Animal Practice* 50 (1): 67–100.
33. Dueland, R.T., K.A. Johnson, S.C. Roe, M.H. Engen, and A.S. Lesser. 1999. Interlocking nail treatment of diaphyseal long-bone fractures in dogs. *Journal of the American Veterinary Medical Association* 214 (1): 59–66.
34. Durall, I., and M.C. Diaz. 1996. Early experience with the use of an interlocking nail for the repair of canine femoral shaft fractures. *Veterinary Surgery* 25: 397–406.
35. Larin, A., C.S. Eich, R.B. Parker, and W.P. Stubbs. 2001. Repair of diaphyseal fractures in cats using

interlocking intramedullary nails: 12 cases (1996-2000). *Journal of the American Veterinary Medical Association* 219 (8): 1098–1104.
36. Raghunath, M., and S.S. Singh. 2003. Use of static intramedullary interlocking nail for repair of comminuted/segmental femoral diaphyseal fractures in four dogs. *Indian Journal of Veterinary Surgery* 24: 89–91.
37. Wheeler, J.L., W.P. Stubbs, D.D. Lewis, and A.R. Cross. 2004. Intramedullary interlocking nail fixation in dogs and cats: biomechanics instrumentation. *Compendium on Continuing Education for the Practising Veterinarian -North American* 26 (7): 519–529.
38. Bellon, J., and P.-Y. Mulon. 2011. Use of a novel intramedullary nail for femoral fracture repair in calves: 25 cases (2008-2009). *Journal of the American Veterinary Medical Association* 238: 1490–1496.
39. Bhat, S.A. H.P. Aithal, P. Kinjavdekar, Amarpal, M.M.S. Zama, P.C. Gope, A.M. Pawde, R.A. Ahmad, and M.B. Gugjoo. 2014. An in vitro biomechanical investigation of an intramedullary interlocking nail system developed for buffalo tibia. *Veterinary and Comparative Orthopaedics and Traumatology* 27: 36–44.
40. Dilipkumar, D., M. Patil, B.V. Shivaprakash, Bhagavantappa B.N. Venkatgiri, D. Jahangir, A. Mahesh, and S. Arunkumar. 2019. Intramedullary interlocking nail fixation for repair of long bone fractures in cattle. *Indian Journal of Veterinary Surgery* 40: 48–51.
41. Madhu, D.N. 2015. Development and evaluation of interlocking nail and tubular locking plate for management of femur fracture in large ruminants. PhD thesis submitted to Deemed University, Indian Veterinary Research Institute, Izatnagar- 243 122 (UP), India.
42. Marturello, D.M., K.M. Gazzola, and L.M. Déjardin. 2019. Tibial fracture repair with angle-stable interlocking nailing in 2 calves. *Veterinary Surgery* 48: 597–606.
43. Nuss, K. 2014. Plates, pins and interlocking nails. *The Veterinary Clinics of North America. Food Animal Practice* 30: 91–126.
44. McClure, S.R., J.P. Watkins, and R.B. Ashman. 1998. An in vivo evaluation of intramedullary interlocking nail fixation of transverse femoral osteotomies in foals. *Veterinary Surgery* 27: 29–36.
45. Watkins, J.P., and R.B. Ashman. 1990. Intramedullary interlocking nail fixation in foals: effects on normal growth and development of the humerus. *Veterinary Surgery* 19: 80.
46. Boudrieau, R.J. 1991. Principles of screw and plate fixation. *Seminars in Veterinary Medicine and Surgery (Small Animal)* 6 (1): 75–89.
47. Brinker, W.O., R.B. Hohn, and W.D. Prieur. 1984. *Manual of internal fixation in small animals*. New York: Springer.
48. Igna, C., and L. Schuszler. 2010. Current concepts of internal plate fixation of fractures. *Bulletin of University of Agricultural Sciences and Veterinary Medicine* 67 (2): 118–124.
49. Muller, M.E., M. Allgower, R. Schneider, and H. Willenegger. 1979. *Manual of internal fixation*. 2nd ed. New York: Springer-Verlag.
50. Allgower, M., R. Ehrsahm, and R. Ganz. 1969. Clinical experience with a new compression plate "DCP". *Acta Orthopaedica Scandinavica. Supplementum* 125: 46–61.
51. Allgower, M., S.M. Perren, and P. Matter. 1970. A new plate for internal fixation-the dynamic compression (DCP). *Injury* 2: 40–47.
52. Ayyappan, S. 2013. AO techniques of dynamic compression plate (DCP) and limited contact dynamic compression plate (LC-DCP) application for fracture management in dogs. *Advances in Animal and Veterinary Sciences* 1 (2S): 33–36.
53. Perren, S.M., M. Russenberger, S. Steinemann, M.E. Muller, and M. Allgower. 1969. A dynamic compression plate. *Acta Orthopaedica Scandinavica. Supplementum* 125: 31–41.
54. Schatzer, J. 1991. Screws and plates and their applications. In *Manual of internal fixation techniques recommended by the AO-ASIF group*, ed. M. Allgower, 3rd ed., 179–199. Cham: Springer.
55. Uhthoff, H.K., P. Poitras, and D.S. Backman. 2006. Internal plate fixation of fractures: short history and recent developments. *Journal of Orthopaedic Science* 11 (2): 118–126.
56. Perren, S.M., K. Klaue, O. Pohler, M. Predieri, S. Steinemann, and E. Gautier. 1990. The limited contact dynamic compression plate (LC-DCP). *Archives of Orthopaedic and Trauma Surgery* 109: 304–310.
57. Nunamaker, D.M., K.F. Bowman, D.W. Richardson, and M. Herring. 1986. Plate luting: a preliminary report of its use in horses. *Veterinary Surgery* 15 (4): 289–293.
58. Nunamaker, D.M., D.W. Richardson, and D.M. Butterweck. 1991. Mechanical and biological effects of plate luting. *Journal of Orthopaedic Trauma* 5 (2): 138–145.
59. Bruese, S., J. Dee, and W.D. Prieur. 1989. Internal fixation with a veterinary cuttable plate in small animals. *Veterinary and Comparative Orthopaedics and Traumatology* 1: 40–46.
60. Theoret, M.C., and N.M.M. Moens. 2007. The use of veterinary cuttable plates for carpal and tarsal arthrodesis in small dogs and cats. *The Canadian Veterinary Journal* 48 (2): 165–168.
61. Lewis, D.D., R.T. van Ee, M.G. Oakes, and A.D. Elkins. 1993. Use of reconstruction plates for stabilization of fractures and osteotomies involving the supracondylar region of the femur. *Journal of the American Animal Hospital Association* 29: 171–178.
62. Anson, L.W., D.J. De Young, D.C. Richardson, and C.W. Betts. 1988. Clinical evaluation of canine

acetabular fractures stabilized with an acetabular plate. *Veterinary Surgery* 17: 220–225.
63. Braden, T.D., and W.D. Trieur. 1986. New plate for acetabular fractures: technique of application and long-term follow-up evaluation. *Journal of the American Veterinary Medical Association* 188: 1183–1186.
64. Brinker, W.O., R.B. Hohn, and W.D. Prieur. 1998. *Manual of internal fixation in small animals*. Berlin: Springer.
65. Barnhart, M.D., and K.C. Maritato. 2018. Locking plates in veterinary orthopaedics. ACVS Foundation, Wiley Blackwell. Onlinelibrary.wiley.com/doi/book/10.1002/9781119380139
66. Frigg, R. 2001. Locking compression plate (LCP). An osteosynthesis plate based on the dynamic compression plate and the point contact fixator (PC-fix). *Injury* 32: 63–66.
67. Frigg, R. 2003. Development of locking compression plate. *Injury* 34: S-B6-10.
68. Gautier, E., and C. Sommer. 2003. Guidelines for the clinical application of the LCP. *Injury* 34: S-B63-76.
69. Kowaleski, M. 2009. Locking plate systems: LCP. In: Proceedings spring scientific meeting, British veterinary Orthopaedic association, Moores A (ed.), 1st April 2009, Austin Court, Birmingham. p 1–3.
70. Kowaleski, M. 2009. Locking plate systems: SOP and ALPS. In: proceedings spring scientific meeting, British veterinary Orthopaedic association. Moores A (ed.), 1st April 2009, Austin Court, Birmingham. pp. 4–9.
71. Wagner, M. 2003. General principles for the clinical use of the LCP. *Injury* 34: S-B31-B42.
72. Wagner, M., and R. Frigg. 2006. *AO manual of fracture management, internal fixators: concepts and cases using LCP and LISS*, 1–57. Clavadelerstrasse: AO Publishing.
73. Aguila, A.Z., J.M. Manos, A.S. Orlansky, R.J. Todhunter, E.J. Trotter, and M.C.H. Van der Meulen. 2005. In vitro biomechanical comparison of limited contact dynamic compression plate and locking compression plate. *Veterinary and Comparative Orthopaedics and Traumatology* 18: 220–226.
74. Egol, K.A., E.N. Kubiask, E. Fulkerson, F.J. Kummer, and K.J. Koval. 2004. Biomechanics of locked plates and screws. *Journal of Orthopaedic Trauma* 18 (8): 488–493.
75. Keller, M., and K. Voss. 2002. AO vet news. UniLock: applications in small animals. AO Dialogue 15: 20–21.
76. Gamper, S., A. Steiner, K. Nuss, S. Ohlerth, A. Fürst, J.G. Ferguson, J.A. Auer, and C. Lischer. 2006. Clinical evaluation of the CRIF 4.5/5.5 system for long-bone fracture repair in cattle. *Veterinary Surgery* 35: 361–368.
77. Reems, M.R., B.S. Beale, and D.A. Hulse. 2003. Use of a clamp-rod construct and principles of biological osteosynthesis for repair of diaphyseal fractures in dogs and cats: 47 cases (1994-2001). *Journal of the American Veterinary Medical Association* 223: 330–335.
78. Zahn, K., and U. Matis. 2004. The clamp rod internal fixator- application and results in 120 small animal fracture patients. *Veterinary and Comparative Orthopaedics and Traumatology* 17: 110–120.
79. Ahmad, R.A. 2013. Development and evaluation of designer locking plates for fixation of tibial and radial fractures in large ruminants. PhD thesis submitted to Deemed University, Indian Veterinary Research Institute, Izatnagar- 243 122 (UP), India.
80. Ahmad, R.A., H.P. Aithal, Amarpal, P. Kinjavdekar, P.C. Gope, and D.N. Madhu. 2021. Biomechanical properties of a novel locking compression plate to stabilize oblique tibial osteotomies in buffaloes. *Veterinary Surgery* 50: 444–454.
81. Hudson, C.C., A. Pozzi, and D.D. Lewis. 2009. Minimally invasive plate osteosynthesis: applications and techniques in dogs and cats. *Veterinary and Comparative Orthopaedics and Traumatology* 3: 175–182.
82. Krettek, C., M. Muller, and T. Miclau. 2001. Evolution of minimally invasive plate osteosynthesis (MIPO) in the femur. *Injury* 32 (Suppl 3): C14–C23.
83. Schmokel, H.G., S. Stein, H. Radke, K. Hurter, and P. Schawalder. 2007. Treatment of tibial fractures with plates using minimally invasive percutaneous osteosynthesis in dogs and cats. *The Journal of Small Animal Practice* 48: 157–160.
84. Tong, G., and S. Bavonratanvech. 2007. *AO manual of fracture management: minimally invasive plate osteosynthesis (MIPO)*, 3–7. Clavadelerstrasse: AO Publishing.
85. Morshead, D. 1982. Fracture fixation with Kirschner wires. *Compendium on Continuing Education for the Practicing Veterinarian* 4: 491–501.
86. Gambardella, P.C. 1980. Full cerclage wires for fixation of long bone fractures. *Compendium on Continuing Education for the Practicing Veterinarian* 2: 665–671.
87. Withrow, S.J. 1978. Use and misuse of full cerclage wires in fracture repair. *The Veterinary Clinics of North America. Small Animal Practice* 8: 201–212.
88. Birchard, S.J., and R.M. Bright. 1981. The tension band wire for fracture repair in the dog. *Compendium on Continuing Education for the Practising Veterinarian* 3: 37–41.
89. Petit, G.B., and D.H.J.S. Slatter. 1973. Tension band wiring for fixation of avulsed canine tibial tuberosity. *Journal of the American Veterinary Medical Association* 163: 242–244.
90. Corr, S.A. 2005. Practical guide to linear external skeletal fixation in small animals. *In Practice* 27 (2): 76–85.
91. Bilgili, H. 2004. Circular external fixation system of Ilizarov: part V. fracture treatment by the Ilizarov technique. *Veteriner Cerrahi Dergisi* 10 (1–2): 75–89.

92. Carnmichael, S. 1991. The external fixator in small animal orthopaedics. *The Journal of Small Animal Practice* 32: 486–493.
93. Egger, E.L. 1998. External skeletal fixation. In *Current techniques in small animal surgery, Bojrab,* ed. M.J., 4th ed., 941–950. Philadelphia.
94. Harari, J., T. Bebchuk, B. Segun, and J. Lincoln. 1996. Closed repair of tibial and radial fractures with external skeletal fixator. *Compendium on Continuing Education for the Practising Veterinarian* 18: 651–657.
95. Ilizarov, G.A. 1992. The apparatus: components and biomechanical principles of application. In *Transosseous Osteosynthesis*, ed. S.A. Green, 63–136. Berlin: Springer-Verlag.
96. Johnson, A.L., and C.E. DeCamo. 1992. External skeletal fixation- linear fixation. *The Veterinary Clinics of North America. Small Animal Practice* 29: 1135–1143.
97. Lewis, D.D., A.R. Cross, S. Carmichael, and M.A. Anderson. 2001. Recent advances in external skeletal fixation. *The Journal of Small Animal Practice* 42: 103–112.
98. Marcellin-Little, D.J. 1999. Fracture treatment with circular external fixation. *The Veterinary Clinics of North America. Small Animal Practice* 29: 1153–1170.
99. Ozsoy, S., and K. Altunatmaz. 2003. Treatment of extremity fractures in dogs using external fixators with closed reduction and limited open approach. *Veterinary Medicine Czech* 48: 133–140.
100. Aron, D.N., J.P. Toombs, and S.C. Hollingworth. 1986. Primary treatment of severe fractures by external skeletal fixation: threaded pins compared with smooth pins. *Journal of the American Animal Hospital Association* 22: 659–670.
101. Toombs, J.P. 1992. Trans articular application of external skeletal fixation. *The Veterinary Clinics of North America. Small Animal Practice* 22: 181–194.
102. Morshead, D., and E.B. Leeds. 1984. Kirschner-Ehmer apparatus immobilization following Achilles tendon repair in six dogs. *Veterinary Surgery* 13: 11–14.
103. Bilgili, H., and B. Olcay. 1998. Circular external fixation system of Ilizarov: part I. history, components, indications and principles of system. *Turkish Journal of Veterinary Surgery* 4: 62–67.
104. Johnson, A.L., J.A.C. Eurel, J.M. Losonsky, and E.L. Egger. 1998. Biomechanics and biology of fracture healing with external skeletal fixation. *Compendium on Continuing Education for the Practising Veterinarian* 20: 487–500.
105. Toombs, J.P. 1991. Principles of external skeletal fixation using the Kirschner-Ehmer splint. *Seminars in Veterinary Medicine and Surgery (Small Animal)* 6 (1): 68–74.
106. Egger, E.L., D.G. Lewallen, and R.W. Norrdin, et al. 1988. Effect of destabilizing rigid external fixation on healing of unstable canine osteotomies. Transactions of the 34th Annual Meeting of Orthopedic Research Society 13: 302.
107. Aron, D.N., and J.P. Toombs. 1984. Updated principles of external skeletal fixation. *Compendium on Continuing Education for the Practicing Veterinarian* 6: 845–858.
108. Green, S.A. 1991. The Ilizarov method. Rancho technique. *The Orthopedic Clinics of North America* 22: 677–688.
109. Hierholzer, G., R. Kleining, G. Horster, and P. Zemenides. 1978. External fixation- classification and indications. *Archives of Orthopaedic and Trauma Surgery* 92: 175–182.
110. Egger, E.L. 1990. Biomechanics and fracture healing with external fixation. In Proceedings 18th annual veterinary surgical forum, Chicago, IL. p 321–323.
111. Kummer, F.J. 1992. Biomechanics of the Ilizarov external fixator. *Clinical Orthopaedics* 280: 11–14.
112. Kürüm, B., H. Bilgili, and C. Yardımcı. 2002. Circular external fixation system of Ilizarov. Part IV: biomechanical properties of the system. *Turkish Journal of Veterinary and Animal Sciences* 8: 107–115.
113. Lewis, D.D., D.G. Bronson, M.L. Samchukov, R.D. Welch, and J.T. Stallings. 1998. Biomechanics of circular external skeletal fixation. *Veterinary Surgery* 27: 454–464.
114. Paley, D. 1991. Biomechanics of the Ilizarov external fixator. In *Operative principles of Ilizarov*, ed. A. Bianchi-Maiocchi and J. Aronson, 33–41. Milan: Medi Surgical Video.
115. Kraus, K.H., H.M. Wotton, R.J. Boudrieau, L. Schwarz, D. Diamond, and A. Minihan. 1998. Type-II external fixation, using new clamps and positive-profile threaded pins, for treatment of fractures of the radius and tibia in dogs. *Journal of the American Veterinary Medical Association* 212: 1267–1270.
116. Aron, D.N., and C.W. Dewey. 1992. Application and postoperative management of external skeletal fixators. *The Veterinary Clinics of North America. Small Animal Practice* 22 (1): 69–98.
117. Egger, E.L. 1990. Principles of fracture management-the use of external skeletal fixation. In *Canine orthopedics*, ed. W.G. Whittick, 2nd ed., 248–264. Philadelphia: Lea & Febiger.
118. Ramakumar, V., M. Manohar, and R.P.S. Tyagi. 1973. Hanging pin cast for oblique fracture of tibia in a cow-A disadvantage. *The Indian Veterinary Journal* 50: 714–716.
119. Lescun, T.B., S.R. McClure, M.P. Ward, C. Downs, D.A. Wilson, S.B. Adams, J.F. Hawkins, and E.L. Reinertson. 2007. Evaluation of transfixation casting for treatment of third metacarpal, third metatarsal, and phalangeal fractures in horses: 37 cases (1994-2004). *Journal of the American Veterinary Medical Association* 230: 1340–1349.
120. Lozier, J.W., A.J. Niehaus, A. Muir, and J. Lakritz. 2018. Short- and long-term success of transfixation pin casts used to stabilize long bone fractures in

ruminants. *The Canadian Veterinary Journal* 59: 635–641.
121. Aithal, H.P. 2015. Management of fractures. In *A handbook on field veterinary surgery*, ed. M.M.S. Zama, H.P. Aithal, and A.M. Pawde, 145–154. New Delhi: Published by Astral.
122. Aithal, H.P., Amarpal, P. Kinjavdekar, A.M. Pawde, K. Pratap, P. Kumar, D.K. Sinha, and H.C Setia. 2009. A novel bilateral linear external skeletal fixation device for treatment of long bone fractures in large animals: A report of 12 clinical cases. 33rd Congress of ISVS held at Veterinary college, GADVASU, Ludhiana (Punjab), 11–13 Nov. 2009, Abst: OR-1.
123. Dubey, P., H.P. Aithal, P. Kinjavdekar, Amarpal, P.C. Gope, D.N. Madhu, Rohit Kumar, T.B. Sivanarayanan, A.M. Pawde, and M.M.S. Zama. 2021. A comparative in vitro biomechanical investigation of a novel bilateral linear fixator vs. circular and multiplanar epoxy-pin external fixation systems using a fracture model in buffalo metacarpal bone. *World Journal of Surgery and Surgical Research* 4: 1331.
124. Singh, G.R., H.P. Aithal, Amarpal, P. Kinjavdekar, S.K. Maiti, M. Hoque, A.M. Pawde, and H.C. Joshi. 2007. Evaluation of two dynamic axial fixators for large ruminants. *Veterinary Surgery* 36: 88–97.
125. Singh, G.R., H.P. Aithal, R.K. Saxena, P. Kinjavdekar, Amarpal, M. Hoque, S.K. Maiti, A.M. Pawde, and H.C. Joshi. 2007. In-vitro biomechanical properties of linear, circular and hybrid external skeletal fixation devices developed for use in large ruminants. *Veterinary Surgery* 36: 80–87.
126. Nash, R.A., D.M. Nunamaker, and R. Boston. 2001. Evaluation of a tapered-sleeve transcortical pin to reduce stress at the bone-pin interface in metacarpal bones obtained from horses. *American Journal of Veterinary Research* 62: 955–960.
127. Nunamaker, D.M., and R.A. Nash. 2008. A tapered sleeve transcortical pin external skeletal fixation device for use in horses: development, application, and experience. *Veterinary Surgery* 37: 725–732.
128. Nunamaker, D.M., D.W. Richardson, D.M. Butterweck, M.T. Provost, and R. Sigafoos. 1986. A new external skeletal fixation device that allows immediate full weight bearing: application in the horse. *Veterinary Surgery* 15: 345–355.
129. Aithal, H.P., G.R. Singh, M. Hoque, S.K. Maiti, P. Kinjavdekar, Amarpal, A.M. Pawde, and H.C. Setia. 2004. The use of circular external skeletal fixation device for the management of long bone osteotomies in large ruminants: an experimental study. *Journal of Veterinary Medicine* A51: 284–293.
130. Farese, J.P., D.D. Lewis, A.R. Cross, K.E. Collins, G.M. Anderson, and K.B. Halling. 2002. Use of IMEX SK-circular external fixator hybrid constructs for fracture stabilization in dogs and cats. *Journal of the American Animal Hospital Association* 38: 279–289.
131. Rao, J.R., V.G. Kumar, T.M. Rao, D.P. Kumar, K.C.S. Reddy, and K.B.P. Raghavender. 2016. Use of hybrid external fixation technique in the repair of long bone fractures in dogs. *International Journal of Current Microbiology and Applied Sciences* 5 (11): 579–586.
132. Aithal, H.P., G.R. Singh, P. Kinjavdekar, Amarpal, M. Hoque, S.K. Maiti, A.M. Pawed, and H.C. Setia. 2007. Hybrid construct of linear and circular external skeletal fixation devices for fixation of long bone osteotomies in large ruminants. *The Indian Journal of Animal Sciences* 77: 1083–1090.
133. Shah, M.A., Rohit Kumar, P. Kinjavdekar, Amarpal, H.P. Aithal, Mohammad Arif Basha, and Asif Majid. 2022. The use of circular and hybrid external skeletal fixation systems to repair open tibial fractures in large ruminants: a report of six clinical cases. *Veterinary Research Communications* 46: 563–575.
134. Marcellin-Little, D.J., A. Ferretti, S.C. Roe, and D.J. Deyoung. 1998. Hinged Ilizarov external fixation for correction of antebrachial deformities. *Veterinary Surgery* 27: 231–245.
135. Aithal, H.P., Amarpal, P. Kinjavdekar, A.M. Pawde, G.R. Singh, and H.C. Setia. 2010. Management of tibial fractures using a circular external fixator in two calves. *Veterinary Surgery* 39: 621–626.
136. Bilgili, H., B. Kurum, and O. Captug. 2008. Use of a circular external skeletal fixator to treat comminuted metacarpal and tibial fractures in six calves. *The Veterinary Record* 163: 683–687.
137. Gulaydin, A., and M. Sarierler. 2018. Treatment of long bone fractures in calves with Ilizarov external fixator. *Veterinary and Comparative Orthopaedics and Traumatology* 31 (5): 364–372.
138. Olcay, B., H. Bilgili, and B. Kürüm. 1999. Treatment of communitive diaphyseal metacarpal fracture in a calf using the Ilizarov circular external fixation system. *Israel Journal of Veterinary Medicine* 54: 122–127.
139. Aithal, H.P., Amarpal, P. Kinjavdekar, A.M. Pawde, G.R. Singh, M. Hoque, S.K. Maiti, and H.C. Setia. 2007. Management of fractures near carpal joint of two calves by transarticular fixation with a circular external fixator. *The Veterinary Record* 161: 193–198.
140. Roe, S.C., and T. Keo. 1997. Epoxy putty for free-form external skeletal fixators. *Veterinary Surgery* 26 (6): 472–477.
141. Tyagi, S.K., H.P. Aithal, P. Kinjavdekar, Amarpal, A.M. Pawde, and J. Singh. 2014. Comparative biomechanical evaluation of acrylic- and epoxy- pin external skeletal fixation systems with two- and three- point fixation per segment under compressive loading. *Advances in Animal and Veterinary Sciences* 2: 212–217.
142. Tyagi, S.K., H.P. Aithal, P. Kinjavdekar, Amarpal, A.M. Pawde, and I.P. Sarode. 2014. Physical

characters and economics of acrylic and epoxy polymers as frame components of external skeletal fixator. *The Indian Journal of Animal Sciences* 84: 1261–1264.
143. Tyagi, S.K., H.P. Aithal, P. Kinjavdekar, Amarpal, A.M. Pawde, T. Srivastava, K.P. Tyagi, and S.W. Monsang. 2014. Comparative evaluation of *in vitro* mechanical properties of different designs of epoxy-pin external skeletal fixation systems. *Veterinary Surgery* 43: 355–360.
144. Tyagi, S.K., H.P. Aithal, P. Kinjavdekar, Amarpal, A.M. Pawde, T. Srivastava, J. Singh, and D.N. Madhu. 2015. In vitro biomechanical testing of different configurations of acrylic external skeletal fixator constructs. *Veterinary and Comparative Orthopaedics and Traumatology* 28: 227–233.
145. Willer, R.L., E.L. Egger, and M.B. Histand. 1991. Comparison of stainless steel versus acrylic for the connecting bar of external fixators. *Journal of the American Animal Hospital Association* 27: 541–548.
146. Aithal, H.P., P. Kinjavdekar, Amarpal, A.M. Pawde, Rohit Kumar, Rekha Pathak, P. Kumar, S.K. Tyagi, P. Dubey, and D.N. Madhu. 2019. Treatment of open bone fractures using epoxy-pin fixation in small ruminants: a review of 26 cases. *Rum Science* 8: 103–114.
147. Aithal, H.P., P. Kinjavdekar, Amarpal, A.M. Pawde, M.M.S. Zama, Prasoon Dubey, Rohit Kumar, S.K. Tyagi, and D.N. Madhu. 2019. Epoxy-pin external skeletal fixation for management of open bone fractures in calves and foals: a review of 32 cases. *Veterinary and Comparative Orthopaedics and Traumatology* 32: 257–268.
148. Bennet, R.A., and A.B. Kuzma. 1992. Fracture management in birds. *Journal of Zoo and Wildlife Medicine* 22: 5–38.
149. Kumar, P., H.P. Aithal, P. Kinjavdekar, Amarpal, A.M. Pawde, K. Pratap, Surbhi, and D.K. Sinha. 2012. Epoxy-pin external skeletal fixation for treatment of open fractures or dislocations in 36 dogs. *Indian Journal of Veterinary Surgery* 33: 128–132.
150. Tyagi, S.K., H.P. Aithal, P. Kinjavdekar, Amarpal, A.M. Pawde, and Abhishek Kumar Saxena. 2021. Acrylic and epoxy-pin external skeletal fixation systems for fracture management in dogs. *Indian Journal of Animal Research*. https://doi.org/10.18805/IJAR.B-4265.

# Management of Specific Fractures in Small Animals

# 3

**Learning Objectives**

You will be able to understand the following after reading this chapter:

- Surgical approaches and techniques of fixation for fractures at different locations of long bones such as humerus, radius-ulna, femur, tibia-fibula, metacarpus, and metatarsus
- Principles, indications, surgical approaches, and techniques of fracture stabilization in mandible, pelvis and spine

**Summary**

- Fractures of humerus can be better treated using internal fixation techniques such as intramedullary (IM) pin/nail fixation or bone plating. Plate should be properly contoured to the curved cranial surface and applied securing radial nerve. ESF using half pins is often used in severely comminuted fractures along with IM pinning.
- Bone plate and screw fixation is ideal to provide rigid stabilization in radius-ulna fractures. Distal third of radius-ulna has a poor blood supply, hence more prone to delayed union and nonunion. ESF is preferred not only in open fractures but also in closed fractures of radius-ulna as it can provide rigid fixation with minimal soft tissue and vascular damage.
- Femur bone is more often fractured than any other bone in dogs and cats, and middle and distal femur is more commonly fractured than the proximal femur, while condylar/supracondylar fractures are more frequent in young animals. Most of the femoral diaphyseal fractures are amenable to IM pin fixation. Interlocking nail (ILN) or bone plate (DCP or LCP) and screw fixation is ideal for comminuted fractures in large breed dogs. For distal fractures, cross IM pinning is ideal in most cases. Most of the transverse or short oblique fractures of the tibial diaphysis can be easily immobilized using IM Steinmann pinning in normograde fashion from proximal end. Plate and screw fixation or interlocking nail may be preferred in unstable tibial fractures in heavy dogs and ESF in open fractures.
- In most cases of metacarpal/metatarsal fractures, external immobilization using splints or cast will provide satisfactory results, especially when all the bones are

(continued)


H. P. Aithal et al., *Textbook of Veterinary Orthopaedic Surgery*,
https://doi.org/10.1007/978-981-99-2575-9_3

not fractured. IM pegs or bone plates can be used to achieve stable internal fixation in heavy animals.

- Orthopedic wiring is the most frequently used internal fixation technique for treatment of fractures of mandible in dogs and cats. It is often difficult to align the fracture segments with IM pin fixation; bone plating can provide perfect anatomical reduction and stability with minimal occlusion. Acrylic-pin or epoxy-pin fixation can also be used effectively as pins can be inserted in different planes by avoiding the root structures and the mandibular canal.
- A large number of pelvic fractures can be managed adequately with conservative treatment. Most ilial fractures can be stabilized by plate fixation, and sacroiliac fractures can be stabilized using lag screws. Ischium and pubis fractures generally do not need surgical fixation.
- Spinal fractures/luxations in the dog occur most frequently in the lumbar region and in cats in the sacrococcygeal region and are often associated with spinal cord injury. The cases with minimal or no displacement of vertebrae are generally managed conservatively. The objectives of surgical fixation are decompression of the spinal cord, reduction of the fracture/luxation, and stabilization using fixation techniques like plating of vertebral body or dorsal spinous processes, PMMA and pin composite fixation, cross-pinning, and stapling. The prognosis generally depends on preservation of neurological integrity.

## 3.1 Fractures of Scapula

Fractures of scapula are uncommon in dogs and cats (1–1.5% of all bone fractures). Adequate soft tissue cover normally protects the bone from getting injured. The incidence of scapular fractures is more in young, medium to large breed dogs [1]. Vehicular trauma is the most common cause, and a large number of scapular fracture cases (about 60–70%) are associated with concurrent injuries such as thoracic trauma. Because of the anatomical location of the scapula and its association with fore limb function, it is required to treat a scapular fracture.

Scapula is a flat bone with a large body, a longitudinal spine, a neck, and an articular surface or glenoid cavity. In flat body of scapula lack medullary cavity, fixation of standard IM pins is not feasible, whereas scapular neck, which is oval in shape, has adequate medullary bone to receive pins and screws [2]. The fossae, cranial, and caudal to the scapular spine are the sites from where the supraspinatus and infraspinatus muscles, respectively, originate. The acromion process, the prominence at the end of spine, is the origin of the acromial head of the deltoideus muscle, and the supraglenoid tubercle is the origin of the biceps brachii muscle. The glenoid cavity articulates with the humeral head. The suprascapular nerve crosses cranially from the scapular notch toward distal to the scapular spine caudally, deep into the acromion. The axillary nerve emerges from the caudal border of the subscapularis muscle and crosses the caudal aspect of the scapulohumeral joint.

Most often, fractures are seen in the scapular body (about 50% cases), spine, or neck, as well as the supraglenoid tuberosity and the glenoid cavity (Fig. 3.1). The animals with scapular fractures show varied signs of lameness, dropped shoulder, extended elbow, carrying of the limb with carpal flexion, and loss of limb function. On palpation, pain may be elicited, and asymmetry can be detected. Injury to supraspinatus nerve may result in atrophy of supraspinatus and infraspinatus muscles. Articular fractures of glenoid may result in severe lameness and functional disability of the limb, crepitation of bone fragments, and unstable shoulder. Radiography will help to confirm the location, type, and extent of fracture.

Many stable extra-articular fractures of scapular body can be treated conservatively, by closed reduction and fixation. Normally, the fractured segment of scapula is displaced minimally toward the body wall and remains stable in position. Traction along

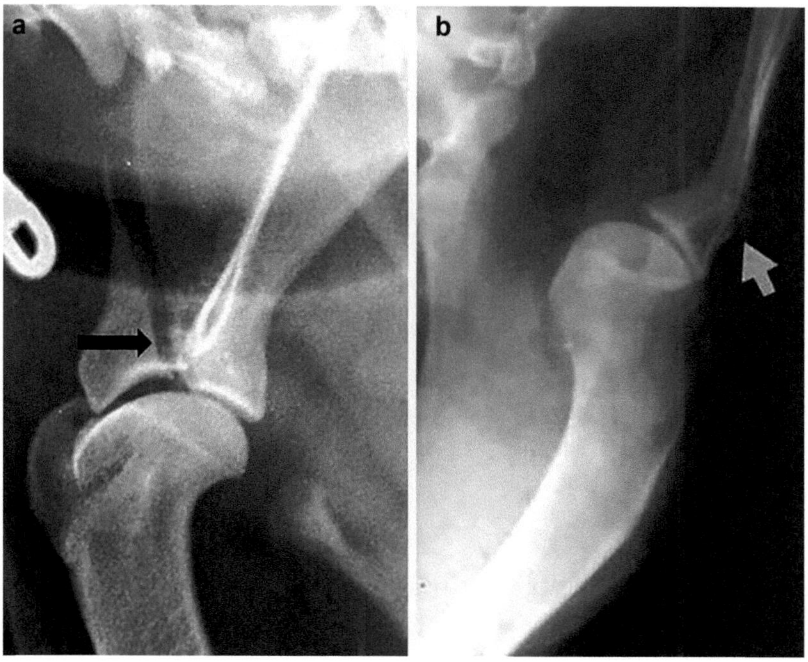


**Fig. 3.1** Fracture involving the glenoid (**a**) and neck (**b**) of scapula in dogs

the limb can help to facilitate reduction and alignment. Application of Velpeau sling can help to relieve load bearing on the limb and immobilize the fractured bone, 3–4 weeks of immobilization, which is usually enough (prolonged immobilization leads to muscle atrophy and limb dysfunction). Fracture of scapular spine can also be treated conservatively using a Velpeau sling. Prognosis is generally excellent, as healing normally occurs quickly with restoration of shoulder function.

Open reduction and internal fixation is advised for unstable fractures of scapular body, spine, fractures of the acromion, and most fractures of the scapular neck, supraglenoid tuberosity, and glenoid cavity [3]. Surgical treatment is challenging due to small fracture fragments and difficult approach owing to extensive soft tissue wrap. The scapular body and spine can be surgically exposed laterally by incising the dense fascia along the cranial and caudal edges of the spine and retracting the omotransversarius and trapezius muscles cranially and deltoideus muscle caudally [4]. The supraspinatus and infraspinatus muscles are elevated from the scapular spine (using a periosteal elevator) and the cranial and caudal fossae, respectively (during the closure of the incision, the fascia is sutured over the scapular spine). Scapular neck is surgically exposed by acromial osteotomy and retracting of supraspinatus and infraspinatus muscles and transaction of their tendons. The surgical approach to the scapular tuberosity is difficult due to its presence below the supraspinatus muscle; it can be approached laterally by osteotomy of greater tubercle of humerus and cranially by transaction of insertion of the superficial and deep pectoral muscles. The surgical approach to glenoid cavity requires acromion osteotomy and infraspinatus tenotomy along with arthrotomy; osteotomy of greater tubercle of humerus provides wider cranial exposure.

Different internal fixation techniques such as wire suture, K-wire, lag screw, tension band wire, and bone plate have been used to treat fractures of scapula [2, 3]. Scapular body fractures can be treated by internal fixation using interfragmentary wiring; however, it generally cannot prevent medial displacement of the fractured segment. Locking plate fixation over the body or attached to the scapular spine provides rigid immobilization (Fig. 3.2). For fracture of spine, placement of wire/plate on cranial surface of the spine can provide good fixation; K-wire can also be fixed through the spine into the scapular body. Fracture of acromion results in displacement of the fractured segment; hence, orthopedic wire sutures or

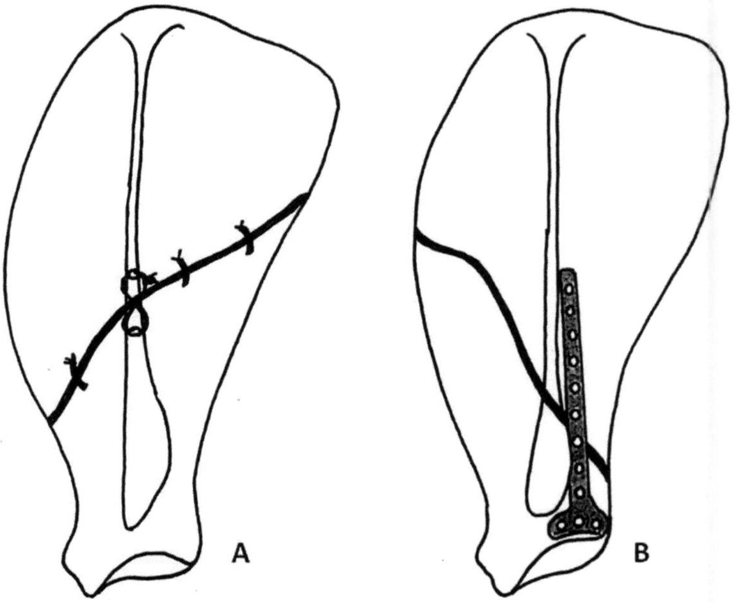


**Fig. 3.2** Fixation of scapular body fracture using interfragmentary wiring (**a**) and locking compression plate just beside and along the scapular spine (**b**)

tension band wiring can be used to provide rigid fixation. In scapular neck fractures, cross pinning can be done: one pin can be inserted through the supraglenoid tubercle and another caudal to the glenoid (Fig. 3.3). Two lag screws can also be fixed in similar fashion. More rigid fixation can be achieved using T- or L-plate (with locking head screws) fixed cranial to the scapular spine. Supraglenoid tubercle fracture can be treated using two K-wires, or lag screw fixation or tension band wiring. The fractured rim of the glenoid cavity should be anatomically reconstructed and fixed using K-wires, lag screws, cross pins, or locking/reconstruction plate and screw fixation. Salvage procedures like excision arthroplasty, partial scapulectomy, glenoidectomy, and shoulder arthrodesis are rarely required but are recommended when the joint is severely injured and difficult to reconstruct and stabilize.

Postoperatively, external immobilization is generally not needed, if required Velpeau sling may be provided for 2–3 weeks in fractures of scapular body and spine treated with less rigid wire sutures/K-wires. With rigid fixation such as plating, external stabilization is not needed. Normal limb movement should be encouraged early in the postoperative period, to prevent ankylosis of joint due to bony callus, especially in fractures near the joint. The prognosis following repair of scapular body/spine fracture is generally excellent, and for scapular neck fractures, it is good to excellent. The prognosis for unstable articular fractures is generally poor, with persistence of lameness in spite of regaining near normal functional recovery. Complications related to nerve injury or entrapment by bony callus may also occur.

## 3.2 Fractures of Humerus

Fractures of humerus are less commonly recorded as compared to other long bones in dogs and cats (7–8% of total long bone fractures in dogs). Although fracture can occur at any location of the bone, more number of fractures are seen at the middle and distal third of the bone [5]. Condylar-supracondylar fractures are often encountered in young growing animals. Oblique/spiral fractures are more frequently recorded than comminuted and transverse fractures.

### 3.2.1 Fractures of the Proximal Humerus

Fracture of the humerus head is somewhat unusual. In young animals, there may be separation at the physeal level with little displacement

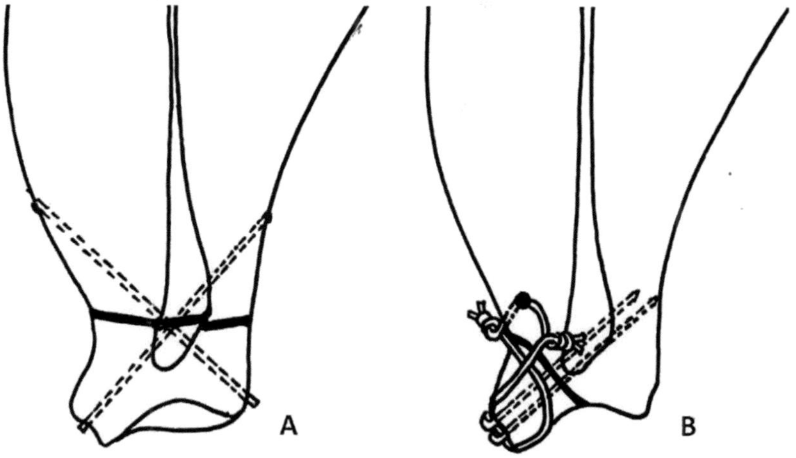


**Fig. 3.3** Schematic presentation of scapular neck fracture fixation using cross pinning done by inserting a pin through the supraglenoid tubercle and another caudal to the glenoid (**a**) and supraglenoid tubercle fracture treated using tension band wiring (**b**)

of the bone fragments. Such fractures may be treated using external fixation method such as a Velpeau sling or coaptation to the body wall placed in situ for about 2–3 weeks [6]. If there is complete separation of the head or greater tubercle, an internal fixation technique may be needed. In case of fracture of humerus head, the proximal humerus is approached through an anterior incision (made in front of, through the middle of or behind the deltoid muscle depending of the fracture location), and small K-wires/Steinmann pins can be inserted across the metaphyseal region into the humeral head. Whereas in fractures of greater tubercle, K-wires may be introduced from the tubercle down through the fracture line into the metaphyseal region. Generally, external immobilization is not needed, and the animal's movement is restricted for a few days. As such fractures are seen mostly in young animals, they heal faster with good functional recovery of the limb.

### 3.2.2 Diaphyseal Fractures of Humerus

Fractures can occur along the length of diaphysis, however, more common in the middle and distal third of humerus [7]. The animals with humerus fracture generally exhibit characteristic knuckling sign (Fig. 3.4), often leading to confusion among less experienced clinicians in localizing the fracture. Other cardinal signs such as swelling, pain, crepitation, and abnormal movement at the injured site may help locate the fracture. Radiography will help confirm the fracture and determine the exact configuration and the extent of fracture.

Complete fractures of humeral diaphysis are difficult to reduce by close method and maintain reduction by any external fixation technique. Fresh transverse fractures with little displacement may sometimes be reduced by external manipulation (by simultaneous traction, counter traction and toggling method) and fixed by closed method of IM pinning. Holding the reduced fracture firmly in one hand (left), an appropriate size Steinmann pin may be introduced by another hand (right) in a normograde manner from the proximal end (curved metaphyseal region distal to the head) down into the distal metaphyseal/epiphyseal region. Most of the diaphyseal fractures need open reduction and fixation.

Surgical approach to the shaft of humerus should be made with great care to locate and protect the radial nerve, which courses along the superficial surface of the brachialis muscle (which is superficial in cats) (Fig. 3.5). For the purpose, the brachialis muscle is identified and fully mobilized, and the nerve is protected by maintaining the contact between the nerve and the muscle belly. The muscle along with the nerve is looped and retracted away from the site of manipulation during fracture reduction. To expose the proximal humerus (especially during

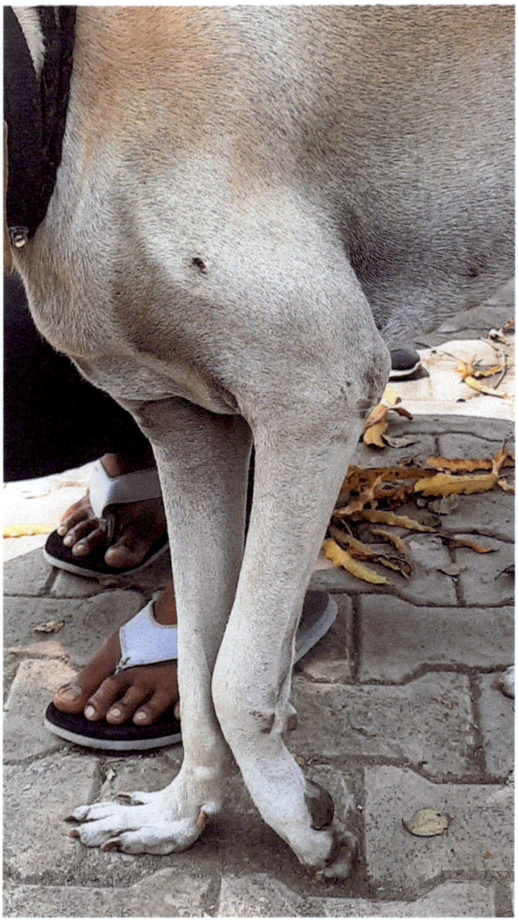

**Fig. 3.4** A dog with humerus fracture shows typical sign of knuckling

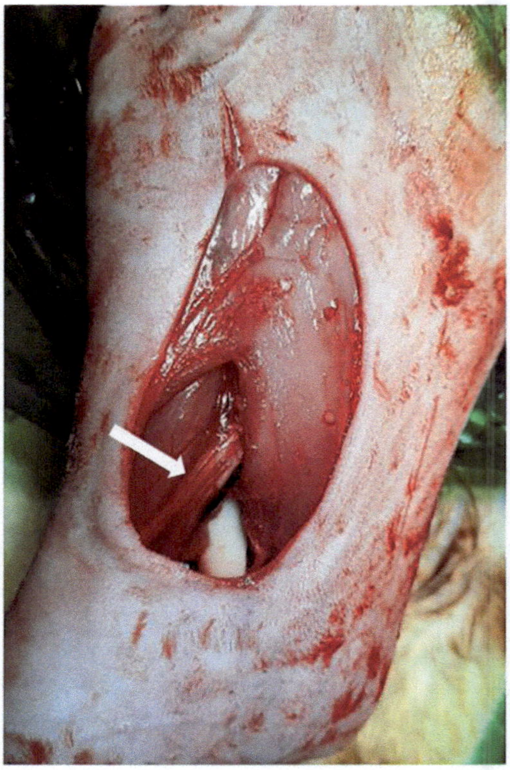

**Fig. 3.5** Radial nerve, coursing along the superficial surface of the brachialis muscle, is very superficial in cats

plating), the deltoid tuberosity may be severed, or the deltoid muscle may be elevated from the tuberosity (which can easily be reattached later).

IM pinning in the humerus can be done by normograde technique from either end or retrograde into either segment. Generally, the pin is passed from the shorter segment first to allow adequate purchase of the shorter segment. The pin can be positioned in the supracondylar region of the distal segment or in the medial epicondylar region. Seating the pin in the supracondylar region allows for the use of a larger diameter pin and is usually suitable for fractures in the proximal diaphysis. Seating the pin in the medial epicondylar region necessitates the use of a much smaller pin but allows much greater distal purchase, which is desirable for fixation of distal humeral fractures. The medial epicondyle has a characteristic square face, which can be used as a landmark for entering and exiting the pin distally. Care should be taken not to protrude any portion of the pin in the distal epicondyle into the surrounding soft tissues, which can cause discomfort and impede elbow range of motion. Generally, single IM pin will suffice to provide stable fixation of simple diaphyseal fractures of humerus [7] (Fig. 3.6). Use of end-threaded pin (Schanz pin) can help to better anchor at the distal metaphysis (Fig. 3.7). However, ILN will provide more stable fixation in comminuted fractures (Fig. 3.8). A suitable size Steinmann pin can be used as reamer to make track in the proximal bone cortex. The nail is inserted from the proximal end in a normograde manner and is seated distally in the supracondylar region.

In comminuted fractures, where intramedullary pin/nail is difficult to be used, bone plating can be done [8] (Fig. 3.9). In the

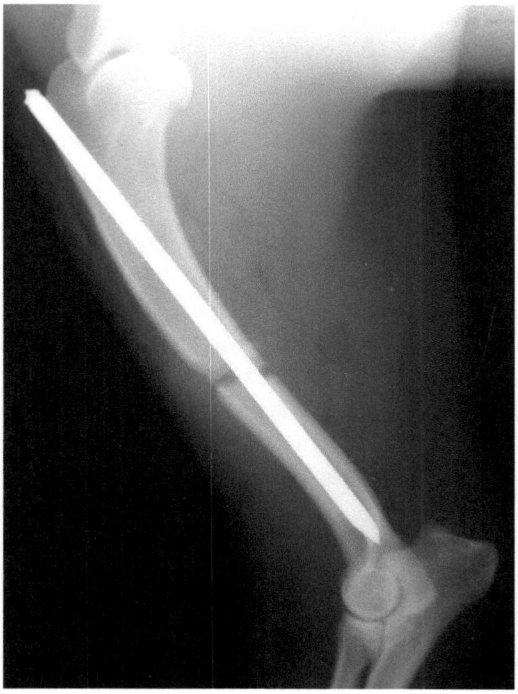

**Fig. 3.6** Intramedullay pin fixation in a mid-diaphyseal fracture of humerus in a dog. Note three point fixation at the proximal and distal ends of the bone, and at the fracture site

shaft of humerus, plate can be fixed in lateral, cranial, or caudal surface. In cranial approach, it is easier to visualize and protect the radial nerve, but the plate needs to be properly contoured to the curved cranial surface for stable fixation. The plate may extend from near the medial condyle distally and up to proximal to the greater tubercle. Generally, plate osteosynthesis provides rigid fixation, and often, the plate may fail by pulling out from the proximal end; hence, more screws may be fixed in the proximal humerus, by aiming the proximal screws toward the humerus head for greater purchase. Distal fractures may be better immobilized by fixing the plate on the caudal surface. External skeletal fixation is generally not indicated for repair of fractures of humerus. However, ESF using half pins and hybrid ESF can be applied in unstable severely comminuted fractures and in open fractures with infection. Often, it is used along with internal fixation such as IM pinning (Tie-in configuration), to provide stable fixation [9].

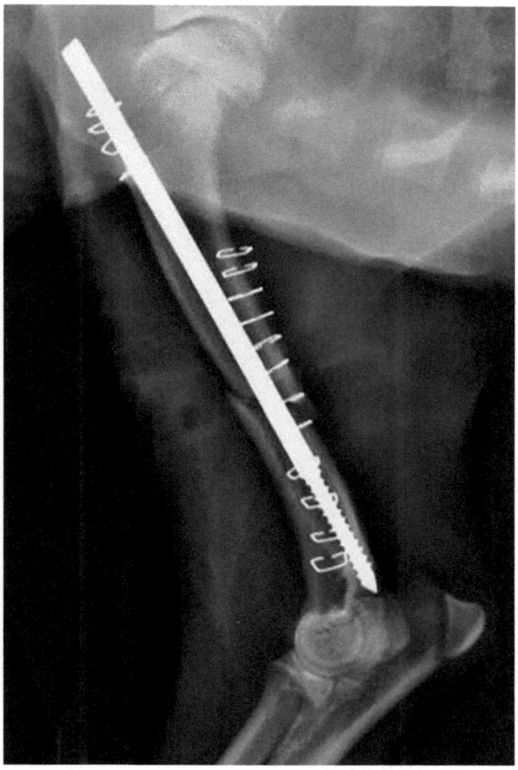

**Fig. 3.7** Use of end threaded pin (Schanz pin) for fixation of diaphyseal fracture of humerus in a dog. Threaded pin end provides better anchorage at the distal end (Courtesy: Dr. Tarunbir Singh, GADVASU, Ludhiana, India)

### 3.2.3 Fractures of the Distal Humerus

Distal humeral fractures may include supracondylar fractures, intercondylar (T/Y type) fractures, and condylar (lateral/medial) fractures or fractures involving the articular surface. These fractures are generally caused due to extension/flexion or shearing injuries. Though these fractures can often be reduced by closed method, it is difficult to retain the bone fragments in alignment using external fixation techniques. Healing with malunion may hamper the joint mobility. Hence, for stable fixation, internal fixation is generally preferred. Nevertheless, Modified Thomas splint has been widely used as external fixation technique of choice to treat fractures of the distal humerus, often with favorable outcome.

Supracondylar fractures of humerus may be caused either by extension injuries (where the

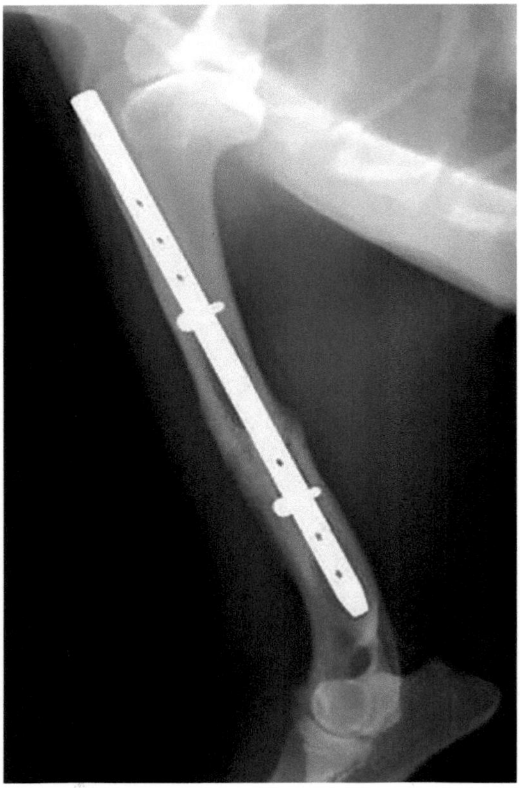

**Fig. 3.8** Static fixation of interlocking nail in diaphyseal fracture of humerus in a dog (Courtesy: Dr. SP Tyagi, Dr. GC Negi College of Veterinary and Animal Sciences, CSKHPKV, Palampur)

distal bone segment lies caudal to the proximal segment) or flexion injuries (where distal bone segment lies cranial to the proximal segment). Fracture can be reduced through a lateral incision made through the anconeus muscle at the joint level, which is then advanced proximally through the distal aspect of lateral head of the triceps. If needed, for better visualization of the condyles, olecranon osteotomy may be performed. Cross IM pinning is the most accepted treatment method in such cases (Fig. 3.10), with the K-wires/Steinmann pins introduced from the epicondylar area of the distal humerus, one each from the lateral and medial side. Medial pin is inserted after making a small stab incision below the medial epicondyle. Radial nerve is not usually affected, but it is taken care not to injure the ulnar nerve that lie caudo-lateral to the medial epicondyle while passing the medial pin. Generally, cross pinning provides stable fixation with good functional recovery.

Lateral condylar fracture of humerus is more common (than that of medial condyle) and usually results from a shear force transmitted along the radial head, shearing off the lateral condyle (common during a fall). In the process, the medial condyle attached with the shaft moves caudally and distally causing an abnormal swelling on the caudomedial aspect of the elbow joint. Palpation of elbow reveals crepitation with movement of lateral condyle. This can be treated by open reduction and placement of an intercondylar

**Fig. 3.9** Fixation of comminuted fracture of humerus in a dog with bone plating. Note the contouring of plate to adequately fix at the distal end of the bone

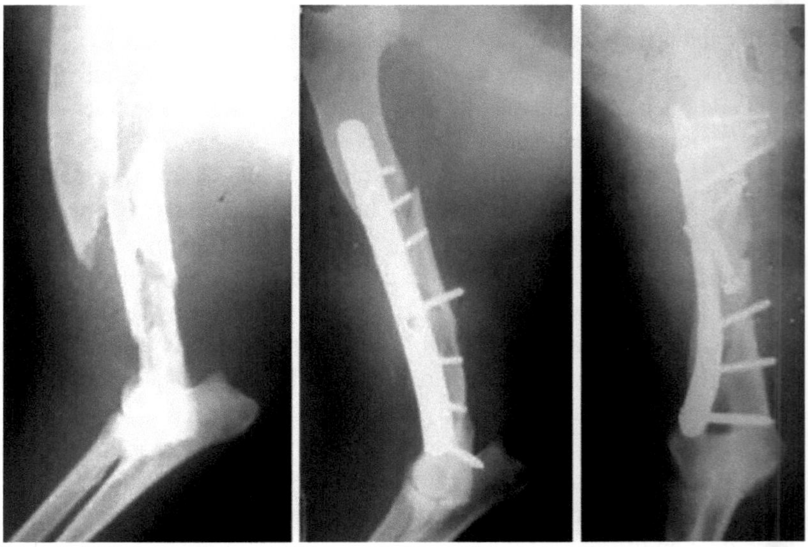

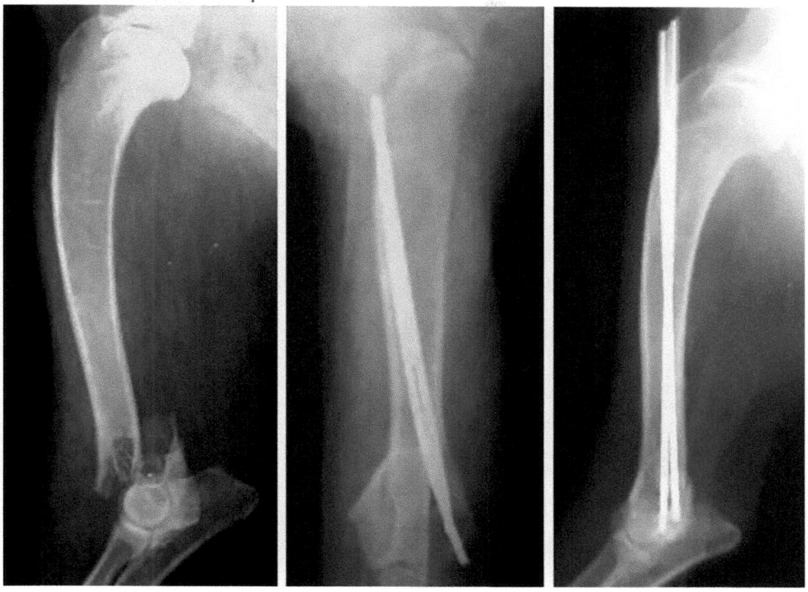

**Fig. 3.10** Supracondylar fracture of humerus stabilized with modified cross pin fixation in a dog. Note both the pins are passed from lateral surface of distal humerus

screw between the condyles (in lag screw fashion) to compress the lateral condyle with the medial condyle (Fig. 3.11). Insertion of a small K-wire through the proximal end of the condyle into the shaft of humerus may prevent rotation of the smaller fragment (Fig. 3.12). If properly reduced and fixed, good results are obtained. Alternatively, two K-wires/Steinmann pins may be fixed by introducing them through the lateral epicondyle (one from the cranial and another from the caudal aspect, alternatively) and then inserting into the proximal fragment to exit at the proximal end of humerus (cross IM pinning). The distal ends of the pins are countersunk beneath the condylar surface, and proximally, the pins are cut short close to the bone. This technique provides rigid fixation of lateral condylar fracture with good functional outcome. However, care should be taken while inserting the pins into the proximal fragment, as the condyles of humerus are clearly bifurcated and the lateral condyle is smaller and is positioned slightly away from the long axis of the diaphysis than the medial condyle, which is positioned more along the axis of the shaft.

In medial condylar fracture, almost similar technique is used to stabilize the fracture. Distal humerus is approached through medial approach by incising through the fascia just cranial to the medial head of triceps. The ulnar nerve and collateral ulnar artery are retracted caudally, and an intercondylar screw is fixed across the condyles (from medial to lateral) to bring about compression between the medial and lateral condyles. If the fracture line is extended proximally, another screw (or a K-wire) is fixed from the medial condyle into the shaft to provide rotational stability. This technique generally works well. Alternatively, 2 K-wires can be fixed in cross manner from the medial condyle into and through the proximal major bone segment as described above.

Intercondylar fractures of humerus (T/Y types) are less common (relatively more common in cats) but are more difficult to deal with than the lateral/medial condylar fractures. Using the standard lateral approach, the bone segments are reduced, and internal fixation is done in combination with olecranon osteotomy. After osteotomizing the ulna just proximal to the interosseous ligament, the annular ligament is laterally transected, and the proximal ulna is medially dislocated to expose the humeral condyles. Both condyles should be stabilized first using interfragmentary compression screws. This can be followed by cross IM pin fixation. In an unstable fracture, additional external support

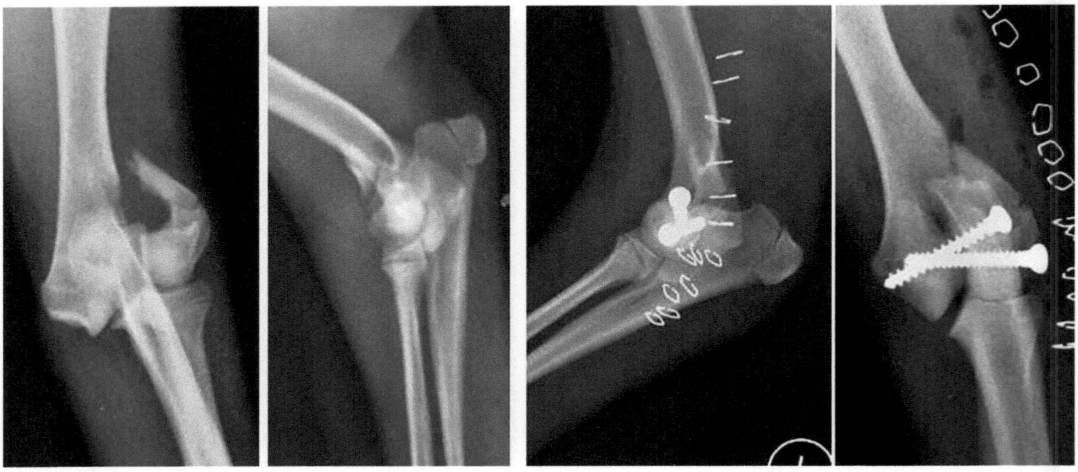

**Fig. 3.11** Lateral condylar fracture of humerus immobilized with two cross lag screws in a dog (Courtesy: Dr. Tarunbir Singh, GADVASU, Ludhiana, India)

may be given for a couple of weeks using a modified Robert Jones bandage or a modified Thomas splint.

The shape of the distal humerus makes bone plate and screw fixation difficult, but it is indicated in severely comminuted fractures, especially in heavy animals. The uneven surface makes it difficult to fix a standard bone plate; hence, plates that can be easily contoured such as SOP locking plates or reconstruction plates

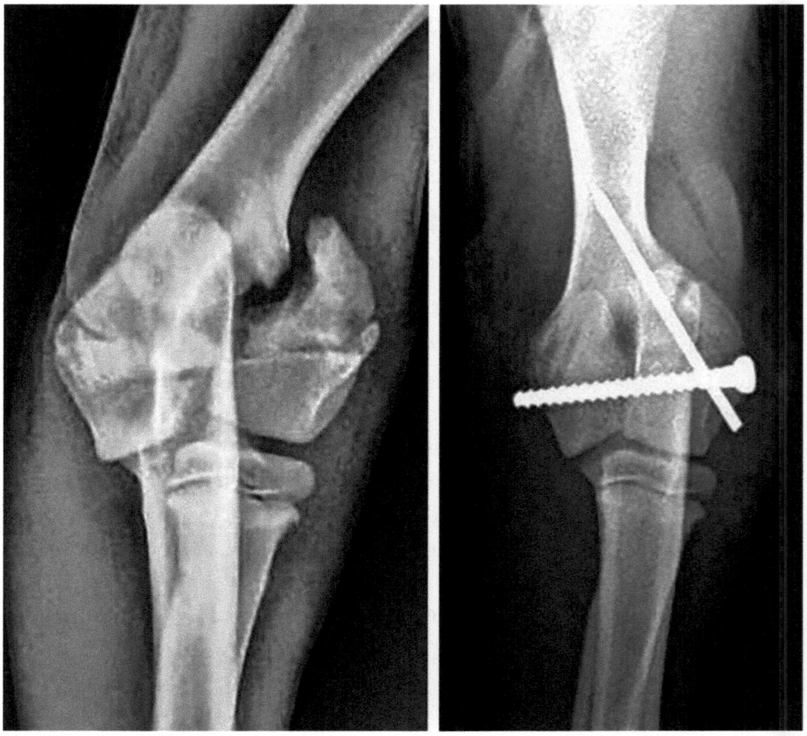

**Fig. 3.12** Intercondylar fracture in a pup stabilized with fixation of a lag screw across the condyles and K-wire (Courtesy: Dr. S. Ravikumar, Bangalore, India)

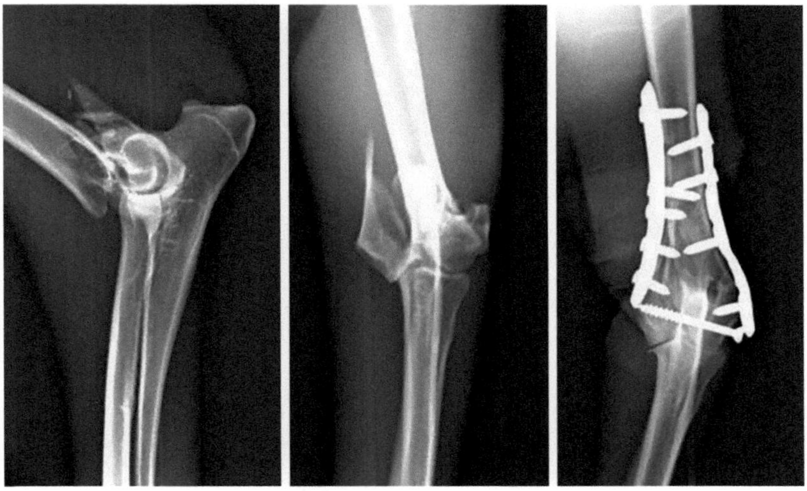

**Fig. 3.13** Comminuted fracture of humerus condyles stabilized with lag screw and double plate fixation with unicortical screws (Courtesy: Dr. Uddhav Sable, Pune, India)

with unicortical screws can be used to provide rigid fixation [10] (Fig. 3.13). Hybrid (combination of linear and circular) external skeletal fixation systems can also be used to stabilize short, juxta-articular fractures of humerus [11]. Fixation of plates and screws or ESF can be successfully used to treat distal and supracondylar humeral fractures in both dogs and cats [12].

## 3.3 Fractures of Radius-Ulna

The incidence of radius-ulna fracture is about 16–18% of all fractures in dogs. In most cases, both radius and ulna are affected; however, in isolated cases, only radius or ulna may get fractured. Radius-ulna fracture can occur along the whole length of the bones; however, most of the fractures are recorded at the middle and distal third of diaphysis. Among different types of fractures, transverse and short oblique fractures are more common [5, 13]. In small breed dogs, landing on the front limbs from a fall (simple fall from owner's arms or jump from height chasing a cat or monkey, etc.) is the most common cause of fracture, and in large breed dogs, usually substantial trauma is needed to break the bone, such as an automobile accident. Closed fractures are more common, but at times, open fractures are also seen, mostly at the distal radius-ulna due to least soft tissues around. Distal third of radius and ulna has a poor blood supply; hence, it is more susceptible to being fractured and is more prone to delayed union and nonunion, especially in small breed dogs [14, 15].

Animals with fracture of radius-ulna are generally presented with non-weight-bearing lameness with carrying of limb. Palpation may reveal crepitation, and the animal may exhibit pain. Bending at the site of fracture and flexion of carpus can also be noticed.

### 3.3.1 Fractures of the Proximal end of Radius/Ulna

Fractures of the head of the radius are uncommon, but when they occur, they are accompanied with fractures of surrounding bones such as ulna or humerus. Generally, there will not be much displacement of bone segments, which can be stabilized using any of the external fixation techniques such as cast immobilization or by internal fixation technique using small K-wires. In case of fracture of olecranon, tension band wire or orthopedic wire fixation (Fig. 3.14) may be used for stabilization [16]. For tension band wiring, two K-wires are inserted in normograde manner from the proximal end of ulna, either cranial or caudal to the attachment of triceps tendon (Fig. 3.15). The proximal cut end of the K-wires is bent cranially to prevent any injury to the tendon and to help secure the orthopedic wire for fixation in figure of 8 fashion

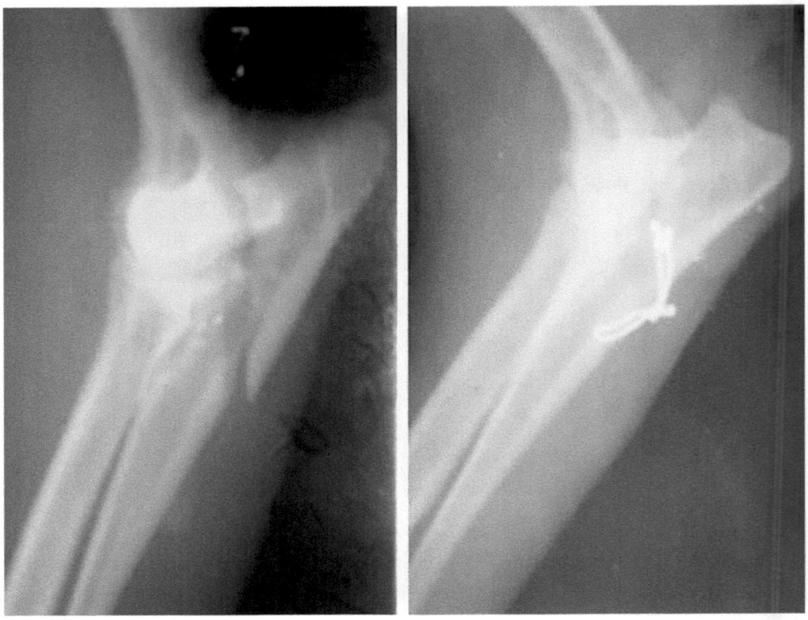

**Fig. 3.14** Orthopedic wire fixation (in figure of 8 fashion) for proximal ulnar fracture in a dog

[17]. Comminuted fractures of olecranon or proximal ulna can be stabilized by fixation of bone plate on the caudal aspect of the bone underneath the extensor carpi ulnaris or flexor carpi ulnaris. If radial fracture is concurrent with fracture of proximal diaphysis of ulna, bone plating can be undertaken to immobilize both the fractured bones. Fracture of upper third of ulnar diaphysis along with cranial luxation of the radial head, commonly referred to as a Monteggia fracture, can often be treated by closed reduction and external immobilization using modified Thomas splint. However, open reduction and internal immobilization provides more stable fixation. IM pin can be introduced by normograde technique through the olecranon process into the ulnar diaphysis (Fig. 3.16) [17]. Bone plate and screws fixed along the caudal (Fig. 3.17) or lateral surface (Fig. 3.18) of ulna can provide rigid fixation, especially in comminuted fractures often accompanied with proximal radial fracture.

### 3.3.2 Diaphyseal Fractures of Radius-Ulna

Diaphyseal fractures of radius-ulna are common and are mostly located at the distal third. As these, fractures are mostly transverse or short oblique in nature, and there is limited soft tissue covering, and such fractures can be easily reduced by closed method (traction, counter traction, and toggling). However, during bone reduction, it should be ensured that the skin is not damaged leading to open fracture.

External immobilization of closed fractures can be achieved by using either splints or casts [14, 18]. Splints and bandage can provide adequate fracture stability in young and small breed dogs, and in adult or heavy animals, cast immobilization should be preferred. But one should also remember that small breeds of dogs are more prone to delayed or nonunion; hence, stable immobilization is needed in small breeds of dogs too. During cast application, the animal is positioned with its injured leg down to prevent the placement of leg in a valgus position leading to external rotation of the limb during bone healing. Cast can be of plaster of Paris or synthetic fiberglass molded to the particular animal, which can be a double half cast or fully encircling cast. A fully encircling cast is the strongest and is preferred in large breeds of dog. On the other hand, a double half cast is preferred when the condition of soft tissues does not permit the placement of permanent encircling cast, like in cases of

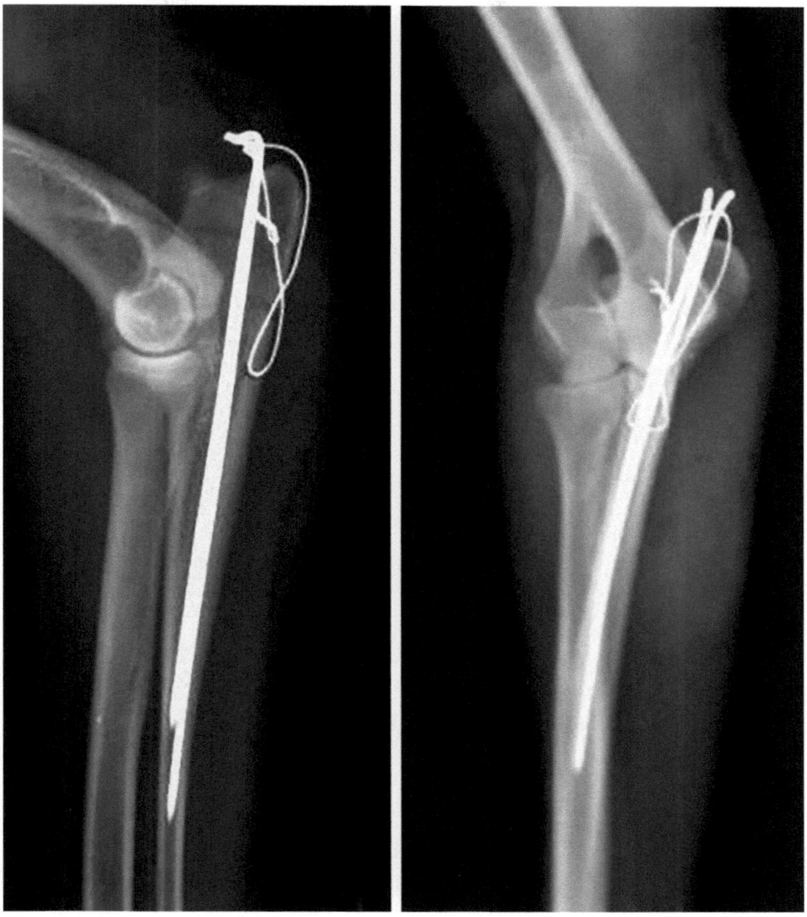

**Fig. 3.15** Tension band wiring for fixation of olecranon fracture in a dog (Courtesy: Dr. Tarunbir Singh, GADVASU, Ludhiana, India)

inflammatory swelling or in open fracture environment, where half cast can be removed for examination and reapplied frequently. Once the swelling subsides, or the open wound heals, if needed, it can be replaced with fully encircling cast.

Internal fixation in radius is done when the fracture is severely comminuted and inherently unstable. Intramedullary pin is seldom used in radius. The shape and position of radius precludes safe placement of pins using standard retrograde or normograde techniques [19]. The exit of the pin through retrograde placement and removal of the pin disrupts the radiocarpal joint and hence not recommended. The small diameter IM pin inserted through the fracture site and toggled into the opposite bone fragment (IM peg) is not enough to resist weight-bearing loads in most cases (Fig. 3.19). Further, as the radius is flattened, it is not amenable to effective use of full cerclage wires. Often, radius and ulna fractures can be treated by inserting a pin in the ulna (by normograde technique through the olecranon), which will help reduce the radial fracture as well. However, in heavy animals, it should be supplemented with a radial plate or an ESF. Hence, most of the times, if surgical fixation is required, the radius-ulna fractures are better treated with fixation of either a bone plate and screws or an external skeletal fixator.

The bone plate (DCP/LCP) is applied on the relatively flat cranial (tension) surface of radius, which will also immobilize the ulna (no need to stabilize ulna separately) (Figs. 3.20 and 3.21) [20]. The skin incision is made in the craniomedial surface, so as to cover the plate with the skin flap. Bone plate and screw fixation provide stability to radius-ulna fractures both in

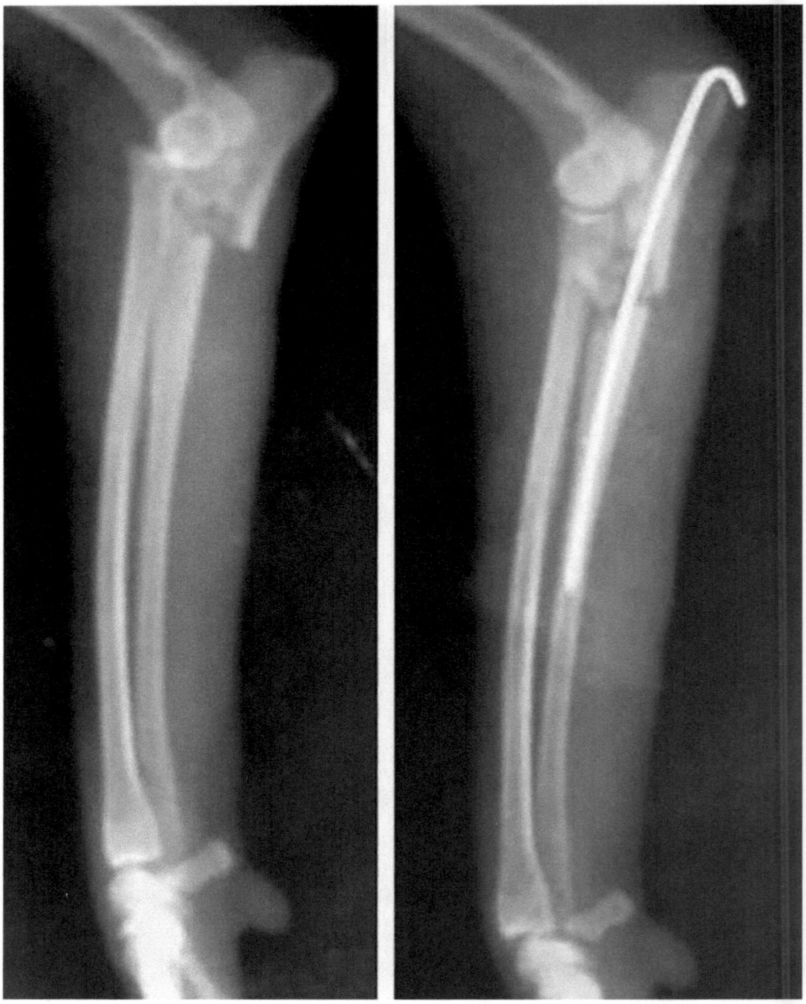

**Fig. 3.16** Normograde pinning for proximal ulnar fracture repair in a dog

small and large breeds of dogs [21–23]. It should be remembered that bone healing takes relatively more time at the distal radius-ulna even with plate and screw fixation, and healed bone does not regain its full strength for some time after plate removal. It is not necessary to remove the plate after fracture healing, unless situation warrants. If removed, the limb should be temporarily splinted to avert the chances of any re-fracture. Another complication that may arise with plating of radius-ulna is the lack of surrounding soft tissues for covering the plate. At times, wound dehiscence leading to exposure of the plate may occur. In such cases, when it is not possible to appose the skin edges, it may be treated as open wound with additional external support with application of splint and bandages. In young animals (< 6–8 month old), application of plate and screws at the distal end may damage the growth plate causing limb shortening and/or deformity. Due to these problems, often radius-ulna fractures are treated using external skeletal fixation (ESF), which is becoming more popular.

ESF is ideally suited for treatment of radius-ulna fractures, as it is easy to palpate the bone and insert the pins due to little soft tissue interference [24, 25]. ESF is preferred not only in open fractures but also in closed fractures of radius-ulna as it can provide rigid fixation with minimal soft tissue and vascular damage. Uniplanar and unilateral fixation systems are used in small animals, whereas in heavy large breeds, bilateral

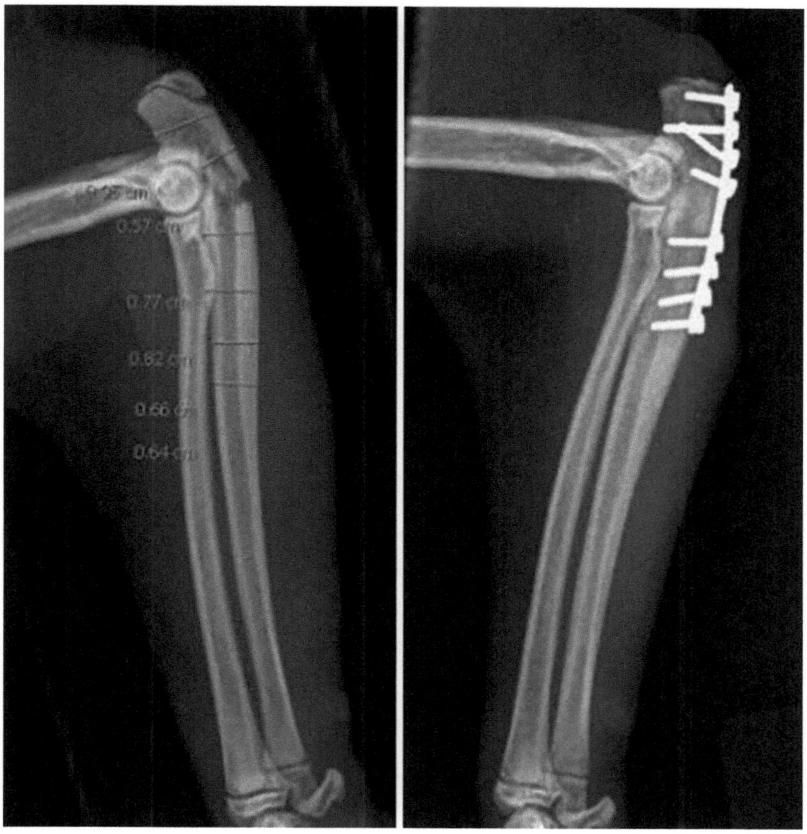

**Fig. 3.17** Rigid fixation of alecranon fracture by plating on the caudal surface of ulna (Reproduced with permission from: Russell Yeadon; External Skeletal Fixation in Small Animal Fracture Repair Vets Now Referrals, Swindon, www.vets-now.com)

or multiplanar systems are used. In unilateral designs, threaded pins are preferred, and in bilateral designs, threaded or smooth pins may be used (Fig. 3.22). Circular and hybrid fixation systems have also been used with success (Fig. 3.23). Acrylic or epoxy-pin fixation systems are versatile and have been found to provide stable fixation of radius-ulna fractures, especially in open fracture environment (Figs. 3.24 and 3.25) [26].

### 3.3.3 Fractures at the Distal Radius and Ulna

Distal epiphyseal fractures may be seen in young dogs and cats. The distal epiphysis typically deviates laterally with external rotation (valgus deformity) of the limb. Such fractures are often managed by closed reduction and external immobilization. If treatment is not done early, permanent lateral deviation may be seen due to fibrosis and callus formation. Any injury to the growth plate may cause premature closure of distal radial or ulnar physis leading to angular deformities. Distal ulnar styloid fracture may also be treated by closed reduction and external immobilization. However, distal radial styloid fracture, which is intraarticular, needs perfect reduction and alignment using an internal fixation, either K-wire or tension band wire, along with external coaptation. In adult animals, bone plate and screw fixation can be done to provide stable fixation (Fig. 3.26). Use of T-plate can provide greater purchase at the small distal bone segment (Fig. 3.27 and 3.28) [27]. Open fractures may be treated using any of the ESF techniques by trans-articular fixation (Fig. 3.29).

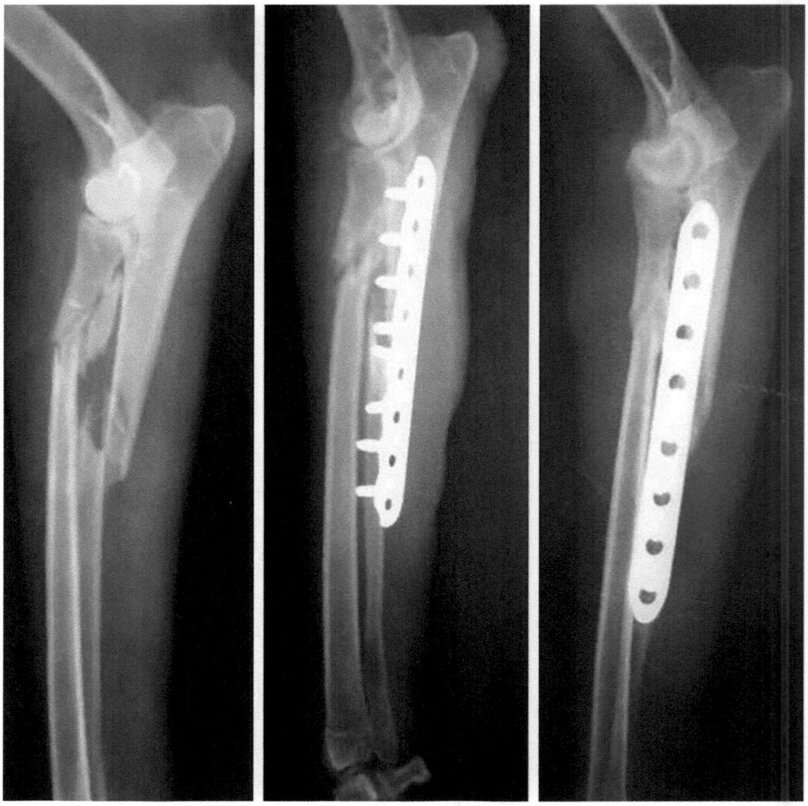

**Fig. 3.18** Locking Compression Plate fixation in comminuted fracture of proximal radius-ulna in a dog. Note that plating of ulna adequately stabilized proximal radial fragments

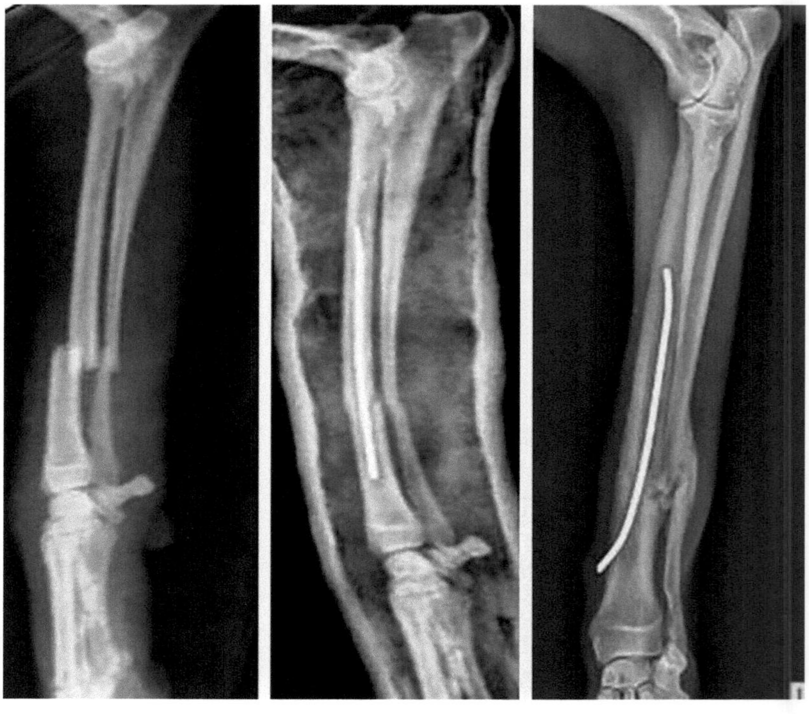

**Fig. 3.19** Stabilization of radial fracture by pegging a small IM pin. As fixation is less stable, the technique can be used only in light weight animals and should be provided with external support during early post-fixation days (Source: M.D. Prabhukumar et al., Elastic stable intramedullary nailing for fixation of distal diaphyseal fracture of radius in two dogs. Indian J. Vet. Surg. 41(2): 134–136, 2020)

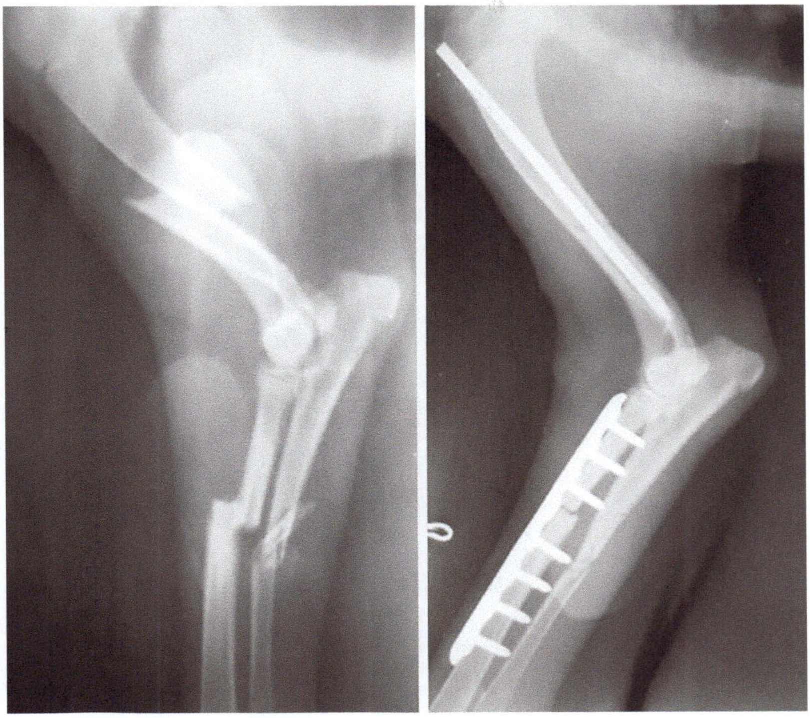

**Fig. 3.20** Comminuted fracture of radius-ulna immobilized with fixation of locking compression plate on the cranial surface of radius, and oblique mid-diaphyseal fracture of humerus stabilized with IM pinning. Note that fixation of radius with plate and screws stabilized ulnar fracture automatically

## 3.4 Fractures of Femur

Fractures involving the pelvic limb are more common than that of pectoral limb. Further, femur bone is more often fractured than other long bones both in dogs and cats [5, 28]. In femur, fracture can occur along the length of the bone. The incidence of fractures at middle and distal end is more than the fractures at the proximal femur. Automobile accident is the common

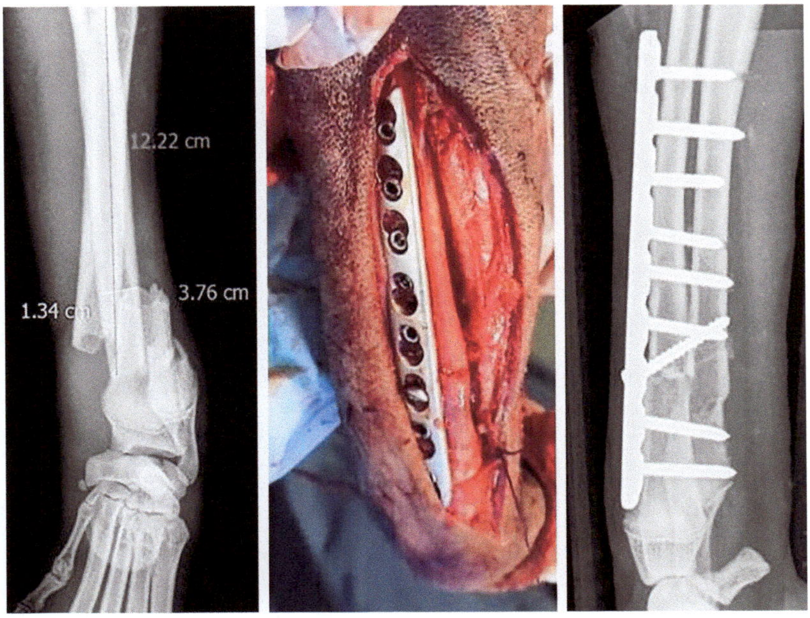


**Fig. 3.21** Fracture of radius and ulna at the distal diaphysis stabilized with locking compression plate. Note the compression at the fracture site due to fixation of a lag screw

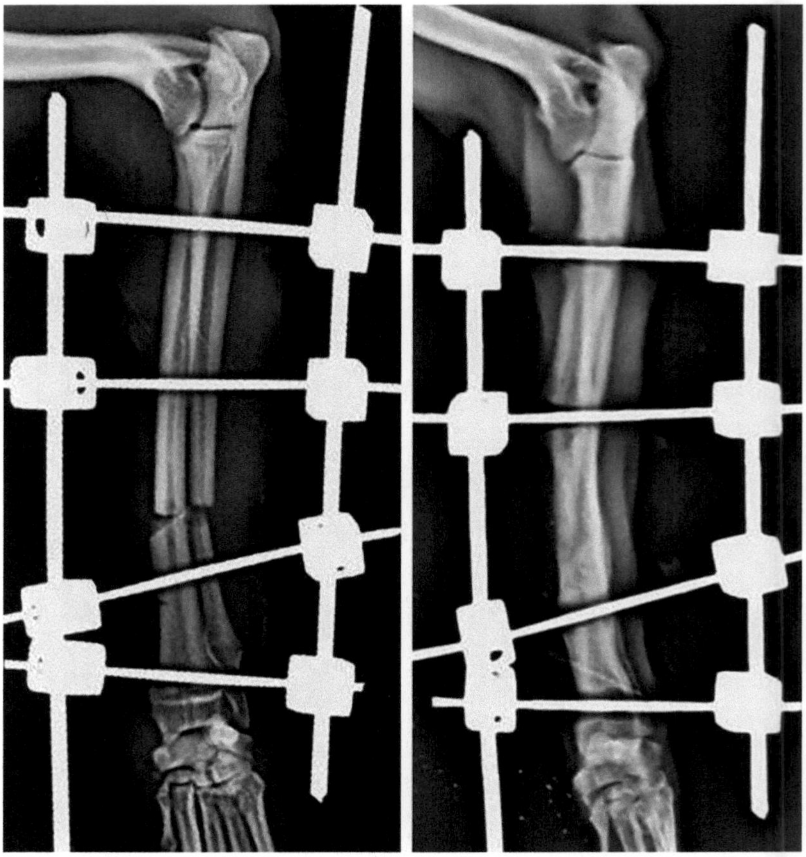

**Fig. 3.22** Bilateral linear ESF applied for fixation of radius-ulna fracture in a dog (Courtesy: Dr. Remala Sridhar, Tanuku, Andhra Pradesh, India)

cause of fractures, while falling/jumping from a height may also lead to fractures, more often at the distal end of femur bone [13]. Though femur fracture is recorded in animals of all age groups,

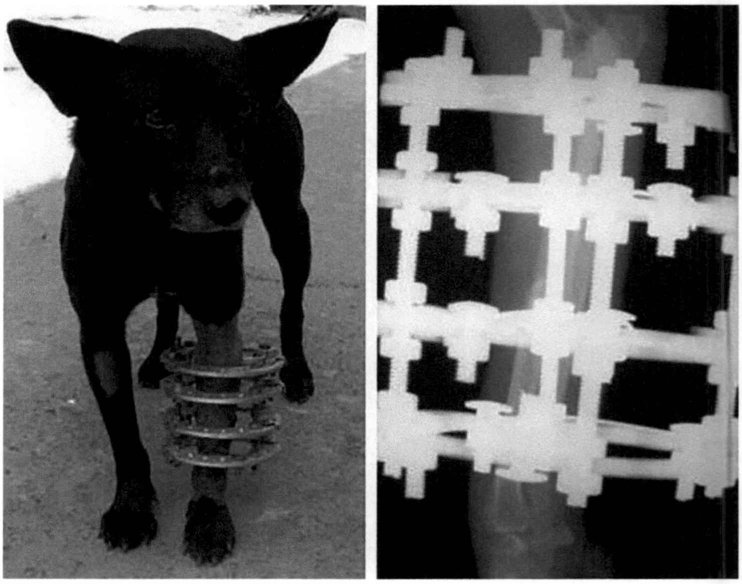

**Fig. 3.23** CEF application for radius-ulna fracture repair in a dog

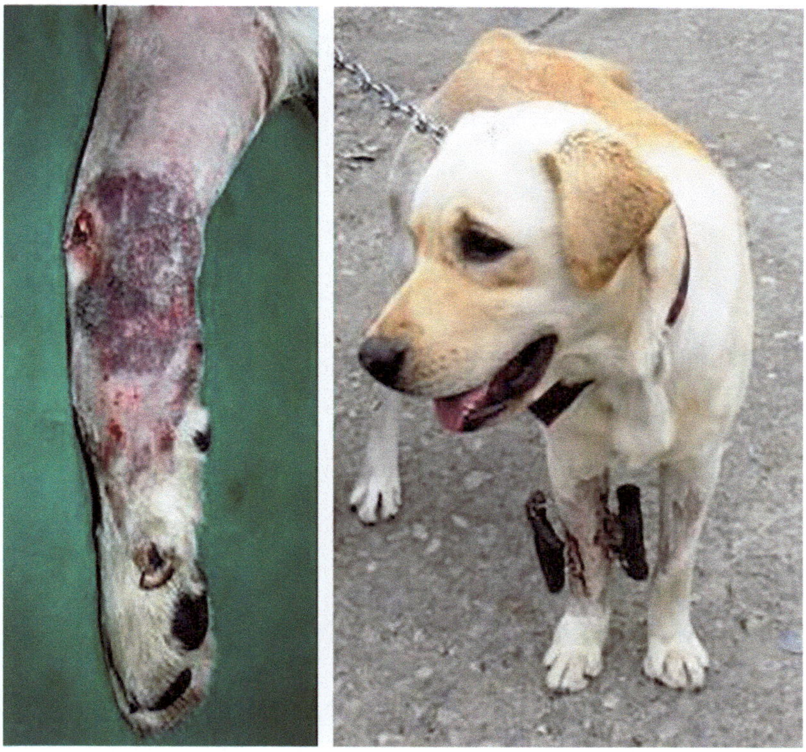

**Fig. 3.24** Multiplanar epoxy-pin fixation for repair of an open fracture of radius-ulna of a dog

young animals aged less than 1 year are more prone. Supracondylar and condylar fractures are more frequent in young animals. Femur fractures are mostly oblique or comminuted in nature. In young and osteoporotic bones, often green stick fractures are recorded [29].

As the femur bone is proximally located more close to the body and is surrounded by heavy musculature, external fixation techniques do not provide stable bone fixation. Hence, internal fixation is generally preferred and more often practiced. For practical purpose, femoral fractures can be categorized as (i) femoral head-neck and sub trochanteric fractures, (ii) diaphyseal fractures, and (iii) distal femoral (distal diaphyseal, condylar, and supracondylar) fractures.

### 3.4.1 Femur Head-Neck and Subtrochanteric Fractures

Femoral head-neck and subtrochanteric fractures constitute about 10–15% of total femoral fractures (Fig. 3.30). Most of the femur head-neck (intracapsular) fractures are encountered in young animals, due to shearing force [30]. Fractures at the base of neck (extracapsular) sometime occur in older animals. Most of such fractures result from vehicular accidents (typically fracture line is perpendicular to the long axis of neck) or sometimes occur due to the animal falling from a height, wherein shearing force act to separate the femur head from the shaft as the axial compression force is transmitted along the long axis of the bone (usually fracture line is parallel to the long axis of weight bearing). The simultaneous fractures of the femur head-neck and the greater trochanter (separation of apophysis) are also not uncommon. Often, fractures are seen at the proximal femur, at the subtrochanteric region.

Clinical signs include non-weight bearing, dragging, and dysfunction of the involved limb and variable degree of soft tissue swelling (generally no soft tissue swelling is seen in cases of hip joint luxation). Radiographic examination may reveal completely severed femoral head and/or

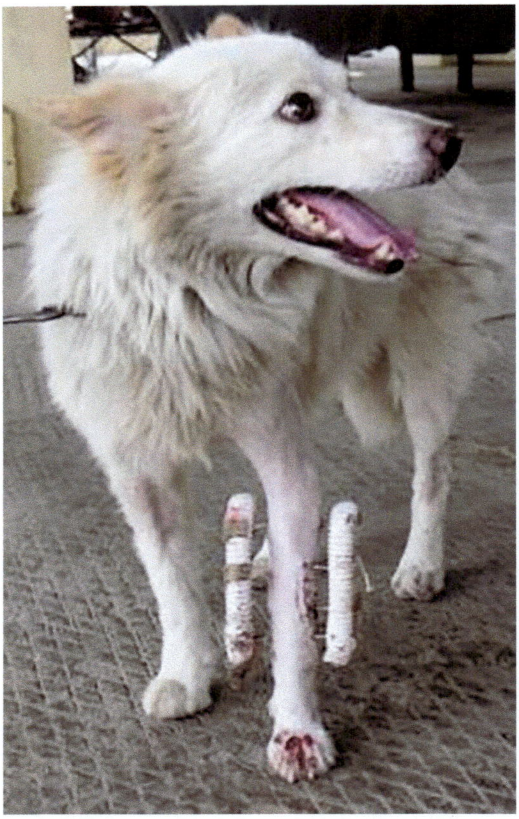

**Fig. 3.25** Multiplanar ESF prepared from dental acrylic for fixation in radius-ulna fracture in dog

neck with the long distal bone fragment displaced proximally or medially.

Fractures of the femur head and neck or subtrochanteric fractures are challenging to stabilize using any of the fixation techniques. Heavy musculature and proximal medial attachment of the femur head within the acetabular cavity make closed reduction of such fractures nearly impossible. Similarly, external fixation is also neither possible nor provide adequate stability at the fracture site, except maybe in incomplete fractures. Plaster cast or Modified Thomas splint should never be applied, as they may act as fulcrum and further disturb the fracture site. Internal fixation with multiple pins or interfragmentary screw fixation is an ideal method for femur neck fractures [31] and more rigid bone plate fixation for subtrochanteric fractures. Surgical treatment of femoral head and neck fractures should be undertaken at the earliest. If delayed or left alone, fibrous nonunion and resorption of femoral neck may result leading to degenerative changes.

#### 3.4.1.1 Surgical Approach

Femoral head and neck may be approached through a cranial incision, to preserve the blood circulation to the joint capsule and femoral head. Dorsal approach through trochanteric osteotomy should be avoided, as it will disrupt the blood flow to the femoral neck coming via gluteal muscle mass and lateral circumflex vessel coming from dorsal side. Further, as femoral head-neck fractures occur mostly in young animals with open physes, trochanteric osteotomy may lead to untimely closure of that physis causing permanent valgus deformity of femoral head and neck.

A cranially curved skin incision is made starting from just above the greater trochanter and further taking around it distal to the proximal one third of the femur. The tensor fascia lata is incised, and the biceps femoris is retracted caudally. Bluntly, the gluteal muscle is pushed dorsally, the rectus femoris and tensor fasciae latae cranially, and the lateral circumflex femoral artery retracted distally, which exposes the acetabular rim and the joint capsule. A small incision is given over the capsule (perpendicular to the acetabular rim) to expose the joint and locate the intracapsular fracture. Opening the joint will also help in extracapsular fractures as well for better visualization of the fracture site.

Surgical approach to the proximal femur (for subtrochanteric fracture repair) can be achieved through routine fascia lata incision. The incision may stretch from the greater trochanter (proximally) up to the mid femur (distally). The femur bone is exposed by retracting the biceps femoris muscle bundle caudally and the vastus lateralis cranially. If the proximal end of femur needs to be accessed, the incision may be extended up to the level of origin of the vastus lateralis. Complete severing of the origin of the muscle (vastus lateralis) may provide access to the proximal medial aspect, but it should be avoided whenever possible.

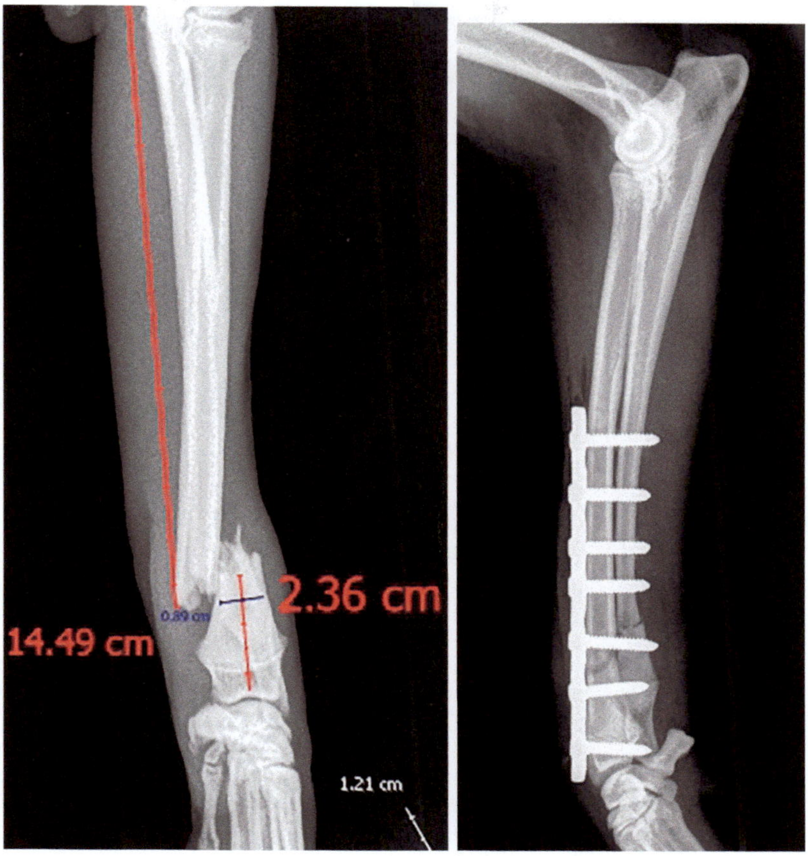


**Fig. 3.26** Distal radius-ulna fracture repair using locking compression plate and locking head screws. Note good fracture reduction and alignment

#### 3.4.1.2 Surgical Fixation

Femoral head-neck fracture is stabilized with an interfragmentary compression technique [32]. A large (gliding) hole is first drilled through the proximal femur, and the femoral head-neck segment is then reduced and fixed temporarily using a small K-wire. The fracture reduction and the range of joint motion is ensured. Following fracture reduction, by inserting the drill through the large hole in the proximal femur, a small threaded hole is drilled along the neck into the head of femur. The hole is then measured and tapped, and a fully threaded cortical screw is drilled from the proximal femoral shaft into the femoral head, making sure that the screw tip has not protruded into the joint. Once the screw is tightened, the K-wire is removed. The joint is then checked for crepitation and the range of motion to make sure that the screw has not entered the joint space. It is not normally necessary to use additional K-wires for rotational stability. However, two to three K-wires can also be used to stabilize the fracture instead of screw fixation (Fig. 3.31). During fixation of fractures at the femur head-neck, care should be taken to see that there is no valgus deformity at the fracture site. Fracture reduction should be either perfect (normal) or in slight varus position. This varus deformity will resolve itself during the course of healing.

Small chip fractures of femoral head are treated by removing the small bony fragments from the acetabular cavity. If allowed to remain in place, it may lead to degenerative changes. Chip fractures on the weight-bearing dorsal surface should be treated with resection of head and neck or total hip arthroplasty.

The simultaneous fractures of femur head-neck and separation of apophysis of greater trochanter can be treated relatively easily, through

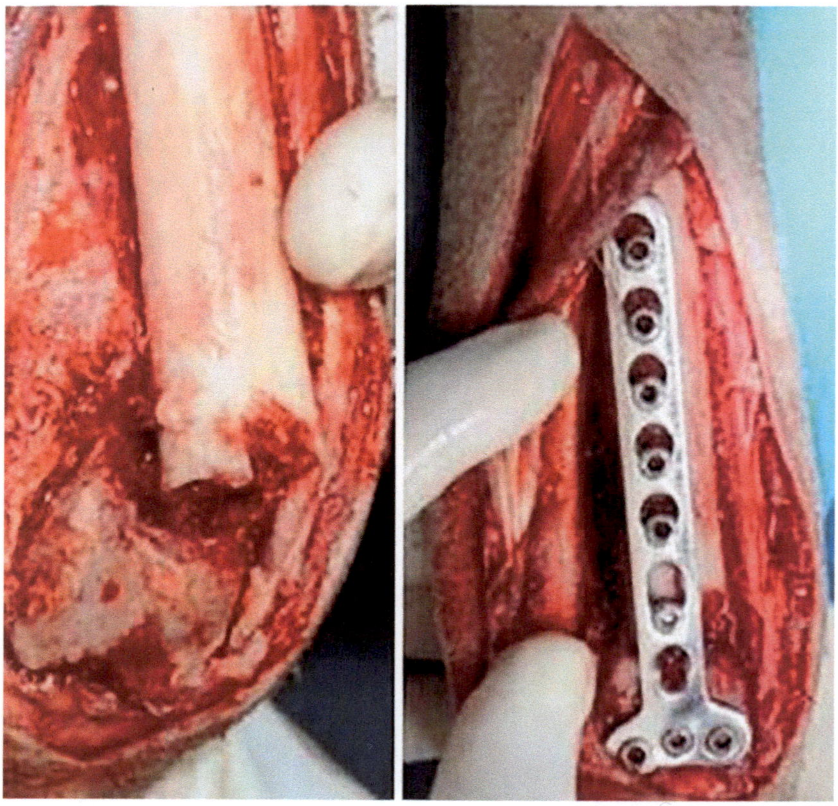

**Fig. 3.27** Surgical fixation of distal radius-ulna fracture using a T-plate (LCP) (Source: Taranjot Kaur Sran et al, Use of locking T-plate for repair of distal third radius-ulna fractures in 12 dogs. Indian J. Vet. Surg. 42 (2), Dec 2021)

an anterior approach. A screw is fixed to bring interfragmentary compression between the head-neck and the femoral shaft, whereas one or two K-wires can be used in the greater trochanter.

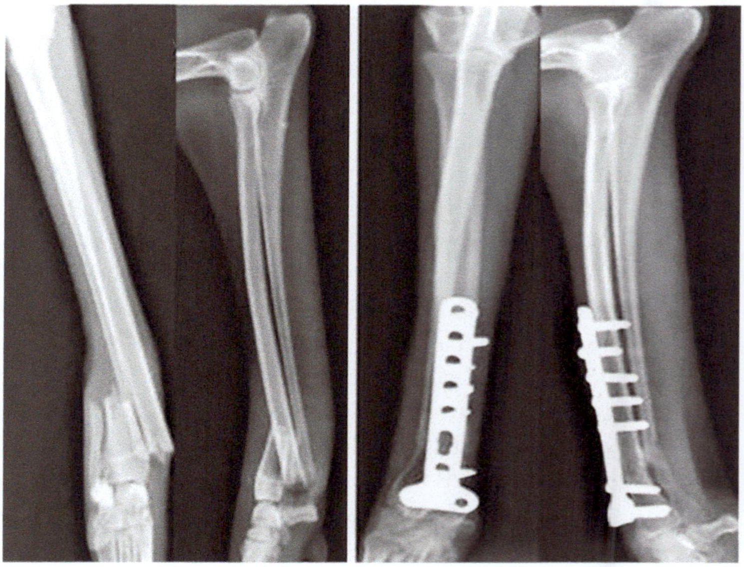

**Fig. 3.28** Radiographs shows distal radius-ulna fracture stabilized with a T-plate. Note good reduction and alignment of bone segments. T-plate allows better purchase at small distal bone segment with more number of screws (Source: Taranjot Kaur Sran et al., Use of locking T-plate for repair of distal third radius-ulna fractures in 12 dogs. Indian J. Vet. Surg. 42 (2), Dec 2021)

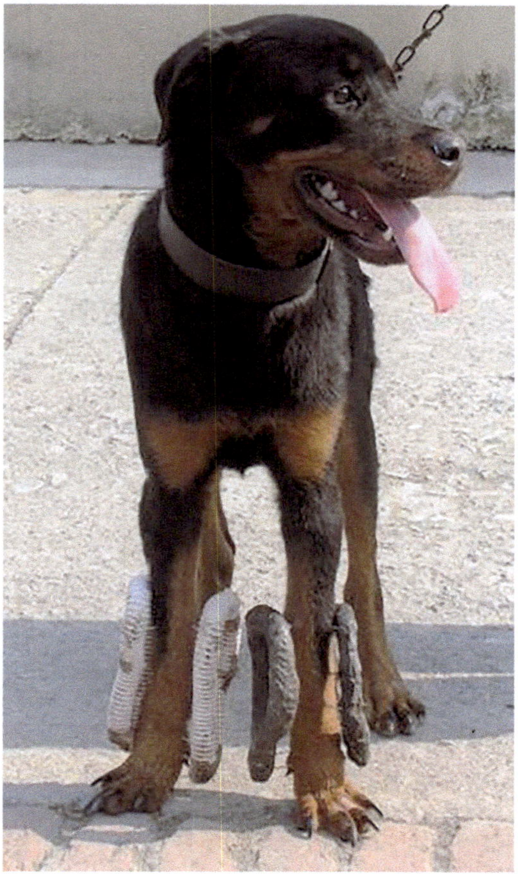

**Fig. 3.29** Bilateral distal radius-ulna fractures repaired using acrylic-pin (right) and epoxy-pin (left) ESF fixation (transarticular)

In cases of subtrochanteric femoral fractures, the fracture site is approached through the proximal surgical approach. Through traction and manipulation, fracture reduction and alignment are achieved. As the subtrochanteric region is subjected to maximum bending stress, any fixation technique used should provide rigid bone fixation. Hence, these fractures can be better stabilized using bone plates, either contoured standard bone plates or angle blade plates. The standard plate must be bent and contoured before fixing on the lateral surface of the proximal femur (tension side), including the greater trochanter. At least one or two screws in the proximal fragment should be directed into the femoral neck/head to achieve greater purchase. The plate should run the maximum length of the diaphysis distally, but at least three screws should be fixed in the distal bone segment. Angle blade plate is also fixed in similar manner, such that the blade of the plate is driven into the femoral neck through the greater trochanter to achieve adequate purchase (Fig. 3.32). Subsequently, the side plate is fixed to the distal segment using adequate number of screws.

In certain cases, if the proximal bone segment has some length to provide purchase for the pin, a Steinmann pin can be inserted first through the proximal segment (normograde or retrograde)

**Fig. 3.30** Femoral head fractures in dog: a case of fresh fracture (**a**) and an old fracture with degenerative changes (**b**)

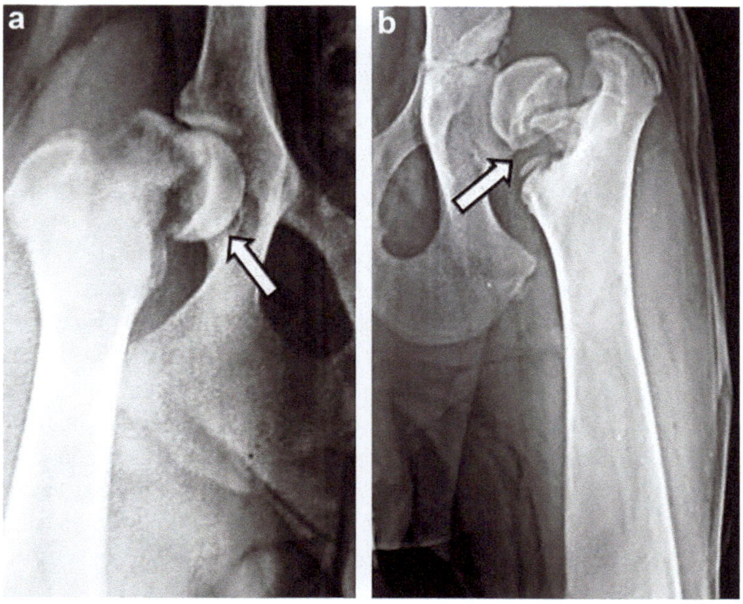

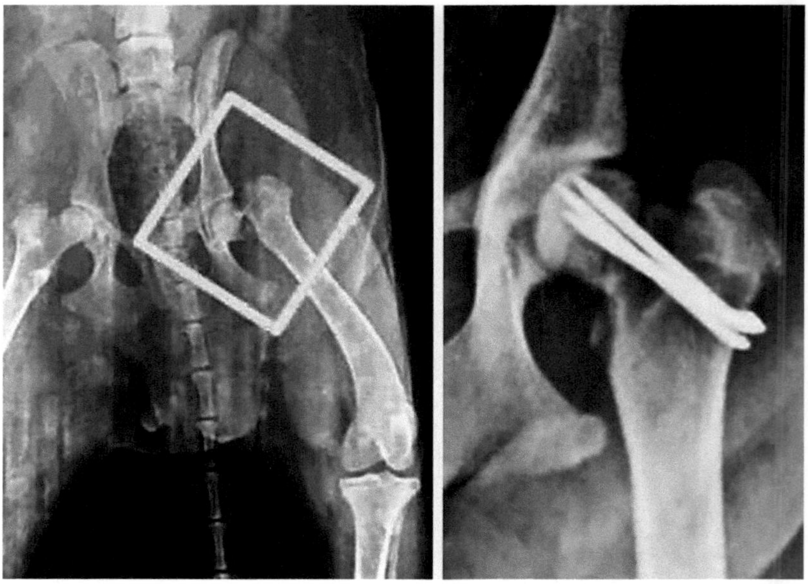

**Fig. 3.31** Surgical fixation of femoral head fracture using K-wires (Courtesy: Dr. Drona Patil, Mumbai, India)

and, then after reducing the fracture, driven into the distal segment to seat in the distal metaphysic (Fig. 3.33). However, utmost care should be taken while inserting the pin in the small proximal segment and while reducing and aligning the bone segments so that there will not be further splintering/comminution of the fractured bone. If done carefully, IM pin can provide adequate stability till the bone heals (generally, healing occurs quickly in the metaphyseal region).

#### 3.4.1.3 Postoperative Care and Possible Complications

Postoperatively, the animals are not placed in any form of external bandage or splint. The animals should be confined to cages and allowed only limited activity. It should be ensured that the normal motion of the hip joint is maintained without putting any undue stress at the fracture site. During weight bearing, the surgical site is subjected to bending and torsional forces, which may lead to bending of the implant and fixation failure. Failure of surgical fixation is often seen during the first 2 weeks of repair; hence, extra care has to be taken during this period. At times, if the motion at the fracture site persists, nonunion may occur. It is not imperative to remove the fracture fixation implants, unless they cause some complication or infection occurs. If IM pin is used, then it is recommended to remove after complete fracture healing as it can be easily done, and prolonged presence of pin may lead to pin loosening and migration.

### 3.4.2 Femoral Diaphyseal Fractures

Diaphyseal fractures constitute about 60–65% of total femoral fractures. Further, more number of fractures are seen in the middle and distal third of shaft than the proximal third. Oblique and comminuted fractures are more common than other types. The animals with femoral diaphyseal fractures are normally presented with non-weight bearing and dragging of the affected limb. Variable degree of soft tissue swelling is seen, sometimes extending downward toward the stifle (more common in distal femoral fractures). Palpation shall reveal crepitus at the site of fracture. Radiography will help to know the type and extent of fracture and help to preplan the fixation.

Closed reduction and blind intramedullary pin fixation [33, 34] of fresh, incomplete fractures with bending at the fracture site can be easily brought about in fresh cases by exerting gentle pressure at the fracture site using a thumb finger along with simultaneous pulling of the leg (Fig. 3.34). Closed reduction of femoral

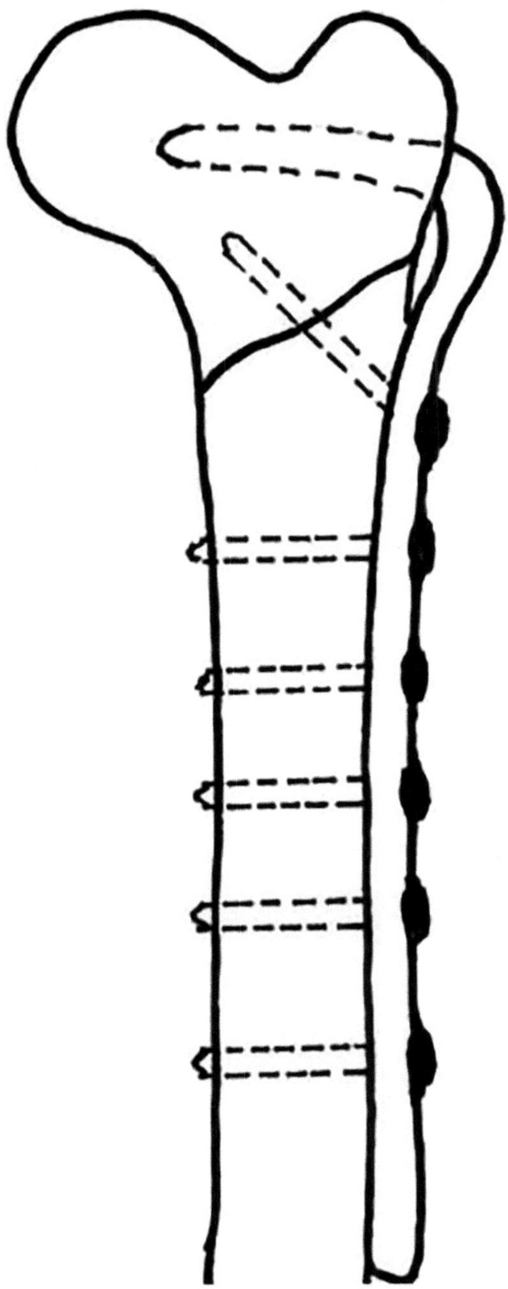

**Fig. 3.32** Schematic presentation of fixation of subtrochanteric fracture of femur using angle blade plate with the blade of the plate driven into the femoral neck through the greater trochanter to achieve adequate purchase

diaphyseal complete fracture is difficult to achieve as there will be severe overriding of bone fragments subsequent to muscular contraction (proximal fragment tends to rotate externally due to the iliopsoas muscle). It can be attempted, especially when an external fixation technique is chosen to immobilize the fracture, under general anesthesia. Pulling the leg manually or by hanging the limb, muscle fatigue can be achieved, which would facilitate fracture reduction. Under complete muscle relaxation, reduction can be attempted by toggling method or by simple manipulation by bringing the fracture ends closer and by aligning and approximating the long oblique or spiral fragments.

External fixation of femoral diaphyseal fractures is generally not advised due to severe overriding of bone segments and the difficulty in immobilizing the hip joint. Plaster of Paris cast is not usually preferred; if done, it should immobilize the hip joint using a spica applied around the animal's body. Complications such as inadequate reduction and stabilization, joint stiffness, heavy weight, soaking with urine, and decubital ulcers are common. The modified Thomas splint may be of use in certain types of fractures, as it will provide traction to keep the bone fragments in alignment. One should make sure that the ring of the splint will lie proximal to the fracture. Hence, Thomas splint is not indicated for proximal femoral fractures and is more suited for middle or distal diaphyseal fractures. During the application, the distal limb is fixed to the splint bar by rotating it externally (outwardly) to bring the fracture fragments in alignment. Further, at the proximal end, it can be secured by bandaging it around the animal's body to stabilize the hip joint. Common complications with modified Thomas splint include inadequate fracture stability leading to large callus formation, malunion or nonunion, and quadriceps muscle atrophy, apart from frequent loosening of the splint leading to fracture site mobility. Hence, it is advised to readjust the splint at least once a week. If properly applied and taken care of, modified Thomas (Schroeder-Thomas) splint may be useful to treat incomplete fractures where internal fixation may not be needed and in certain severely comminuted fractures, which are difficult to treat by internal fixation techniques.

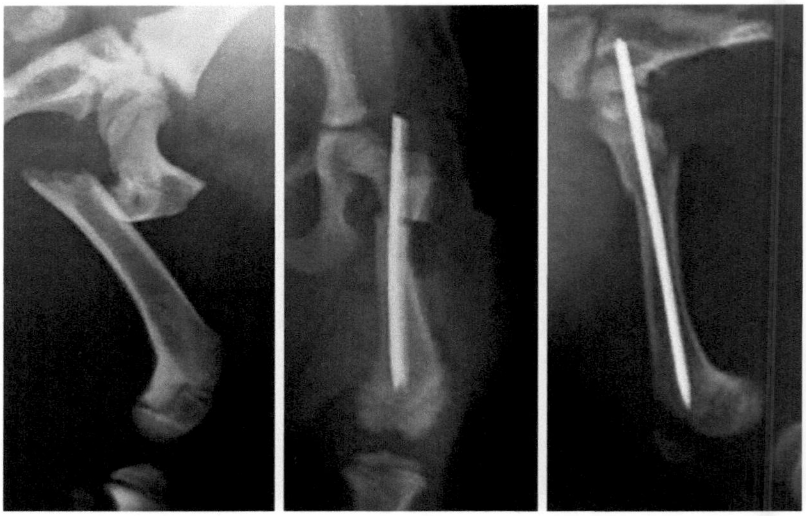

**Fig. 3.33** Proximal femoral (sub-trochanteric) fracture immobilized with IM pin fixation. Such fractures need to be carefully handled to prevent intraoperative and postoperative complications. (Courtesy: Dr. S. Ravikumar, Bangalore, India)

#### 3.4.2.1 Surgical Approach

Surgical access to the femoral diaphysis can be achieved through a standard cranio-lateral approach [4]. An incision is made along the length of femur bone. In proximal diaphyseal fractures, the incision may be extended more toward the proximal end and in distal fractures more distal. The fascia lata is incised, and vastus lateralis muscle is retracted cranially and biceps femoris muscle caudally. The femur bone should be approached and reduced with minimal soft tissue manipulation. The attachment of muscles,

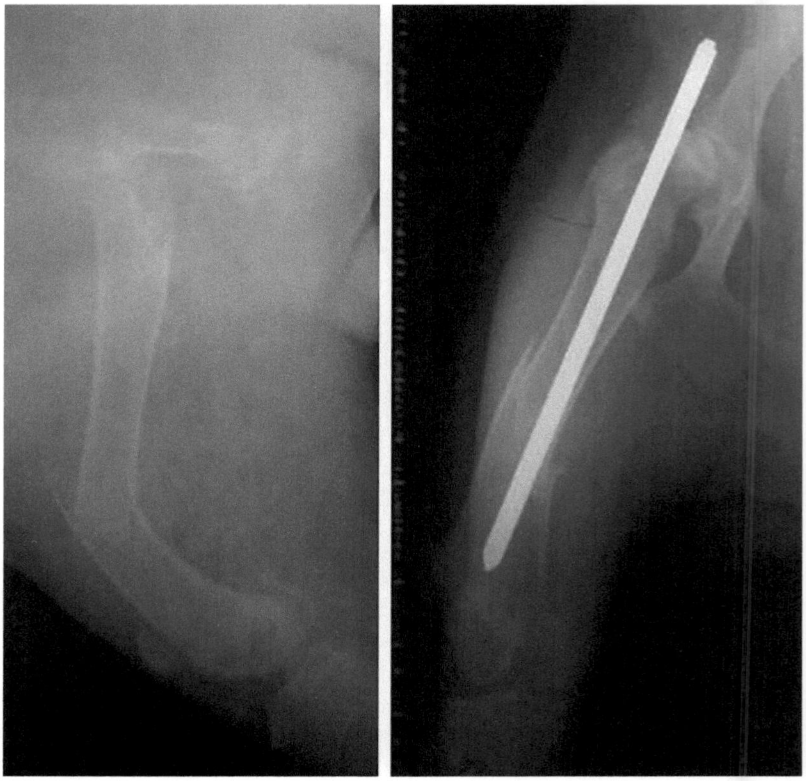

**Fig. 3.34** Normograde pin fixation by close method in minimally displaced femoral diaphyseal fracture in a dog

such as the insertion of adductor to the bone fragments, should be preserved as far as possible, which is a significant source of blood supply, especially in young animals. In femoral diaphyseal fractures, the proximal end of the distal segment often tends to displace medially and proximally, at times with severe overriding. In fresh cases of transverse or short oblique fractures, during fracture reduction, the cut ends of the bone should be protected using the index finger (to avert any injury to the femoral artery and/or nerve) while dragging the fracture end toward the incision. Use of a curved artery forceps or bone holding forceps will facilitate the reduction. Subsequently, the fracture ends can be reduced by toggling method. In long-standing cases, if the muscle contraction is considerable or if the fracture is long oblique/spiral, it may require more time and manipulation for reduction. In comminuted fractures, it is often difficult to reduce and reconstruct the shaft using all the bony pieces. Only the large bony pieces that can be secured with wire/screw fixation may be retained, and all the very small bone pieces, which are free of soft tissue attachment, should be removed. It is taken care not to damage the soft tissue attachment to the bone segments, which would help in early incorporation of the bone and healing of fracture.

#### 3.4.2.2 Surgical Fixation

Several surgical techniques like intramedullary (IM) pins alone or along with cerclage wires, bone plates and screws, tie-in configuration, and interlocking nails have been used to repair femoral diaphyseal fractures [28, 35–42]. Most of the femoral diaphyseal fractures are amenable to intramedullary (IM) pin fixation. Transverse, slightly oblique, or minimally comminuted fractures can be treated using IM fixation. Pin fixation in femur can be done either by retrograde or normograde technique. During retrograde pinning, the pin is inserted through the fracture site into the medullary cavity of the proximal main segment. Retrograde pinning is technically easier to perform, but many times, it is difficult to determine where the pin exits the proximal end of the bone. Retrogradely placed pin tends to be placed much closer to the sciatic nerve than normogradely placed pins, especially in distal femoral fractures. During retrograde pinning, the proximal segment should be positioned such that the hip is in an adducted, extended, and internally rotated position. If the hip is held in abducted, flexed, and externally rotated position, the pin may proximally exit at the medial side of the trochanteric fossa possibly injuring the sciatic nerve [19]. Even if the pin does not directly contact and traumatize the nerve, the motion of the pin through the gluteal musculature during ambulation can cause scar tissue formation entrapping the nerve. Similarly, retrograde pinning in young animals may cause damage to the femoral neck causing abnormal proximal femur.

In femur, although normograde pinning can be done from either end of the bone; in diaphyseal fractures, pinning is normally done from the proximal end. During the normograde insertion of pin from the proximal end of the bone, the pin should be placed on the tip of the greater trochanter and gently pushed craniomedially until the tip slips into the craniolateral aspect of the trochanteric fossa. Once seated in the trochanteric fossa, pin is inserted through the bony cortex. As the pin is advanced, the long axis of the pin should align with the long axis of the femur to avoid accidental penetration of the bone cortex of the proximal fracture segment. Once the pin tip reaches the fracture site, the bone segments are reduced, and the pin is further progressed into the distal segment.

Generally, the IM pin should tightly but comfortably fit in the medullary cavity (60–70%) to provide stable fixation [19, 43] (Fig. 3.35). The narrowest part of femoral diaphysis is isthmus (proximal third of diaphysis), which should be taken into account while selecting the pin diameter [44]. In young animals with thin bony cortex, it is not needed (not possible also) to snugly fit the pin in the medullary cavity. Fixation of fracture with relatively small diameter pin can provide adequate fixation. Fracture healing can occur with relatively large external callus formation in a short period of time (2–3 weeks), provided the pin is not severely migrated and fracture alignment maintained. End threaded pins (Schanz

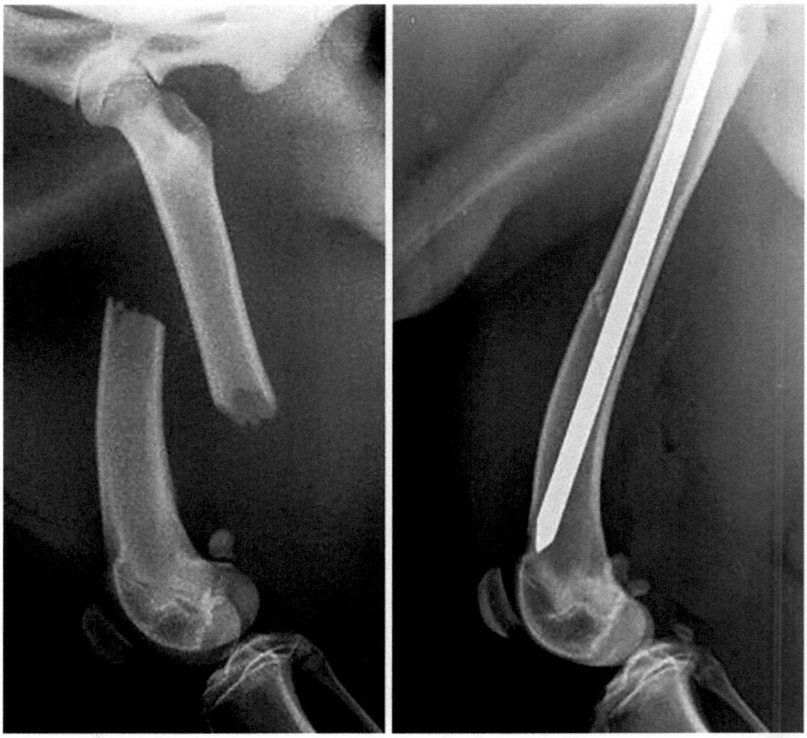

**Fig. 3.35** Retrograde IM pin fixation after open reduction of femoral diaphyseal fracture. Note alignment of dentated fracture ends provides adequate rotational stability (Courtesy: Dr. Anil Deshpande, Deputy Commissioner of Animal Husbandry, Pune, Maharashtra, India)

pins) have also been used to provide better anchorage at the distal end. End threaded positive profile "Admit pin" has been shown to firmly engage the distal bone segment and thus provide stable fixation in a variety of femoral diaphyseal fractures [45, 46] (Fig. 3.36). In cases of instability, and to counteract the rotational forces, multiple small diameter pins may be used (stack pinning) in transverse or short oblique fractures [47] (Fig. 3.37). In comminuted femoral fractures (having large butterfly fragments), hemi-cerclage or full-cerclage wires can be used effectively (Fig. 3.38). Half-pin external skeletal fixation using a K-E splint may also be used in heavy adult animals to provide additional stability along with bone pinning. IM pin can also be made more stable by Tie-in fixation with an external fixation device.

The Kuntscher nail has also been used for the fixation of femoral diaphyseal fractures in heavy adult animals. Only the proximal bone segment should be reamed to open the medullary cavity, and reaming through the entire medullary cavity can be avoided to prevent damage to the cortex. K-nailing should be avoided in young, osteoporotic bones and also in cases where longitudinal crack exists in the diaphysis. The use of interlocking nail has in recent years replaced K-nailing to a large extent, due to mechanical advantages.

Interlocking nail (ILN) is being most widely used for fixation of femur fractures in small animal practice (Figs. 3.39, 3.40 and 3.41). It provides stable fixation even in comminuted diaphyseal fractures of femur [37, 48–51]. The diameter of ILN may vary from 6 to 10 mm, with variable length. ILN is always inserted in normograde fashion through the trochanteric fossa for fixation of diaphyseal fractures. A Steinmann pin is passed in a retrograde manner to establish an intramedullary channel in the proximal femur segment before reaming. Just like in IM pinning, the proximal segment should be held with hip in standing position (no flexion, abduction, or external rotation) during retrograde pinning. The nail is seated distally in such a way that the proximal end remains below the tip of the greater trochanter and the most proximal

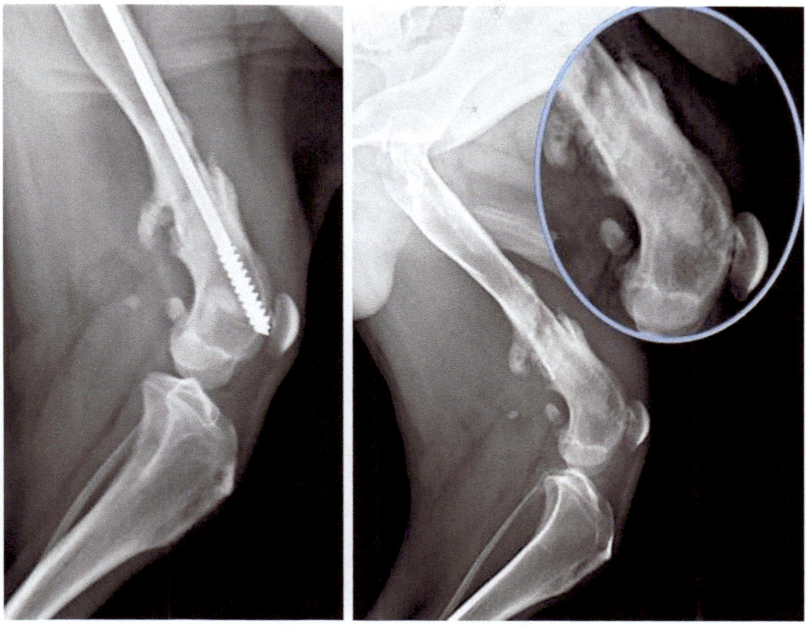

**Fig. 3.36** Use of Admit pin (positive profile end threaded pin) for fixation of distal femoral fracture in a dog (Source: Dr Adarsh Kumar, Dr. GC Negi College of Veterinary and Animal Sciences, CSKHPKV, Palampur)

transfixation screw/bolt is fixed near the lesser trochanter. In transverse or short oblique fractures, dynamic fixation (fixation of bolt at only one end of bone) can be done, and in comminuted fractures or fractures with a gap filled with bone graft, static fixation (fixation of

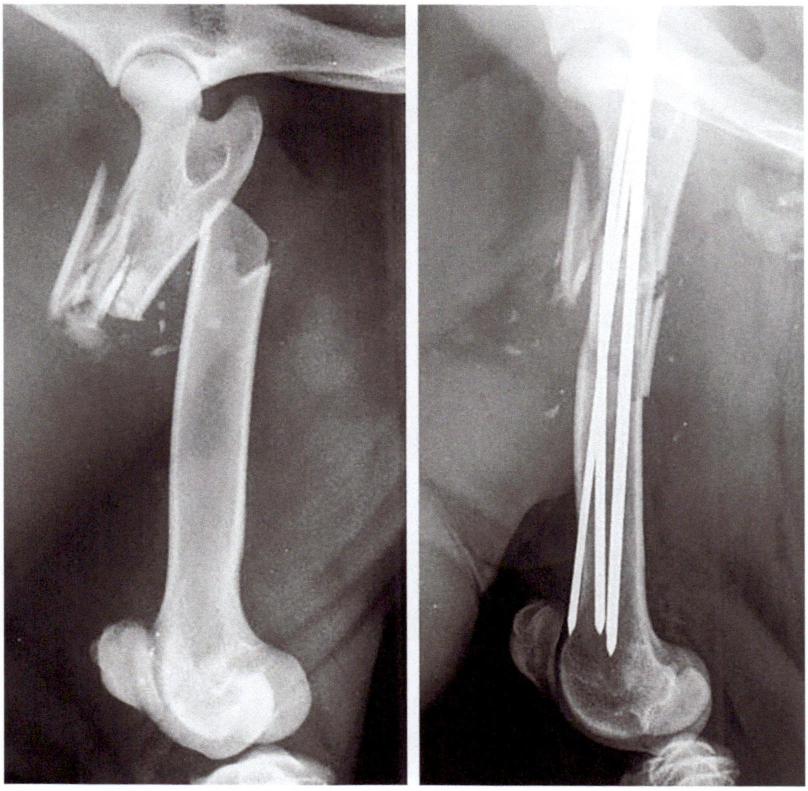

**Fig. 3.37** Comminuted fracture of proximal femur in a goat treated with stack pinning. Small bone fragments at fracture site were secured with absorbable sutures with minimal manipulation

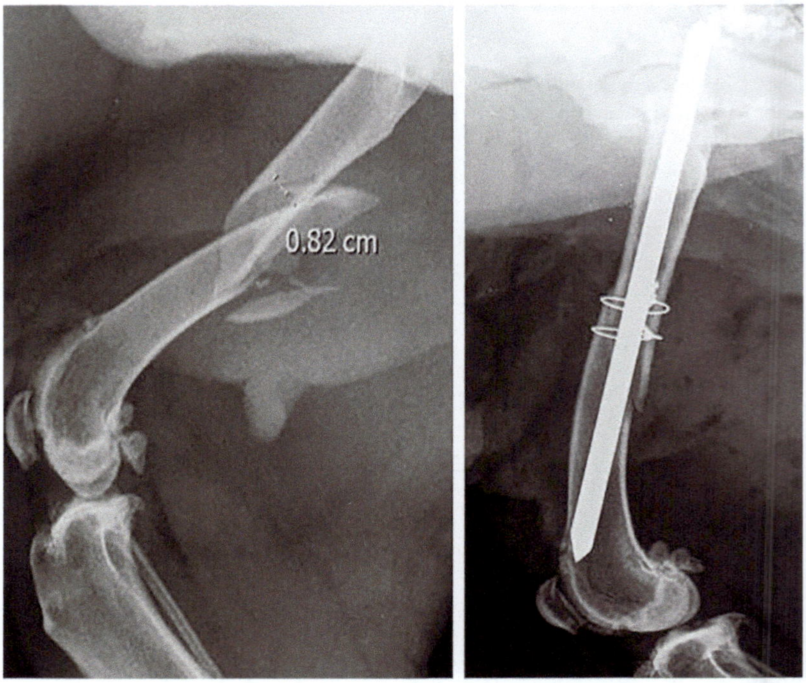


**Fig. 3.38** IM pinning with cerclage wiring for fixation of comminuted femoral diaphyseal fracture in a dog

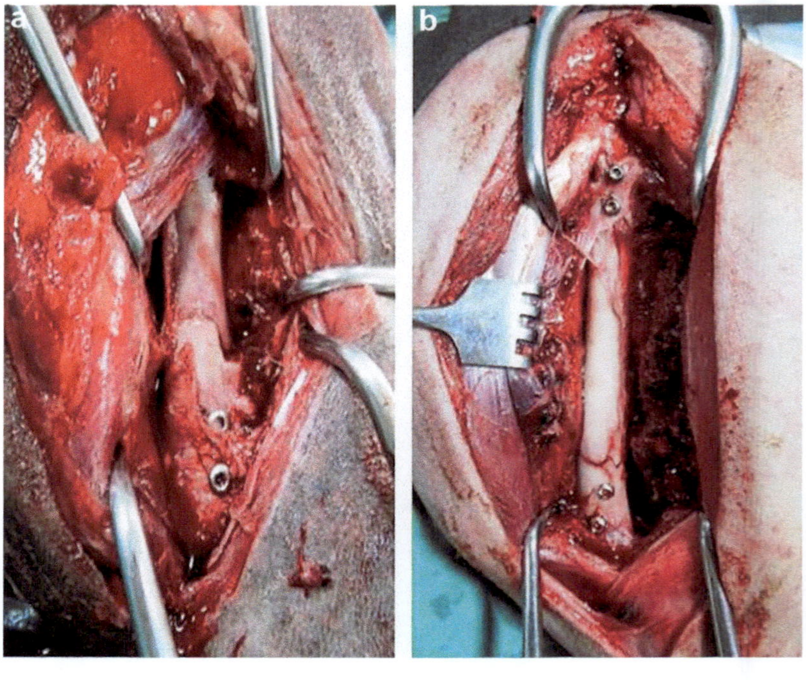


**Fig. 3.39** Dynamic (**a**) and static (**b**) ILN fixation in a dogs' femur (Courtesy: Dr. Tarunbir Singh, GADVASU, Ludhiana, India)

bolt at both ends) is recommended. Generally, one to two fixation bolts are fixed in each fracture segment. In comminuted fractures, cerclage wiring is generally used as an ancillary fixation device to retain the bone fragments. Use of anatomically contoured interlocking nail can

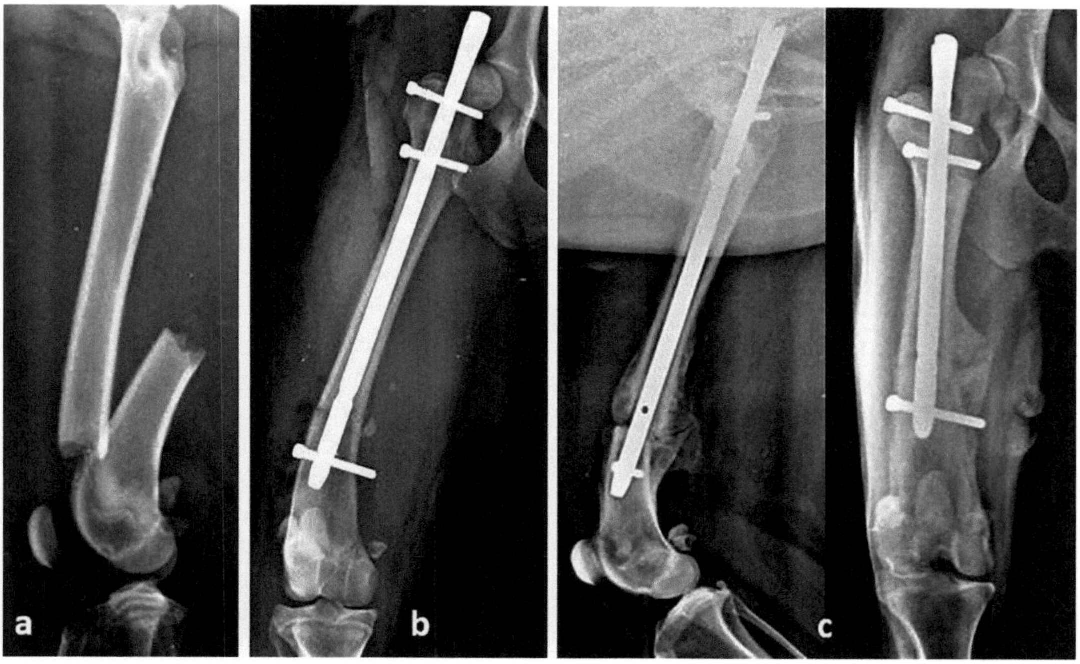


**Fig. 3.40** Static interlocking nailing of femoral diaphyseal fracture in a dog using two fixation screws in the proximal bone segment and one screw in the distal segment (Courtesy: Dr. Kiranjeet Singh, Indian Veterinary Research Institute, Izatnagar, Bareilly, India)

**Fig. 3.41** Mid-diaphyseal fracture of femur (**a**), immobilized with static ILN fixation in a dog using two fixation screws each bone segment (**b**), and good healing at the fracture site at 60 days (**c**) (Courtesy: Dr. Kiranjeet Singh, Indian Veterinary Research Institute, Izatnagar, Bareilly, India)

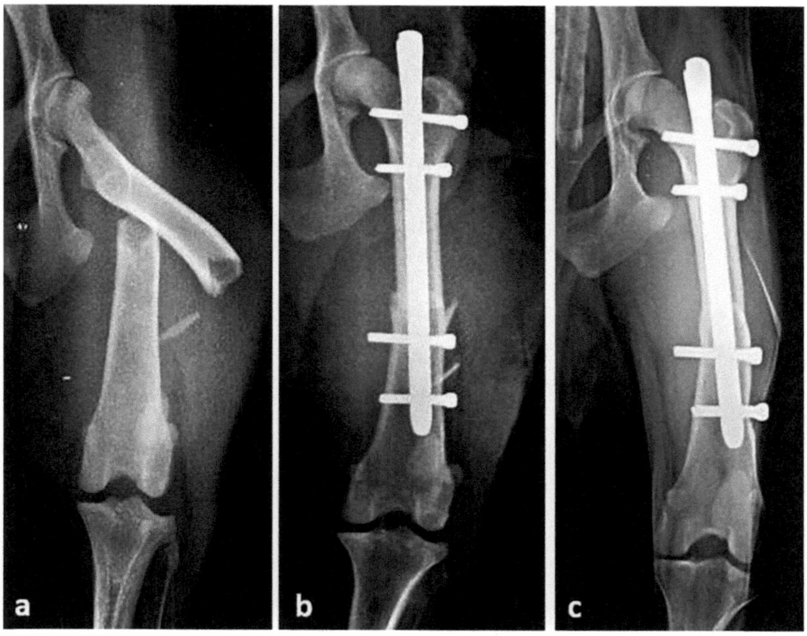

provide stable fixation by maintaining the contour of the bone (Fig. 3.42). Use of ILN fixation should be avoided in very young animals.

ILNs can be combined with external skeletal fixation (ESF) for stabilization of unstable femoral diaphyseal fractures. ILN locked with a type I ESF in femoral diaphyseal fractures can be used to provide dynamization and achieve early limb function [52]. One such technique is the use of long locking screws (partially threaded ILN pins) inserted into the ILN holes. The ILN pin has a short threaded portion for engaging the bone cortices and the long non-threaded part, which projects outside the skin as ESF fixation pin. Two to four such ILN fixation pins are connected to form a rigid frame, which can be a metal or an epoxy (Fig. 3.43). In other words, the transfixation pins of the ESF interlock within the nail. The addition of the ESF to the ILN improves its resistance to torsional forces. However, postoperative care and management of the animal is difficult, as any movement of the ESF pins may cause motion at the ILN-pin interface, causing damage to the fragile healing fracture environment.

Bone plate (DCP) and screw fixation can be undertaken in any type of femoral diaphyseal fractures but is ideal for comminuted fractures in large breed dogs, as it provides rigid and stable fixation [53, 54]. In femur bone, bone plate is fixed on the lateral (tension band) surface, extending the whole length of the bone. In transverse fractures, pre-stressed/contoured plate is fixed under tension, so that the bone segments are compressed on the medial side. In long oblique or spiral fractures, bone fragments are first fixed under compression using interfragmentary screws (lag screws), before fixation of plate (neutralization plate). If possible, based on the fracture line, compression/lag screw may also be fixed initially through the plate itself, and subsequently, the remaining screws are fixed. In comminuted fractures, the fracture is first anatomically reconstructed by securing the bone pieces using compression screws or cerclage wires before fixing the plate. Relatively strong plates have to be used (buttress type), and at least two screws should be fixed in the normal portion of the diaphysis. If a gap persists after plate fixation, there is every chance of bending of plate at the gap site and failure of fixation. In severely comminuted fractures with considerable loss of cortical bone, the use of cortical allograft (frozen)/tissue-engineered bone scaffold may be

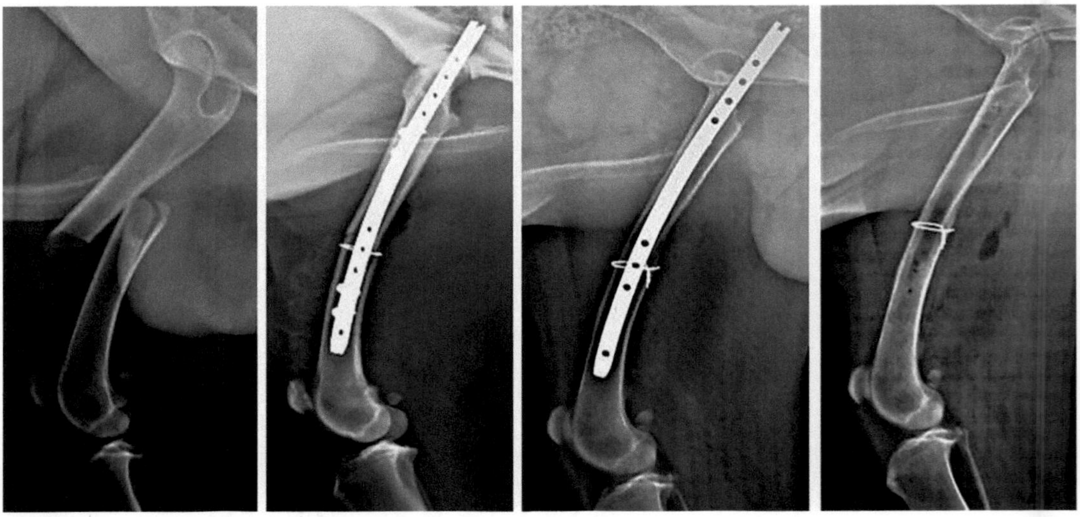

**Fig. 3.42** Comminuted fracture of femoral diaphysis in a dog stabilized using angularly contoured ILN immediately after fixation, and on 200th day after fixation and after removal of the nail (Courtesy: Dr. SP Tyagi, Dr. GC Negi College of Veterinary and Animal Sciences, CSKHPKV, Palampur, India)

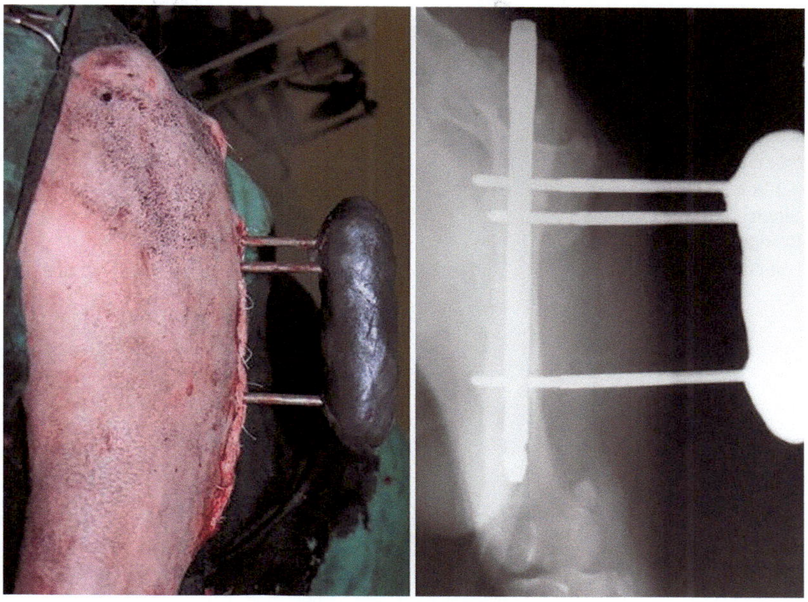

**Fig. 3.43** Modified ILN with epoxy-pin ESF used for fixation in a femoral diaphyseal fracture. Note the long fixation bolts joined outside the skin to construct the connecting bar

considered. In that case, an appropriate size cortical bone graft/scaffold is first fixed to the plate using screws, and then the plate with the graft is fixed to the femoral diaphysis using additional screws. In case of only a small gap at the fracture site after plate fixation, a cancellous graft may be used to fill the gap.

In recent years, the locking compression plate (LCP) is becoming more popular, especially for the fixation of comminuted femoral diaphyseal fractures, as it provides greater fixation rigidity [41, 55] (Fig. 3.44). It has the advantage of more stable plate-screw interface, and hence, chances of screw loosening are minimal even in comminuted fractures. String of Pearls (SOP) locking plates can also be used for successful management of femoral diaphyseal fractures in dogs [56]. Plate-pin constructs (Fig. 3.45) or SOP plate-pin constructs (Fig. 3.46) have also been used successfully for the fixation of femoral diaphyseal fractures, especially comminuted fractures.

In very young animals with thin cortices or in osteoporotic bones, tubular plate (thin curved plate without screws) may be fixed using cerclage wires or synthetic absorbable sutures. The fixation is generally stable if used along with a small diameter IM pin to resist bending stress.

#### 3.4.2.3 Postoperative Care and Possible Complications

Apart from routine anti-inflammatory and antibiotic drug administration, the restriction of

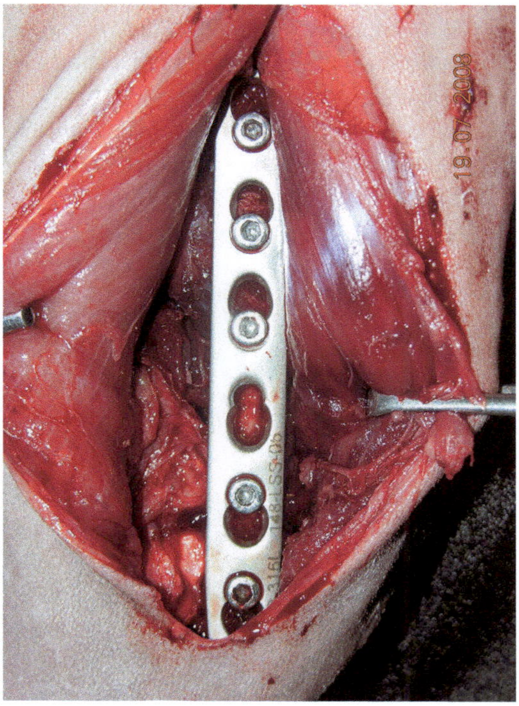


**Fig. 3.44** Fixation of femoral diaphyseal fracture using a LCP

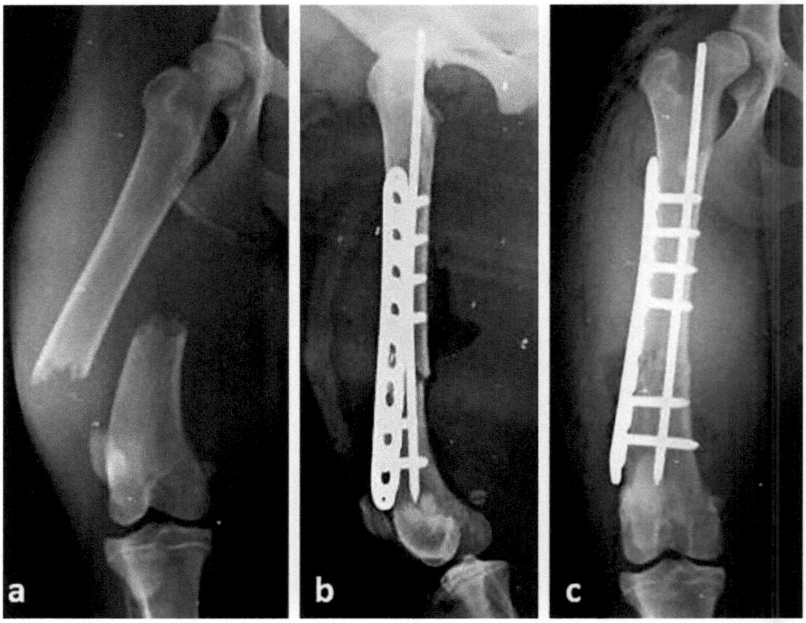


**Fig. 3.45** Plate-pin construct used for repair of femoral diaphyseal fracture. Note that the IM pin used with plate construct is of relatively small diameter (Courtesy: Dr. Kiranjeet Singh, Indian Veterinary Research Institute, Izatnagar, Bareilly, India)

animal's movement is needed during the initial postoperative period. Only limited weight bearing is allowed, especially in severely comminuted fractures. External coaptation along with internal fixation may not provide additional stability. Instead, if improperly applied, it may act as fulcrum at the fracture site causing further damage to healing fracture.

Complications with external fixation techniques may include decreased range of motion of different joints, quadriceps tie-down leading to knee joint stiffness, ulceration at the groin, decubital ulcers, and paw devitalization apart from delayed union, malunion, and nonunion. With internal fixation, pin loosening, and migration, or fixation failure may occur if the fracture site remains unstable, especially in severely comminuted fractures or fractures with a gap between the bone segments. Delayed union is common if very rigid fixation is employed

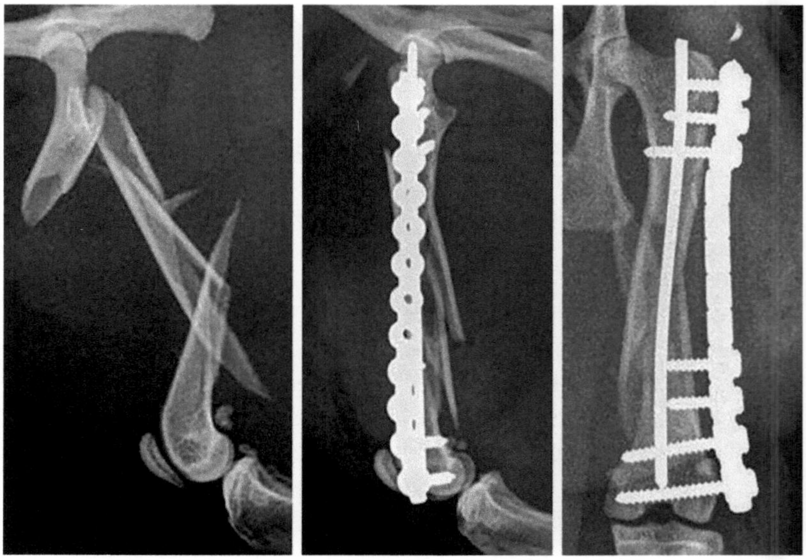

**Fig. 3.46** Reconstruction of comminuted femoral diaphyseal fracture using SOP plate and pin construct (Reproduced with permission from: Russell Yeadon; www.vets-now.com)

(with either very large diameter snugly fitting IM pin or rigid plate). Though uncommon, sciatic nerve entrapment may cause knuckling of paw and hyperalgesia. Prognosis in femoral diaphyseal fracture repair is generally good if the fracture is adequately fixed with good functional recovery of the limb.

### 3.4.3 Distal Femoral Fractures

Fractures at the distal femur (distal diaphysis, supracondylar, and condylar regions) constitute about 18–20% of femoral fractures and 7–8% of total fractures recorded in dogs. Distal femoral fractures are most often seen in young animals aged less than 1 year (about 80%), due to incomplete ossification of the growth plate situated between the diaphysis and metaphysis/epiphysis [5]. Such fractures are generally of transverse or short oblique type and are caused by shear force, as seen during a fall from height. These fractures are occasionally accompanied with ligament injuries of the knee joint.

The animals with distal femoral fractures may show different signs such as variable amounts of lameness and swelling, which are severe in comminuted fractures and fractures involving the stifle joint. The distal end of proximal fracture fragment may prominently project cranially (with the distal fragment displaced caudally) with free movement often giving an impression as the patella and the knee joint. There will be laxity of quadriceps muscles with clear crepitation. Radiography will help determine the type and extent of fracture and plan for fracture fixation.

Closed reduction of distal femoral fractures may be undertaken only in fresh cases in small dogs and cats. This may be achieved either through traction and digital manipulation to "pop" the distal fragment into alignment, or through flexion and toggling of fracture fragments into reduction. Fracture reduction needs to be perfect in distal femoral fractures, as they are very close to the stifle joint, and improper reduction and fixation may lead to large callus formation involving the adjacent stifle joint. Hence, closed reduction and fixation is more successful only in cases of physeal separation in young ones, where the fracture fragments may interdigitate and tend to stay reduced, than in transverse, oblique, comminuted fractures, or those involving the articular surface of the joint.

External fixation by closed method may be undertaken using different techniques in stable reductions. Flexion bandages may be applied by keeping the stifle in flexed position so that the femoral condyles are locked between the tibial plateau, the patella, and the quadriceps. The flexion bandage, however, should be removed as early as possible, and the limb is rehabilitated to prevent development of joint stiffness and impairment in the motion. Well-constructed coaptation splint immobilizing the whole limb and the hip immobilized with a spica may also be successful to stabilize a stable fracture. Modified Thomas splints (Schroeder-Thomas splint) have been traditionally used for the fixation of distal femoral fractures. In this technique, the tongs are placed around the condyles and are incorporated into the splint to maintain continued traction with the knee placed in normal anatomical position. This method can be successful only in young animals, and in adults, to maintain traction, the whole limb has to be pulled into extension, which may lead to reduced range of stifle joint motion.

#### 3.4.3.1 Surgical Approach

The distal femur is approached through standard lateral incision to femur and stifle [4]. The skin incision is started from about the middle of femur extending downward in curvilinear fashion (Fig. 3.47). The incision on the fascia lata is extended distally over the lateral side of stifle to make an arthrotomy incision lateral to the patellar ligament. The stifle joint and hence the fracture site are exposed by effecting the complete medial patellar luxation and quadriceps retraction. The severed caudal femoral artery on the way may be sutured. The fracture is reduced through digital manipulation by flexion, traction, and toggling. Fracture through the growth plate is relatively easy to reduce and retain in position. When it is difficult to reduce the bone segments to normal anatomical position, slight over reduction of the distal segment is generally preferred (than under

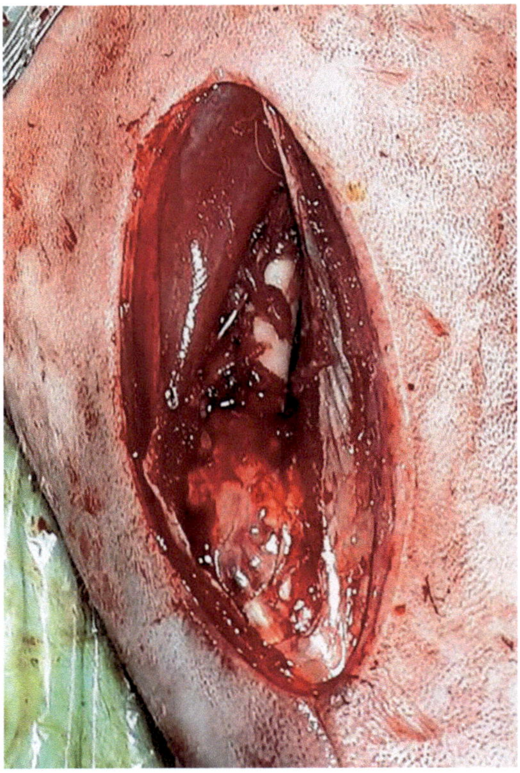

**Fig. 3.47** Surgical approach to distal femur: A curvilinear skin incision is made from the middle of femur extending downward, the incision on the fascia lata is extended distally over the lateral side of stifle to make an arthrotomy incision

reduction) for better anchorage of fixation implants at the small distal segment.

#### 3.4.3.2 Surgical Fixation

Surgical fixation of distal femoral fractures can be brought about by different techniques such as single IM pinning, cross pinning, Rush pinning, cross IM pinning, interlocking nailing, and bone plating (reconstruction plate, supracondylar plate), etc. [57–66]. Single IM pinning provides adequate fixation if fracture configuration ensures rotational stability (dentated fracture-separation at physeal plate). IM pin is placed in a normograde manner from the distal end, by inserting it in the nonarticular surface of the intercondylar fossa, just cranial to the cranial cruciate ligament taking care not to disrupt the origins of the cruciate ligaments (Fig. 3.48). The pin is directed in such a way that it emerges at the fracture line slightly toward the caudal cortex. The bone segments are then reduced, and the pin is pushed into the proximal bone segment until it exits through the intertrochanteric fossa. The distal end of the pin is countersunk beneath the articular surface to prevent any damage from the cut ends (it is preferred to use Steinmann pins with one end smooth). The extra length of the pin is cut close to the skin from the proximal end.

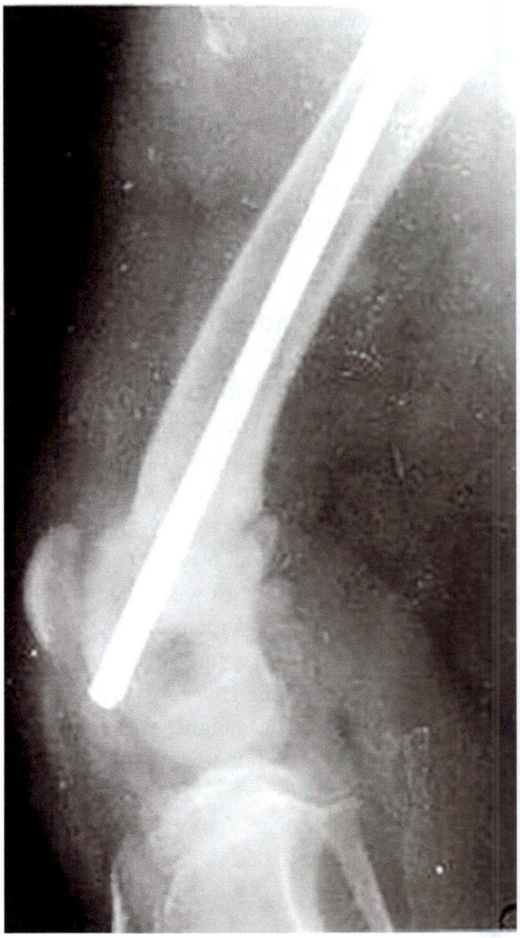

**Fig. 3.48** Normograde fixation of IM pin through intercondylar fossa for fixation of supracondylar femoral fracture

Rush pins were earlier used to provide stable fixation of supracondylar fractures. A pair of Rush pins are inserted one each through the medial and lateral condyles (about 30° to the long axis of the bone) using a reamer (Fig. 3.49). The point of pin insertion on the

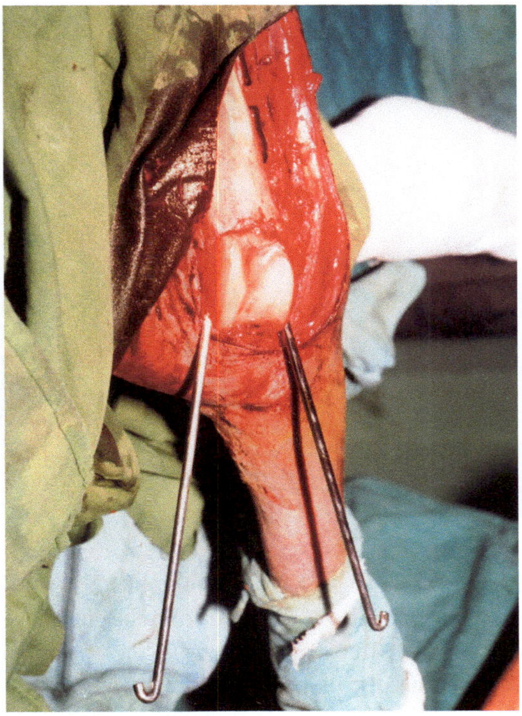

**Fig. 3.49** Rush pin fixation for supracondylar femoral fracture repair

lateral condyle is just cranial to the origin of long digital extensor muscle tendon and symmetrically on the medial condyle. Once the pin ends reach the fracture line, the bone segments are reduced, and the pins are driven through the proximal fragment alternatively by hammering them. In young animals, the pins are driven carefully (too much hammering should be avoided) to prevent splintering of condyles and growth plate damage leading to fixation failure or subsequent premature growth plate closure.

The technique of cross IM pinning using Steinmann pins or Kirschner wires done the same way as Rush pinning is more frequently used nowadays to treat condylar/supracondylar femoral fractures [67] (Figs. 3.50 and 3.51). Unlike Rush pins, the cross IM pins are allowed to exit proximally through the trochanteric fossa, which facilitates removal of pin subsequently. The distal ends of pins are countersunk beneath the cartilaginous surface (Fig. 4.52). As relatively small diameter pins are used, the damage to the growth plate is negligible, and the chances of tearing of condyles are also less. The technique of cross pinning, wherein the wires/pins are crossed through the fracture site and are exited through the opposite cortex, has also been used to treat condylar/supracondylar fractures. This technique may provide adequate stability in young dogs and cats but may not be adequate for adult large dogs. Interlocking nail could be used to stabilize distal femoral fractures in adult heavy animals, especially for comminuted fractures, provided the distal fragment has enough length to place at least one fixation bolt. ILN fixation should not be done in immature animals to avoid possible damage to the growth plate. To achieve greater purchase at the small distal bone fragment, the ILN could be inserted through the intercondylar fossa, just cranial to the cruciate ligament similar to single Steinmann pinning (Fig. 3.52).

Bone plate and screw fixation is indicated for distal femoral fractures in heavy/large animals, or in severely comminuted fractures. The uneven surface and small distal fragment make fixation of standard plate difficult. Use of plate very close to the stifle joint may lead to reduced joint motion. It has to be ensured that the plate is properly contoured to the lateral surface of the femur, and at least two screws are fixed across both the cortices for adequate fixation stability. As the distance between the plate holes is smaller in a DCP than in a LC-DCP, a standard DCP can accommodate more screws for a given length potentially increasing stabilization in small fragments. Reconstruction plate, which can be readily contoured to the bone surface, can be used [61] (Fig. 3.53). Locking plate systems due to their greater fixation stability compared to traditional plates minimize the number of screws needed for adequate stabilization and do not require anatomic contouring of the plate simplifying application of plate at the condylar region of femur. Newly developed veterinary LCP plates have some improvement in the plate design such as rounded hole at one end of the plate with small distance between the screw holes, which allows placement of plate very close to the joint minimizing the impingement of soft tissues associated with the joint and range of motion. Veterinary cuttable plates with very small inter-screw distance or T-pates, which

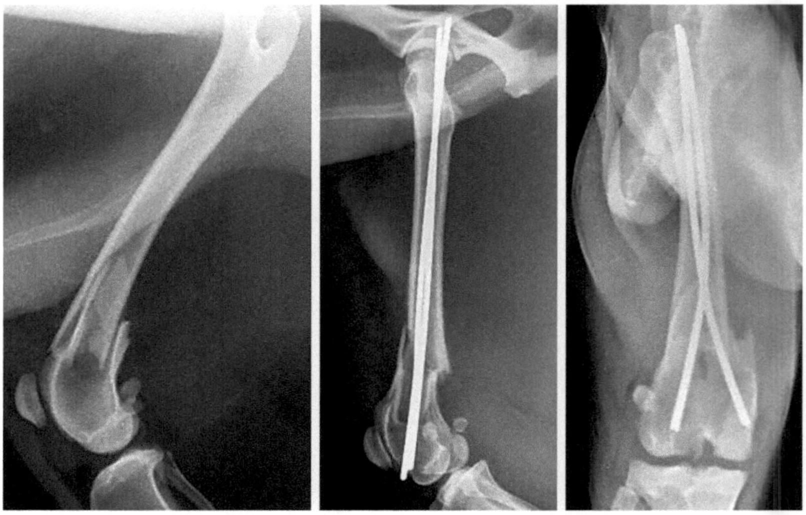

**Fig. 3.50** Cross IM pin fixation for comminuted supracondylar femoral fracture repair

allow placement of more number of screws in small fragment, may be ideal choice to treat distal femoral fractures. Specially developed supracondylar plate [65] and femoral condylar plate [68] have also been used for stabilization of distal femoral or supracondylar fractures.

In condylar fractures (separation of one condyle or intercondylar fractures-T/Y type), either lag screws or small K-wires are used [69, 70]. If only one condyle is separated from the shaft, one or two lag screws inserted from the separated condyle into the main fracture fragment will suffice to bring about adequate reduction and compression between the bone fragments. In T/Y fractures, the separated condyles are first reconstructed using either lag screws or multiple

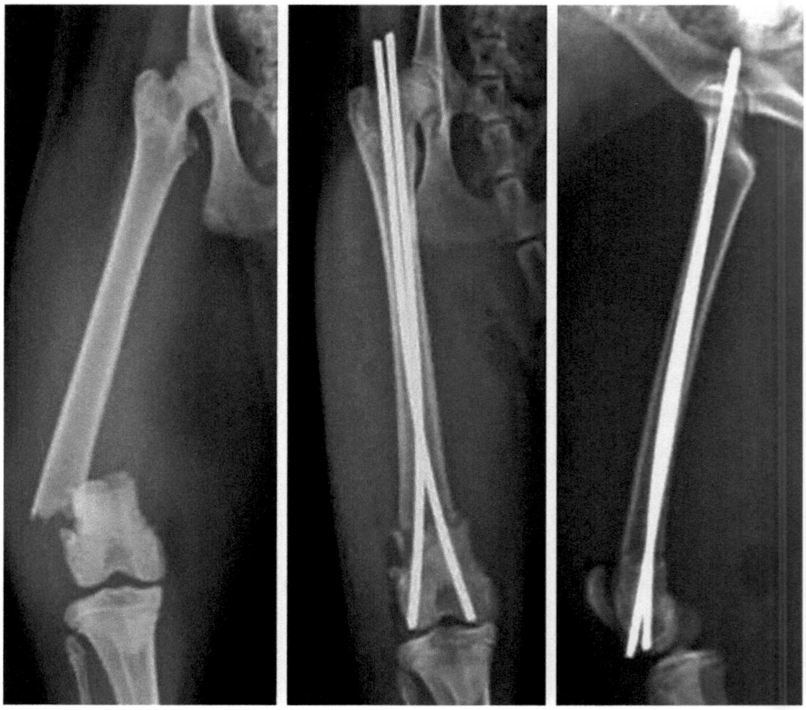

**Fig. 3.51** Cross IM pin fixation of supracondylar femoral fracture in a cat (Courtesy: Dr. S. Ravikumar, Bangalore, India)

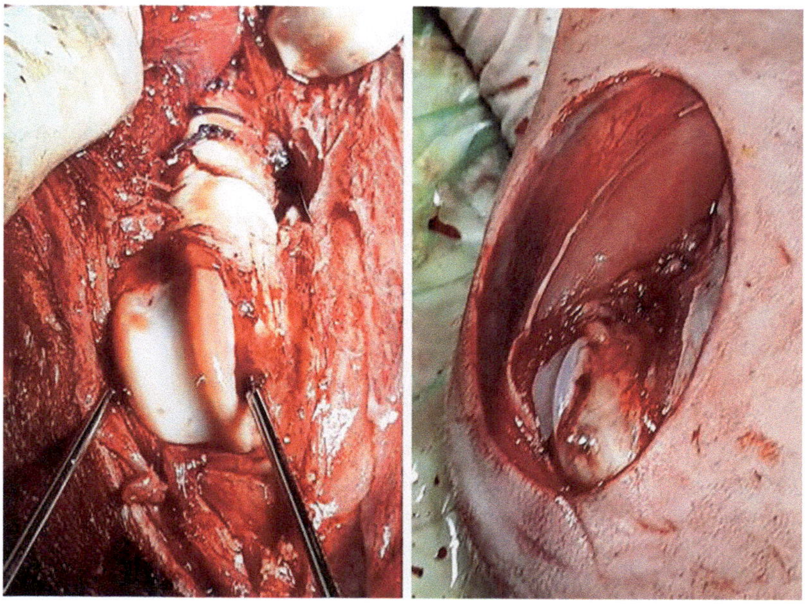

**Fig. 3.52** Cross IM pinning in distal femoral fracture: see the location of pin insertion on medial and lateral surfaces of the condyles and seating of pin ends below the articulating surface

K-wires fixed across the condyles (lateromedial), before reducing and stabilizing the reconstructed condyles with the femoral shaft using any of the techniques (cross IM pinning or plating) described above.

#### 3.4.3.3 Postoperative Care and Possible Complications

With external fixation technique, it is advised to examine the animal frequently during the first few days to ensure proper fracture reduction and any

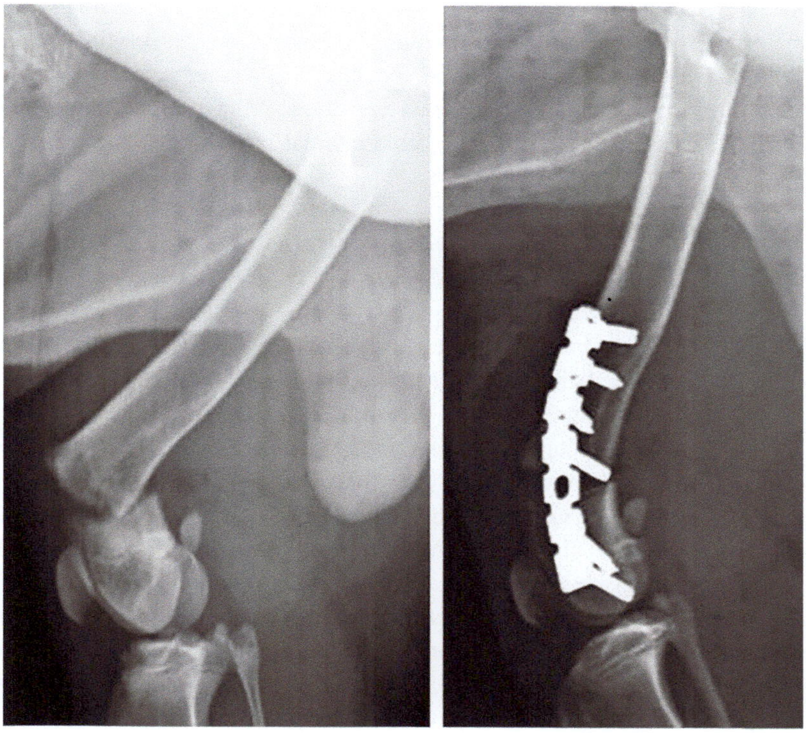

**Fig. 3.53** Use of reconstruction plate for fixation of supracondylar femoral fracture in a dog (Source: Amit Kumar et al., Surgical management of supracondylar femoral fracture using reconstruction bone plate in dogs. Indian J Vet Surg. 40(2): 131–133, 2019)

complications like groin injury, skin bite wounds, and loosening of fixation device etc. It is also advised to observe for fracture union and remove the fixation device as early as possible, as prolonged immobilization of the limb may lead to quadriceps tie-down and affect the knee joint mobility. After removal of the external device, physiotherapy (extension and flexion of the joint) is advised for early regaining of normal limb function.

Animals with internal fixation should be allowed only minimum weight bearing in the immediate postoperative period, especially in unstable comminuted fractures. With intramedullary pin fixation, common complication is migration of the pin mostly distally causing lameness and affecting the stifle joint motion. Hence, it is advised to remove the pin through an incision in the trochanteric fossa immediately after the bone union. Often, proximal migration of the pin is also observed; if it is not affecting the fracture reduction and alignment (most often), the migrated pin may be reinserted by gently tapping the cut end back into the medullary cavity. Chances of nonunion are rare in the distal metaphyseal/epiphyseal region. However, if the fracture stability is not adequate, sometimes, it may lead to malunion and osteoarthritis of the stifle joint. Complications can be reduced by adopting proper technique of fracture fixation. Prognosis is generally good with stable internal fixation.

## 3.5 Fractures of Tibia-Fibula

Fractures of tibia-fibula are frequently seen in dogs and cats, constituting about 17–22% of total long bone fractures in dogs. Mostly, both tibia and fibula are fractured together, but in about one third of cases, only tibia may be fractured (mostly caused due to fall), and occasionally (2–3% cases), only fibula is fractured. Most of the tibial fractures are seen in the diaphysis, proximal and middle third frequently involved [5]. Incomplete fractures are common in young growing dogs, mostly seen in the diaphysis or metaphysis. In young animals, physeal fractures are also often seen. Among different types of fractures, long oblique/spiral fractures are common in tibia, apart from comminuted and transverse fractures. Automobile accident is the most common cause of tibial fractures, and fractures due to fall are typically located at the proximal tibia near the stifle joint.

### 3.5.1 Proximal Physeal Fractures

Proximal physeal fractures of the tibia are commonly seen in young animals and are mostly Salter type I and II [71]. Many of these fractures can be reduced by closed manner and immobilized adequately with external fixation technique such as Modified Thomas Splint or lateral coaptation splint. Internal fixation can be done using multiple small K-wires. Intramedullary pinning (single or cross) can also be undertaken (by closed method) to provide stable fixation in heavy animals if there is minimal displacement of bone segments, and the fracture can be reduced by close method (Fig. 3.54). Opening the fracture site is rarely needed for IM pin fixation except in cases of severe displacement of bone fragments or in old cases. Avulsion fractures of tibial crest are also often seen in young animals, which require open reduction and internal fixation. Tension band wiring is the method of choice for treating avulsion of tibial crest [72] (Fig. 3.55). When used in immature animals, the implants should be removed as early as possible after fracture healing [73].

### 3.5.2 Diaphyseal Fractures

Diaphyseal fractures of tibia can often be immobilized using functional cast (cranial half cast) applied below the knee, or using modified Thomas splint application. However, due to difficulty in immobilizing the stifle joint by external fixation and due to the mechanical advantage of internal fixation techniques, tibial diaphyseal fractures are better treated using either IM pinning/IL nailing or bone plating. Most of the transverse or short oblique fractures of the tibial

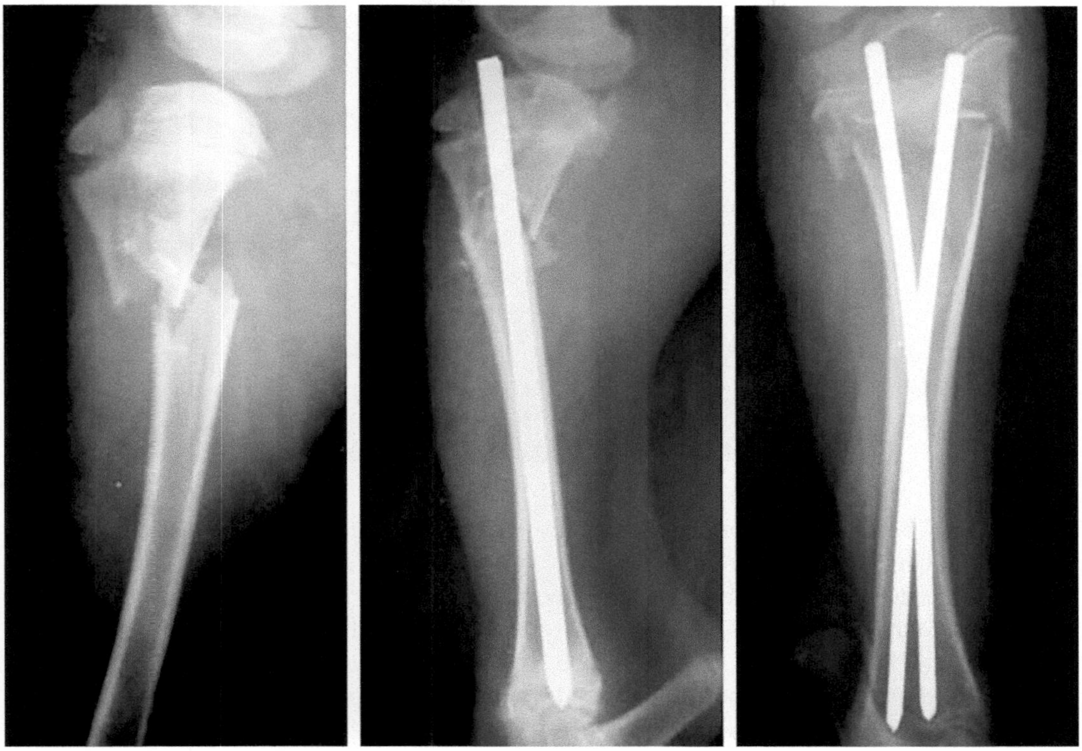

**Fig. 3.54** Single (**a** and **b**) and cross (**c**) IM pin fixation for stabilization of comminuted fractures of proximal tibia in goat

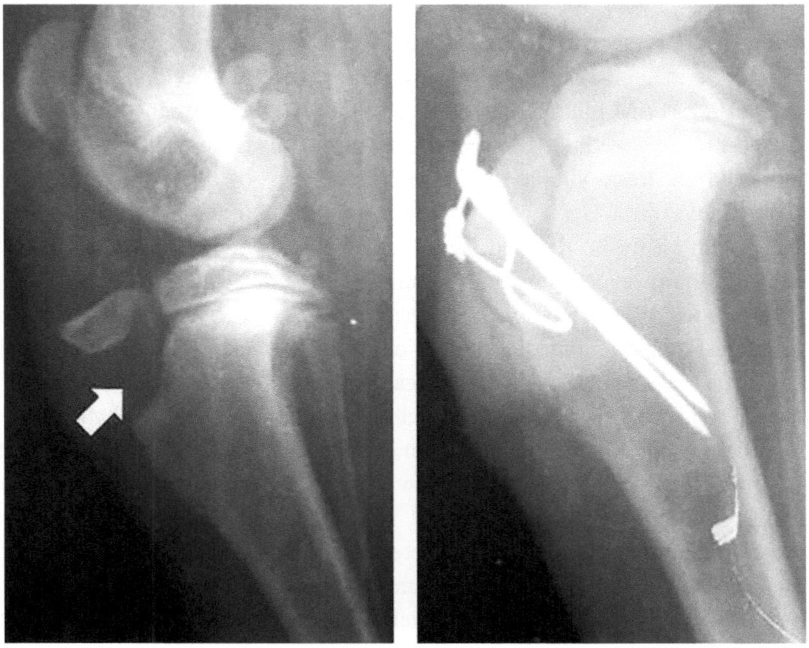

**Fig. 3.55** Tension band wiring for fixation of avulsion fracture of tibial crest

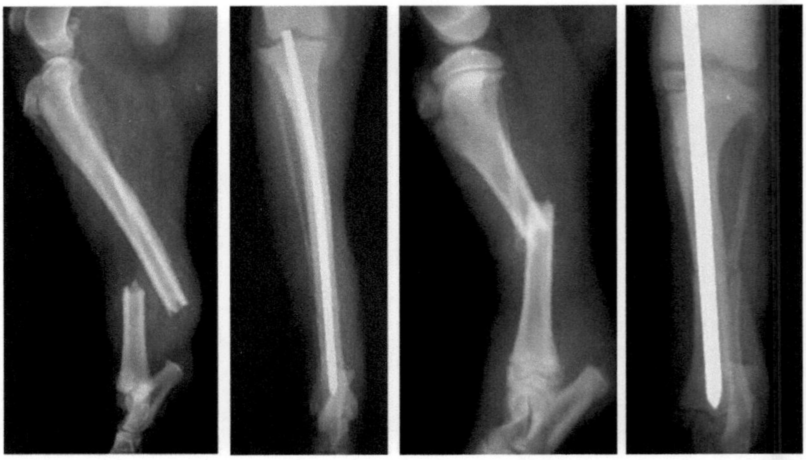

**Fig. 3.56** Transverse fractures of tibial diaphysis immobilized with close method of normograde IM pinning

diaphysis can be easily immobilized using IM Steinmann pinning. As tibia does not have heavy musculature around the cranio-medial aspect, many times in fresh cases, fracture can be reduced closely by traction and toggling and IM pin fixed by close method easily [34] (Fig. 3.56). However, much effort should not be made to reduce a fracture closely, and similarly repeated attempts should not be made to insert the pin by close method, as it may injure the surrounding soft tissues including vessels and nerves, often leading to comminution of bone fragments.

In tibia, IM pin is always passed by normograde method from the proximal end, as retrograde method will cause injury to the stifle joint [19, 74]. IM pinning can be done either by closed or open method. Closed/blind pinning is indicated in fresh simple diaphyseal fractures (incomplete, transverse, or slight oblique), which can easily be reduced by closed method [33]. In spiral or comminuted fractures, always open reduction and fixation is done. IM pin is inserted on the craniomedial margin of the tibia, half-way between the patellar ligament and medial collateral ligament (between the tibial tuberosity and the medial collateral ligament). At this site, generally, the pin will remain extracapsular; even if intracapsular, it will be extra-articular and does not interfere with the menisci or the cranial cruciate ligament at its insertion. During pin insertion, initially the pin end must be angled somewhat laterally to ensure proper fixing of the trocar point. Once anchored, the pin angle is flattened out to enter the medullary cavity and directed along the medullary canal. It is always advised to start with a relatively small diameter pin because in most instances the pin will have to "bounce off" the lateral endosteal surface of the intramedullary canal as it courses distally. The use of large diameter pin may lead to splintering of bone. As the tibial medullary canal is slightly curved in "S" shape, fixation of straight pin through the shaft generally provides stable fixation due to multiple points of pin contact. Hence, external support is generally not needed, but cerclage or hemi-cerclage wires can be used to provide rotational stability in long oblique or comminuted fractures (Fig. 3.57). But one should remember that the proximal and distal diaphysis of tibia is not well suited for full cerclage wire fixation because of the triangular shape of the bone proximally and the attachment of fibula distally.

Tibial diaphyseal fractures can also be treated using interlocking nail fixation, especially in large dogs with comminuted fractures [48, 75, 76]. A Steinmann pin is passed in normograde fashion to establish an intramedullary channel in the proximal segment similar to IM pinning. The nail is inserted through a point about half-way between the tibial tuberosity and the medial collateral ligament by making a medial parapatellar arthrotomy incision. Similar to Steinmann pin, a

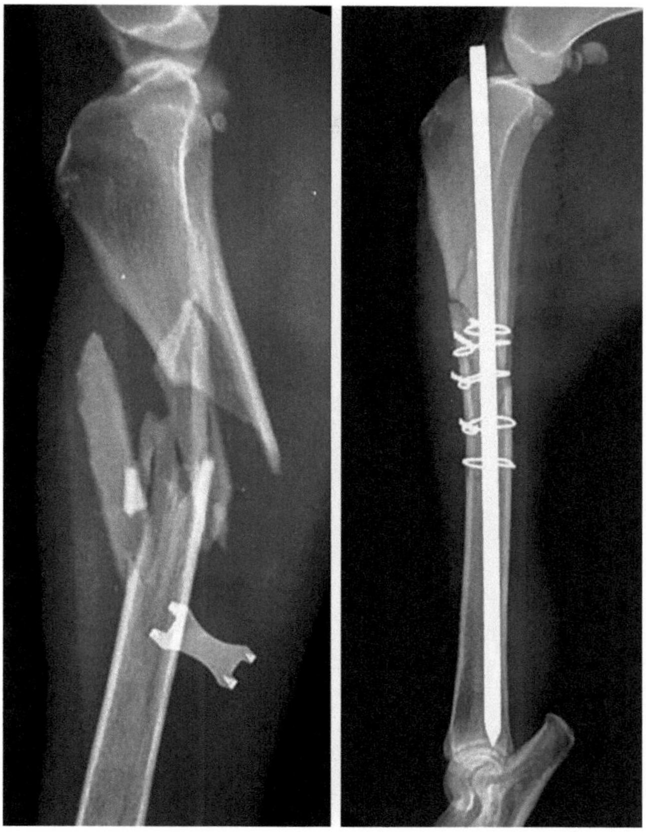

**Fig. 3.57** Comminuted fracture of tibial diaphysis stabilized with IM pinning and cerclage wiring

reamer or interlocking nail should never be passed in retrograde manner in tibia. Make sure to seat the nail distally so that the proximal end of the nail does not protrude into the stifle joint.

Plate and screw fixation is often preferred for repair of unstable tibial fractures in heavy dogs (Figs. 3.58 and 3.59). After giving skin incision on the cranial or cranio-lateral surface, a properly contoured plate is fixed on the cranio-medial surface of the bone, so that the skin incision does not directly lie over the plate. Hemi-cerclage wires or lag screws may be used to reduce and reconstruct a comminuted fracture before bone plate and screw fixation. More recently, introduced locking compression plate (LCP) systems provide greater fixation stability in tibial fracture repair [77]. The LCP or String of Pearls (SOP) plate [78], a unique and versatile design of locking plate system, which allows two plane bending and torsion, can also be applied by minimally invasive percutaneous plate osteosynthesis (MIPO) technique to achieve biological bone healing in comminuted fractures of tibial diaphysis [79–81] (Fig. 3.60).

External skeletal fixation (ESF) systems (half pin or full pin) have also been used extensively for both closed and open diaphyseal fracture repair in tibia [74, 82–85]. The presence of least soft tissues around the tibia make pin placement easy. Half-pin device is usually placed with the connecting frame on the medial or cranial surface of the bone, whereas full-pin frame (bilateral) is placed mediolaterally. Circular fixator was used for repair of tibial fractures with the tranfixation pins passed from cranio-lateral to caudo-medial and caudo-lateral to cranio-medial directions or vice versa. Freeform epoxy-pin or acrylic-pin fixation systems have also been successfully used for the treatment of tibial fractures (Fig. 3.61).

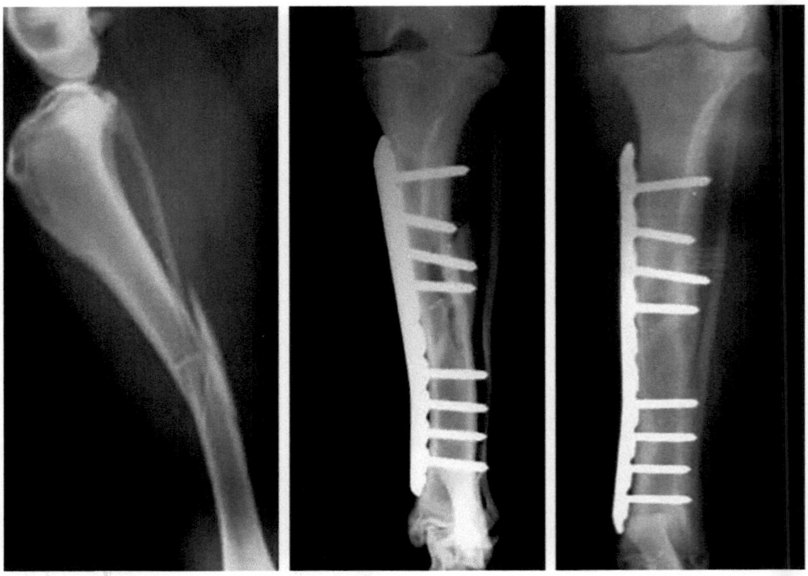

**Fig. 3.58** Spiral fracture of tibia stabilized with locking compression plate. (Source: S Sahu et al., Evaluation of locking compression plate in wedge and complex fractures of long bones in dogs. Indian J Vet Surg. 38 (2): 81–85, 2017)

These ESF systems are ideal for treatment of open infected tibial diaphyseal fractures [26, 86].

### 3.5.3 Distal Tibial/Malleolar Fractures

Fracture at the distal end of tibia close to the hock joint is sometimes seen in dogs and cats. Such fractures can be treated by either external fixation (MTS) or internal fixation using K-wires. Crossed K-wires generally provide stable fixation (Fig. 3.62); however, it has to be reinforced with external bandaging (e.g., Robert-Jones bandage). Instability of hock joint due to fracture of medial or lateral malleolus is often encountered in dogs. In such cases, tension band wiring done using two small diameter K-wires along with external application of Robert Jones bandage may prove successful. Special bone plates such as T-plate can also be used to provide stable fixation (Fig. 3.63).

Fracture-dislocation of tibio-tarsal joint is common in dogs and cats mostly caused due to

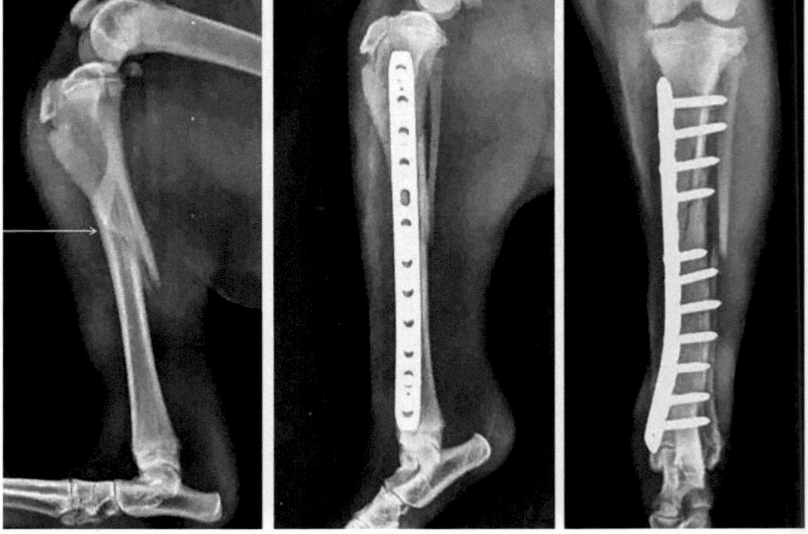

**Fig. 3.59** Spiral fracture of tibia stabilized with locking compression plate. Note that fixation of long plate helps to distribute the load along the length of the bone (Courtesy: Dr. Dharamraj, R., Bangalore, India)

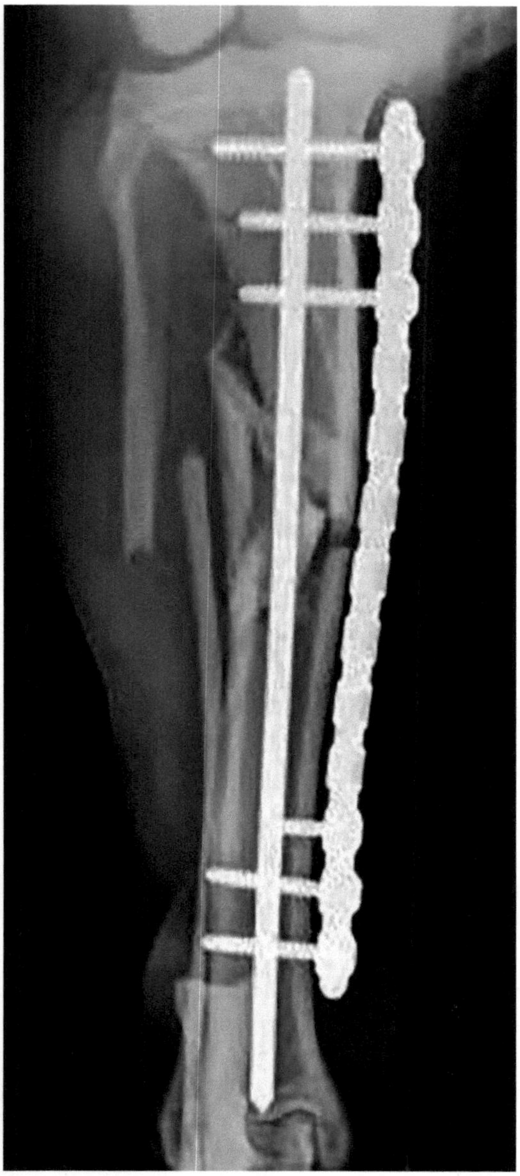

**Fig. 3.60** Comminuted tibial fracture repair by minimally invasive technique using SOP plate-pin construct (Reproduced with permission from: Michael Kowaleski, Cummings School of Veterinary Medicine at Tufts University; British Vet Association, Spring Scientific Meeting: Advances in Fracture Management, Birmingham, first April 2009)

severe twisting/scrape injuries or hyperextension of the joint. This is often accompanied with rupture of one or both collateral ligaments and fracture of one or both malleoli and/or tibial tarsal bone. Clinically, the animal is presented with carrying of limb with swinging of the limb distal to the joint, often accompanied with crepitation and joint swelling. Though close reduction can be achieved in most cases, closed fixation generally does not yield favorable results. Hence, open reduction and fixation is preferred. After reduction of the joint, malleolar fracture if present should be rigidly fixed (by tension band wiring) [71], and the collateral ligament tear should be repaired as far as possible. The joint is immobilized for 5–6 weeks using splint and bandaging. In cases of severe instability and fracture, arthrodesis may be undertaken. In open infected cases, the joint may be immobilized using any of the ESF techniques such as epoxy-pin fixation (Fig. 3.64). The prognosis is generally favorable in most cases with adequate stabilization of fracture and the joint; however, in cases of arthrodesis, some degree of gait abnormality may persist.

## 3.6 Fractures of Metacarpus and Metatarsus

The incidence of metacarpal (MC) and metatarsal (MT) fractures is about 2–3% each (together 4–6%) of all bone fractures in dogs and cats. Fractures of MC and MT are generally seen in young puppies or kittens, most often caused by fall from a height or by crush injuries (stepped upon). If caused by automobile accidents, they are often accompanied by fractures of other bones. Fractures may be incomplete or complete with involvement of one or more bones. The animal is presented with carrying of the affected limb with soft tissue swelling and pain on palpation over the site. If only one or two MC or MT bones are broken, there will be little deviation of fragments. Generally, the surrounding soft tissues are not affected much except in major traumatic cases where laceration of tendons and vessels may occur.

Treatment of MC/MT fractures is relatively easy. In most cases, external immobilization using splints or cast will be effective, especially when one or two bones are involved. If more than two or three bones are fractured with

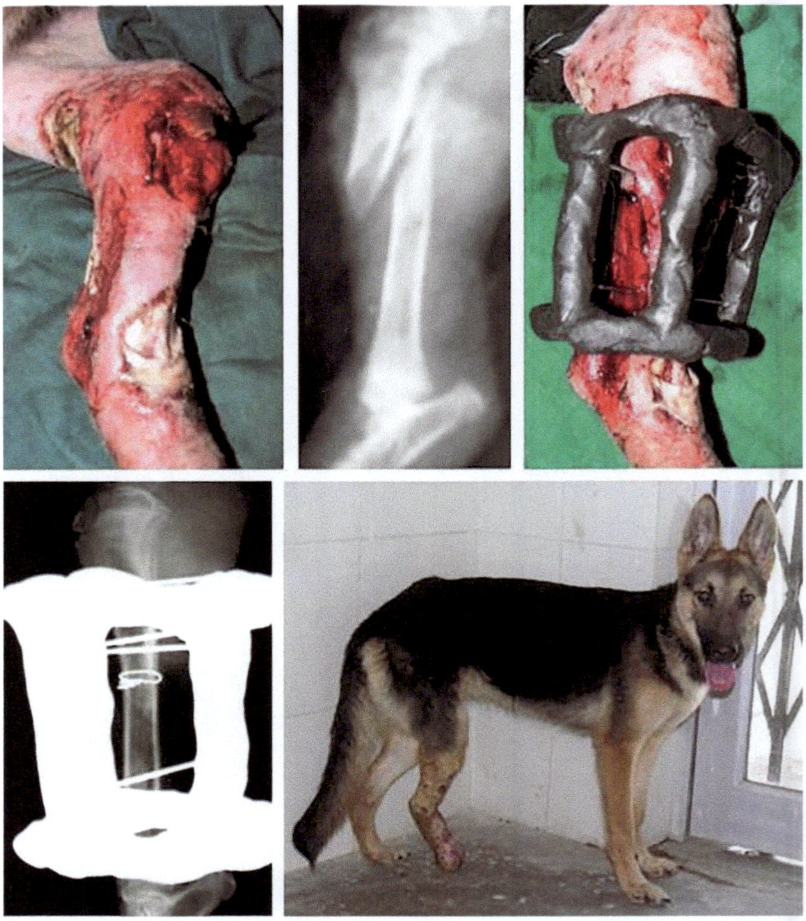

**Fig. 3.61** Epoxy-pin fixation with cerclage wiring of an open infected tibial diaphyseal fracture. Note the good bone healing and satisfactory functional recovery of the limb in spite of severe soft tissue damage and infection

displacement of bone fragments, internal or external skeletal fixation may be preferred [87].

Internal fixation may be accomplished by intramedullary fixation (Dowel pinning) [88] using Steinmann pin/K-wire or orthopedic wire (Fig. 3.65). IM pins can be introduced through II and V MC/MT bones, dorsal to the metacarpo/metatarso-phalangeal joints and then driven

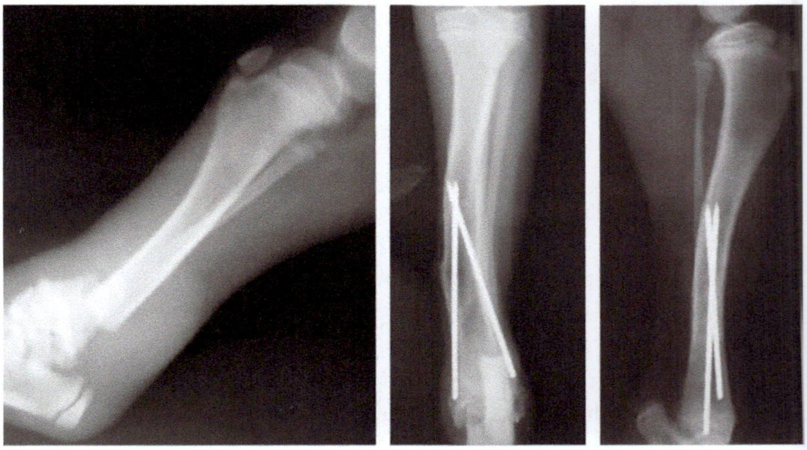

**Fig. 3.62** Cross pinning for distal tibial fracture repair

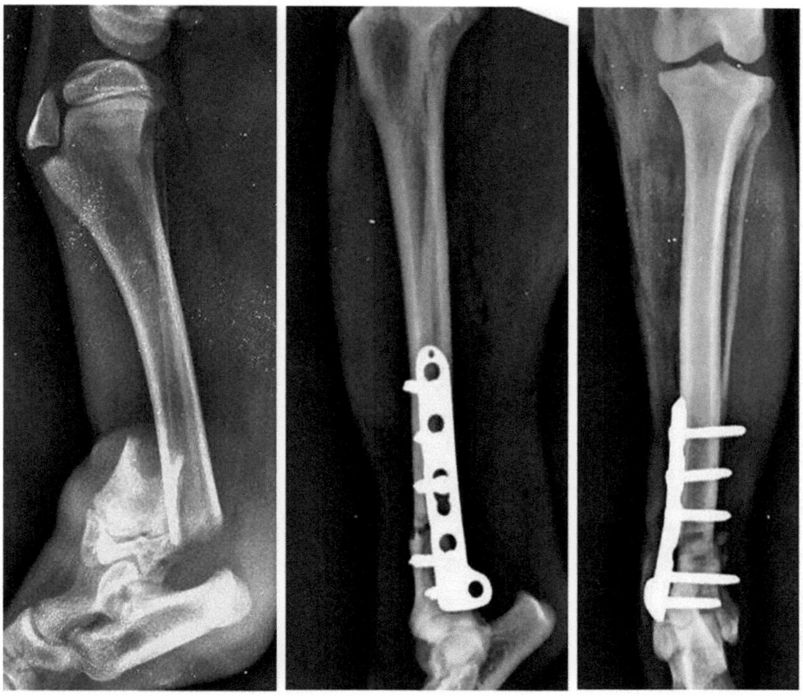

**Fig. 3.63** Stabilization of distal tibial fracture using a mini plate

through the proximal bone fragments. The exposed distal end of the pin is bent carefully so that they will not interfere with the joint function. Normally, immobilization of II and V bones will stabilize III and IV MC/MT bones as well. Subsequently, external coaptation is provided to protect the small diameter pins from direct weight bearing. Small lightweight plates (such as titanium 1.5 mm LCP) can also be used for internal fixation of MC/MT fractures (Fig. 3.66) [89]. Four to six hole plates are fixed on the dorsal surface of the II or/and V MC/MT bones to provide rigid fixation. Care should be taken to see that the screws are of optimum size, such that the tips of the screws just come out of the opposite cortex after tightening, to prevent pricking of soft tissues/skin on the palmar/plantar surface. External support should be provided to prevent screw loosening and bending of plates/pins or refracture of bones at the sites of screw insertion.

External skeletal fixation can also be used for fixation in MC/MT, especially in open fractures [90]. K-wires introduced through the medullary cavity can be extended externally, bent toward each other, and fixed using an epoxy mold. Or else 3–4 small diameter (1.2–1.5 mm) K-wires may be transfixed on either side of fracture and are externally bent and joined to make a frame, over which epoxy dough is applied to construct epoxy-pin side bars (Fig. 3.67). The transfixation pins passed mediolaterally/lateromedially should penetrate through at least two MC/MT bones to provide stable fixation. In large heavy animals and in cases where the proximal radius-ulna/tibia-fibula is also fractured, the transcortical pins are also fixed in the radius-ulna/tibia-fibula to provide more stable trans-articular fixation.

If proper technique is used, complications are rare, and generally, MC/MT fractures heal uneventfully with excellent functional recovery. Open fractures with severe crush injury may lead to vascular compromise and necrosis often leading to sloughing of paw, or injury to flexor or extensor leading to digital malfunction.

## 3.7 Fractures of Mandible

Fractures of the mandible are very common in dogs and cats, which constitute about 4–5% of total fractures in dogs. Common causes of trauma leading to mandibular fractures are road traffic

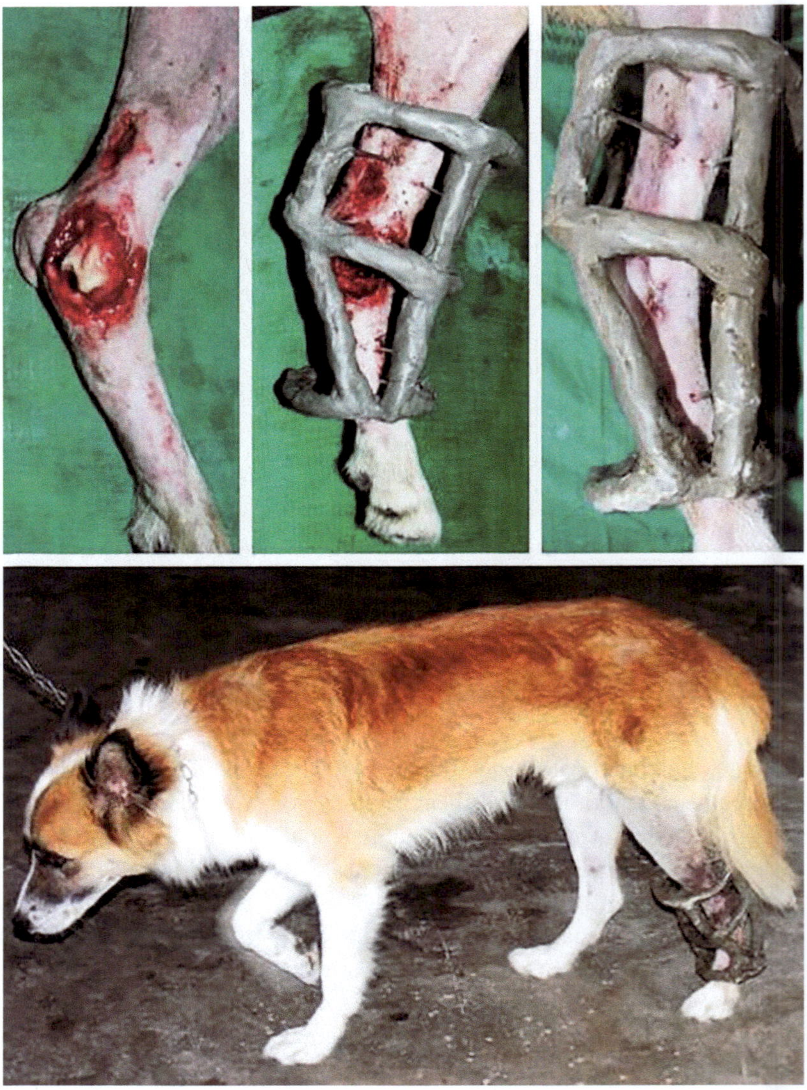

**Fig. 3.64** Epoxy-pin fixation (circular) for open fracture-luxation of tarsal joint. Note the fixation of hock joint in normal angulation and good functional recovery of the affected limb

accidents, falls, kicks, bites, and gunshot injuries, and they occur more frequently in young male dogs. Other causes may include neoplasia, severe periodontitis, metabolic disorders such as secondary hyperparathyroidism, and iatrogenic tooth extractions.

The mandible contains two separate bones (hemimandibles), which are joined cranially with each other at the symphysis and caudally with the temporal bones at the temporomandibular joints. Each hemimandible includes a horizontal part (body) and a vertical part (ramus). The body of the mandible accommodates the teeth, and the ramus includes many important structures like parotid glands, nerves, and muscles. The incisor and canine teeth (with single alveoli per tooth) occupy the rostral part of the mandible, and the premolar, molar teeth (with two alveoli per tooth), and the third molar (with single alveoli) are positioned caudally. In dogs, the mandibular fractures are most commonly open and located in the premolar region, that is, between the canine and first molar teeth, often involving the alveolus. In cats, fractures are common in the symphyseal region. The incidence of open fractures in the caudal mandible is lower, which is probably attributed to heavy musculature in the area.

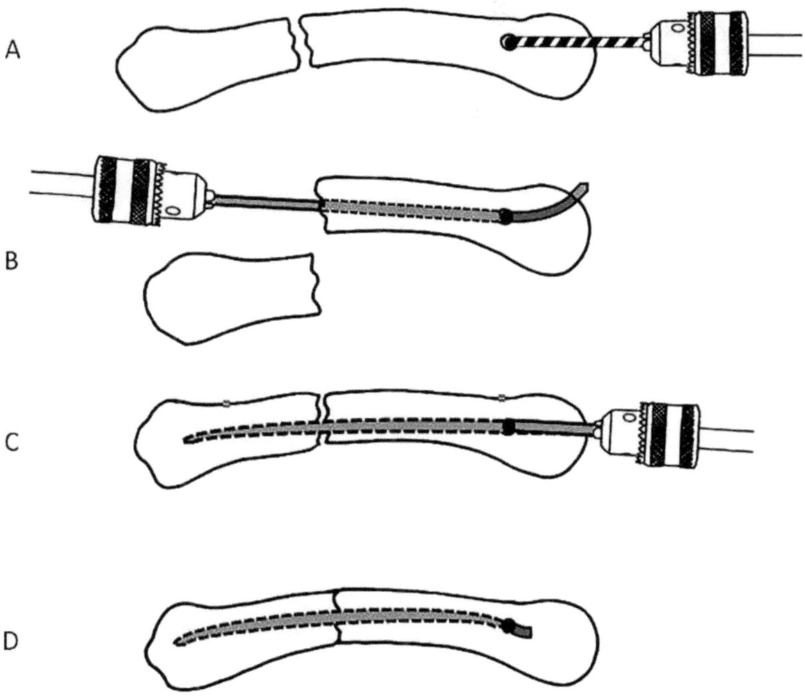


**Fig. 3.65** Schematic diagram showing intramedullary pinning in metacarpus and metatarsus: A small hole is drilled in the dorsal surface of the distal end of distal bone segment (**a**); an adequate diameter pin with slightly bent tip is inserted from the fracture site and taken out though the predrilled hole (**b**); the pin is withdrawn till the distal end reaches the fracture site, and then the bone is reduced, and the pin is directed into the proximal bone segment (**c**); once the pin is properly seated at the proximal end of proximal bone segment, the extra length pin is cut short at the level of insertion hole (**d**)

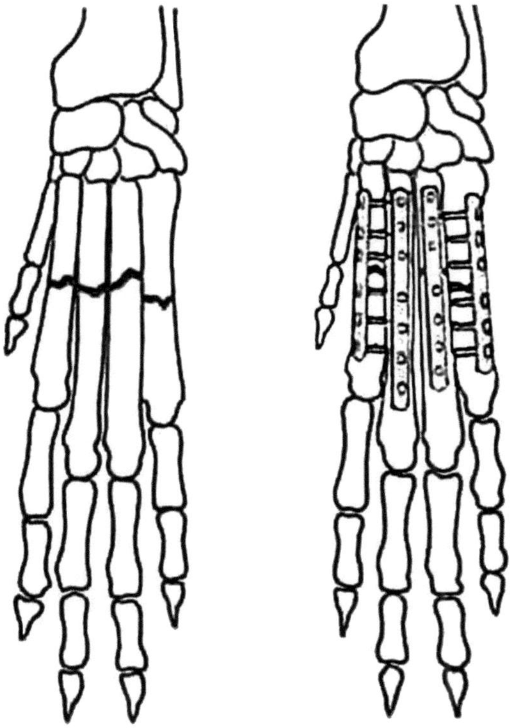

**Fig. 3.66** Schematic diagram showing bone plating of metacarpus and metatarsus: small 4/6-hole plates (preferably 1.5 mm titanium plates) are fixed across the major fractured bones with at least two screws fixed across the fracture site

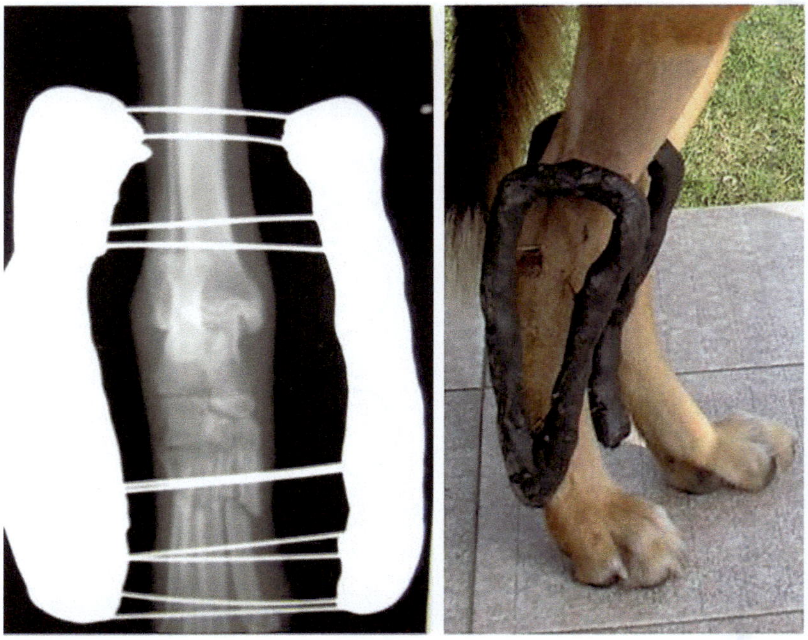

**Fig. 3.67** Multiplanar transarticular epoxy-pin fixation for immobilization of metatarsal fractures in dog

Clinical signs of mandibular fracture may include dropping of jaw, asymmetry, hemorrhage, and drooling of saliva. Radiography (extraoral and intraoral radiographs) may help confirm the diagnosis of fractures, especially in the body of the mandible, whereas fractures near the temporo-mandibular joint area may require CT scan to provide confirmatory diagnosis.

The mandible, due to its unique shape, presents inherent limitations for surgical repair. The curvature of the bone, the presence of dental structures leaving limited bone stock for purchase of fixation implants, and heavy musculature make surgical repair of mandibular fractures challenging. The goal of mandibular fracture treatment, like any other fracture, is early return to normal function. It includes establishing of the normal dental occlusion and immediate regaining of most important function of feeding. The location and orientation of the fracture line determine the technique and outcome of surgical fixation. Fractures running in caudoventral direction have the tendency for distraction and are unfavorable, whereas those with caudodorsal fracture line are favorable as they assist compression of fracture segments due to muscular contraction. By uniting the occlusal surface (biting surface of the teeth), that is, the tension side of the mandible, compression can be achieved on the ventral surface during closure of the jaw. External fixation (use of muzzle), internal fixation (orthopedic wire, Steinmann pin, plate, and screw, etc.), or external skeletal fixation (KE splint, acrylic, or epoxy-pin fixation) can be employed for effective treatment of mandibular fractures as per the case [91–96].

### 3.7.1 External Fixation

Application of tape muzzles is the routine method used to immobilize simple undisplaced or easily reducible fractures of the mandible such as unilateral body fractures and separation of symphysis. Muzzles are typically made of a tape, having an encircling band around the mandible and maxilla with attachments connecting both sides going behind and secured by tying behind the ears (Fig. 3.68). The muzzle is placed in such a way that the dog can open its mouth enough to eat soft foods like gruel with its tongue (to allow about 1.0 cm space between the incisors). It can be used as a first aid option to provide temporary stabilization and also as an adjunct to internal fixation to spare the fracture site from undue distraction. To prevent removal of muzzle by the animal itself, an Elizabethan collar can be used temporarily.

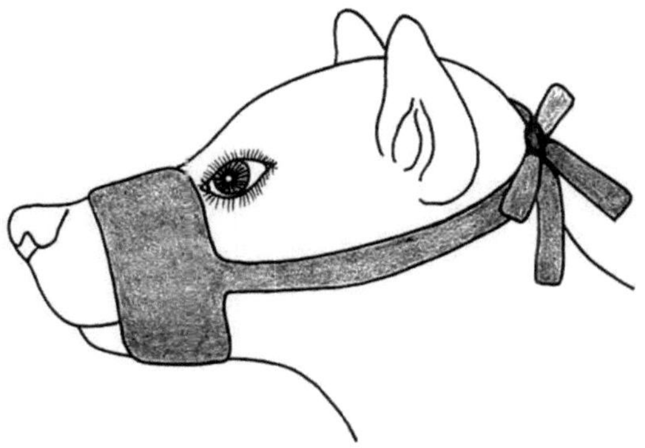

**Fig. 3.68** Tape muzzle applied around the mandible and maxilla and secured by tying behind the ears can provide stability to undisplaced mandibular fracture. It can be used to provide temporary stabilization or as an adjunct to internal fixation

Rostral fractures are generally treated conservatively with muzzles since the presence of numerous alveoli will compromise fixation device attachment. Since mandibular fractures do not require very rigid fixation (as load bearing long bones), muzzle can be acceptable to accomplish healing in most cases. However, complications such as malocclusion, breathing difficulty, and aspiration may often occur, especially when the muzzle is applied improperly.

### 3.7.2 Internal Fixation

Most of the mandibular fractures are open fractures, and it is usually not possible to maintain strict aseptic procedures during an internal fixation procedure due to the location of the bone. However, as mandible is relatively resistant to infection, internal fixation can achieve an early satisfactory healing within 4–6 weeks of time. Though mandible can be approached through an extraoral (incision through the skin) incision, intraoral approach should be preferred (for less postoperative complications), and whenever possible, the implant (e.g., plate and screws) should be covered by the mucosa. External implants should always be removed after the bone union.

Orthopedic wiring is the most frequently used internal fixation technique in mandibular fractures. It can be used as cerclage wire, suture, interdental wire, or tension band wire (Fig. 3.69a–d). Interdental cerclage wire can be used for oblique fractures of the horizontal ramus and also in symphyseal separation, and suturing technique may be used for transverse fractures of the horizontal ramus. These techniques are not the strongest but, when combined with application of muzzles, can be successful. Also, tension band wiring done over the dental arcade provides more stable fixation of the horizontal ramus.

Intramedullary fixation of Steinmann pin or K-wire is often employed for fixation of fractures in the horizontal body part of the mandible (Fig. 3.70a, b). However, due to the peculiar shape of the marrow space in the mandible, it is very difficult to align the fracture fragments, often leading to malalignment and fracture instability. Further as the roots of the canine teeth occupy a large space, IM fixation in rostral fractures would be difficult. Similarly, the vertical ramus is a thin bone with minimal space for fixation of intramedullary pins.

Bone plating can provide perfect anatomical reduction and stability of the mandibular fracture with minimal occlusion and early restoration of function. When bone plate is used to stabilize fractures of the mandible, it is preferred to place the screws monocortically to minimize injury to the tooth roots. However, it is technically difficult to apply a standard plate in the rostral mandible, as it is difficult to contour the plate. Hence, special plates like reconstruction plates may be more useful (Fig. 3.71a, b). At the caudal mandibular region, application of a plate may require more soft tissue dissection, which may affect bone healing adversely. Similarly, it is difficult to approach and reduce fractures near the temporomandibular joint and to achieve absolute joint conformity. Hence, fractures of the caudal mandible are generally treated by conventional methods.

### 3.7.3 External Skeletal Fixation

External skeletal fixation has often been used to treat mandibular fractures in dogs and cats (Fig. 3.72). Typically, KE splints are the method of choice. Threaded pins or long cortical screws can be used as fixation elements (instead of smooth pins) in the mandible for greater purchase

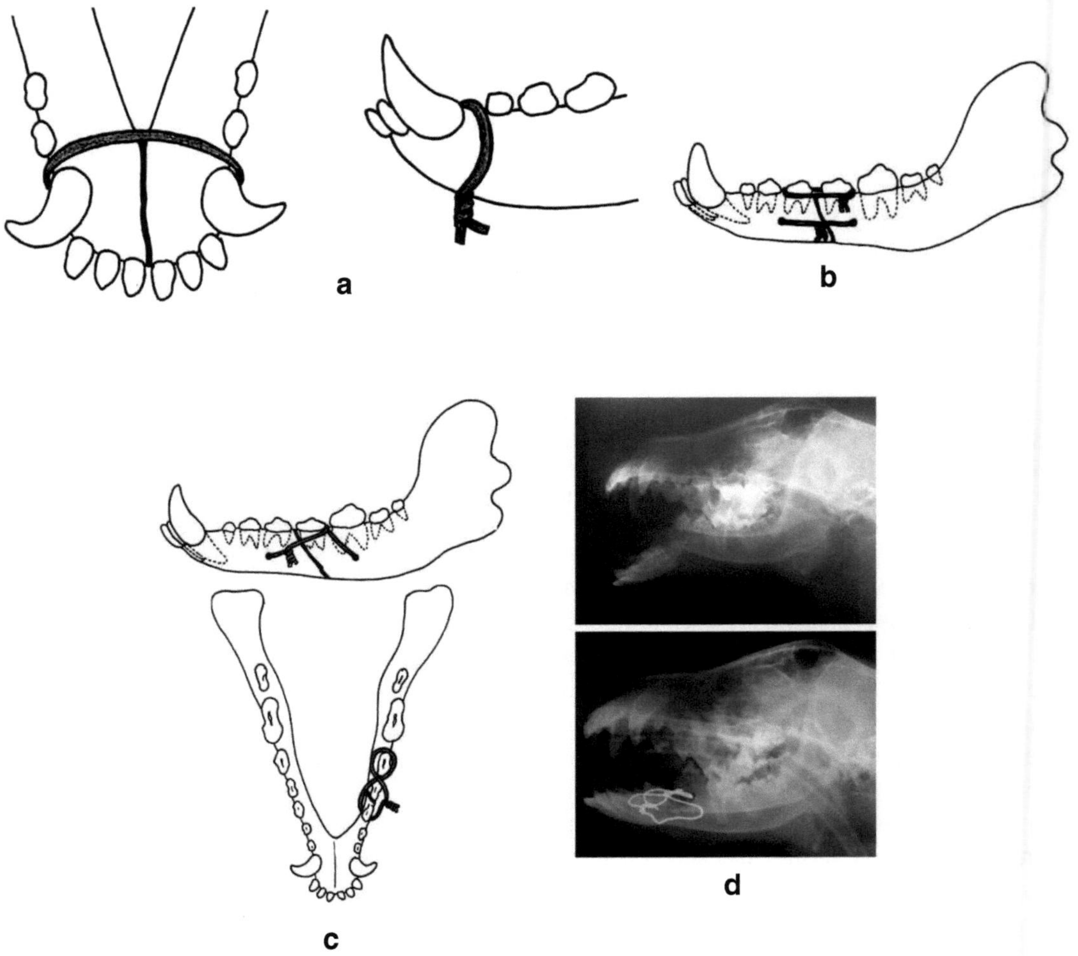


**Fig. 3.69** (**a**) Orthopedic wire fixation for repair of mandibular symphyseal fracture; (**b**) interdental wiring in the form of mattress suture to stabilize fracture at the horizontal ramus; (**c**) interdental wiring in the form of figure of 8 over the dental arcade provides more stable fixation; and (**d**) mandibular fracture behind the canine teeth in a dog treated with simple interdental wire fixation

in the thin soft bone. The fixation pins can then be attached to a metallic side bar. On the other hand, the transfixation pins or screws can be connected using a wire to make a scaffold over which an acrylic or epoxy column can be constructed. Such acrylic-pin or epoxy-pin fixation is very versatile, as the pins can be inserted in different planes by avoiding the root structures and the mandibular canal, to achieve satisfactory reduction and fixation in difficult cases. Transfixation, however, is not advocated cranial to the first molar to avert injury to the sublingual structures.

### 3.7.4 Complications and Prognosis

Complications with mandibular fractures are common, which include malocclusion, malunion, nonunion, infection, and fixation failure. In cases of malocclusion, the fixation should be rechecked and corrected when possible. In osteomyelitis cases, infection should be first treated as per the culture and sensitivity tests. Bone graft (autogenous cancellous or rib graft) may be used to treat nonunions (after the fracture ends are freshened) and osteomyelitis (after controlling infection). In severe cases of infection or nonunions, partial

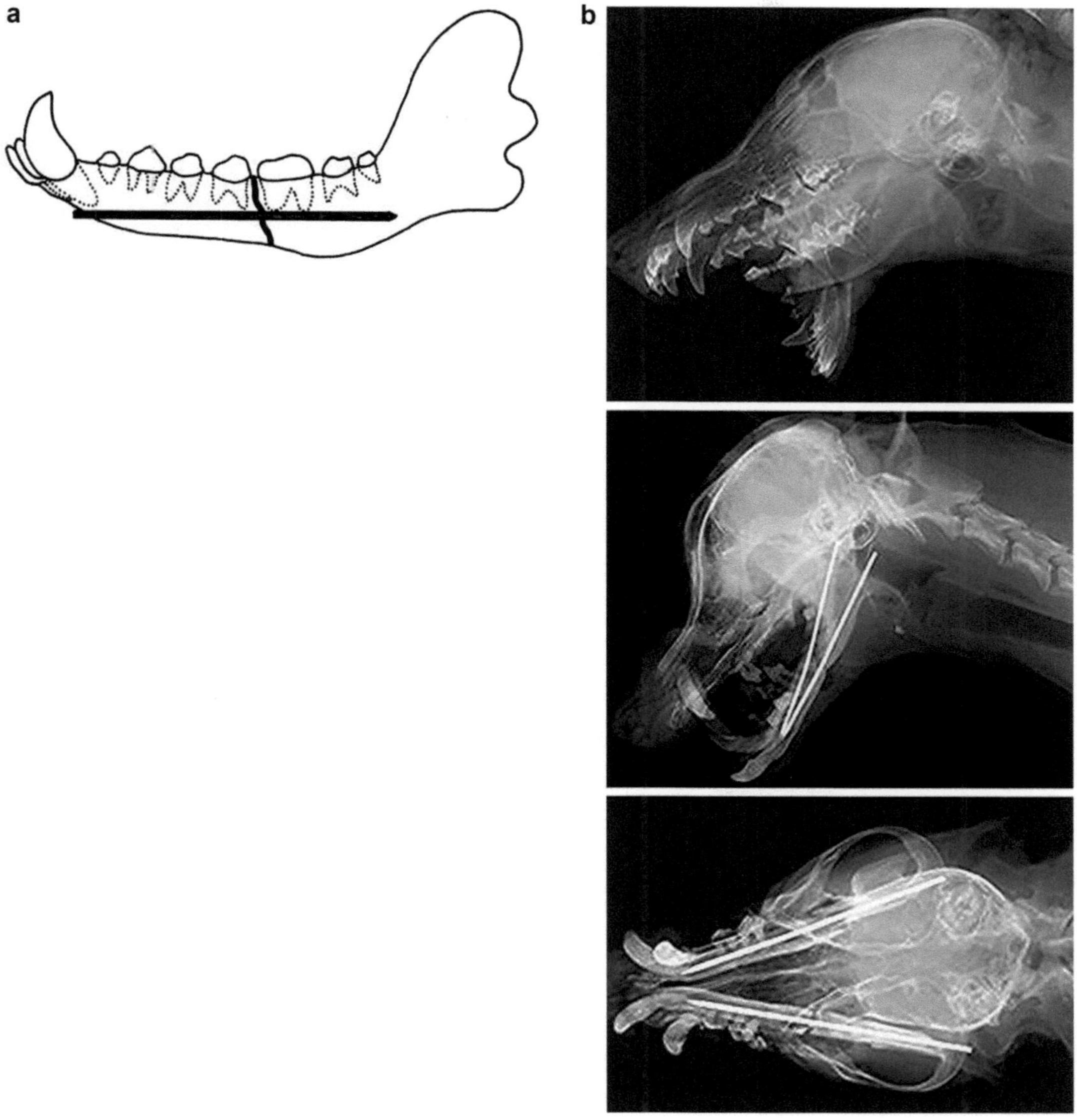

**Fig. 3.70** (**a**) Intramedullary pinning for fixation of mandibular fracture at the horizontal ramus; (**b**) bilateral mandibular fracture stabilized using IM pinning in dog (Source:: S. Purohit et al., Intraoral approach of retrograde intramedullary pin fixation for repair of mandible fractures in 4 dogs, Indian J Vet Surg. 40 (1): 66–67, 2019)

mandibulectomy is indicated. With ESF, most common complications are pin tract infection and premature loosening of pins; these complications can be reduced by using proper pin insertion techniques.

Prognosis of mandibular fracture repair is generally favorable. Healing is generally faster, and functional outcome is more favorable in fractures cranial to the first molar (than caudal fractures), maybe because rigid fixation can be achieved in these fractures more easily.

## 3.8 Fractures of Pelvis

The pelvis is made up of three major bones: ilium, ischium, and pubis, and young immature animals have a fourth bone, the acetabular bone. The

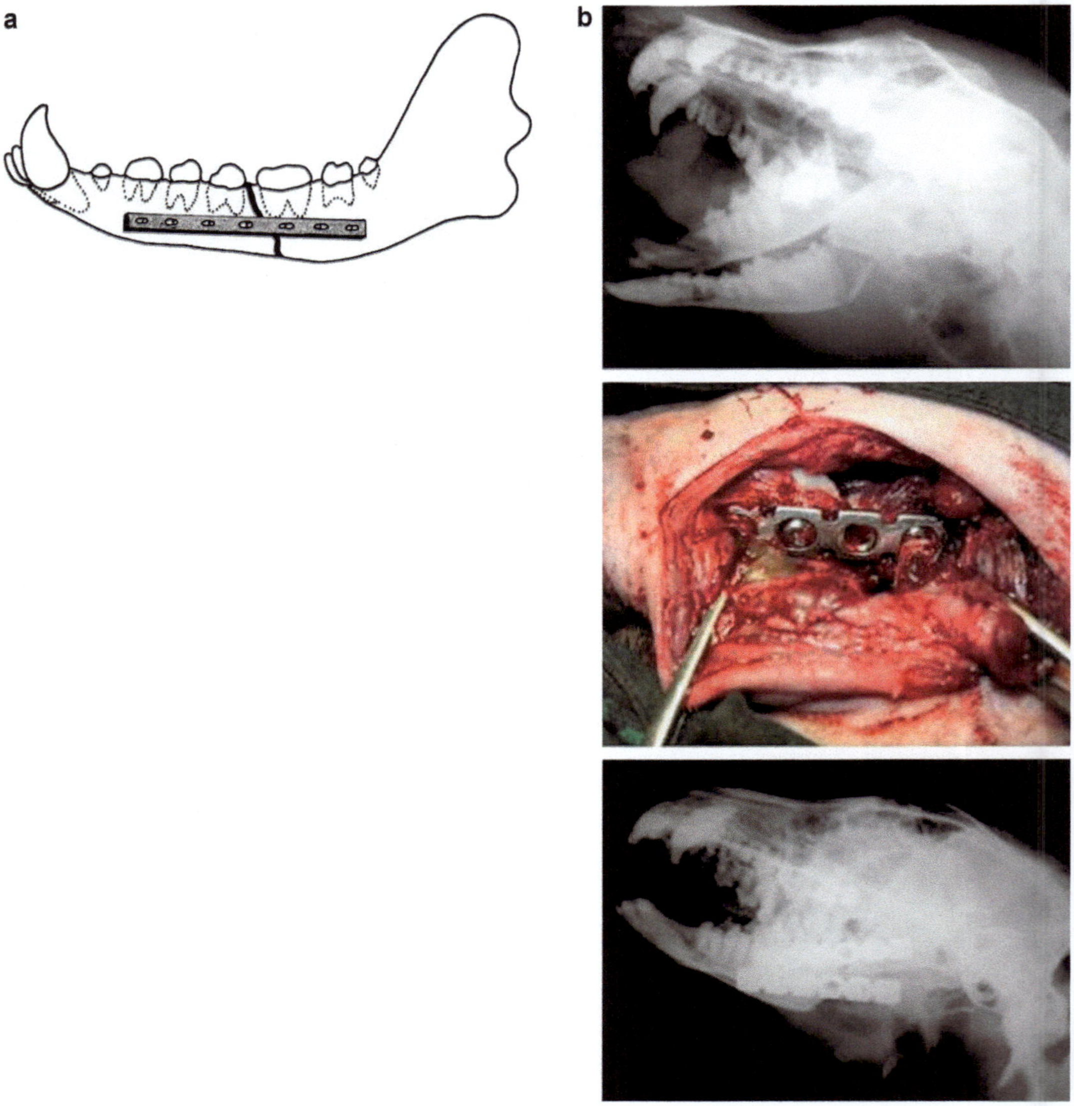


**Fig. 3.71** (**a**) Fixation of bone plate for mandibular fracture- plate should be fixed below the teeth roots to prevent possible damage; (**b**) application of reconstruction plates for bilateral fracture at the caudal mandibular region in a dog

pelvis is attached to the sacrum, which connects the pelvic (hind) limbs to the axial skeleton. The acetabulum, the pelvic component of the hip joint, is attached to the hind limbs through the femur head. Fractures of the pelvic girdle are very common (about 20–25% of all fractures) in dogs and cats and generally affect multiple sites of the pelvis [97]. Pelvic fractures are common in young animals, caused mostly by automobile accidents. When the dogs and cats are hit from behind, the pelvis usually sustains injury leading to multiple comminuted fractures of more than one bone, although the incidence of ilial fractures is relatively higher than others. Fractures of the pelvis are often associated with dislocation of sacro-iliac joint, dislocation of hip joint, and fracture of femur bone.

Dogs and cats with pelvic fractures are typically presented with varied degrees of lameness with history of trauma. Occasionally, they may be recumbent with multiple injuries. In animals with pelvic fracture, concurrent injuries such as

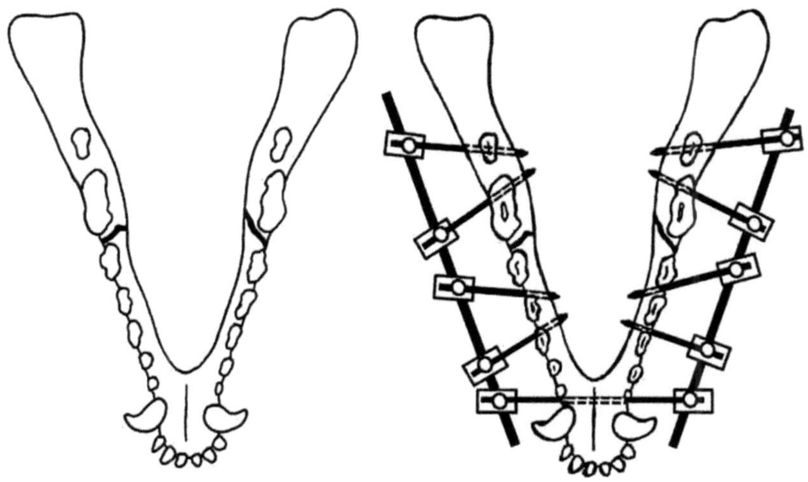

**Fig. 3.72** Bilateral ESF application for fractures at the body of mandible

thoracic trauma (in about 50% cases), urinary tract trauma (in about 30% cases), and diaphragmatic hernia are common [98, 99]. A thorough physical examination of the vital organs should be conducted before addressing the specific management of pelvic fracture. Pelvis should be examined for pain on palpation to localize the site of injury, the animal's ability to stand, pelvic symmetry, and instability at sacroiliac joint. Rectum may be examined to determine the possible perforation of rectal wall and narrowing of pelvic canal. In pelvic fractures with urinary incontinence (seen in about 10% cases), a complete neurological examination of peripheral nerve and nerve roots is advised to detect any abnormality. Although most neurological deficits are mild and transient, signs suggesting loss of sensation and tone in the perineal region and deep pain in hind limbs may indicate prolonged recovery and poor prognosis.

The pelvis is surrounded by heavy musculature along with important nerves (sciatic nerve, which runs along the inner side of the ilium and over the top of the ischium behind the acetabulum) and vessels (internal iliac vessels) supplying to the hind quarters; hence, the surgical approach to the pelvic bones is difficult [100]. However, due to a large muscle mass, pelvis provides an optimal environment for biological healing of fracture, and a large number of pelvic fractures including those with minimally displaced segments can be managed adequately with conservative treatment alone, without surgery [97, 101]. Nevertheless, surgical fixation relieves discomfort quickly and hastens bone healing and functional recovery.

A ventrodorsal radiographic view will help to plan for treatment. Fractures in weight-bearing bones (segment that transfers load from the hind limb to the spine) such as acetabular fractures and markedly displaced ilial fractures and sacroiliac luxations (>50%) need surgical fixation. Surgical repair is also indicated in cases with pronounced narrowing (>40%) of pelvic canal, bilateral pelvic fractures, and those associated with multiple limb fractures. And conservative treatment is recommended for most ischial and pubic fractures and minimally displaced ilial fractures and sacroiliac luxations with only slight narrowing of pelvic canal. In short, stable fractures that do not involve the acetabulum or compromise the pelvic canal diameter can be managed conservatively. Stabilization of pelvic fractures within 2–3 days of injury is easier and results in better outcome, and about 7 days after the trauma, primary surgical repair may not be possible.

Conservative treatment of pelvic fractures can be done by close reduction and immobilization. Heavy musculature covering the pelvic bone normally protects the fracture fragments, often leading to satisfactory healing. Manual reduction of fractured segments by close method can be done only to a limited extent. Dorsally displaced ileal wing can be reduced to some extent by pushing it ventrally, and some ilial shaft fractures may be aligned by forced adduction of the pelvic limbs. Similarly, through rectal palpation, it is often possible to realign the ischial fragments to some extent. Closed immobilization can be accomplished by confining the animal in a cage or small enclosure for 2–4 weeks. Normally, the animals may begin to stand and walk in about 1–2 weeks; however, they should not be allowed normal activity for 6–8 weeks until the fracture is healed completely.

### 3.8.1 Surgical Approach

Various approaches have been used to access different pelvic bones. The ilium can be accessed either through a lateral or dorsal approach. Through lateral approach, the ilium may be exposed by giving an incision between the fascia lata and middle gluteal muscles and elevating the latter from its origin on the ilial wing. Through dorsal approach, the ilium may be exposed by elevating and ventrally retracting the middle gluteal muscle by taking care to protect the cranial gluteal artery and nerve. It is difficult to approach the acetabulum due to crossing over of gluteal tendons that insert on the greater trochanter of the femur. Elevation of the gluteal muscles dorsally and dissection between the middle and deep gluteal heads can give access to the cranial acetabulum. Dorsally, the acetabulum can be approached by either gluteal muscle tenotomy or trochanteric osteotomy that can help to retract the gluteal muscles completely resulting in better exposure of the acetabulum. However, osteotomy is a better technique than tenotomy (as a bone can heal better and faster than a tendon). The caudal acetabulum can be accessed by retracting the biceps femoris muscle carefully by protecting the sciatic nerve. Retraction of biceps along with gemellus and internal obturator tenotomy can expose the ischium. Pubic bone is approached by positioning the animal in dorsal recumbency and making an incision directly over the pubic symphysis and elevating the adductor and gracilis muscles at their origin.

### 3.8.2 Surgical Management

#### 3.8.2.1 Ilial Fractures

Ilial fractures can be categorized into two types, fractures of the ilial wing and fractures of ilial shaft. As the ilial wing is situated cranial to the sacrum, wing fractures rarely cause any significant instability requiring internal fixation. Fractures of the ilial shaft are most common pelvic fractures. Ilial shaft fractures are mostly oblique (cranioventral to caudodorsal fracture line) with the caudal segment displaced medially and cranially often resulting in narrowing of the pelvic canal.

The ilium is accessed through standard lateral approach by elevating the gluteal muscles dorsally. The fracture is reduced manually by traction, levering and dragging the caudal ilial shaft caudolaterally. Holding the greater trochanter using a bone forceps may help to achieve proper bone reduction.

Fracture of the wing of the ilium is stabilized using orthopedic wire sutures, K-wire, or Steinmann pin fixation. Use of lag screws or small finger plate shall provide more rigid fixation. In ilial shaft fractures, internal fixation can be achieved through intramedullary pin or plate and screw fixation. Relatively flexible Steinmann pin/K-wire is inserted into the ilial wing on the cranio-medial surface and passed straight down the ilial axis. Use of two pins and/or additional orthopedic wire may help to achieve better fracture reduction and fixation. In small breeds of dogs and cats having very thin bone with nonexistent medullary cavity, orthopedic wire sutures or small K-wire fixation with orthopedic wiring is the only option. In long oblique fractures, lag screws (directed ventrodorsally) or K-wires with hemicerclage wires can be used for bone fixation. Otherwise, most ilial fractures, especially in large breeds of dogs, can be better immobilized by bone plating [98, 99, 102] (Figs. 3.73 and 3.74). The plate is contoured to the concave surface of the ilium and fixed using two to three screws on either side of the fracture line. Reconstruction plate or SOP plates can be a better option as it can be easily contoured to the desired shape [44]

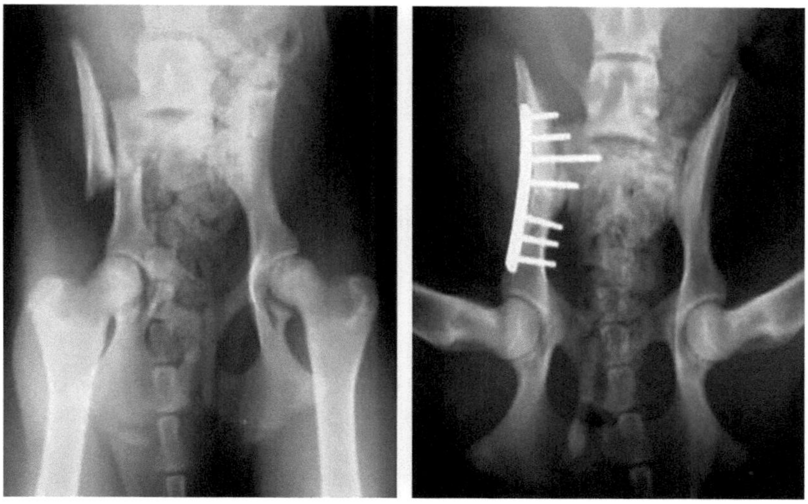

**Fig. 3.73** Bone plating for repair of ilial fracture in a dog (Reproduced with permission from: Fractures of the pelvis. www.animalsurgicalcenter.com)

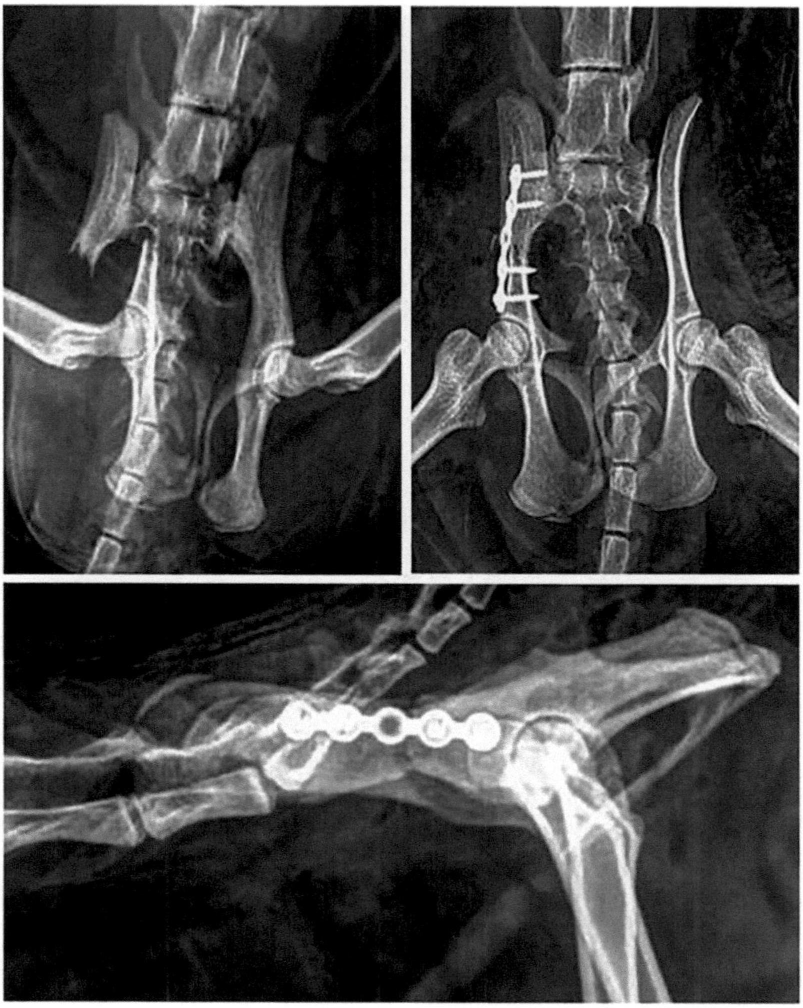

**Fig. 3.74** Stabilization of ilial fracture in a cat using reconstruction plate (Courtesy: Dr. Shashank Tripathi, Kolkatta, West Bengal, India)

**Table 3.1** Choice of plate size in pelvic bones in relation to animal's body weight

| Body weight | | | | | | |
|---|---|---|---|---|---|---|
| Type of long bone | Type of bone plate | ≤10 kg | 10–20 kg | 20–30 kg | 30–40 kg | > 40 kg |
| Ilium | MP | MP | | | | |
| | RP | | 2.7 | 2.7/3.5 | 3.5 | |
| | VCP | 2.0 | 2.0/2.7 | | | |
| | DCP/LC-DCP/LCP | 2.0 | 2.7 | 2.7/3.5 | 3.5 | 3.5 |
| Acetabulum | MP | MP | | | | |
| | RP | 2.0 | 2.0 | 2.7 | 2.7/3.5 | 3.5 |
| | AP | 2.0 | 2.7 | 2.7 | 2.7/3.5 | 3.5 |
| | DCP/LC-DCP/LCP | | 2.7 | 2.7 | 2.7/3.5 | 3.5 |

*MP* mini plate, *RP* reconstruction plate, *VCP* veterinary cuttable plate, *DCP* dynamic compression plate, *LC-DCP* limited contact dynamic compression plate, *LCP* locking compression plate, *AP* acetabular plate

(Table 3.1). One or two cranial screws can be fixed deep into the sacrum to achieve more stable fixation. Care should be taken to prevent pelvic narrowing while reducing and fixing the caudal iliac segment. The postoperative care includes restricted activity with limited weight bearing on the limb for 2–4 weeks. Possible complications may include injury to the vessels and nerves, entrapment of sciatic nerve, implant loosening, fixation failure, and narrowing of the pelvic canal. The use of locking compression plate and screws should provide more stable fixation with reduced complications.

#### 3.8.2.2 Acetabular Fractures

Acetabular fractures, comprising about 10–12% of pelvic fractures in dogs and 6–8% in cats, are very challenging to repair. They require accurate anatomic reduction and stable fixation to avoid the development of degenerative changes in the hip joint. Difficulty in accessing and visualizing the acetabular cavity makes it further demanding to accomplish this. As the cranial two third of the acetabulum is the weight-bearing surface in dogs and cats, fractures at this location require rigid stabilization. Whereas fractures at caudal and middle acetabulum are commonly treated conservatively with successful outcomes, however, conservative treatment may often lead to degenerative joint disease. Usually, acetabular fractures with minimal displacement, especially in young animals, respond well to conservative treatment.

Surgical access to acetabulum is usually achieved either through a dorsal or a caudal approach based on the location of fracture. The fracture reduction can be achieved by maneuvering of the tuber ischii or the greater trochanter, if the round ligament is still connected with the caudal segment. The reduced bone segments can be briefly maintained in alignment by using bone holding forceps and K-wires. Fracture fixation can be accomplished by using diverse bone plates, or composite fixation of screws, orthopedic wire, and polymethyl-methacrylate [98, 102, 103]. While standard bone plates are difficult to contour to the dorsal rim of acetabular, more specific acetabular plates, reconstruction plates, or SOP plates may be easier to contour and align; nevertheless, fixation of any bone plate in acetabulum is a challenge without compromising the bone alignment. Hence, malunion, fixation failure, and degenerative joint disease are the common complications of acetabular fracture fixation. Post fixation, the fracture stability can be better assessed by stress radiography, wherein a radiograph is made with the affected side of the hip placed down against the radiographic cassette, while the femoral head is pressed dorsally against the acetabular rim with the stifle in flexed position.

When surgical fixation is not feasible, femoral head and neck ostectomy may be done to alleviate pain and restore the limb function [97].

#### 3.8.2.3 Fracture of Sacroiliac Joint

Sacroiliac joint fracture can be unilateral or bilateral. It may occur alone or along with fracture of any of the pelvic bones, most often during an automobile accident. In sacroiliac fractures, the

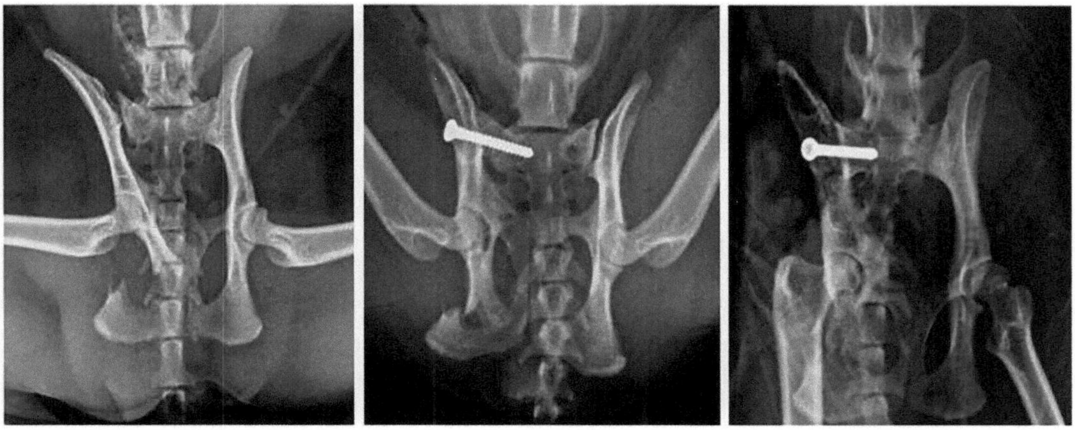

**Fig. 3.75** Fixation of sacroiliac joint luxation using a lag screw (Courtesy: Dr. Pampapathi Multi Specialty, Bangalore, India)

ilium is usually displaced craniodorsally in relation to the sacrum. In cases with >50% override and/or hip instability, open fixation is advised [100]. In unilateral fracture, with the patient in lateral recumbency, the sacroiliac joint is usually approached from dorsally. Sternal recumbency preferred if bilateral repair is necessary, and ventral approach is advocated if the ipsilateral ilium needs to be approached. The fractured ilium is manually reduced by pushing it ventrally. If needed, two vertical K-wires may be used to achieve proper bone alignment; one K-wire passed in the sacrum and another in the ilium are superimposed to align the fracture [104]. Fracture reduction can be facilitated by pulling the greater trochanter or ischial tuberosity caudally using a bone clamp. Once reduced, fixation can be achieved by using two cancellous screws or two crossed pins, or a combination of pin and screw [105–107]. For screw fixation, threaded holes are first drilled in the body of the sacrum just cranial to the c-shaped cartilage, and then the glide holes are drilled in the ilium using the landmarks on the lateral surface. Subsequently, long lag screws are fixed across the ilium toward the sacrum achieving compression (Fig. 3.75). When the sacroiliac fracture is accompanied with ilial shaft fracture, which is stabilized using a plate and screws, sacroiliac joint can be secured using one or two relatively long screws fixed through the plate [108]. Care should be taken not to penetrate the spinal canal while placing the screw/pin. In bilateral fractures, the same technique can be repeated on the opposite side. Common complications of sacroiliac joint stabilization include fixation failure (mostly seen when only one pin or screw is used), misdirection of the screw (fixation of L6 or L7), or nerve damage (sciatic entrapment).

#### 3.8.2.4 Fractures of the Ischium and Pubis

Fractures of the ischium or pubis rarely occur independently and are usually accompanied by ilial fractures. Reduction and fixation of these fractures are generally not needed, as the bone segments are usually aligned during the stabilization of ilium. However, in cases of severe fragment displacement (medial), fragment involving the acetabulum or in cases of expected sciatic entrapment, internal fixation of ischial fracture is indicated [100]. Ischium is surgically approached through a caudal incision to the hip, wherein the retraction of biceps femoris and tenotomy of internal obturator and gemellus can expose the ischium. Internal fixation can be achieved by use of IM pins, wires, or small plate and screws. Placement of a single IM pin in the ischial shaft normally provides stable fixation. Pubic fractures, if necessary, are accessed through a ventral midline incision directly over the symphysis carefully dissecting the adductor and gracilis muscles.

Orthopedic wire fixation in the form of an interrupted loop is sufficient for stability.

### 3.8.3 Postoperative Care and Complications

Possible complications of pelvic fracture fixation include sciatic nerve damage, difficulty in urination (due to entrapment of urethra), and chronic constipation and difficulty in parturition (due to development of large scar or callus in the pelvic canal), apart from fixation failure, infection, non-healing of fracture, and narrowing of pelvic canal. In acetabular fractures, degenerative arthritis leading to chronic pain, lameness, and limb deformity may occur.

## 3.9 Fractures of Spine

Fractures or luxations of the spine occur when dogs and cats are met with road traffic accidents or suffer other major trauma such as a fall or jump from a height. Spinal fractures are often associated with varying degrees of spinal cord injury. Although many animals may be paralyzed as a result of the fracture due to nerve injury, they often recover, provided they retain their sensation (ability to feel pain) and are managed appropriately. Some cases may recover after medical treatment, but it is often necessary to stabilize a fractured spine. The treatment and prognosis of spinal fractures and luxations depend on the extent of neurologic injury and presence or absence of nociception [109]; hence, its precise evaluation is essential. The patients preserving pain sensation before treatment generally have better prognosis and functional restoration after medical treatment or surgical fixation [110].

Spinal fractures and luxations can be diagnosed by thorough physical and neurologic examination along with radiographic evaluation. Radiography can assist in detecting the location and type of fracture or luxation and the extent of fragment displacement. Radiographic evaluation, however, may not reveal the full extent of spinal cord trauma; hence, modern imaging techniques like CT scan or MRI can be more useful [109].

In dogs, spinal injuries are commonly recorded in the lumbar region (35–40%), followed by sacrococcygeal (25–30%) and thoracic (20–25%) parts; cervical region is least affected (4–6%). In cats, fractures and luxations are most frequently recorded in sacrococcygeal region (about 40% cases). A typical compression fracture of vertebra causes vertebral body shortening without any displacement of fragments.

In spinal fracture/luxation cases accompanied with neural deficit, it is difficult to determine whether they need surgical intervention or can be better managed conservatively with cage rest or/and external fixation. The choice of treatment is determined by several factors such as the site, nature and extent of the spinal cord injury, and the duration since trauma. In general, patients having only paresis or paralysis (grade I and II) are given conservative medical therapy initially along with strict cage rest and external fixation, if needed. If the condition does not improve or gets worse and if there is definite indication of vertebral instability, surgical fixation can be considered. Surgical treatment is also indicated in paralyzed patients with diminished deep pain perception (grade III) if the vertebral instability is obvious, and there is continuous deterioration in the condition. And in animals with no deep pain sensation and paralysis (grade IV), surgical treatment is not recommended as in such patients, the prognosis is generally poor irrespective of the choice of treatment. In such cases, if there is no progress in neurologic status within a few days of conservative management, euthanasia may be considered.

In patients with spinal cord trauma, the primary objective of treatment should be to stabilize the life-threatening cardiovascular and pulmonary status. This should be followed by measures to stop or minimize further damage to the spinal cord by restricting the animals' movement. Extra attention should be given while moving the patients by employing deep sedation or general anesthesia. Glucocorticoids such as dexamethasone (2 mg/kg two to three times a day) and a hyperosmolar agents such as mannitol (2 g/

kg, i.v.) may be administered initially. The animals in the early phase (3–4 weeks) of spinal trauma should be handled with utmost care, until adequate stability is attained through fibrous union. They should be protected from developing decubital ulcers by providing soft beds and frequent side changes. In patients with urinary dysfunction, urinary bladder should be regularly checked and evacuated manually or by using an indwelling urinary catheter. Broad spectrum antibiotics may be administered to prevent cystitis, and steroid therapy may be gradually withdrawn over a period of 7–10 days.

### 3.9.1 Nonsurgical Stabilization of the Spine

Conservative method of stabilization should be undertaken in fractures/luxations of the spine that are significantly stable with only mild displacement (<1/3 the spinal canal), minimal neurologic deficits (grade I and II), and stable cardiovascular status. In fractures/luxations with firm intrinsic stability, confinement of the animal to a cage can be an effective method of management. The animal should be confined to a small cage having enough space allowing the animal to stand and lie down comfortably with the limbs extended.

Splint and cast application is also employed to stabilize an animal with spinal fracture/luxation. The cast or splint should be adapted as per the fracture location and secured on both sides. In small dogs and cats, contoured splints prepared from either plaster cast or thermoplastic may be used to secure along the dorsum, and in large dogs, aluminum sheet typically shaped as a sloped roof may be used to perfectly fit the animal's back. Adequate padding should be provided for splints and casts to prevent pressure sores. Cast and splint can be secured to the body using an elastic bandage. Splints firmly secured between two points across the injured part can stabilize the area. For immobilizing a fracture at thoracic or lumbar region, a splint spanning from the cranial thorax up to the pelvis is fixed on the dorsum and firmly secured.

Cage rest or/and application of splints and casts is not only useful as a primary treatment option for certain fractures and luxations of the spine, but it is also useful as an adjunct to internal fixation techniques.

### 3.9.2 Surgical Stabilization of the Spine

The objectives of surgical fixation of spinal fractures/luxations are to decompress the spinal cord and to reduce and immobilize the spinal segments [111].

Decompression refers to relieving pressure on the spinal cord by removing the dorsal or lateral components of the vertebral arch. The commonly used decompression techniques are hemilaminectomy and dorsal laminectomy, as used in cases of intervertebral disc prolapsed [112, 113]. The choice of technique may depend on the extent of fracture, the neurological signs and the proposed method of spinal fixation. In general, hemilaminectomy is less destabilizing but allows only limited visualization of injured spinal cord than dorsal laminectomy; however, hemilaminectomy preserves the dorsal spinous processes for subsequent spinal fixation.

The technique used for surgical fixation of the spine varies with the anatomical site of injury. As thoraco-lumbar spine is most prone to fracture and luxations in canines, the surgical techniques commonly employed at this site is described below.

### 3.9.3 Thoracic and Lumbar Fracture/Luxations

#### 3.9.3.1 Hemilaminectomy

For hemilaminectomy, the thoracolumbar spine can be approached through a dorsolateral or a lateral approach; however, the exposure is better with dorsolateral access. Through a skin incision just over the site of injury, the muscle is dissected down to reach the transverse processes of the vertebrae. By taking transverse process of L1 and the 13th rib as guide, the site of suspected

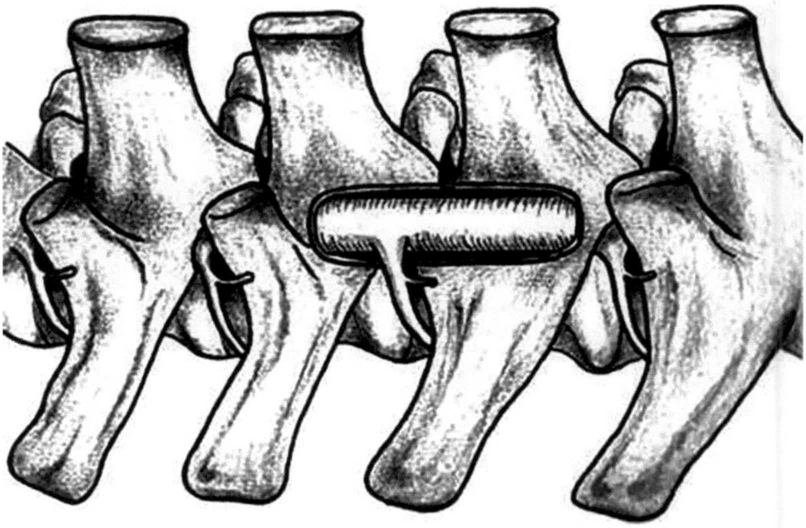

**Fig. 3.76** Schematic presentation of hemilaminectomy

fracture/luxation or intervertebral disc protrusion is identified. After ascertaining the involved vertebrae, the articular processes are removed using a bone drill or a rongeur (Fig. 3.76). The intervertebral space can be increased by gently elevating the dorsal spinous process of the vertebra just cranial to the affected site using a Backhaus towel clamp. The exposure to the spinal cord can be further increased by widening the space using a Lampert rongeur. Alternatively, a Michele trephine can be used to remove a circular core of the lateral lamina and expose the spinal cord. This technique is effectively used in small dogs and cats. In large dogs, hemilaminectomy can be performed using a surgical drill.

The length of hemilaminectomy should extend one vertebral length cranial and caudal to the injured site, or at least till the normal appearance of the cord, and ventrally, it should stretch up to the floor of the spinal canal. After making the bony defect, the thin stiff endosteal layer is pierced carefully using a dural hook to enter the spinal canal. The necrotic tissue often seen at the site of injury, along with epidural fat and extruded disc material if any, is removed from the site. Using a probe, the spinal cord is carefully freed from any adhesion with the surrounding tissues. Often, it becomes difficult to detach the tightly adhered necrotic tissue or disc material from the cord resulting in hemorrhage, which may be controlled by applying digital pressure or using an absorbable gelatin sponge. The bilateral hemilaminectomy can be performed if greater exposure of the spinal canal is necessary. Flushing with saline solution can help to remove most of the tissue debris. Once the spinal canal is free of all the tissue debris and complete hemostasis is achieved, a layer of sublumbar fat or

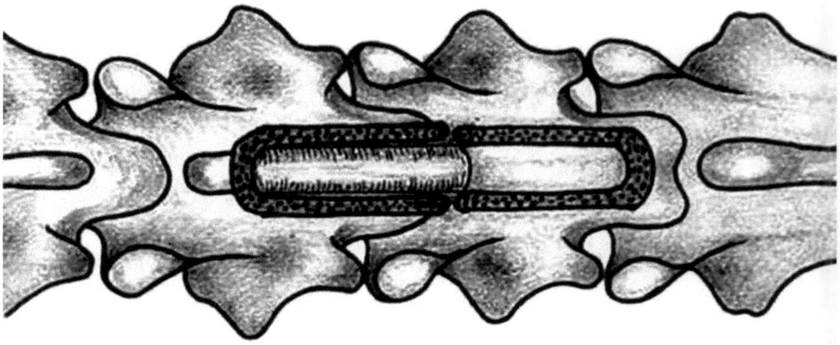

**Fig. 3.77** Schematic presentation of dorsal laminectomy

gelatin sponge is placed over the exposed spinal cord for protection, before closing the incision.

The main advantage of hemilaminectomy is that the spinal cord and nerve roots can be clearly visualized, and the tissue debris can be easily removed from the spinal canal. However, it requires more muscle dissection, and there is need for protecting the nerve roots and vessels while dissecting. With hemilaminectomy, it is also difficult to expose the thoracic vertebrae.

#### 3.9.3.2 Dorsal Laminectomy

The surgical preparation for dorsal laminectomy is identical to hemilaminectomy. By positioning the patient in sternal recumbency, a dorsal midline skin incision is made extending between two vertebrae cranial and caudal to the injured site. Using retractors (Gelpi retractor), the thoracolumbar muscles are retracted on either sides of the vertebrae to reach up to the base of transverse processes. The dorsal spinal processes of involved vertebrae along with one cranial and one caudal vertebra are then cut and removed using bone rongeurs (Fig. 3.77). As the dorsal laminae are very thin, they can also be removed easily using a surgical drill. The laminectomy and decompression are continued on both sides till the detection of normal epidural fat. During the process of cutting and removal of spinous processes, one should be careful not to exert undue pressure on the vertebral bodies and incite further damage.

Following a dorsal laminectomy, complications such as compression of spinal cord due to scarring and disfiguration of the dorsum at the surgical site can develop. To prevent these problems, 20–22 G orthopedic wire can be used to secure the injured site by looping around the dorsal spinous processes of cranial and caudal vertebrae. The wire loop can be applied in a figure of eight manner and slightly tightened to provide support at the site of instability. Alternatively, two K-wires of suitable size can also be placed on either sides of the vertebrae and secured to the transverse processes cranial and caudal to the injury using orthopedic wire. Subsequently, the thoracolumbar muscles, fascia, and the skin are sutured over the wire. In cases of fracture/luxation of vertebrae, any of the surgical fixation technique can be used to fix the site of instability. Selective regional spinal cord hypothermia can be used along with dorsal laminectomy procedure to achieve better results by applying cold lactated Ringer's solution directly over the spinal cord tissue, especially in acute spinal cord trauma cases.

The advantage of dorsal laminectomy is adequate visualization and decompression of the spinal cord, but it requires considerable muscle dissection. It also allows fenestration of discs is required, but it may lead to further muscle damage. It is difficult to remove the debris and the extruded disc material from the floor of the spinal canal, which requires additional manipulation of the spinal cord.

### 3.9.4 Reduction and Surgical Fixation

Many surgical techniques have been described to immobilize the fractures/luxations in the thoracolumbar spine, including plating of vertebral bodies or dorsal spinous processes, combination of pin and polymethylmethacrylate (PMMA) fixation, cross-pinning, stapling, transilial pinning, etc. [110, 114–116]. The selection of technique depends on the type and extent of spinal structures involved. The spinal injuries can involve the dorsal structures (the neural arch, processes and ligaments), the ventral structures (the vertebral bodies and discs), or both the dorsal and ventral components. The loss of dorsal stabilizing structures is treated by the application of fixation dorsally, and injury and loss of ventral stabilizing element involving vertebral body may be managed by vertebral body plating. Damage and collapse of both dorsal and ventral parts may result in extreme instability causing angular, rotational, and translational displacements, often leading to intense narrowing of the spinal canal and compression of spinal cord. In such cases, surgical fixation of both dorsal lamina/spines and ventrally the vertebral bodies is indicated.

#### 3.9.4.1 Spinal Process Fixation

Fixation of spinal process by plate and screws/bolts is probably the earliest method used for

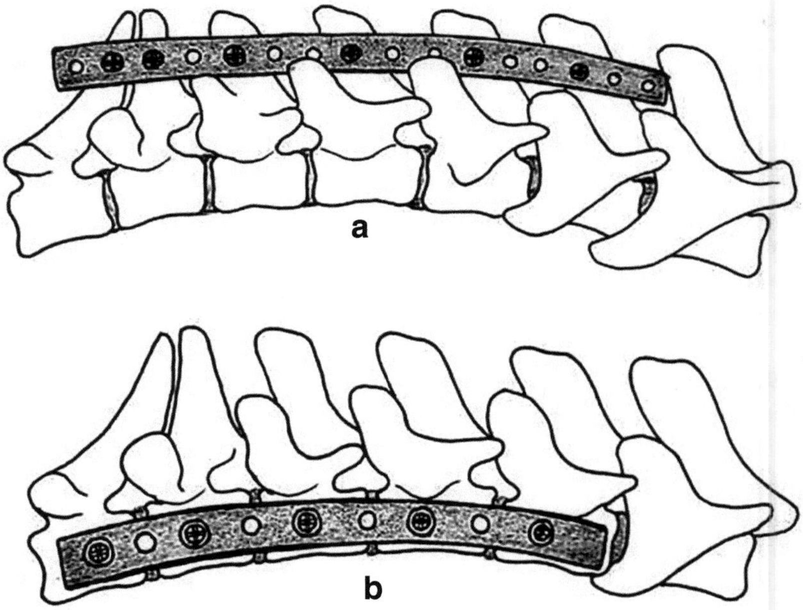


**Fig. 3.78** Schematic presentation of spinal plating: (**a**) plating of spinal processes, (**b**) vertebral body plating

spinal stabilization (Fig. 3.78). Plates are generally applied in pairs on either side of spinal processes (unilateral fixation of a single plate to the dorsal spinous processes does not provide adequate stability), extending at least two to three vertebrae beyond the site of fracture/luxation. The standard surgical approach includes a skin incision on the dorsal lumbar region and bilateral parallel deep incisions through the deep fascia on both sides of the midline. The muscles attached to the dorsal spines (multifidus, interspinalis, and longissimus muscles) are carefully separated up to the point of the articular facets, taking care to preserve the attachments of the muscles to the articular processes. The dorsal lamina may be grooved with a drill or rongeur to ensure optimum plate-to-bone contact and to allow placing of plates near the base of the spines. Either metal or plastic plates may be used for spinal fixation. Metal plates are tightly secured by fastening bolts through predrilled holes in the spinous processes. Care should be taken to select proper size bolts (if long, extra length should be trimmed) and not to use excessive force while tightening the bolts (to prevent fracture or crushing of the spine). On the other hand, plastic plates are fixed by placing the friction-grip surface facing the spine and tightening the bolts inserted between the spinous processes until the paired plates come in firm contact. This also allows better plate-to-bone contact with least chance of spinous process fractures and loosening of screws. Once the adjacent vertebrae are reduced and stabilized adequately, fracture segments may be secured to the plate using fixation of orthopedic wires (18–20 G). The fascia and subcutaneous tissue are sutured to cover the plate, and the skin is closed in routine manner. Post-plate stabilization, it is advised to protect the injured spine by providing ancillary fixation in the form of splint or cast for 3–4 weeks.

Stabilization of spinal processes can also be done using spinal stapling. In this technique, a small diameter pin (K-wire) is secured to the dorsal spines by orthopedic wire suturing. The surgical approach is similar to plating of spinous processes. A small hole is drilled at the base of the dorsal spinal processes of two to three vertebrae on either side of the site of instability. A small diameter (1.2–2.0 mm) stainless steel pin bent on either ends is fixed through the most cranial and caudal holes. The pin is then secured to the intervening dorsal spinous processes using 22–24 G orthopedic wire sutures. Alternatively, two pins can be used on either side of the midline (or a U-shaped pin that runs bilaterally) and are

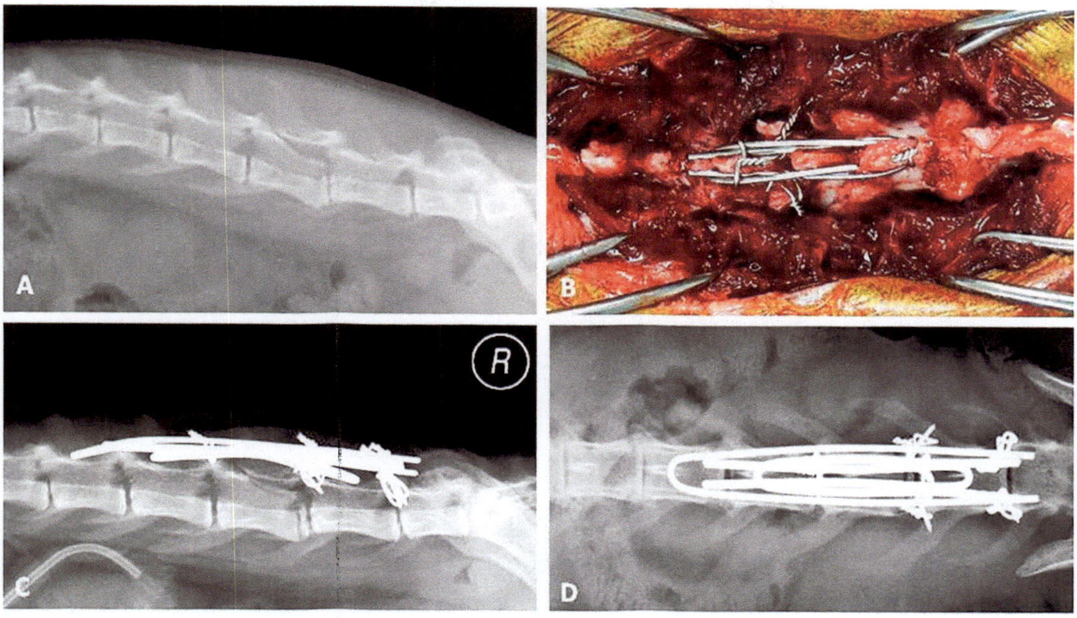


**Fig. 3.79** Lateral radiograph showing fracture–luxation of L5-L6 in a cat (**a**), tension band stabilization (**b**), lateral (**c**) and ventrodorsal (**d**) radiographs showing adequate stabilization (Courtesy: Dr. S Ayyappan, Madras Veterinary College, Chennai, Tamil Nadu, India)

secured to the intervening spinous processes by orthopedic wiring (Figs. 3.79 and 3.80). The fascia, subcutaneous tissue, and skin over the dorsum are closed routinely. An external support by applying splint or cast is indicated for 2–3 weeks. This technique can provide stable fixation of spinal instability in small dogs and cats.

#### 3.9.4.2 Vertebral Body Fixation

Vertebral body fixation is easier and can provide more stable fixation than spinous process fixation due to the availability of sufficient bone tissue for purchase of screws or pins, and hence, the accompanying complications are also relatively less. Although several techniques of vertebral body fixation have been described, only cross pinning, dorsolateral plating, and a combination of pin and PMMA fixation are commonly used in routine clinical practice.

***Vertebral Body Cross-Pinning***: In this technique, the injured spine is immobilized by using small stainless steel pins inserted into the vertebral bodies across the site of instability. The site of injury is approached through a dorsolateral incision made on the dorsum. The muscular attachments along the dorsal processes are bluntly dissected and laterally retracted to reach up to the level of transverse processes/rib heads, while taking care not to damage the spinal nerves and vessels while dissecting deep. In case of spinal cord compression, hemilaminectomy may be executed as described before.

Proper diameter pin is selected based on the weight of the patients. Generally, 0.5–1.0 mm diameter pins are adequate for animals weighing up to 15 kg. In larger dogs, 1–2 mm pins may be needed. The placement of pins is determined by the nature of injury. Injuries at or near the intervertebral space are stabilized by crossing two pins diagonally through the vertebral bodies cranial and caudal to the site of instability. In vertebral body fractures, pins are placed spanning three vertebral bodies, including the injured vertebra and the adjacent two vertebrae on either sides. One pin is inserted through the vertebra just cranial to the injured vertebra and pushed caudally, and another pin is directed from the caudal vertebra cranially. In both cases, the pins are inserted

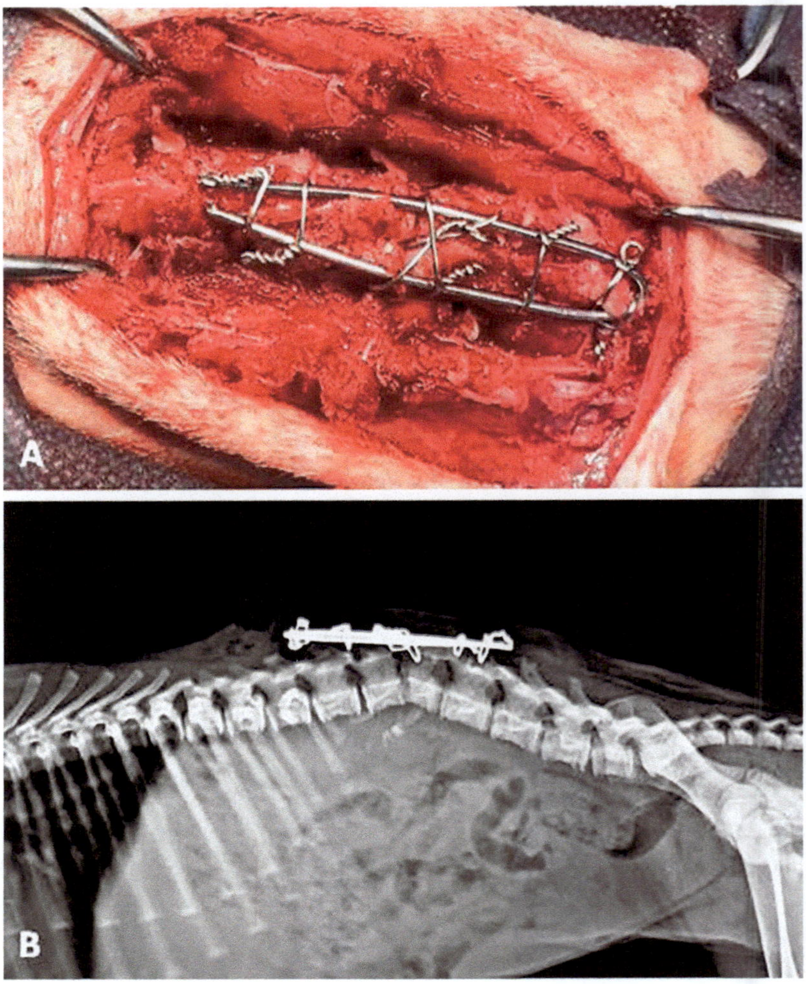


**Fig. 3.80** Modified tension band wiring technique for stabilization of L2-L3 fracture luxation in a pup; gross photograph (**a**) and radiograph made soon after fixation (**b**) Courtesy: Dr. S Ayyappan, Madras Veterinary College, Chennai, Tamil Nadu, India)

from the middle of the vertebral body (just dorsal to the lateral process in lumbar vertebra, and dorsal aspect of the rib in thoracic vertebra) inclined diagonally and ventrally (to avert damaging the venous sinuses) across the site of instability. Extra length of pins is then cut close to the body of vertebrae. The surgical incision is closed routinely. Externally, splint application is advised for 3–4 weeks to protect the injured site.

The application of cross pinning in thoracic region is difficult due to the presence of ribs. While placing the pins, the vital structures beneath the spinal column such as aorta, vena cava, and lungs should be well protected. The cross pins are good in resisting the shear force and translational movement, but not suitable to restrict the angular deformities of the spine. Additional support in the form of external fixation can resist bending and provide sufficient spinal stability. However, the technique is not advocated for treating comminuted fractures of vertebral body, which can crumble.

***Vertebral Body Plates:*** For plating of vertebral body, similar surgical approach used for cross pinning is used barring a relatively long incision and deep muscle dissection to precisely visualize the transverse processes of the lumbar vertebrae or the costovertebral junctions of the thoracic spine. Extreme care should be taken to isolate and protect the vital nerve roots and spinal vessels emanating from the intervertebral foramens. A hemilaminectomy may be performed if needed.

In the lumbar region, the plate can be easily and precisely applied on the dorsolateral surface

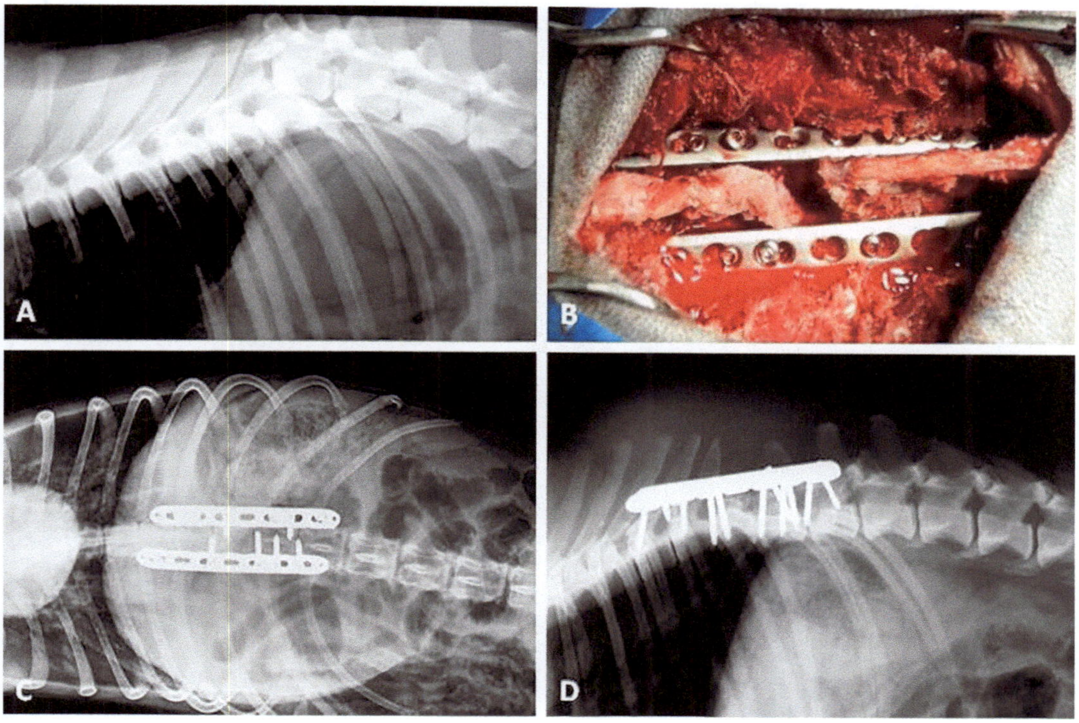


**Fig. 3.81** Lateral Radiograph demonstrating a T1-T12 fracture-luxation in a dog (**a**), stabilized bilaterally with 8-hole 3.5 mm LCPs (**b**), ventrodorsal (**c**) and lateral (**d**) radiographs made on 30th postoperative day shows implant stability and callus formation Courtesy: Dr. S Ayyappan, Madras Veterinary College, Chennai, Tamil Nadu, India)

of the vertebral bodies without much difficulty. Whereas in thoracic region, due to the interference from the rib heads, vertebral body plating is more difficult. It is required to retract the ribs ventrally, often by cutting the rib heads using a rongeur or bone cutter. Subsequent to bone plating, the ribs can be secured firmly to the dorsal processes of the spine by fastening orthopedic wires inserted through predrilled holes in the rib heads.

A suitable plate with correct size and length is selected depending on the patient's size and length of the spinal defect. Primarily, the principles of plate and screw fixation in thoracolumbar spine are the same as practiced in long bone fractures. Ideally, two screws should be fixed in each vertebral body engaging four cortices, occasionally involving more than two vertebral segments. The screws are drilled on the dorsolateral surface of the vertebral body, directed perpendicular to the spinal axis and a little ventrally so as to exit the opposite cortex on the ventrolateral surface. Alternatively, double plates can be fixed bilaterally (Figs. 3.81 and 3.82). If structural deficit is evident, bone grafting can be done. Plate and screw fixation provides excellent stability against angular, rotational, and translational movements.

The stability of vertebral body plating is determined by the region of vertebral column. It is difficult to expose the vertebral bodies in the cranial thoracic area; hence, plating should be avoided in this region. The major advantage of plate fixation is its resistance against compression force transmitted along the axis of spine; hence, it is the method of choice for fixation of fractures/luxations with collapse and shortening of vertebral body.

***Pin-PMMA Composite Fixation:*** It is the method of spinal stabilization wherein the pins

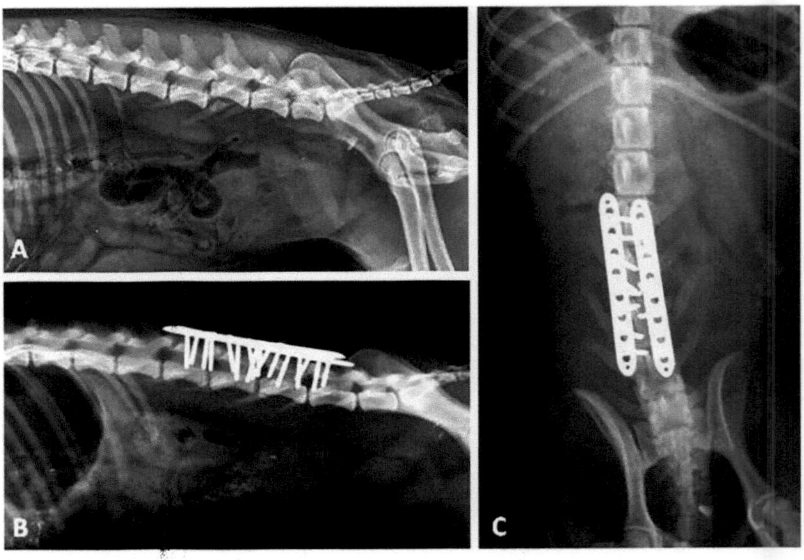


**Fig. 3.82** Lateral radiography demonstrating a fracture-luxation between L4 and L5 vertebrae in a dog (**a**), lateral (**b**) and ventrodorsal (**c**) radiographs show stabilization of fracture-luxation using 8-hole 2.7 mm locking compression plates applied bilaterally Courtesy: Dr. S Ayyappan, Madras Veterinary College, Chennai, Tamil Nadu, India)

passed through the vertebral bodies are connected to an interconnecting frame of polymethylmethacrylate (PMMA). It overcomes some of the constraints of vertebral body plating (difficulty in fixing in thoracic area) and cross pinning (difficulty in pin placement). It is easy to apply and can be adapted to any location. The injured site is first accessed through a standard dorsal approach. In cases of spinal compression, dorsal laminectomy can be performed. The fixation technique involves angular placement of two bilateral pins on the dorsolateral surface by securing them into the cranial and caudal vertebral bodies (similar to cross pinning), spanning the site of instability. Pins can also be fixed by crossing through the spinal processes (Fig. 3.83). The site of injury is adequately exposed, and the fracture/luxation is reduced and aligned. The spinal cord is carefully protected by covering with gauze soaked in saline. The PMMA is mixed (for 4–5 min) and allowed to harden (10–12 min), and while in dough stage, it is molded into the shape of a long cylinder of 1–1.5 cm diameter and laid along the site of instability incorporating the pins. PMMA mold is further contoured to the shape of the spinal column by incorporating the articular processes. Care is taken to prevent thermal damage and necrosis of the surrounding tissues from exothermic reaction during the process of polymerization of PMMA by irrigating with cold normal solution. The surgical incision is then closed in routine manner.

The stability provided by pin-PMMA composite fixation is comparable with plating of dorsal processes with additional rotational stability. It, however, neither provides as rigid fixation as vertebral body plating nor withstands large compressive forces in cases with structural deficits/loss in the vertebral bodies.

### 3.9.5 Lumbosacral Fractures

In small animal, fractures and luxations of the lumbosacral region of vertebral column are more often observed, mostly due to direct trauma such as road traffic accidents. The most common luxation is the cranio-ventral displacement of caudal sacral segment with respect to the cranial lumbar segment. Injuries in this location frequently lead to gross displacement of segments; however, neurological deficit is least, and such animals commonly respond well to conservative management.

The common surgical technique used to restrict the cranio-ventral displacement in lumbosacral fracture/luxation is trans-ilial pinning [117]. In this technique, the caudal aspect of the last (seventh) lumbar vertebra (including spinous processes and articular facets) and cranial part of the sacrum (including medial crest, and cranial

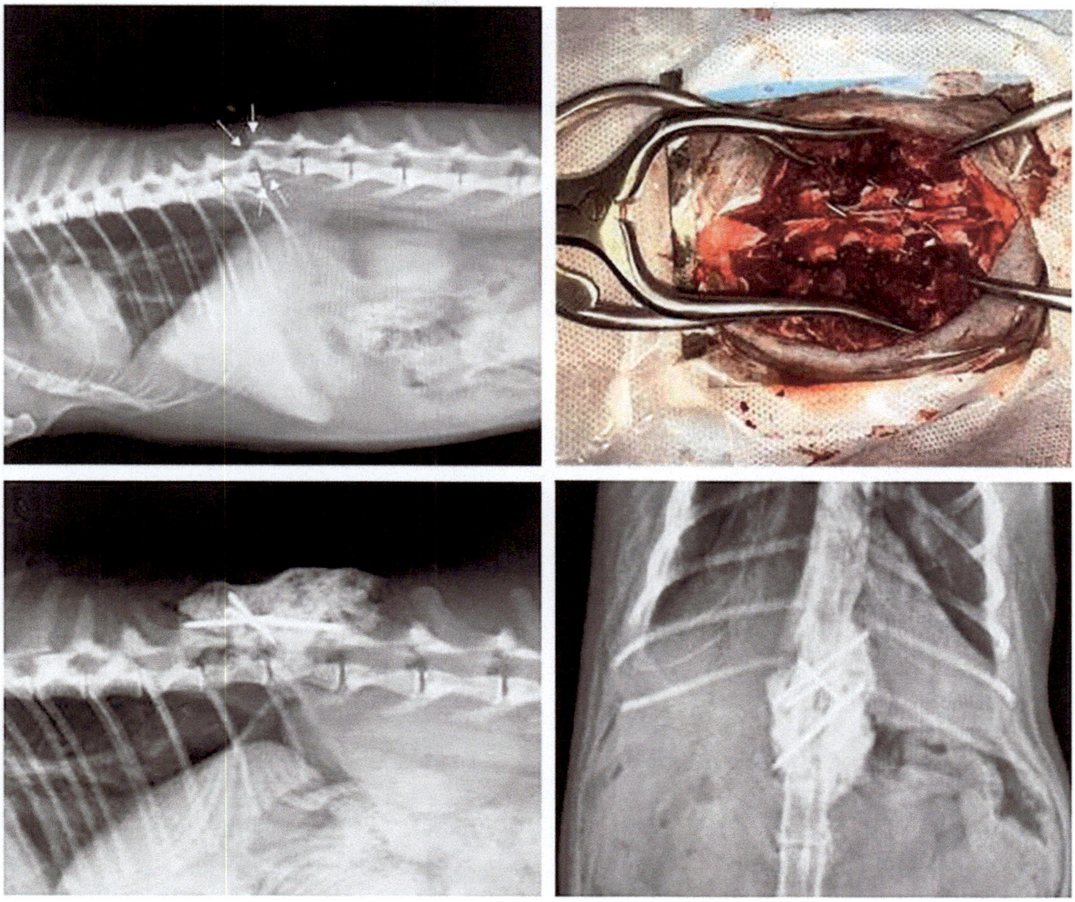

**Fig. 3.83** Spinal stabilization with the pins crossed through the spinal processes across the site of instability and fixed using polymethylmethacrylate (Courtesy: Dr. Drona Patil, Mumbai, India)

articular process and facet) are surgically exposed. The displaced segments are reduced by applying traction along the cranial and caudal vertebral column and lifting the sacrum to its natural position. A trans-ilial pin is then fixed (fixing both wings of the ilium) by directing the pin laterally through the gluteal muscle and above the caudal lamina of L7. This technique can provide adequate reduction and prevent cranioventral displacement of the sacral segment, usually resulting in favorable outcome. The movement of pin can be prevented if threaded pin is used along with nuts.

Use of plate and screw fixation in the lumbosacral region is limited by the small dorsal processes of the sacrum. Combination of spinal plating (steel or plastic plate) with trans-ilial pinning for lumbosacral fracture/luxation has been reported recently. In large dogs, the plate can be fixed directly to the sacrum with long screws passed through the medial sacral crest.

## Chapter 3: Sample Questions

### Q. No. 1: Mark the correct answer

1. Which of the following is not true with respect to radius-ulna fractures.
   (a) common causes are falls or traffic accidents (b) mostly located at middle and proximal third (c) transverse and short oblique

fractures are common (d) both radius and ulna are frequently fractured

2. Monteggia's fracture refers to.
   (a) fracture-dislocation of carpal joint (b) dislocation of the head of the radius with fracture of the upper one-third of the shaft of the ulna (c) fracture of upper third of radius along with dislocation of head of radius (d) dislocation of olecranon process of ulna along with fracture of upper third of radius
3. Severely comminuted femoral diaphyseal fractures can be effectively treated using.
   (a) intramedullary pin (b) external skeletal fixation (c) interlocking nail (d) K-nail
4. Orthopedic wiring can be used for the internal fixation of mandibular fractures as.
   (a) cerclage wire (b) interdental wire (c) tension band wire (d) all the above
5. Spinal fractures/luxations in the dog occur most frequently at.
   (a) cervical region (b) thoracic region (c) lumbar region (d) sacrococcygeal region

**Q. No. 2: State true or false**

1. Complete fractures of humerus and femur are difficult to reduce by close method.
2. Medial condylar fracture of humerus is more common than that of lateral condyle.
3. Intramedullary pinning is usually not indicated in radius.
4. Most of the femoral diaphyseal fractures are amenable to intramedullary pin fixation.
5. During retrograde pinning in femur, the proximal bone segment is held in abducted, flexed, and externally rotated position to avoid injury to the sciatic nerve.
6. Distal femoral fractures are more frequent in young animals aged less than 1 year.
7. Interlocking nail is not indicated for supracondylar fractures in immature animals.
8. It is usually difficult to align the fractured mandibular segments by IM pinning.
9. Pelvis surrounded by a significant muscle mass provides a good biological environment for fracture healing.
10. Fractures in the weight-bearing bones of pelvis generally require surgical repair, whereas most ischial and pubic fractures with minimal pelvic canal narrowing can be managed conservatively.
11. Animals with spinal fracture having no deep pain sensation and paralysis (grade IV) are best subjects for surgical treatment.
12. Hemilaminectomy is less destabilizing and allow wide visualization of the spinal cord as compared to dorsal laminectomy.
13. Semirigid plastic plates allow interspinous fixation of bolts and provide better plate-bone contact, thus reducing the chance of spinous process fractures and screw pull-out from the bone.

**Q. No. 3: Fill up the blanks**

1. The dogs with humerus fracture generally exhibit characteristic sign of ____________ ____________.
2. Surgical approach to the shaft of humerus should be made carefully to protect the ____________________ nerve, which courses along the superficial surface of the ____________________________ muscle.
3. The bone plate is usually applied on the ______________________ surface of radius, so that it can also immobilize the ulna.
4. ________________________ bone is more often fractured than other long bones, and ____________________________ part of the bone is commonly affected.
5. Femur bone is surgically accessed through a standard ________________________ approach, incising the ________________ _____ and by retracting the muscles, ________________________________ and ________________________________.
6. In femur, normograde IM pin fixation can be done from the distal end by inserting it through the ______________________ _____, just cranial to the origin of ________________________________ _.
7. In tibia, intramedullary pinning is always done by ____________________________ __ method to avoid damage to the stifle joint.

8. In tibia, plate and screw fixation is commonly fixed on the _________________________ ______ surface of the bone.
9. The most common location for mandibular fractures in dogs is the ___________________________ region and in cats the _________________________ area.
10. Bone plating in mandibular fractures is done by placing the screws monocortically to _______________________________.
11. Most common complication with mandibular fracture repair is ________________________ __________.
12. The technique of inserting small IM pins into the vertebral bodies, across the site of instability to achieve spinal stabilization is called ___________________________________________.

**Q. No. 4: Write short note on the following**

1. Repair of supracondylar femur fractures
2. Surgical approach to distal humerus
3. Stabilization of distal tibial fractures
4. Hemilaminectomy
5. Orthopedic wiring for mandibular fracture stabilization

## References


1. Cook, J.L., C.R. Cook, J.L. Tomlinson, D.L. Millis, M. Starost, M.A. Albrecht, and J.T. Payne. 1997. Scapular fractures in dogs: epidemiology, classification, and concurrent injuries in 105 cases (1988-1994). *Journal of the American Animal Hospital Association* 33: 528–532.
2. Newton, C.D. 1985. Fractures of the scapula. In *Textbook of small animal orthopaedics*, ed. C.D. Newton and D.M. Nunamaker, 1st ed., 333–342. Philadelphia: J.B. Lippincott.
3. Perry, K.L., and S. Woods. 2017. Fractures of the scapula. *Companion Animals* 22 (6): 340. https://doi.org/10.12968/coan.2017.22.6.340.
4. Piermattei, D.L., and R.G. Greeley. 1980. *An atlas of surgical approaches to the bone of the dogs and cat*. 2nd ed. Philadelphia: W.B. Saunders.
5. Aithal, H.P., G.R. Singh, and G.S. Bisht. 1999. Fractures in dogs: A survey of 402 cases. *Indian Journal of Veterinary Surgery* 20: 15–21.
6. Nunamaker, D.M. 1985. Fractures of the humerus. In *Textbook of small animal orthopaedics*, ed. C.D. Newton and D.M. Nunamaker, 1st ed., 357–363. Philadelphia: J.B. Lippincott.
7. Bardet, J.F., R.B. Hohn, R.L. Rudy, and M.L. Olmstead. 1983. Fractures of humerus in dogs and cats: a retrospective study of 130 cases. *Veterinary Surgery* 12: 73–77.
8. Simpson, A.M. 2004. Fractures of the humerus. *Clinical Techniques in Small Animal Practice* 19: 120–127.
9. Yardimci, C., T. Önyay, K.S. İnal, B.D. Özbakir, and A. Özak. 2018. Management of humeral fractures in dogs by using semicircular external fixator and intramedullary pin tie-in combination. *Kafkas Universitesi Veteriner Fakultesi Dergisi* 24: 295–300.
10. Ness, M.G. 2009. Repair of Y-T humeral fractures in the dog using paired 'string of pearls' locking plates. *Veterinary and Comparative Orthopaedics and Traumatology* 22: 292–297.
11. Kirkby, K.A., D.D. Lewis, M.P. Lafuente, R.M. Radasch, N. Fitzpatrick, J.P. Farese, J.L. Wheeler, and J.A. Hernandez. 2008. Management of humeral and femoral fractures in dogs and cats with linear- circular hybrid external skeletal fixators. *Journal of the American Animal Hospital Association* 44: 180–197.
12. Longley, M., D. Chase, I. Calvo, J. Hall, S.J. Langley-Hobbs, and M. Farrell. 2018. A comparison of fixation methods for supracondylar and distal humeral shaft fractures of the dog and cat. *The Canadian Veterinary Journal* 59: 1299–1304.
13. Aithal, H.P., and G.R. Singh. 1999. Pattern of bone fractures caused by road traffic accidents and falls in dogs: A retrospective study. *The Indian Journal of Animal Sciences* 69: 960–961.
14. Lappin, M.R., D.N. Aron, H.L. Herron, and G. Manati. 1983. Fractures of the radius and ulna in the dog. *Journal of the American Animal Hospital Association* 189: 643–650.
15. Welch, J.A., R.J. Boudrieau, L.M. Dejardin, and G.J. Spodnick. 1997. The intraosseous blood supply of the canine radius: implications for healing of distal fractures in small dogs. *Veterinary Surgery* 26 (1): 57–61.
16. Tyagi, S.P., I.V. Mogha, G.R. Singh, H.P. Aithal, and Amarpal. 2002. Management of olecranon fracture using different internal fixation techniques in dog. *Indian Journal of Veterinary Surgery* 23: 16–18.
17. Nunamaker, D.M. 1985a. Fractures and dislocations of the elbow. In *Textbook of small animal orthopaedics*, ed. C.D. Newton and D.M. Nunamaker, 1st ed., 365–372. Philadelphia: JB Lippincott.
18. Frost, R.C. 1965. The closed reduction and repair of radio-ulna fractures in the dog. *The Journal of Small Animal Practice* 6: 197.
19. Howard, P.E. 1991. Principles of intramedullary pin and wire fixation. *Seminars in Veterinary Medicine and Surgery (Small Animal)* 6: 52–67.

20. Nunamaker, D.M. 1985b. Fractures of the radius and ulna. In *Textbook of small animal orthopaedics*, ed. C.D. Newton and D.M. Nunamaker, 1st ed., 373–379. Philadelphia: JB Lippincott.
21. Gibert, S., G.R. Ragetly, and R.J. Boudrieau. 2015. Locking compression plate stabilization of 20 distal radial and ulnar fractures in toy and miniature breed dogs. *Veterinary and Comparative Orthopaedics and Traumatology* 28 (06): 441–447.
22. Piermattei, D.L., and G.L. Flo. 1997. Fractures of the radius and ulna. In *Handbook of small animal orthopaedics and fracture repair*, 3rd ed., 321–343. Philadelphia: Saunders.
23. Ramírez, J.M., and C. Macías. 2016. Conventional bone plate fixation of distal radius and ulna fractures in toy breed dogs. *Australian Veterinary Journal* 94 (3): 76–80.
24. McCartney, W., K. Kiss, and I. Robertson. 2010. Treatment of distal radial/ulnar fractures in 17 toy breed dogs. *The Veterinary Record* 166: 430–432.
25. Piras, L., F. Cappellari, B. Peirone, and A. Ferretti. 2011. Treatment of fractures of the distal radius and ulna in toy breed dogs with circular external skeletal fixation: a retrospective study. *Veterinary and Comparative Orthopaedics and Traumatology* 24 (03): 228–235.
26. Kumar, P., H.P. Aithal, P. Kinjavdekar, Amarpal, A.M. Pawde, K. Pratap, Surbhi, and D.K. Sinha. 2012. Epoxy-pin external skeletal fixation for treatment of open fractures or dislocations in 36 dogs. *Indian Journal of Veterinary Surgery* 33: 128–132.
27. Hamilton, M.H., and S.L. Hobbs. 2005. Use of the AO veterinary mini 'T'-plate for stabilisation of distal radius and ulna fractures in toy breed dogs. *Veterinary and Comparative Orthopaedics and Traumatology* 18 (01): 18–25.
28. Roberts, V.J., and R.L. Meeson. 2022. Feline femoral fracture fixation: what are the options? *Journal of Feline Medicine and Surgery* 24 (5): 442–463.
29. Kumar, K., I.V. Mogha, H.P. Aithal, P. Kinjavdekar, Amarpal, G.R. Singh, A.M. Pawde, and R.B. Kushwaha. 2007. Occurrence and pattern of long bone fractures in growing dogs with normal and osteopenic bones. *Journal of Veterinary Medicine A* 54: 484–490.
30. Nunamaker, D.M. 1985c. Fractures and dislocations of the hip joint. In *Textbook of small animal orthopaedics*, ed. C.D. Newton and D.M. Nunamaker, 1st ed., 403–414. Philadelphia: JB Lippincott.
31. Daly, W.R. 1978. Femoral head and neck fractures in dog and cat: a review of 115 cases. *Journal of Veterinary Surgery* 7: 29–38.
32. Lovric, L., M. Kreszinger, and M. Pecin. 2020. Surgical treatment of canine femoral fractures- A review. *World's Veterinary Journal* 10 (2): 137–145.
33. Martin, R.A., J.L. Milton, P.K. Shires, et al. 1988. Closed reduction and blind pinning of selected fractures and luxations in dogs and cats. *Compendium on Continuing Education for the Practicing Veterinarian* 10: 784–799.
34. Newmann, M.E., and J.L. Milton. 1989. Closed reduction and blind pinning of 29 femoral and tibial fractures in 27 dogs and cats. *Journal of the American Animal Hospital Association* 25: 61–68.
35. Beale, B. 2004. Orthopedic clinical techniques femur fracture repair. *Clinical Techniques in Small Animal Practice* 19 (3): 134–150.
36. DeCamp, C.E. 2015. *Brinker, Piermattei and Flo's handbook of small animal orthopedics and fracture repair*. 5th ed. St. Louis, Missouri: Saunders Elsevier.
37. Dueland, R.T., K.A. Johnson, S.C. Roe, M.H. Engen, and A.S. Lesser. 1999. Interlocking nail treatment of diaphyseal long-bone fractures in dogs. *Journal of the American Veterinary Medical Association* 214: 59–66.
38. Libardoni, R.N., D. Costa, F.B. Menezes, L.G. Cavalli, L.F. Pedrotti, P.R. Kohlrausch, B.W. Minto, and M.A.M. Silva. 2018. Classification, fixation techniques, complications and outcomes of femur fractures in dogs and cats: 61 cases (2015-2016). *Ciência Rural* 48 (6). https://doi.org/10.1590/0103-8478cr20170028.
39. Newton, C.D. 1985b. Fracture of the femur. In *Textbook of small animal orthopaedics*, ed. C.D. Newton and D.M. Nunamaker, 1st ed., 415–431. Philadelphia: JB Lippincott.
40. Roush, J.K. 2005. Management of fractures in small animals. *The Veterinary Clinics of North America. Small Animal Practice* 35: 1137–1154.
41. Sahu, S., Rekha Pathak, M.A. Shah, Santi Jayalekshmi Reetu, G.T. Darshan, Deepti Sharma, H.P. Aithal, Amarpal, P. Kinjavdekar, and A.M. Pawde. 2017. Evaluation of locking compression plate in wedge and complex fractures of long bone in dogs. *Indian Journal of Veterinary Surgery* 38: 81–85.
42. Saravanan, B., S.K. Maiti, M. Hoque, H.P. Aithal, and G.R. Singh. 2002. Management of comminuted femoral fracture by different internal fixation techniques in dogs. *The Indian Journal of Animal Sciences* 72: 1104–1107.
43. DeYoung, D.J., and C.W. Probst. 1985. Methods of fracture fixation. In *Textbook of small animal surgery*, ed. D.H. Slatter, vol. 2, 1949–2014. Philadelphia: PA Saunders.
44. Rudy, R.L. 1975. Principles of intramedullary pinning. *The Veterinary Clinics of North America. Small Animal Practice* 5: 209–228.
45. Chanana, M., Adarsh Kumar, S.P. Tyagi, A.K. Singla, A. Sharma, and U.B. Farooq. 2018. End-threaded intramedullary positive profile screw ended self-tapping pin (admit pin) – A cost-effective novel implant for fixing canine long bone fractures. *Veterinary World* 11 (2): 181–185.
46. Sharma, M., Adarsh Kumar, S.P. Tyagi, and Amit Kumar. 2022. Clinical appraisal of admit pin for

management of femur fractures in canine. *The Indian Journal of Animal Sciences* 92 (5): 560–564.
47. Chaffee, V.W. 1977. Multiple (stacked) intramedullary pin fixation of humeral and femoral fractures. *Journal of the American Animal Hospital Association* 13: 599–601.
48. Arican, M., F. Alkan, S. Altan, K. Parlak, and N. Yavru. 2017. Clinical experience of interlocking nail stabilization of long bone fractures in dogs – a retrospective study of 26 cases. *Isreal J Vet Med* 72: 45–50.
49. Raghunath, M., and S.S. Singh. 2003. Use of static intramedullary interlocking nail for repair of comminuted/segmental femoral diaphyseal fractures in four dogs. *Indian Journal of Veterinary Surgery* 24: 89–91.
50. Wheeler, J.L., W.P. Stubbs, A.R. Cross, and R.B. Parker. 2004. Intramedullary interlocking nail fixation in dogs and cats: clinical applications. *Compendium* 2004: 531–544.
51. Wheeler, J.L., W.P. Stubbs, D.D. Lewis, and A.R. Cross. 2004. Intramedullary interlocking nail fixation in dogs and cats: biomechanics instrumentation. *Compendium on Continuing Education for the Practising Veterinarian -North American* 26: 519–529.
52. Durall, I., C. Falcon, M.C. Diaz-Bertrana, and J. Franch. 2004. Effects of static fixation and Dynamization after interlocking femoral nailing locked with an external fixator: an experimental study in dogs. *Veterinary Surgery* 33: 323–332.
53. Aguila, A.Z., J.M. Manos, A.S. Orlansky, R.J. Todhunter, E.J. Trotter, and M.C.H. Van der Meulen. 2005. In vitro biomechanical comparison of limited contact dynamic compression plate and locking compression plate. *Veterinary and Comparative Orthopaedics and Traumatology* 18: 220–226.
54. Patil, M., and D. Dilipkumar. 2019. Roentgenographic study on DCP, LCP and IILN for femur fracture repair in dogs. *Veterinary Practioner* 20: 227–232.
55. Zhao, X., W. Jing, Z. Yun, X. Tong, Z. Li, J. Yu, Y. Zhang, Y. Zhang, Z. Wang, Y. Wen, H. Cai, J. Wang, B. Ma, and H. Zhao. 2021. An experimental study on stress-shielding effects of locked compression plates in fixing intact dog femur. *Journal of Orthopaedic Surgery and Research* 16: 97. (2021).
56. Kumari, Anita, P. Bishnoi, A.K. Bishnoi, S. Palecha, and Purushottam. 2022. Evaluation of string of pearls (SOP) locking plate system for management of femur fractures in dogs. *Indian Journal of Veterinary Surgery* 2022. (in press): 126.
57. Aithal, H.P., and G.R. Singh. 1998. Evaluation of fixation devices for resistance of bending and rotation in supracondylar femoral fracture fixation in dogs. *The Indian Journal of Animal Sciences* 68: 1121–1125.
58. Aithal, H.P., Singh G.R. Amarpal, P. Kinjavdekar, and M. Hoque. 1999a. Modified pin fixation for distal metaphyseal-epiphyseal fractures of femur in the dog: A review of 7 cases. *The Indian Veterinary Journal* 76: 220–224.
59. Aithal, H.P., G.R. Singh, and Amarpal and Setia, H.C. 1999b. Horn plates in the management of supracondylar femoral fracture in dogs. *The Indian Journal of Animal Sciences* 69: 912–917.
60. Aithal, H.P., G.R. Singh, A.K. Sharma, and Amarpal. 1998. Modified technique of single pin fixation and cross intramedullary pin fixation technique for supracondylar femoral fracture in dogs: a comparative study. *Indian Journal of Veterinary Surgery* 19: 84–89.
61. Lewis, D.D., R.T. Van Ee, M.G. Oakes, and A.D. Elkins. 1993. Use of reconstruction plates for stabilization of fractures and osteotomies involving the supracondylar region of the femur. *Journal of the American Animal Hospital Association* 29: 171–178.
62. Lidbetter, D.A., and R. Glyde. 2000. Supracondylar femoral fractures in adult animals. *Compendium on Continuing Education for the Practicing Veterinarian* 22: 1041–1053.
63. Madhu, D.N., R.A. Ahmad, T.B. Sivanarayanan, R. Kumar, P. Dubey, H.P. Aithal, Amarpal, and P. Kinjavdekar. 2014. Surgical management of supracondylar femoral fracture in dogs. *Indian Journal of Canine Practice* 6: 158–160.
64. Scotti, S., A. Klein, J. Pink, A. Hidalgo, P. Moissonnier, and P. Fayolle. 2007. Retrograde placement of a novel 3.5 mm titanium interlocking nail for supracondylar and diaphyseal femoral fractures in cats. *Veterinary and Comparative Orthopaedics and Traumatology* 20: 211–218.
65. Silveira, F., I.C. Monotti, A.M. Cronin, N.J. Macdonald, S. Rutherford, K. Tiffinger, I. Faux, J. Rincon-Alvarez, E. Kulendra, F. Tavola, B. Santos, and N.J. Burton. 2020. Outcome following surgical stabilization of distal diaphyseal and supracondylar femoral fractures in dogs. *The Canadian Veterinary Journal* 61: 1073–1079.
66. Stigen, O. 1999. Supracondylar femoral fractures in 159 dogs and cats treated using a normograde intramedullary pinning technique. *The Journal of Small Animal Practice* 40: 519–523.
67. Whitney, W.O., and S.C. Schrader. 1987. Dynamic intramedullary crosspinning technique for repair of distal femoral fractures in dogs and cats: 71 cases (1981-1985). *Journal of the American Veterinary Medical Association* 191: 1133–1138.
68. Ahmad, Raja Aijaz, D.N. Madhu, H.P. Aithal, Amarpal, P. Kinjavdekar, and A.M. Pawde. 2018. Use of distal femoral condylar locking plate for management of supracondylar femur fracture in a Saint Bernard. *Indian Journal of Veterinary Surgery* 39: 55–56.
69. Frydman, G.H., L.C. Cuddy, S.E. Kim, and A. Pozzi. 2014. Treatment of bicondylar femoral fractures complicated by concurrent ligament or tendon

injuries in four dogs. *Veterinary and Comparative Orthopaedics and Traumatology* 27: 324–332.
70. Guiot, L.P., R.M. Demianiuk, and L.M. Dejardin. 2012. Fractures of the femur. In *Veterinary surgery: small animal*, ed. K.M. Tobias and S.A. Johnston, 865–905. St. Louis, MO: Saunders.
71. Nunamaker, D.M. 1985d. Fractures of the tibia and fibula. In *Textbook of small animal orthopaedics*, ed. C.D. Newton and D.M. Nunamaker, 1st ed., 439–444. Philadelphia: JB Lippincott.
72. Pettit, G.D., and D.H. Slattet. 1973. Tension-band wires for fixation of an avulsed canine tibial tuberosiry. *Journal of the American Veterinary Medical Association* 164: 242–244.
73. Birchard, S.J., and R.M. Bright. 1981. The tension band wire for fracture repair in the dog. *Compendium on Continuing Education for the Practicing Veterinarian* 3: 37–41.
74. Glyde, M., and R. Arnett. 2006. Tibial fractures in dog and cat: options for management. *Irish Veterinary Journal* 59: 290–295.
75. Duhautois, B. 2003. Use of veterinary interlocking nails for diaphyseal fractures in dogs and cats: 121 cases. *Veterinary Surgery* 32: 8–20.
76. Endo, K., K. Nakamura, H. Maeda, and T. Matsushita. 1998. Interlocking intramedullary nail method for the treatment of femoral and tibial fractures in cats and small dogs. *The Journal of Veterinary Medical Science* 60: 119–122.
77. Haaland, P.J., L. Sjöström, M. Devor, and A. Haug. 2009. Appendicular fracture repair in dogs using the locking compression plate system: 47 cases. *Veterinary and Comparative Orthopaedics and Traumatology* 22: 309–315.
78. Joshi, S., S. Venugopal, S.S. Nair, and N.S. Sunilkumar. 2021. Management of fracture of long bones using string of pearls (SOP) plating technique in dogs. *International of Journal of Science Research* 10: 1086–1091.
79. Alcântara, B.M., B.W. Minto, G.G. Franco, D.V.F. Lucena, and L.G.G.G. Dias. 2021. Bridge plating for simple tibial fractures treated by minimally invasive plate osteosynthesis. *Arq Bras Med Vet Arquivo Brasileiro de Medicina Veterinária e Zootecnia* 73 (03): 589. https://doi.org/10.1590/1678-4162-12261.
80. Baroncelli, A.B., B. Peirone, M.D. Winter, D.J. Reese, and A. Pozzi. 2012. Retrospective comparison between minimally invasive plate osteosynthesis and open plating for tibial fractures in dogs. *Veterinary and Comparative Orthopaedics and Traumatology* 25: 410–417.
81. Cabassu, J. 2019. Minimally invasive plate osteosynthesis using fracture reduction under the plate without intraoperative fluoroscopy to stabilize diaphyseal fractures of the tibia and femur in dogs and cats. *Veterinary and Comparative Orthopaedics and Traumatology* 32: 475–482.
82. Aronsohn, M.G., and R.L. Burk. 2009. Unilateral uniplanar external skeletal fixation for isolated diaphyseal tibial fractures in skeletally immature dogs. *Veterinary Surgery* 38: 654–658.
83. Brinker, W., D. Piermattei, and G. Flo. 1983. *Handbook of small animal orthopedics and fracture treatment*, 110–122. Philadelphia: WB Saunders.
84. Harari, J., B. Seguin, T. Bebchuk, and J. Lincoln. 1996. Closed repair of tibial and radial fractures with external skeletal fixation. *Compendium on Continuing Education for the Practicing Veterinarian* 18: 651–665.
85. Rovesti, G.L., A. Bosio, and D.J. Marcellin-Little. 2007. Management of 49 antebrachial and crural fractures in dogs using circular external fixators. *The Journal of Small Animal Practice* 48: 194–200.
86. Tyagi, S.K., H.P. Aithal, P. Kinjavdekar, Amarpal, A.M. Pawde, and Abhishek Kumar Saxena. 2021. Acrylic and epoxy-pin external skeletal fixation systems for fracture management in dogs. *Indian Journal of Animal Research*: B-4265. https://doi.org/10.18805/IJAR.B-4265.
87. Newton, C.D. 1985c. Fracture and dislocation of metacarpal bones, metacarpophalangeal joints, phalanges, and interphalangeal joints. In *Textbook of small animal orthopaedics*, ed. C.D. Newton and D.M. Nunamaker, 1st ed., 387–381. Philadelphia: J.B. Lippincott.
88. Kornmayer, M., and U. Matis. 2017. Dowel pinning for metacarpal and metatarsal fractures in dogs. *Tierärztliche Praxis. Ausgabe K, Kleintiere/Heimtiere* 45: 154–162.
89. Kornmayer, M., K. Failing, and U. Matis. 2014. Long-term prognosis of metacarpal and metatarsal fractures in dogs. A retrospective analysis of medical histories in 100 re-evaluated patients. *Veterinary and Comparative Orthopaedics and Traumatology* 27: 45–53.
90. Fitzpatrick, N., J.O. Riordan, T.J. Smith, J.H. Modlinska, R. Tucker, and R. Yeadon. 2011. Combined intramedullary and external skeletal fixation of metatarsal and metacarpal fractures in 12 dogs and 19 cats. *Veterinary Surgery* 40: 1015–1022.
91. Basuki, W., J.E. Rawlinson, and R.H. Palmer. 2018. Repair of bilateral comminuted mandibular fractures in a 12-week-old puppy using locking and nonlocking maxillofacial reconstruction plates. *Journal of Veterinary Dentistry* 35 (4). https://doi.org/10.1177/0898756418812818.
92. Bilgili, H., and B. Kurum. 2003. Treatment of fractures of the mandible and maxilla by mini titanium plate fixation systems in dogs and cats. *Australian Veterinary Journal* 81: 671–673.
93. Glyde, M., and D. Lidbetter. 2003. Management of fractures of the mandible in small animals. *In Practice* 25: 570–585.
94. Nunamaker, D.M. 1985e. Fractures and dislocations of the mandible. In *Textbook of small animal*

*orthopaedics*, ed. C.D. Newton and D.M. Nunamaker, 1st ed., 297–305. Philadelphia: JB Lippincott.

95. Owen, M.R., S.J.L. Hobbs, A. Moores, D. Bennett, and S. Carmichael. 2004. Mandibular fracture repair in dogs and cats using epoxy resin and acrylic external skeletal fixation. *Veterinary and Comparative Orthopaedics and Traumatology* 17 (4): 189–197.
96. Oxford, M. 2015. Techniques for intraoral fixation of jaw fractures. Vet Times February 16, 2015. p 21. https://www.vettimes.co.uk
97. Piermattei, D.L., G.L. Flo, and C.E. DeCamp. 2006. Fractures of the pelvis. In *Handbook of small animal orthopaedics and fracture treatment*, 4th ed., 433–460. St. Louis, MO: Saunders Elsevier.
98. DeCamp, C.E. 2005. Fractures of the pelvis. In *AO principles of fracture Management in the dog and cat*, ed. A.L. Johnson, J.E.F. Houlton, and R. Vannini, 161–199. New York: Thieme.
99. Olmstead, M.L. 1998. The pelvis and sacroiliac joint. In *Manual of small animal fracture repair and management*, ed. A. Coughlan and A. Miller, 217–219. Cheltenham: Br. Small Anim. Vet Assoc.
100. Newton, C.D. 1985d. Fractures of the pelvis. In *Textbook of small animal orthopaedics*, ed. C.D. Newton and D.M. Nunamaker, 1st ed., 393–402. Philadelphia: J.B. Lippincott.
101. Bouabdallah, R., F.Z. Meghiref, N. Azzag, C. Benmohand, W. Zenad, and M. Rebouh. 2020. Conservative management of pelvic fractures in dogs and cats in Algiers: incidence and long-term clinical outcomes. *Veterinary World* 13: 2416–2421.
102. Henry, W.B. 1985. A method of bone plating for repairing iliac and acetabular fractures. *Compendium on Continuing Education for the Practicing Veterinarian* 7: 924–938.
103. Lewis, D.D., W.P. Stubbs, L. Neuwirth, S.G. Bertrand, R.B. Parker, J.T. Stallings, and S.T. Murphy. 1997. Results of screw/wire/polymethylmethacrylate composite fixation for acetabular fracture repair in 14 dogs. *Veterinary Surgery* 26: 223–234.
104. Brinker, W.O. 1975. Fractures of the pelvis. In *Current techniques in small animal surgery*, ed. M.J. Bojrab, 414–424. Philadelphia: Lea & Febiger.
105. Déjardin, L.M., D.M. Marturello, L.P. Guiot, L.P. Guillou, and C.E. DeCamp. 2016. Comparison of open reduction versus minimally invasive surgical approaches on screw position in canine sacroiliac lag-screw fixation. *Veterinary and Comparative Orthopaedics and Traumatology* 29: 290–297.
106. Singh, H., M.P. Kowaleski, R.J. McCarthy, and R.J. Boudrieau. 2016. A comparative study of the dorsolateral and ventrolateral approaches for repair of canine sacroiliac luxation. *Veterinary and Comparative Orthopaedics and Traumatology* 29: 53–60.
107. Tonks, C.A., J.L. Tomlinson, and J.L. Cook. 2008. Evaluation of closed reduction and screw fixation in lag fashion of sacroiliac fracture-luxations. *Veterinary Surgery* 37: 603–607.
108. Sadan, M.A., A. Fischer, J. Bokemeyer, and M. Kramer. 2015. Surgical repair of ilial fractures in dogs and cats using string of pearls (SOP) plate. *Indian Journal of Veterinary Surgery* 36: 41–45.
109. Orgonikova, I., J. Brocal, G.B. Cherubini, and V. Palus. 2021a. Vertebral fractures and luxations in dogs and cats, part 1: evaluation of diagnosis and prognosis. *Companion Animals* 26 (2): 1. https://doi.org/10.12968/coan.2020.0027.
110. Bruce, C.W., B.A. Brisson, and K. Gyselinck. 2008. Spinal fracture and luxation in dogs and cats. A retrospective evaluation of 95 cases. *Veterinary and Comparative Orthopaedics and Traumatology* 21: 280–284.
111. Olby, N. 2010. The pathogenesis and treatment of acute spinal cord injuries in dogs. *The Veterinary Clinics of North America. Small Animal Practice* 40: 791–807.
112. Olby, N. 1999. Current concepts in the management of acute spinal cord injury. *Journal of Veterinary Internal Medicine* 13: 399–407.
113. Olby, N., J. Levine, T. Harris, K. Muñana, T. Skeen, and N. Sharp. 2003. Long-term functional outcome of dogs with severe injuries of the thoracolumbar spinal cord: 87 cases (1996-2001). *Journal of the American Veterinary Medical Association* 222 (6): 762–769.
114. Krauss, M.W., L.F.H. Theyse, M.A. Tryfonidou, H.A.W. Hazewinkel, and B.P. Meij. 2012. Treatment of spinal fractures using lubra plates. A retrospective clinical and radiological evaluation of 15 cases. *Veterinary and Comparative Orthopaedics and Traumatology* 25: 326–331.
115. Orgonicova, I., J. Brocal, G.B. Cherubini, and V. Palus. 2021b. Vertebral fractures and luxations in dogs and cats part 2: treatment and surgery options. *Companion Animals* 26 (3): 15–19.
116. Sturges, B.K., A.S. Kapatkin, T.C. Garcia, C. Anwer, S. Fukuda, P.L. Hitchens, T. Wisner, K. Hayashi, and S.M. Stover. 2016. Biomechanical comparison of locking compression plate versus positive profile pins and polymethylmethacrylate for stabilization of the canine lumbar vertebrae. *Veterinary Surgery* 45: 309–318.
117. Dona, F.D., G.D. Valle, B. Lamagna, C. Balestriere, C. Murino, B. Santangelo, F. Lamagna, and G. Fatone. 2016. Percutaneous transilial pinning for treatment of seventh lumbar vertebral body fracture. A retrospective analysis of 17 cases. *Veterinary and Comparative Orthopaedics and Traumatology* 29: 164–169.

# Management of Specific Fractures in Large Animals

# 4

**Learning Objectives**

You will be able to understand the following after reading this chapter:

- Surgical approaches and various techniques of fixation for fractures in long bones such as humerus, radius-ulna, femur, tibia-fibula, metacarpus, metatarsus, and phalanges in large animals
- Principles and techniques of fracture stabilization in mandible and pelvis

**Summary**

- Fracture of the scapula is not common in large animals. However, if recorded, scapular fractures are treated conservatively by stall rest and confinement.
- Fracture of humerus is difficult to reduce due to heavy musculature and fracture configuration. Intramedullary (IM) nail or plate fixation can be used for the repair of diaphyseal fractures with good success, especially in young and light-weight animals. In heavy adult animals, prognosis is guarded, and radial nerve damage caused either due to fracture trauma or during fracture fixation is common.
- The fractures of radius-ulna are most suited for external fixation as bones are fairly straight and surrounded by little soft tissues. For rigid immobilization of radial fractures, internal fixation is advised. Bone plating (either DCP or LCP, double plate in heavy animals) can be used as an ideal internal fixation technique. ESF is indicated in open fractures, and linear systems work well as radius is placed straight.
- Femur fractures are more common in young calves and are relatively uncommon in adult cattle and buffaloes. Femoral diaphyseal fractures can be better treated with open reduction and internal fixation using IM pins/nails or bone plates. Multiple cross IM pin fixation technique can provide stable fixation of distal femoral or supracondylar fractures.
- Fractures of tibia are common in cattle and buffaloes of all age groups. Angular placement of the bone and heavy musculature around the stifle joint make cast application difficult in tibia. Hemi-cerclage wiring is useful to reduce and hold the bone segments in alignment. IM

(continued)


H. P. Aithal et al., *Textbook of Veterinary Orthopaedic Surgery*,
https://doi.org/10.1007/978-981-99-2575-9_4

nail fixed by normograde technique and plate osteosynthesis can provide good immobilization of tibial fractures, but in heavy animals, double bone plate fixation is recommended. Open fractures can be stabilized with circular or hybrid ESF.

- Fractures of metacarpus (MC) and metatarsus (MT) are most common in both equines and bovines. MC and MT bones are placed straight; hence, cast can be easily applied to provide stable fixation. In heavy adult animals, bone plate (DCP or LCP) fixation can provide rigid stabilization of fractures. In open fractures, linear or circular ESF technique can be effective.
- Pelvic fractures usually occur in mature adult animals, and the wing of ilium is the most common site. Due to heavy surrounding musculature, the pelvis is difficult to approach surgically. The prognosis depends on the location of fracture; ilial fractures usually heal well, but the prognosis is generally poor in cases of multiple pelvic fractures.
- Mandibular fractures should not be managed conservatively in cattle. In young calves, bilateral IM pins, cerclage wires, or KE splints can provide good fixation, whereas in adult animals, DCP plating of the ventrolateral aspect of the mandible or type I and II external fixators can provide a stable fixation. The results of surgical fixation are generally acceptable especially with more rostral fractures.

## 4.1 Fractures of Scapula and Humerus

Fracture of the scapula is infrequent in large animals [1], and when occurs, it is usually caused by a vehicular accident or a fall. The animal with scapular fracture shows signs of pain, lameness, and swelling in the shoulder region. Radiography will help confirm the diagnosis.

As scapula is located more proximally close to the body surface, usually, there is less movement and overriding of fractured bone fragments. Generally, scapular fractures are treated conservatively by stall rest and confinement. Application of bandage around the body incorporating the fracture site will provide additional support and reduce fracture site mobility. Scapular fracture generally heals satisfactorily (might be with slight malunion), without adversely affecting the functional usage of limb. Internal fixation of scapular fracture although difficult can be undertaken using either plates, screws, or tension band wires, which may provide better bone alignment leading to early healing and functional recovery.

As humerus is well covered and protected by heavy musculature in large animals, it is not easily predisposed to fracture. However, fracture of humerus may be seen in both young as well as adult ruminants, accounting for about 5–10% of all fractures [2]. More often, humerus fractures are oblique or spiral in nature [3], and condylar/supracondylar fractures are common in young animals [4].

Animals with humerus fracture exhibit cardinal signs of fracture such as lameness, swelling and excessive movements at the fracture, and shortening of the limb, along with characteristic knuckling of fetlock and dropped elbow appearance. The radial nerve, coursing along the musculospiral groove spanning the length of humerus, is likely to get damaged during the fracture of humerus diaphysis, causing the animal to drag the limb in a flexed position. Radiographic examination will help assessing the location and type of fracture and planning treatment.

The treatment of humeral fractures in large animals remains a challenge [5]. Fractures at the proximal end of humerus are very rare. In such cases, external fixation may not be possible because of proximal location of fracture. Conservative treatment with application of coaptation bandage with the body and stall rest may be attempted in heavy adult animals, which may lead to healing with malunion. In young animals, cross pinning may be done. If the proximal fragment is sufficiently long to allow adequate

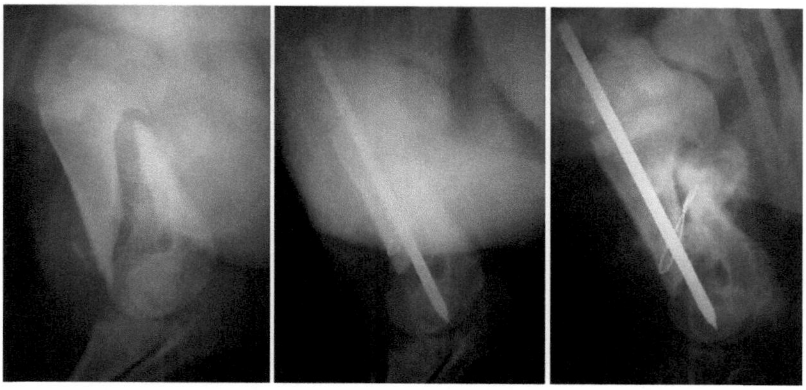

**Fig. 4.1** IM Steinmann pin along with orthopedic wiring for fixation of oblique/spiral fracture of humerus in a calf

purchase of implants, intramedullary pin/interlocking nail may be used to immobilize the fracture.

Diaphyseal fracture of humerus is difficult to reduce due to heavy musculature and fracture configuration. Often, conservative treatment by stall rest can also help to manage humeral diaphyseal fractures [6]. Intramedullary pin fixation has been successful for the repair of humeral fractures [7, 8]. In young animals, single or multiple stack intramedullary pins can be used to immobilize the fracture (Fig. 4.1). Use of hemicerclage/full cerclage wires would help reduce an overriding fracture and temporarily stabilize the bone fragments. K-nail or interlocking nail may also be used for the repair of humeral diaphyseal fractures with good success, especially in young and lightweight animals [9] (Fig. 4.2). Humerus is surgically approached by giving an oblique incision starting at the craniolateral aspect of the shoulder up to the caudolateral aspect of the elbow along the cranial border of the brachialis muscle. The bone is exposed by retracting the brachialis muscle caudally and the brachiocephalicus muscle cranially. The distal third of the humerus is approached by cranial retraction of brachialis and caudal retraction of triceps brachii muscle. While exposing and reducing the bone segments, it is taken care to protect the radial nerve and collateral radial artery by identifying and keeping them away from manipulation. Once the bone is exposed and the fracture segments exteriorized, the medullary cavity of the proximal bone segment is reamed, and a hole is drilled in the proximal bone cortex through which a guide wire is inserted. Along the guide wire, a K-nail or an interlocking nail attached to the jig is introduced in normograde fashion. Once the nail reaches the distal end of proximal fragment, the fracture fragments are reduced by taking help of the nail (the nail exited through the fracture site may be toggled into the distal fragment) and aligned, and then the nail is driven into the distal fragment. In oblique/spiral fractures, hemicerclage wire may be used to reduce and align the bone fragments before nail fixation. Take care not to trap the radial nerve during fracture reduction and fixation. In the interlocking nail, two to four fixation bolts can be fixed in the humerus diaphysis depending on the location and type of fracture. Generally 12–14 mm nail is adequate for humerus in a medium-sized animal. With intramedullary fixation, healing is generally successful in humerus with good callus formation, provided the fragment alignment is maintained. Slight displacement/migration of nail generally does not affect the level of fixation.

Bone plating can also be used for the repair of diaphyseal fracture of humerus in adult cattle [10]. In large ruminants, it is generally difficult to access humerus for plate fixation owing to heavy musculature and attachment of tendons. The radial nerve come across in the surgical area needs to be shielded. This problem can be reduced by approaching the humerus through cranial incision than lateral incision. While lateral fixation of plate is difficult due to the shape of humerus, cranial fixation needs proper contouring of the plate. Broad DCP or LCP (8–10 hole, 4.5/5.5 mm plate) can be used in humerus [8]. In heavy large animals, double plate fixation (cranially and laterally) can be considered to provide

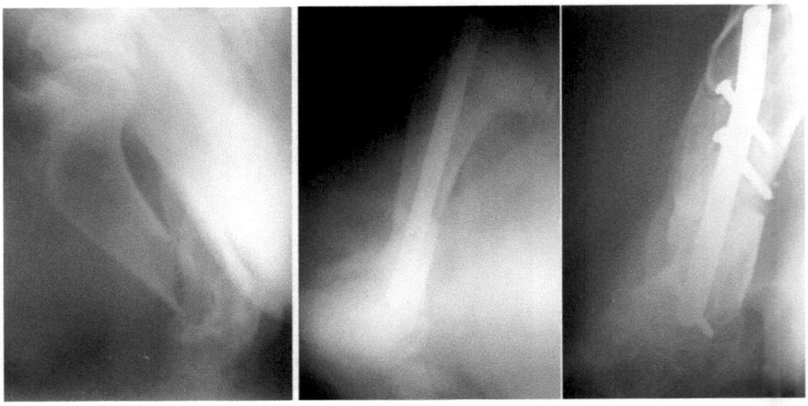

**Fig. 4.2** Interlocking nail fixation for repair of diaphyseal fracture of humerus in a calf

more stable fixation. Often, plate fixation may also fail due to inadequate fixation. However, the use of newly developed LCP may improve the outcome of plate fixation. Clamp rod internal fixation system (CRIF 4.5/5.5 system) has also been used for the repair of humeral diaphyseal fracture in cattle [11]. In young calves, unilateral ESF with epoxy putty has also been used with good success [12].

Fractures of distal humerus (condylar/supracondylar) are often encountered in young animals. Such cases can be managed by external application of modified Thomas splint using steel rods (8–10 mm). However, unstable fracture fixation of condylar or supracondylar fractures may lead to large callus formation resulting in joint stiffness or ankylosis. Hence, rigid fixation using an internal fixation technique is generally preferred.

Internal immobilization of a distal humerus fracture can be undertaken by a modified technique of cross intramedullary pinning (Fig. 4.3). Exposure of the distal humerus is done by a standard lateral incision through the anconeus muscle at the level of joint space. The incision may be extended proximally through the distal aspect of the lateral head of the triceps. While exposing the bone fragments, radial nerve should be protected by gentle handling. From the epicondylar portion of the distal fragment, two K-wires (2.5–3.0 mm) are passed alternatively in crossed manner one from the cranial and another from the caudal aspect of the lateral surface. Once the K-wires reach the proximal end of distal fragment, the bone fragments are reduced and aligned, and then they are progressed alternatively into the proximal fragment. The wires are exited through the cranio-medial aspect of proximal humerus, and the distal ends of wires are concealed below the surface of articular cartilage. At the proximal end, the protruding ends of the wires are cut close to the skin, and the surgical incision is then sutured routinely. This technique generally provides stable fixation of lateral condylar/supracondylar fractures. Distal pin migration is the most common complication; however, it generally does not affect the fixation stability. In intercondylar fractures, both condyles are reduced and immobilized first using one or two lag screws fixed across the condyles before going for IM pin fixation.

The outcome of fracture fixation in humerus is usually good in young calves, and in heavy adult animals, prognosis is guarded. Radial nerve damage caused either due to fracture trauma or during fracture fixation is very common. Further, large callus formation at the site of fracture often traps the radial nerve leading to prolonged and persistent lameness.

## 4.2 Fractures of Radius-Ulna

Radius-ulna fractures are quite common in large animals, and the incidence in cattle and buffaloes may vary from about 10–15%. Ulna is also usually fractured along with radius. Fracture can occur anywhere in the shaft of long bones; however, most radius fractures occur in the middle to

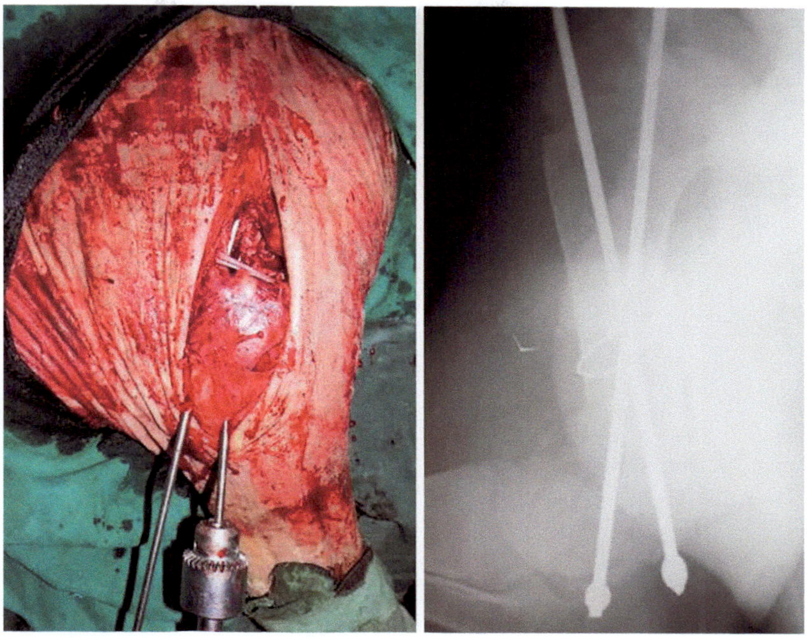

**Fig. 4.3** Modified cross pin fixation for repair of distal humeral fracture in a calf

proximal diaphysis, which are frequently comminuted [13]. Fracture of the olecranon is rare in cattle. The epiphyseal and metaphyseal fractures are more common in young animals, and most often the distal diaphyseal or physeal fractures are open [4]. In open fractures, open wounds are normally seen on the medial surface of the limb, where the bone is more superficial with less soft tissue covering.

Diagnosis of a radial fracture can easily be done by characteristic clinical signs and physical examination. Radiography may not be needed if the fracture is simple (closed) and involves the diaphysis, when external fixation technique such as plaster cast can be used to immobilize the fracture. However, radiographic examination is useful especially when the fracture is comminuted, open, or suspected to have involved the joint, where internal fixation or external skeletal fixation is advised.

Generally, the fractures of radius-ulna are most suited for external fixation as the bones are fairly straight and surrounded by little soft tissues. In young animals (<150 kg), a POP cast spanning only the antebrachium is adequate, which allows free movement of the limb. In heavier patients (>150 kg), a full-limb cast is needed. The walking cast can also be used for successfully treatment of radius-ulna fractures, which protects the fracture site from direct weight bearing. Synthetic fiberglass cast is ideal for fixation of closed radius-ulna fractures even in heavy animals (Fig. 4.4). Modified Thomas splint-cast combination and transfixation pinning alone or along with casting (TPC) have also been used extensively for the repair of closed radial fractures [14, 15].

For rigid immobilization of radial fractures, internal fixation is advised. Intramedullary pin/nail is not indicated in radius [16] due to the presence of joints at both ends of the bone, which does not allow safe placement of pin/nail using standard retrograde or normograde techniques, without damaging the joints. Bone plating, either conventional DCP or LCP (10–14 hole broad 4.5–5.5 mm plates), fixation can be used as an ideal internal fixation technique [17, 18]. Under general anesthesia, the radius is accessed through a cranial approach. The cranio-medial approach provides easier access to the bone, while the lateral approach between the extensor carpi radialis and the common digital extensor muscles allows adequate soft tissue covering of the plate. Plate and screw fixation through the cranial approach also stabilizes the fractured ulna

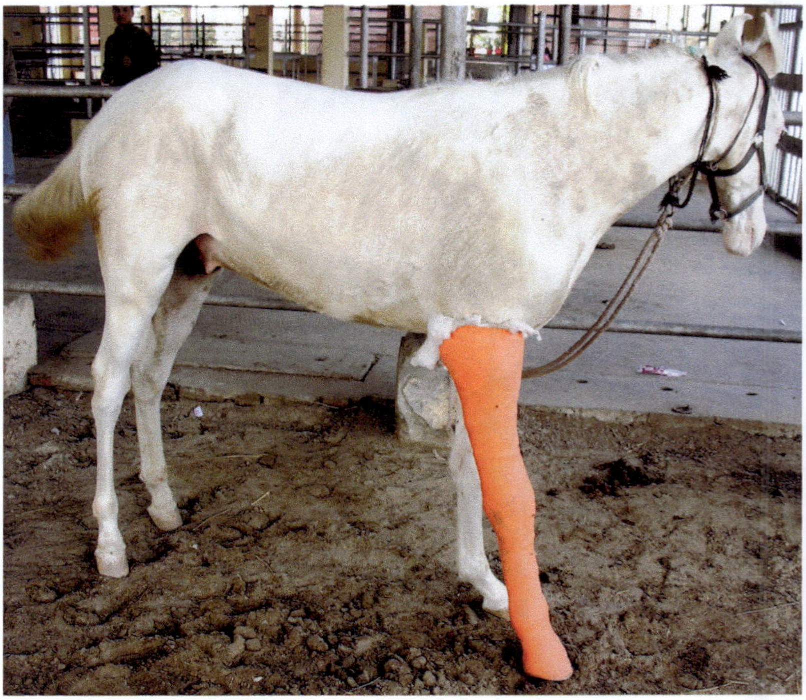

**Fig. 4.4** Fiberglass cast for radius-ulna fracture repair in an adult horse

(no efforts needed to reduce stabilize the ulna separately) (Figs. 4.5 and 4.6). In heavy animals, double plate fixation is undertaken [17], one on the cranial and another on the medial or lateral surface based on the fracture pattern (Fig. 4.7). In some cases, external support such as full limb cast may provide additional support to internal fixation. More recently developed contoured locking plate for bovine radius, fixed on craniomedial surface of radius in cattle and buffaloes, has shown to provide greater stability due to the fixation of locking screws in two rows giving double plate effect [19]. Recent advances such as locking plate and clamp-rod osteosynthesis has improved the outcome of radial fracture repair even in heavy large animals [10, 11] (Fig. 4.8).

Fracture of olecranon/ proximal ulnar diaphysis without the involvement of radius may be treated by tension band wire or orthopedic wire fixation (fixed in figure of "8" or as mattress suture) in young animals. In heavy adult animals, bone plating (DCP/LCP) provides more rigid fixation [20] (Fig. 4.9). While fixing the plate on the caudal surface (through lateral incision), care should be taken to choose appropriate length screws, so that they do not penetrate the joint surface. More distal screws may be fixed in the radius to achieve more rigid fixation. External splint and bandage or cast application may be done for a few days to provide additional support.

Open fractures are often seen in radius-ulna of large animals. In open fractures, if POP/fiberglass cast needs to be applied, an aperture (window) should be left/created in the cast to provide access to the wound. Keeping a window at the level of joint will reduce the strength of fixation to a large extent. Hence, in such cases, metal or wooden splints should be used to provide strength to the fixation. Open fractures of radius-ulna can be better managed using any of the external skeletal fixation techniques [21–24]. The animal may be restrained in dorsal recumbency by holding the limb in suspension from a height or in lateral recumbency with the open skin wound surface facing upward. Fixation of ESF is easier in forelimb than in hind limb as it is relatively straight. Further, as the forelimb is straight, bilateral linear fixators generally provide good fixation [22, 25] (Fig. 4.10). As open fractures are more common in the distal radius, where the short bone fragment

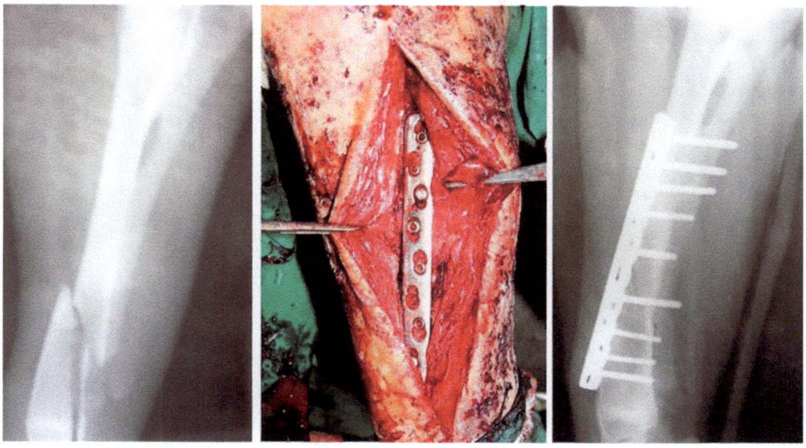

**Fig. 4.5** Radius-ulna fracture repair using 4.5 locking compression plate in a cattle

may not allow two point fixation, transarticular immobilization can be done by fixing a minimum of two pins in the metacarpal bone (Fig. 4.11). The principal nerves and vessels in the region occupy the caudomedial location of the radius; hence, pins can be safely placed in mediolateral of lateromedial direction with least chance of damaging the neurovascular structures. In adult heavy animals, 6–7 mm transcortical pins (usually fully threaded) are placed in the radius through the fascia intervening the *lateral digital extensor* and *ulnaris lateralis* muscles. A circular fixator (3.5–4.0 mm cross pins) can provide more stable fixation of radial fractures (Fig. 4.12), especially in very heavy animals. In young lightweight animals, multiplanar epoxy-pin ESF (pin size-2.5 to 3.0 mm, with 18–20 mm epoxy columns) provides stable fixation [26] (Fig. 4.13).

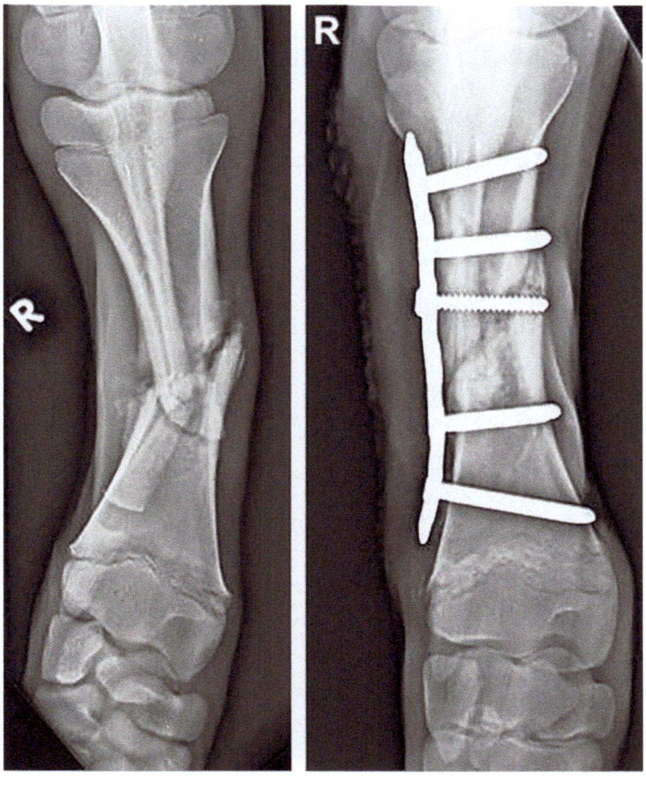


**Fig. 4.6** Fixation of radius-ulna fracture in a 12-day old HF calf using a narrow LCP with a 4.5-mm lag screw (Reproduced with permission from: Karl Nuss, Plates, Pins, and Interlocking Nails. Vet Clin Food Anim 30: 91–126, 2014)

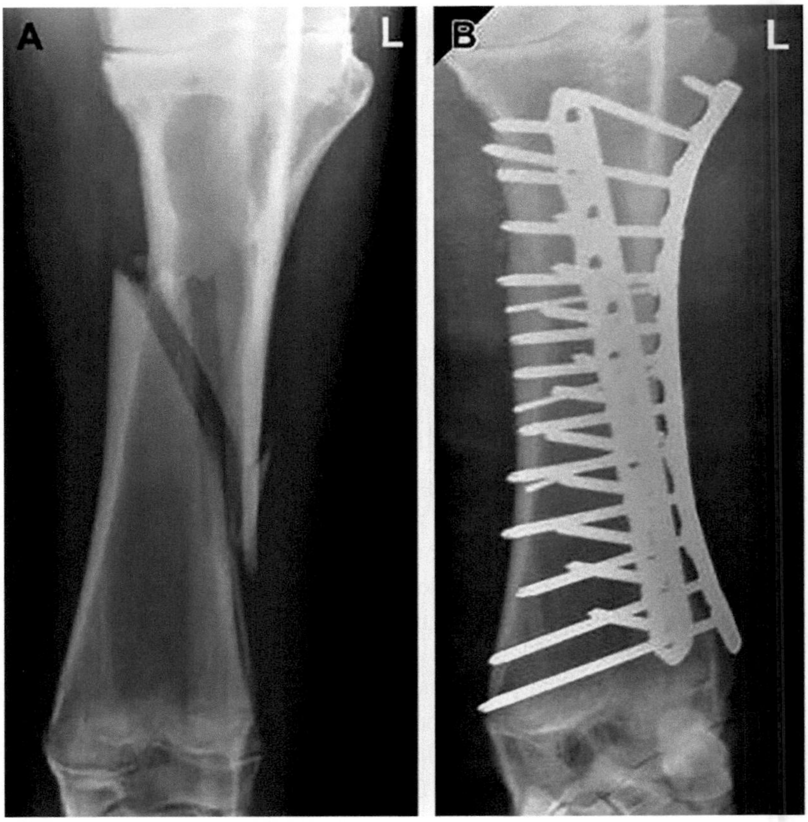


**Fig. 4.7** Double plate (2 LCPs placed 90° to each other) fixation for radius-ulna fracture in a heifer (Reproduced with permission from: Karl Nuss, Plates, Pins, and Interlocking Nails. Vet Clin Food Anim 30: 91–126, 2014)

## 4.3 Fractures of Femur

Femur fractures are more frequent in young calves and are relatively uncommon in adult cattle and buffaloes. However, often femoral capital epiphyseal fractures are seen in adult animals. In young calves, femoral neck and capital femoral epiphyseal and distal femoral fractures are more

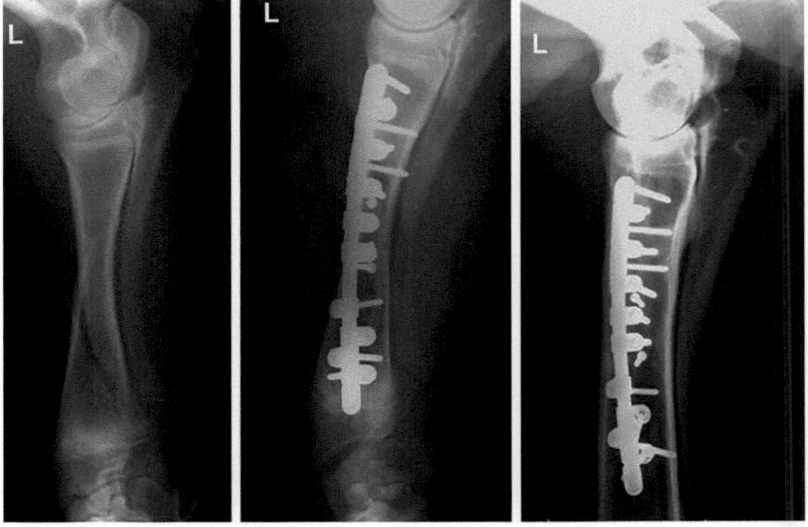


**Fig. 4.8** Clamp-rod internal fixation for radius-ulna fracture (Reproduced with permission from: Karl Nuss, Plates, Pins, and Interlocking Nails. Vet Clin Food Anim 30: 91–126, 2014)

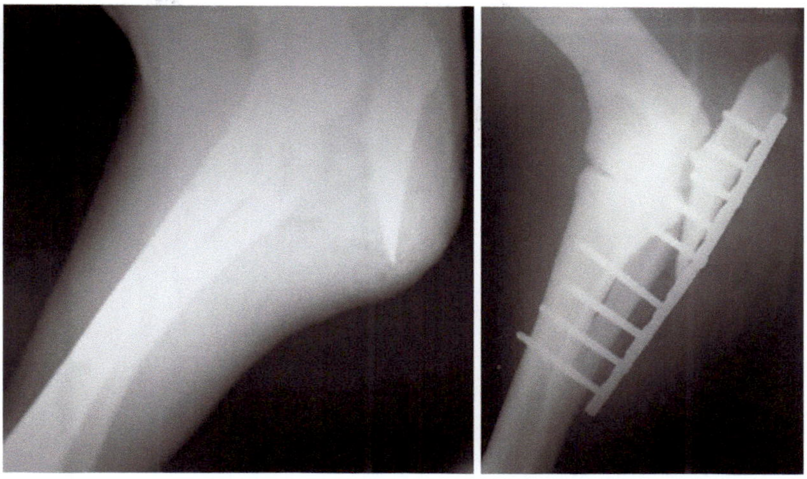

**Fig. 4.9** Fixation of 4.5 LCP for repair of olecranon fracture in a cattle

frequent [27]. In bovines, femoral fractures account for less than 5% of all the fracture cases [4]. Most femoral fractures that occur in new born calves are associated with obstetrical injury. In young calves, crush injury due to stepping by the dam is also reported to be the common cause of femur fracture. Most femoral fractures are transverse or slight oblique. Severe periosteal stripping, soft tissue injury, and overriding of fragments are characteristics of femoral fractures.

Femoral fractures can be diagnosed based on the clinical signs of lameness, swelling, and crepitation in the thigh region and inability to bear weight on the injured limb. Soft tissue swelling is more in distal fractures located near or involving the stifle joint. In case of femoral neck or capital epiphyseal fractures, the animal may be able to bear some weight on the limb with less degree of lameness. Large swelling near the hip joint may create confusion with coxofemoral luxation;

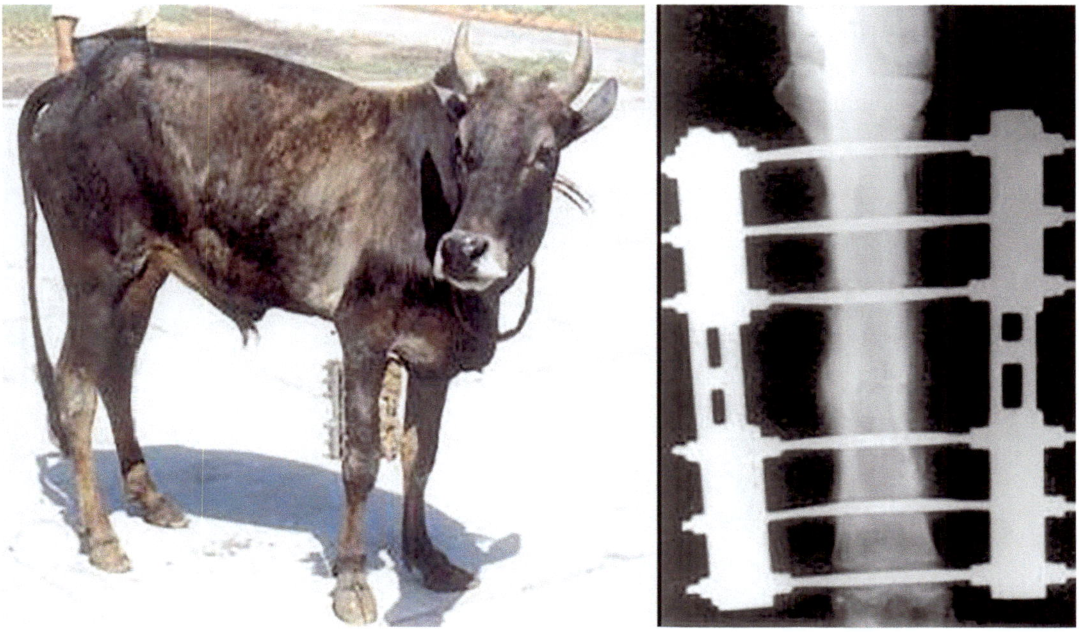

**Fig. 4.10** Mid diaphyseal fracture of radius treated with a bilateral linear fixator

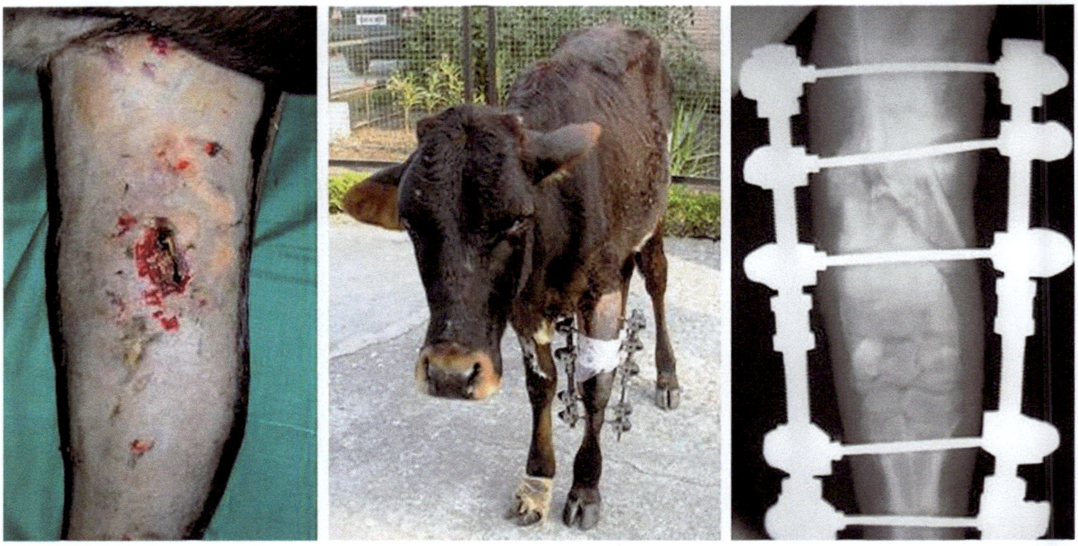

**Fig. 4.11** Repair of open fracture of distal radius by transcarpal fixation using the novel bilateral linear fixator in cattle

however, fracture causes more of inflammatory swelling. Survey radiography can help to affirm the diagnosis and determine the location and pattern of fracture. However, as the femur is located more proximally with lots of soft tissue covering, computer radiography or CT scan would be more diagnostic.

Conservative treatment of femoral fractures is generally unsuccessful due to severe overriding of bone segments [10]. Stall rest may be considered in adult animals as a conservative method of treatment, but malunion or nonunion is common. Successful conservative management of selected femoral diaphyseal fractures has been reported in young foals [28] and cattle [29]. Application of modified Thomas splint with or without cast application has been used especially in fractures of middle or distal diaphysis of femur with little overriding of bone fragments (it is difficult to reduce overriding femoral diaphyseal fracture by close method due to heavy muscular pull). However, complications such as decubitus ulcers and slippage of splints leading to overriding of fragments and large callus formation are common

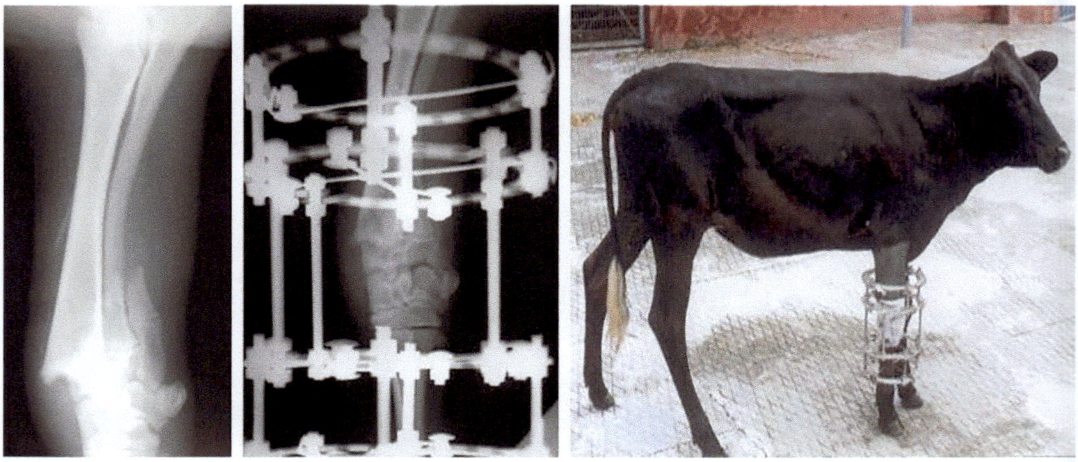

**Fig. 4.12** Repair of open fracture of distal end of radius-ulna using circular external fixator in cattle

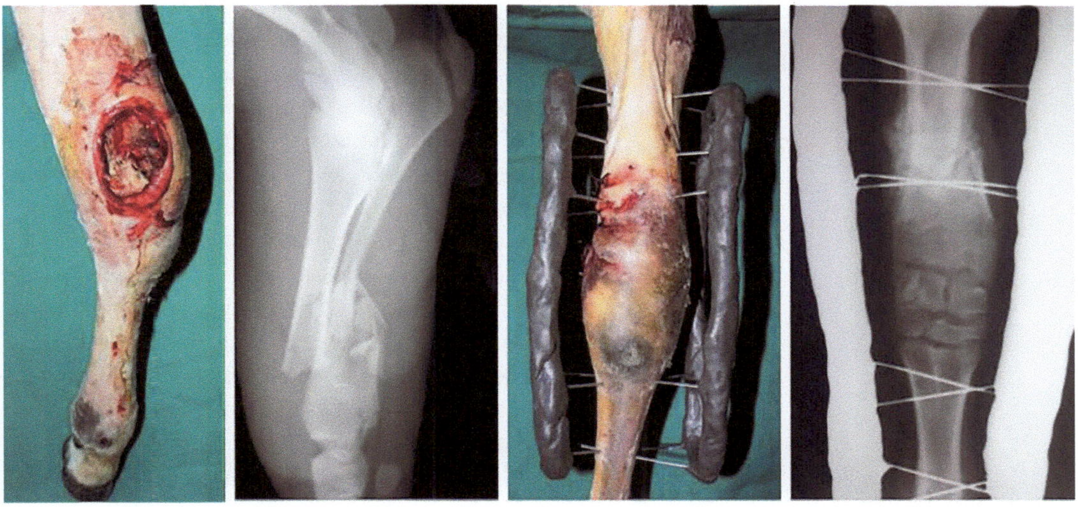

**Fig. 4.13** Repair of open fracture of distal radius-ulna using epoxy-pin external fixator in a calf (using 3 mm pins)

[14]. Modified Thomas splints should never be used in proximal diaphyseal or epiphyseal fractures.

Fractures of femoral capital epiphysis have been treated using multiple pin fixation or large compression screws. The proximal femur including femur head and neck and the cranial aspect of the acetabulum are accessed by a craniolateral approach. The fracture reduction is achieved by internal rotation and abduction of the limb before fixation. Use of cannulated screws (of about 7 mm diameter and 130 mm long) has been shown to provide better interfragmentary compression. However, it is difficult to anatomically reduce the bone fragments, especially in adult animals, and prognosis following femoral neck and epiphyseal fractures is generally guarded. Excision arthroplasty of the femoral head and neck may be done as a salvage procedure for capital femoral epiphyseal fractures. A cranial approach along the ventral border of the middle gluteal muscle and over the greater trochanter is advocated for the procedure. This may lead to formation of pseudoarthrosis and acceptable weight bearing, especially in young animals.

Femoral diaphyseal fractures can be better managed by open reduction and internal fixation using IM pins/nails or bone plates. A craniolateral incision extending from slightly caudal to the greater trochanter up to the lateral femoral condyle is used to approach the femoral diaphysis. The aponeurosis of the tensor fascia lata is incised, and the biceps femoris and vastus lateralis muscles are pulled aside to access the femur. A severely overriding fracture is difficult to reduce, especially when the fracture is of several days old. Careful dissection and use of strong blunt instruments may help reducing the bone fragments. Use of hemi-cerclage wire may help reduce an oblique fracture and temporarily hold the fragments in alignment.

Single intramedullary pin fixation is generally not adequate to provide stable fixation of femoral diaphyseal fractures. Intramedullary stack pinning is the simplest technique, which can provide satisfactory fixation of shaft fractures in calves and foals (Fig. 4.14). A hemicerclage wire is useful to reduce and align the bone fragments before IM pin fixation. The most common complication with the IM pin fixation is pin migration. Modified technique of multiple cross IM pin fixation provides better stability in diaphyseal as well as supracondylar fractures than conventional stack pinning. In this technique, multiple pins are passed in normograde fashion from outer surfaces of medial and lateral condyles. Four or six pins (2.5–3.5 mm diameter) are passed alternatively in crossed manner from either surface of the distal fragment (2–3 pins on either side), from the cranial and caudal aspects (Fig. 4.15). The

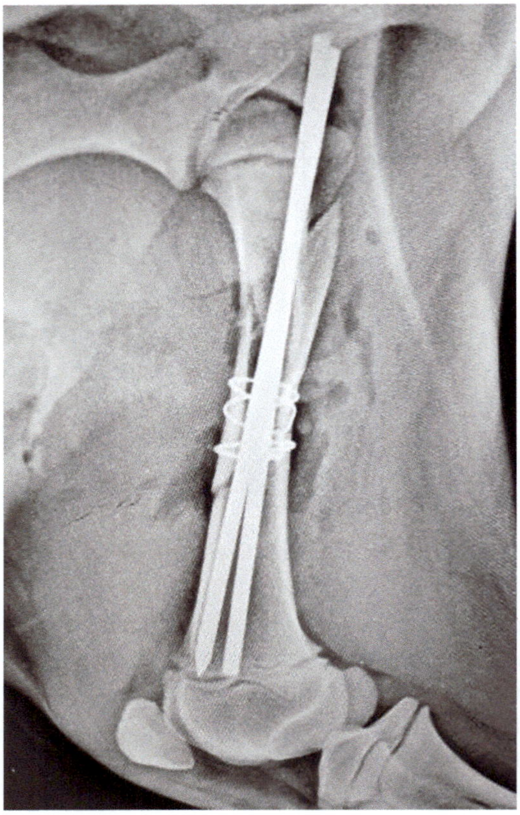

**Fig. 4.14** Stack pinning and wiring for repair of comminuted femoral diaphyseal fracture in a 2-month old foal

pins are passed in about 20–30° angle to the longitudinal axis of the bone (if pins are passed in more acute angle, they may penetrate the opposite cortex). Once the pins reach the proximal end of the distal fragment, the fracture fragments are reduced and aligned, and subsequently, the pins are progressed alternatively in the proximal fragment. The pins are then allowed to exit through the trochanteric fossa proximally. The distal ends of the pins are seated below the level of articular cartilage, and the extra length pins are cut close to the skin proximally. In this technique, as the pins are fixed in spring loaded tension, fixation is more stable, and chances of pin migration are also less. K-nailing can also be used for fixation of femoral diaphyseal fractures in young adult animals (Fig. 4.16). Two K-nails, one slided into another, have been used successfully for repair of mid shaft fractures in adult cattle. In recent years, interlocking nails have replaced K-nails. Novel custom made interlocking nails have been used to achieve good fixation and outcome in calves [30]. Novel interlocking nail system developed specifically for bovine femur has shown to provide stable fixation of diaphyseal fractures [31]. 14–18 mm diameter nail with threaded screw holes spanning the length of the nail is found ideal for fixation in bovine femur. In distal diaphyseal fractures, interlocking nail may be

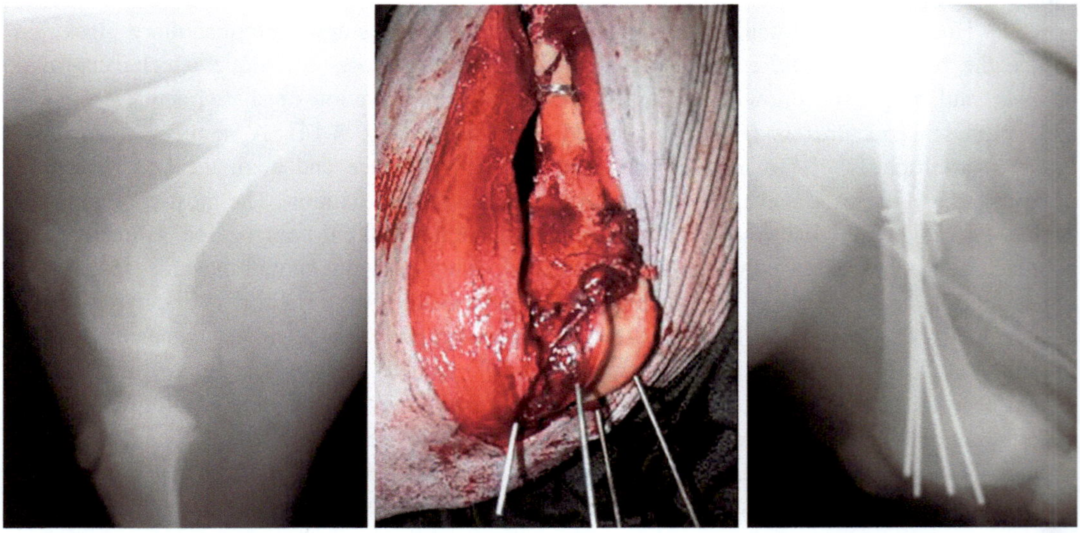

**Fig. 4.15** Multiple cross pin fixation along with cerclage wiring for femoral diaphyseal fracture repair

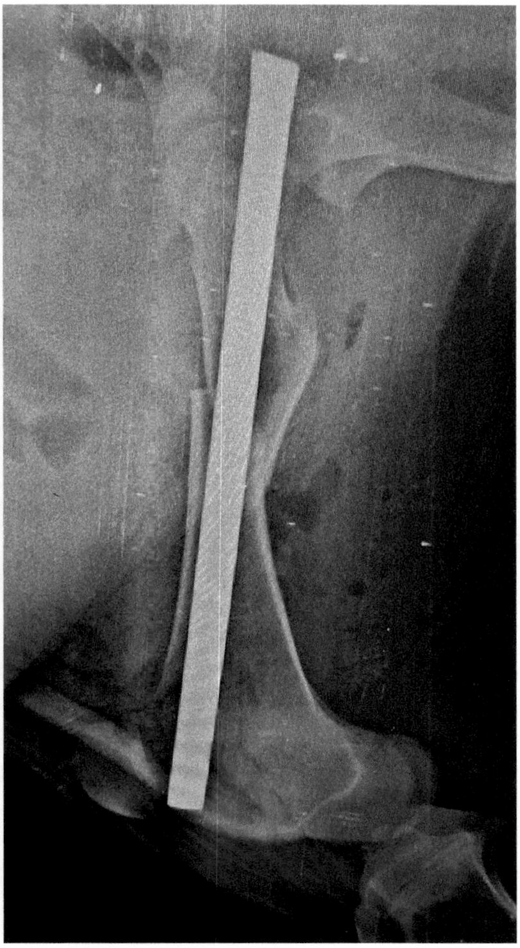

**Fig. 4.16** Fixation of K-nail in mid diaphyseal fracture in a calf (Courtesy: Dr Rohit Kumar, Indian Veterinary Research Institute, Bareilly, India)

introduced between the femoral condyles, and one or two fixation bolts may be placed in the distal fragment (Fig. 4.17).

Plate osteosynthesis has proved successful in some cases of femoral diaphyseal fractures [27, 32]. Failure of the screws to securely hold the bone plate in position is a common problem in young calves. This can be overcome by the use of locking compression plates, which provide better bone-plate anchorage. Double plate fixation (4.5/5.5 DCP or LCP), one on the lateral and another on the cranial surface, has shown to provide more stability to fixation [10] (Fig. 4.18). Novel contoured locking plate developed for fixation of femoral diaphyseal fractures is well contoured to craniolateral surface of femur bone and has two rows of holes for fixation of locking screws in different planes (Fig. 4.19). Both in vitro and clinical studies have shown that these designer plates are better fixed in the femoral diaphysis and provide more stable fixation than conventional plates [31].

Distal femoral fractures in young calves may be treated by application of modified Thomas splint, if there is little or no displacement of bone fragments. However, the outcome of external fixation is not good most of the times, as it may lead to fracture instability and large callus formation leading to joint stiffness [14]. Modified technique of multiple cross IM pin fixation described above can give good fixation of condylar and supracondylar fractures (Fig. 4.20). In supracondylar fractures, interlocking nail could be introduced through the intercondylar fossa (normograde technique) to provide better anchorage in the small distal fragment (Fig. 4.21). However, interlocking nail should be carefully used in young animals with open physes. Further, fixation bolt/s should be fixed in only one of the bone segments, not to affect the longitudinal growth of the bone. Angled blade plates (LCP) have also been used for successful repair of distal femoral fractures [33]. However, during screw fixation, bridging the growth plate cannot be prevented in young animals. Hence, it is advised to remove the plate and screws as early as possible soon after bone healing.

The outcome of femur fracture repair depends on several factors such as the age of animal, location and type of fracture, the degree of fracture reduction and alignment, etc. In general, a fractured femur heals well because of thick vascular periosteum and large soft tissue coverage, especially in young animals.

## 4.4 Fractures of Tibia

Tibial fractures are common in cattle and buffaloes of all age groups, with an incidence of about 25–30% of all fractures [34]. In young animals, proximal epiphyseal fractures are commonly seen, whereas in adult animals, fracture

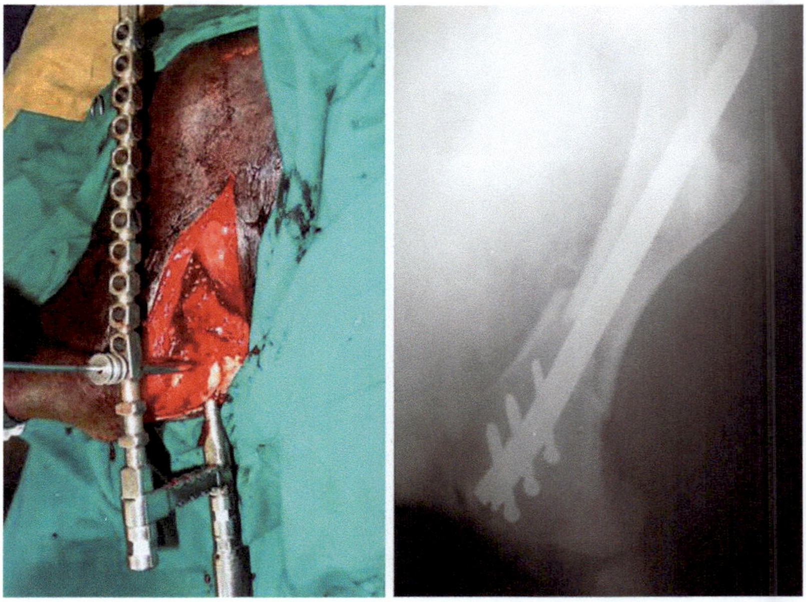

**Fig. 4.17** Interlocking nail fixation through intercondylar fossa for femur fracture repair in a cattle

can be seen all along the length of bone [13]. Vehicular accident is the most frequent direct cause of trauma leading to a fracture. The tibial fracture is frequently comminuted, but spiral and long oblique fractures are also common. Fractures of tibia are often accompanied with severe soft tissue damage. The medial surface of the distal tibia is devoid of any soft tissue coverage; hence, most often, distal tibial fractures get open on the medial surface. Diagnosis of tibial fracture can easily be made based on clinical symptoms of inability to bear weight and carrying of the limb, crepitation, soft tissue inflammation, and swelling at the injured site. Physical examination and radiography will help to know the type and extent of fracture.

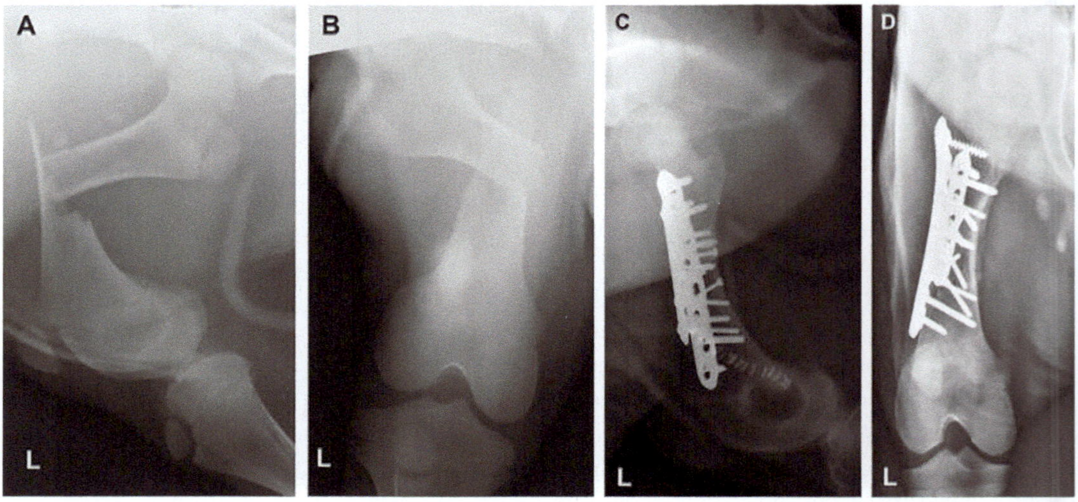


**Fig. 4.18** Repair of femur fracture using double locking compression plate fixation in a calf using 3.5-mm lag screws and a lateral and cranial LCP (with 4.5-mm cortical screws and 5.0-mm locking screws) (Reproduced with permission from: Karl Nuss, Plates, Pins, and Interlocking Nails. Vet Clin Food Anim 30: 91–126, 2014)

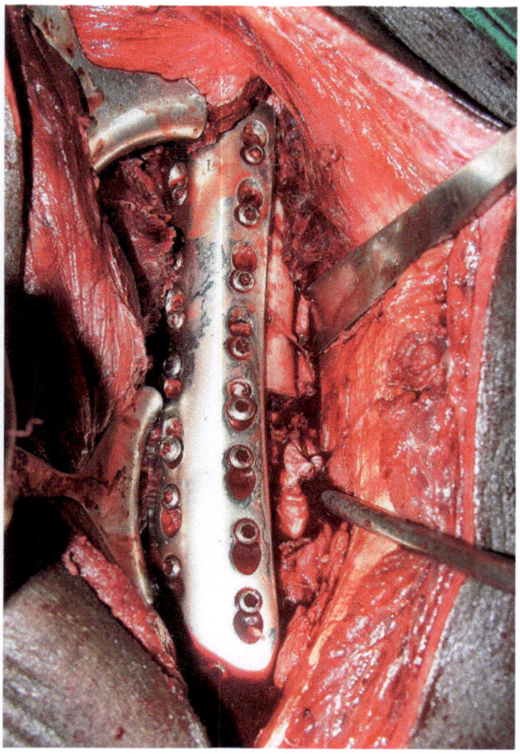

**Fig. 4.19** Use of contoured locking plate in femoral diaphysis

Angular placement of the bone and heavy musculature around the stifle joint make cast application difficult in tibia. In young animals, however, lack of development of quadriceps muscle enables the cast to be extended above the stifle joint and its possible retention (Fig. 4.22). Due to its light weight and greater strength, fiberglass cast is preferred over plaster cast. In heavy animals, hanging limb pin cast may be used to treat middle or distal tibial fractures. One or two Steinmann pins passed latero-medially/mediolaterally in the proximal bone segment will help anchoring the cast and its retention (Fig. 4.23). However, hanging limb pin cast has disadvantages like inadequate fixation stability due to rotation of the distal limb and pin tract infection [35]. Modified Thomas splint alone (in young animals) or along with cast (in heavy adults) can also be used for successful management of closed fractures, especially of distal diaphysis of tibia [36, 37].

Proximal epiphyseal/metaphyseal factures in young animals can be better treated using cross IM pin or Rush pin fixation. As the soft tissue covering is less at the proximal end of tibia and severe displacement of fracture fragments is uncommon, fracture fragments can be easily reduced and immobilized. The pins can be passed through the smaller proximal fragment by normograde technique. Fixation of lateral pin is relatively difficult (due to lateral curvature of proximal tibia), often leading to penetration of pin through the cortex into the soft tissues. Nevertheless, in very young animals, if the pin has

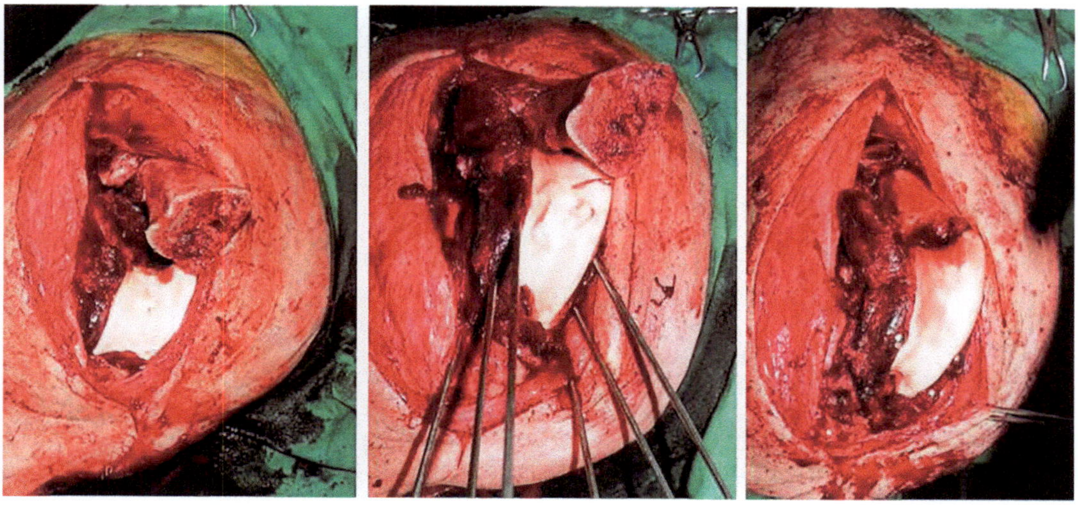

**Fig. 4.20** Supracondylar femoral fracture fixation using multiple cross pins

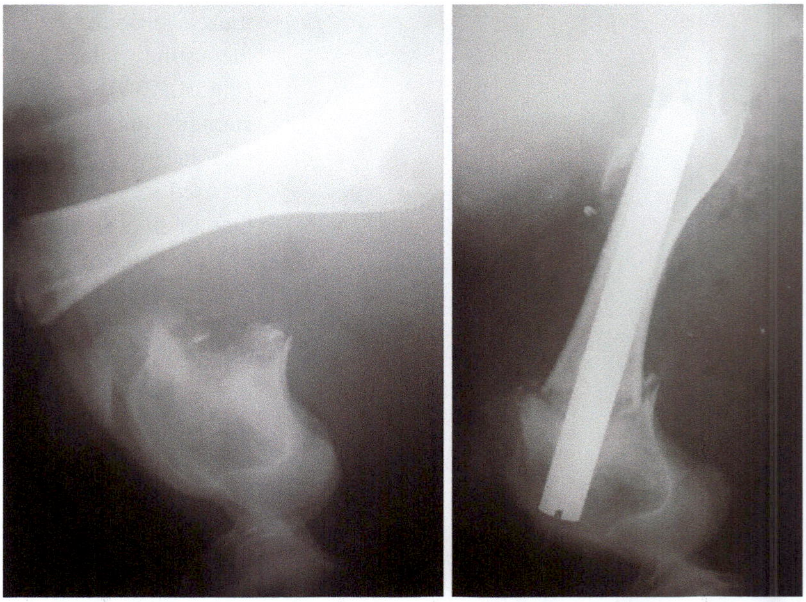

**Fig. 4.21** Repair of supracondylar fracture of femur using interlocking nail (normograde through intercondylar fossa)

passed through the distal fragment up to a certain length, it will not affect the stability of fixation. However, it is advised to fix the pins under fluoroscopic/C-arm guidance. Pin insertion on the craniomedial margin of the tibia, half-way between the middle patellar ligament and medial collateral ligament, is relatively easy, as tibia is relatively straight medially. Single IM pin fixation through cranio-medial approach often provides satisfactory level of fixation, provided additional external support is given in the form of splint and bandage application. T-plate (fixed cranio-medially) can also be used to provide rigid fixation of proximal tibial fractures in young animals [10].

Different internal fixation devices such as intramedullary pins/nails and plates have been used for internal fixation of diaphyseal fractures of tibia. Intramedullary Steinmann pin can at best be used in very young lightweight animals. K-nails have been used for the fixation of tibial diaphyseal fractures [38]. However, more recently introduced interlocking nails provide greater fixation rigidity with fewer complications.

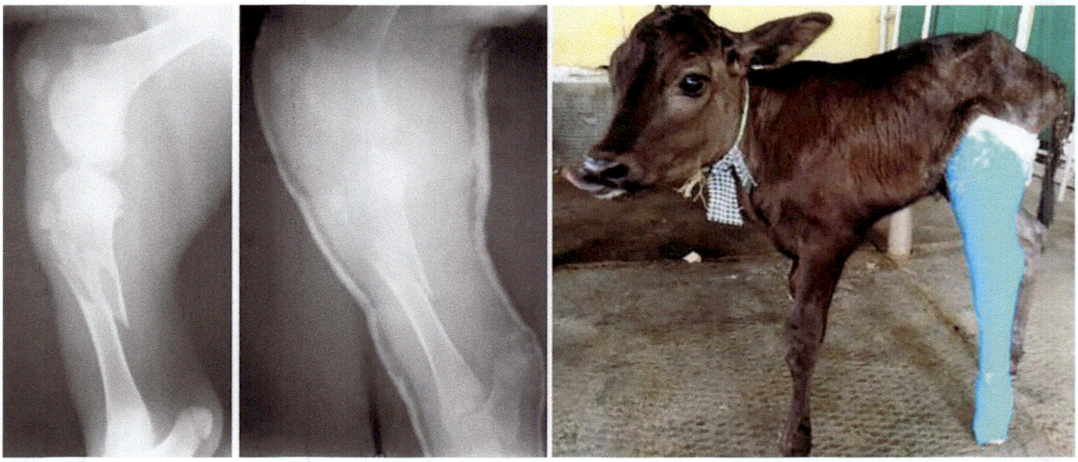

**Fig. 4.22** Fiberglass cast applied to immobilize proximal tibial fracture in a young calf

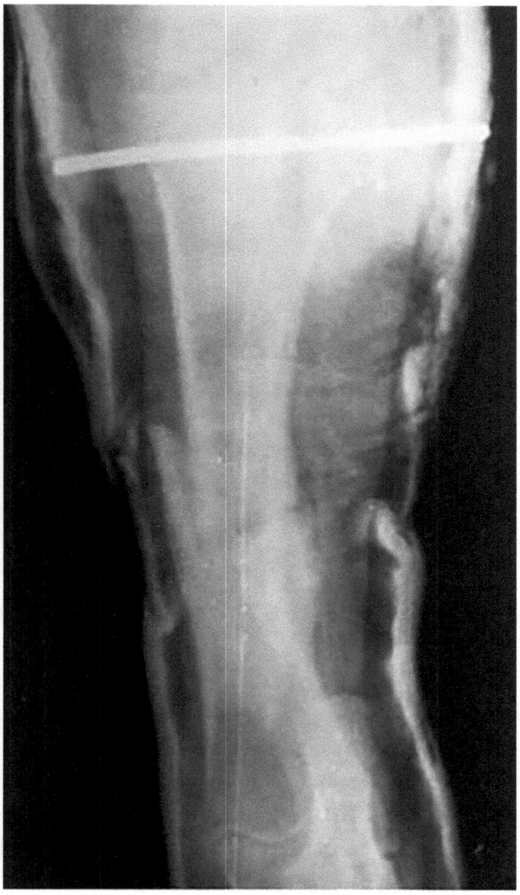

**Fig. 4.23** Hanging limb pin cast for fixation of tibial diaphyseal fracture in an adult cattle

Successful use of both straight and specially designed angular nails has been reported for fixation of tibial fractures in lightweight animals. The angular nail can be placed in the medullary cavity of tibia without damaging the articulating surface of the stifle joint through the cranio-medial surface of proximal tibia [39]. The point of insertion is on the medial condyle slightly above and medial to the tibial tuberosity, cranial to the horn of medial menisci, and below the articular ridge (Fig. 4.24).

The fracture site is approached through a medial incision, and the bone segments are reduced (either manually of using bone holding forceps); hemi-cerclage wiring is useful to reduce and hold the bone segments in alignment. At the nail insertion site in the proximal bone segment, a hole is made in the bony cortex to enter the medullary cavity using a curved bone awl (Fig. 4.24). The medullary cavity along the length of bone is reamed using successively larger size reamers. The interlocking nail attached to the zig is then inserted into the medullary cavity through the proximal segment by normograde technique. Once the distal end of nail reaches the distal end of proximal segment, by using the nail and the zig attached to the proximal segment as a handle, the fracture segments may be reduced by toggling. Subsequently, the nail is driven into the distal segment. The diameter and length of the nail used may vary from case to case. In young medium-sized animals, generally 20–24 cm long nails with 10–12 mm diameter are optimum. Two to four fixation bolts (in proximal and distal bone segments) should be used to fix the nail to the bone cortex (Figs. 4.25 and 4.26). Use of more number of fixation bolts provides greater stability, especially in adult animals. Interlocking nailing provides stable fixation, hence allowing immediate weight bearing and early functional recovery of the limb.

Plate osteosynthesis provides rigid immobilization of tibial fractures, especially in young and lightweight adult animals [17, 27, 38]. Bone plates (8–12 hole, broad 4.5 DCP or LCP) can be applied in fractures of tibial diaphysis using different approaches, such as medial, cranial, or lateral. Medial surface of tibia is easier to approach surgically because of little soft tissue coverage. While exposing the bone through a full length linear incision on the medial surface of the tibia, one should be careful not to damage the medial saphenous artery, vein, and nerve. However, due to lack of adequate soft tissue covering and reduced blood supply on the medial aspect, the implants will have poor protection. In cranial approach, the cranial muscle is reflected laterally from the tibial shaft to expose the bone. In lateral approach, the femorotibial joint structures and the fibular nerve need to be carefully protected. In cranial and lateral approaches, sufficient tissue is available to cover and protect the plate. Further, a cranial approach can be used for either craniomedial or lateral plate fixation, hence better for double plate fixation. Single

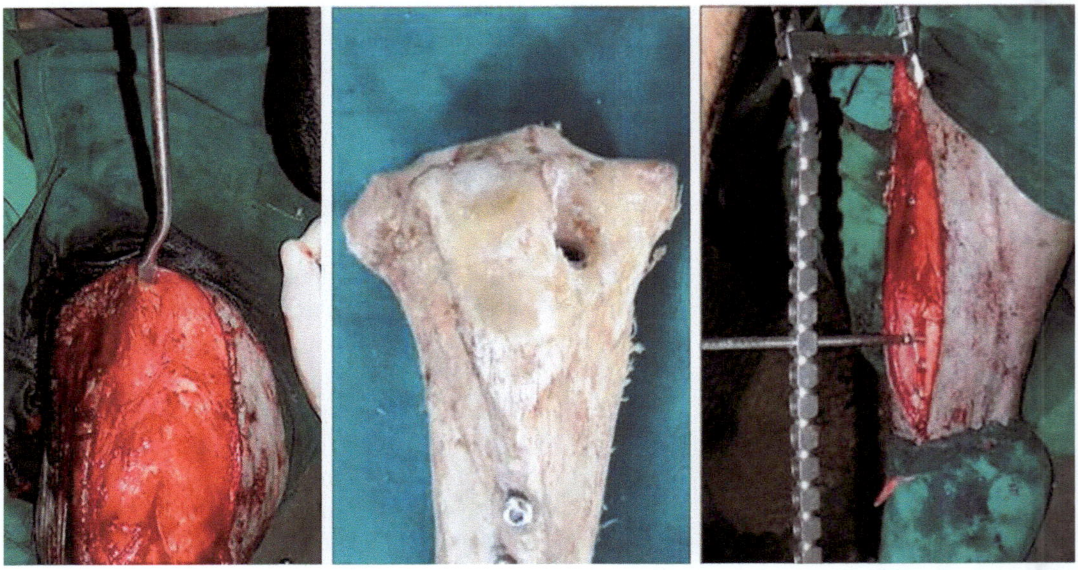

**Fig. 4.24** Interlocking nail fixation in bovine tibia: Note the insertion site on the medial condyle slightly above and medial to the tibial tuberosity, below the articular ridge

bone plate can provide sufficiently stable fixation in lightweight animals (weighing up to about 200–250 kg) (Fig. 4.27); however, in heavy animals, double bone plate fixation is always advised [10, 40] (Fig. 4.28). External splint/cast application provides additional support in heavy animals, especially when single plate is used. Use of locking compression plates can provide more stable fixation of comminuted fractures of tibia. Clamp-rod internal fixation system was also found to provide stable fixation in tibial diaphyseal fractures in cattle [11]. Recently contoured locking plate has been developed specifically for bovine tibia, which can be fixed on the

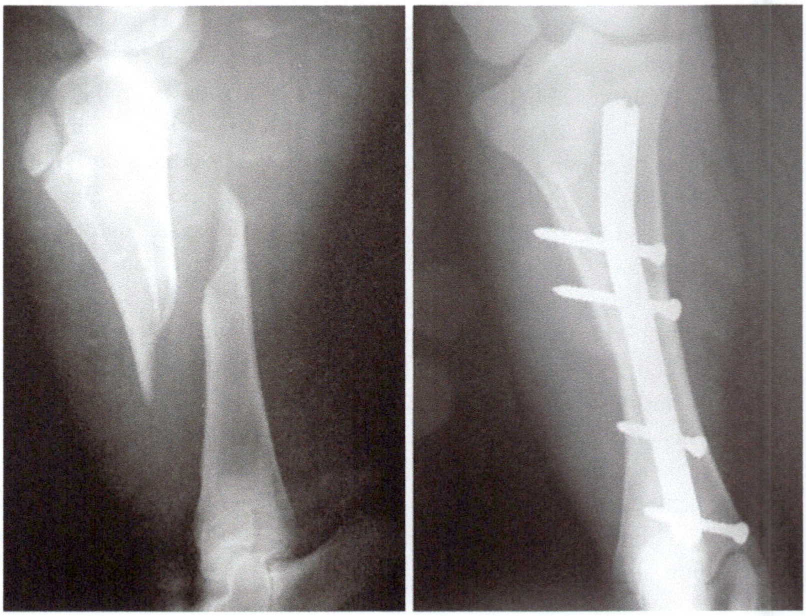

**Fig. 4.25** Repair of tibial diaphyseal fracture in a calf using interlocking nail with four fixation bolts, two each in proximal and distal bone segments

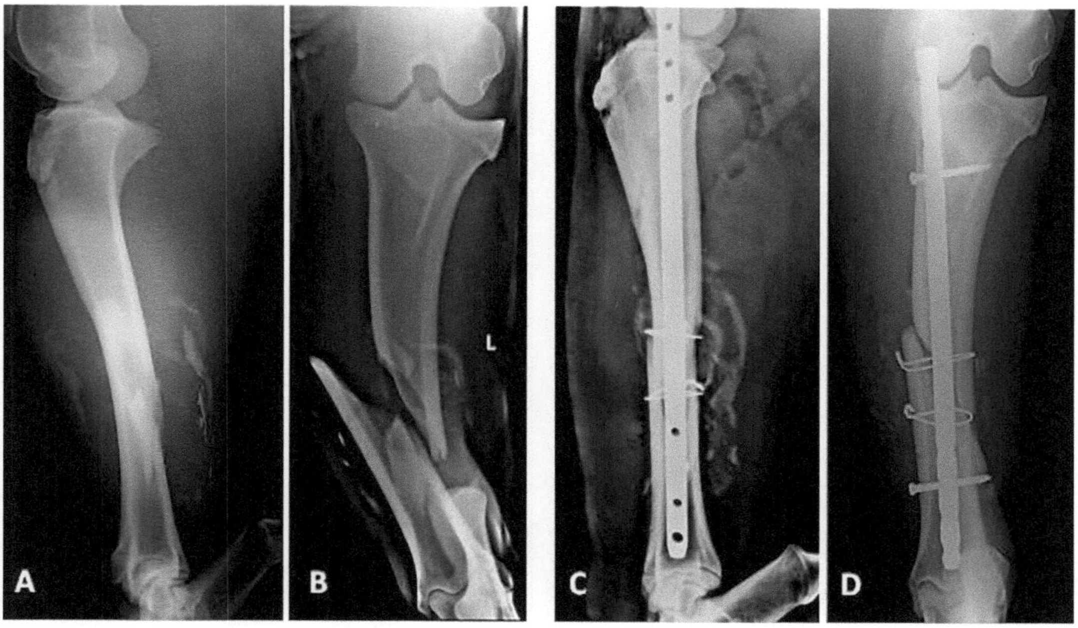


**Fig. 4.26** Comminuted fracture of tibia in a calf treated using straight interlocking nail and with cerclage wiring (Courtesy: Dr. Vijay Kumar and Dr. D. Dilipkumar, Veterinary College, Bidar, Karnataka, India)

craniomedial surface (Fig. 4.29). This contoured plate with two full rows of screws has been shown (both by in vitro mechanical tests and in vivo application) to provide more rigid bone fixation than conventional plates [41]. This plate may be useful to treat certain complex tibial fractures, which are otherwise difficult to treat with conventional methods.

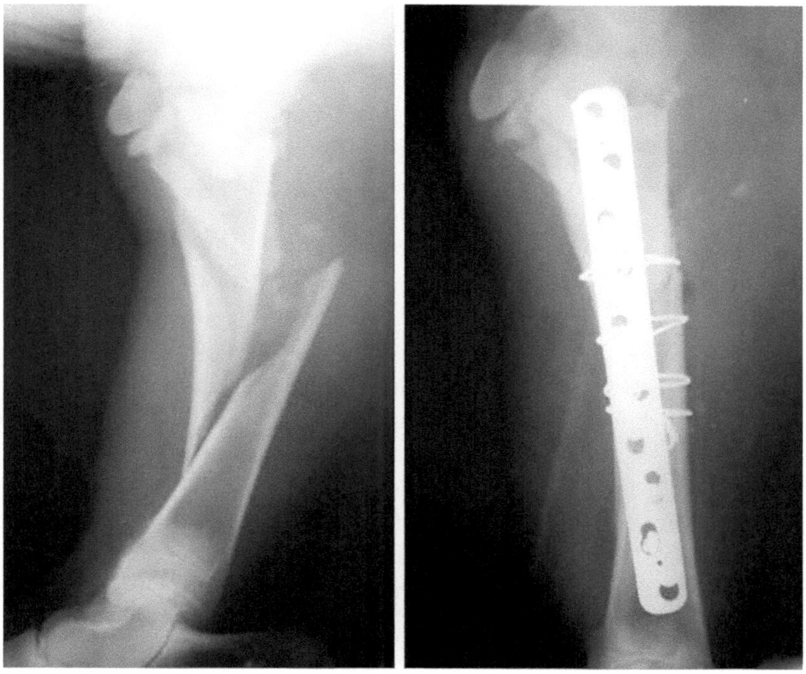

**Fig. 4.27** Repair of comminuted fracture of tibia using 4.5 locking compression plate and cerclage wiring

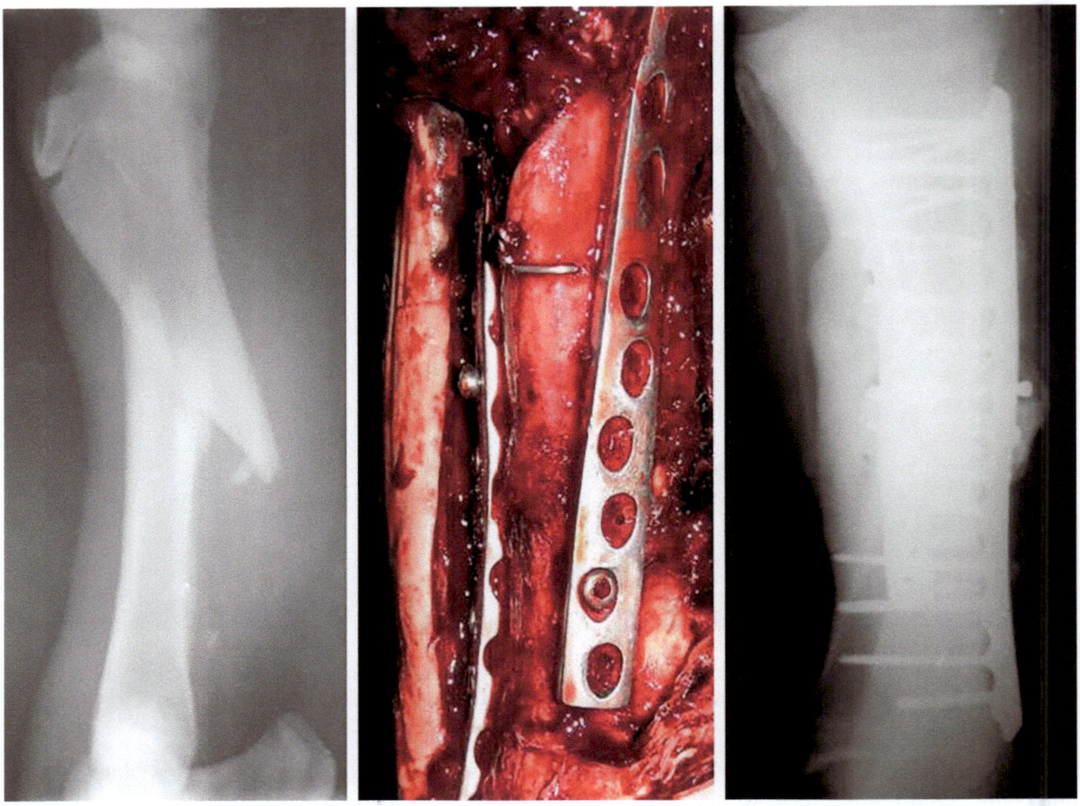

**Fig. 4.28** Use of double plate for repair of comminuted fracture of tibia in an adult horse

Open fractures of tibia are most difficult to treat in large animals. However, the advent of external skeletal fixation has made it possible to treat many such fractures. Angular placement of the bone and the hind limb make fixation of linear fixators difficult. However, linear fixator may be used successfully in relatively young lightweight animals along with cerclage wiring, which will help reduce and retain the bone fragments in alignment. Circular ESF is ideal for treatment of tibial fractures, especially of middle and distal diaphysis [4, 21, 42–44] (Fig. 4.30). For proximal diaphyseal fractures (where it is difficult to use full rings), hybrid ESF can be useful [24, 45] (Fig. 4.31). As distal tibial open fractures are more common in large ruminants, circular ESF can be employed to provide stable fixation by transtarsal application. At the level of tarsal joint, two-third circular/incomplete rings (open at caudal aspect) are chosen, which will not only allow the use of relatively smaller diameter rings but also avoid inflicting pressure wounds at the level of tuber-calcis. Similarly, multiplanar or circular designs of epoxy-pin fixation can be effectively used in similar fashion in young, lightweight animals (Fig. 4.32). They are very effective for transtarsal fixation, as the side bars can be angled as per the requirement of the case to maintain the normal angulation of the hock joint [26].

Fracture of the distal tibial physis, which is often seen in young animals, is difficult to treat. It is generally difficult to stabilize small distal bone fragment. Cross pinning (Krischner wires) can be done along with external cast immobilization for management of such fractures. Due to devoid of soft tissue covering on the medial aspect of hock, most often such fractures are open in nature, which may be treated by transtarsal application of an ESF.

The postoperative care and management is critical for successful outcome of a tibial fracture repair. The prognosis can be favorable in young

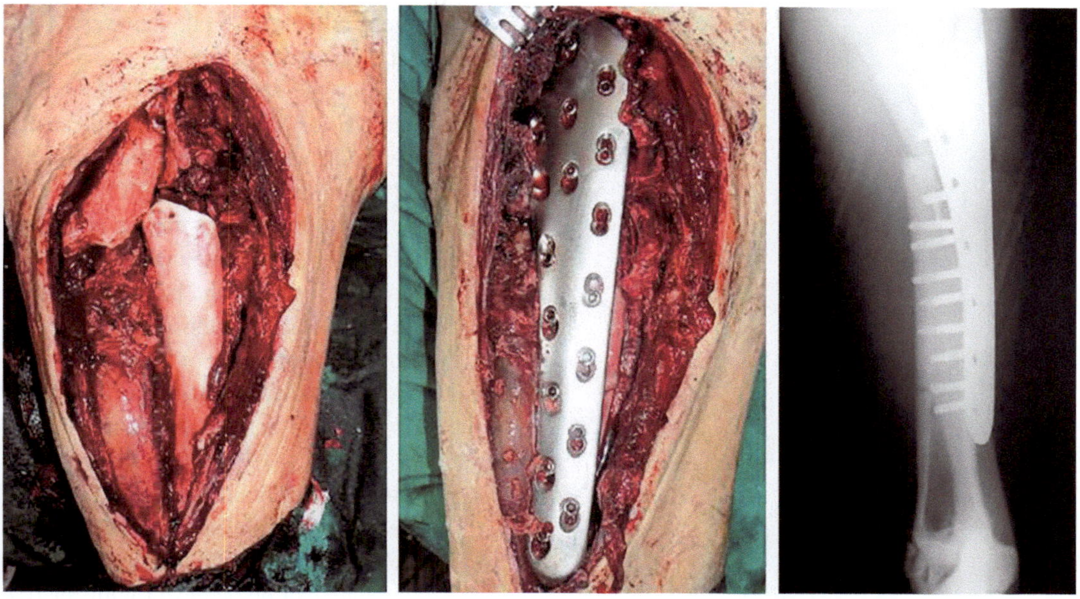

Fig. 4.29 Use of contoured locking compression plate for repair of tibial fracture in cattle

animals; however, in heavy adult animals, it is generally unfavorable, especially if the fracture is open and contaminated. However, the advent of newer internal fixation implants like interlocking nails and locking plates and ESF techniques has improved the outcome of tibial fracture repair in large animals to a great extent.

## 4.5 Fractures of Metacarpus, Metatarsus, and Phalanges

The fractures of metacarpus (MC) and metatarsus (MT) are very often seen in large animals, both in equines and bovines (10–20%) [46]. In calves, the incidence of metacarpal fractures is higher and is mostly related to injuries caused due to dystocia

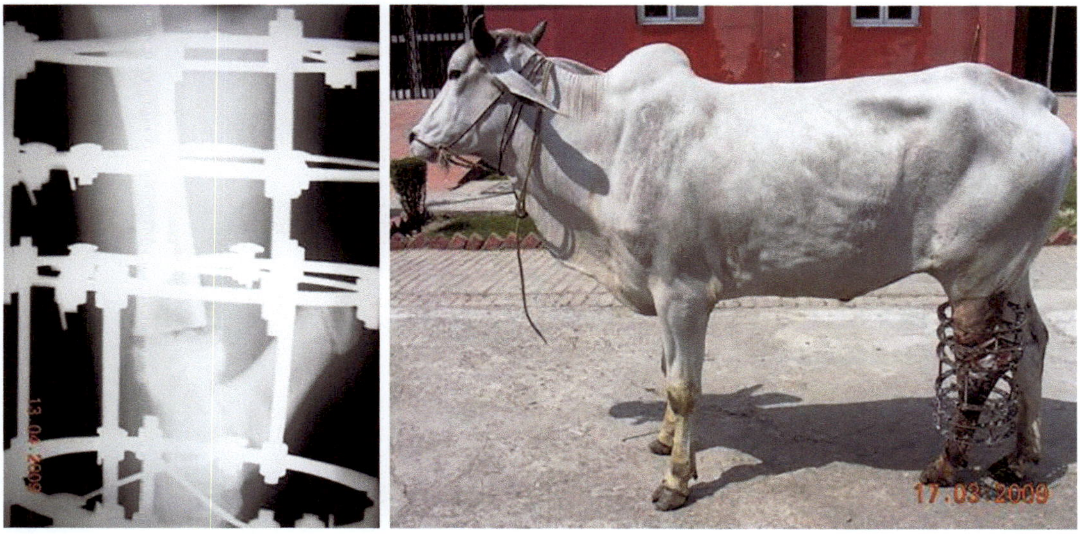


Fig. 4.30 Use of CEF for repair of distal tibial fracture in adult cattle using 3.5 mm transfixation pins

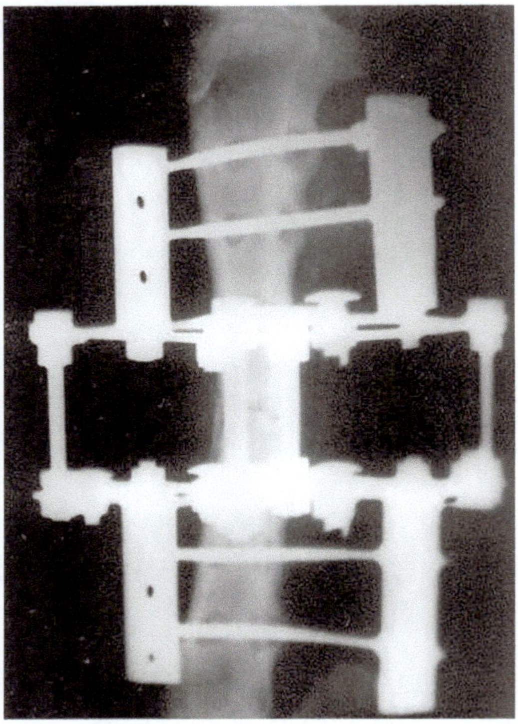

**Fig. 4.31** Use of Hybrid ESF in tibial diaphyseal fracture repair in cattle

and obstetrical manipulation at the time of calving. Comminuted fractures of MC and MT are most common, although spiral, transverse, and oblique fractures are often seen [4]. Fracture can be recorded along the whole length of the bones. Animals with MC or MT fractures are presented with non-weight-bearing lameness with lifting of the affected limb. Diagnosis of MC and MT fractures is easy, as the fracture site can be readily palpated. Most often, open fractures occur due to little soft tissue covering of the bones, and many times, if not treated early, a closed fracture may become open with protruding of bone fragments. A plain radiograph may be obtained to determine the nature of fracture and to decide the line of treatment.

As the MC and MT bones are placed straight, their fractures are relatively easy to repair even in heavy animals. Alignment and positioning of the fracture fragments can be achieved with relative ease following closed reduction (favored by least soft tissue coverage). Most simple fractures in young animals can be treated by splint and bandage application. Application of a cast will provide more rigid fixation [47, 48], and in heavy large animals, fiberglass cast is preferred, which is lightweight and stronger (Fig. 4.33). Comminuted or overriding fractures may be better treated using a transfixation cast in both cattle

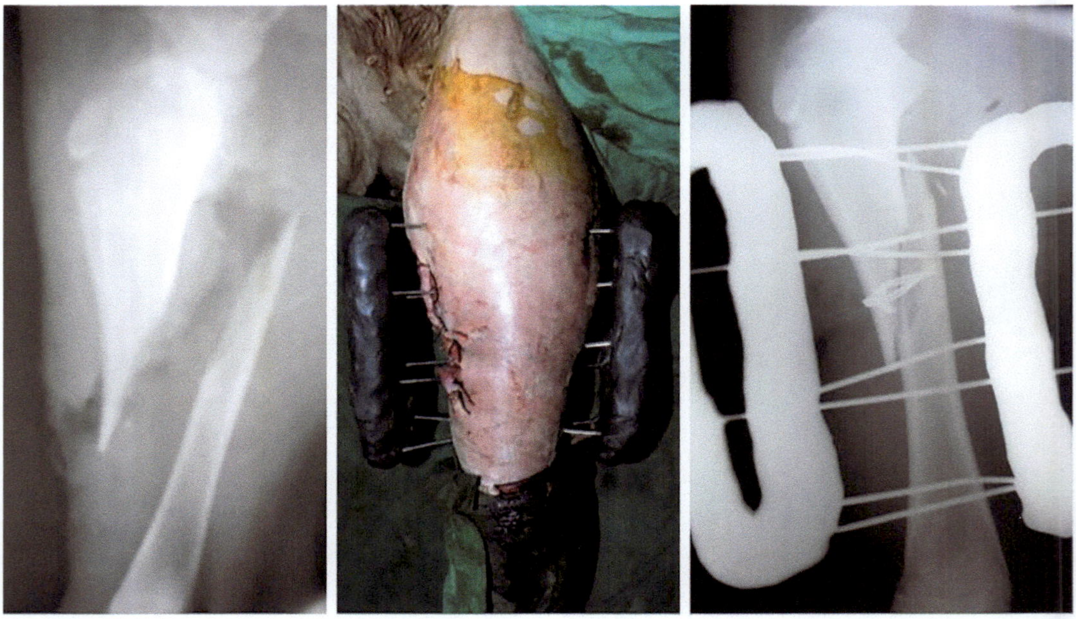

**Fig. 4.32** Cerclage wiring with epoxy-pin fixation (3 mm pins) for repair of open tibial fracture in a calf

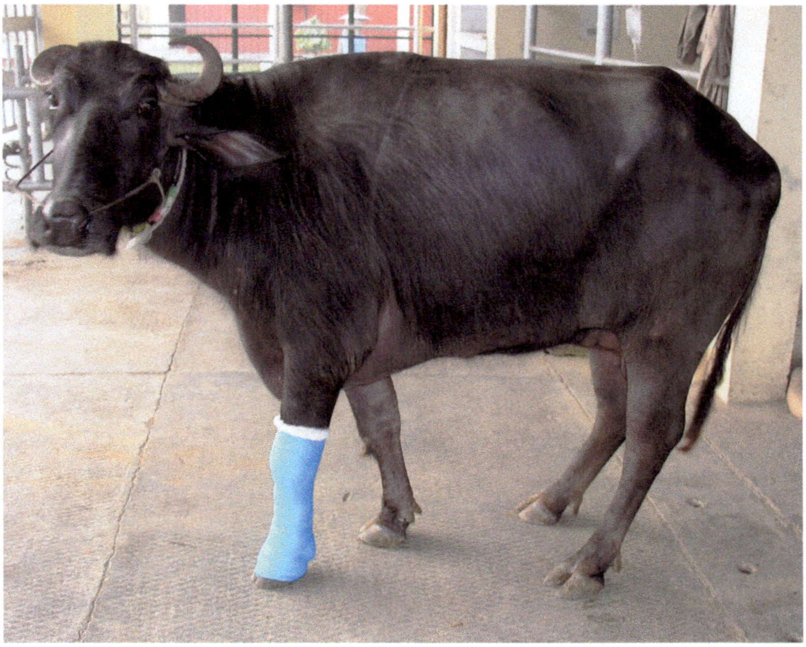

**Fig. 4.33** Fiberglass cast application for metacarpal fracture repair in an adult buffalo weighing about 500 kg. Note good weight bearing on the limb immediately after bone fixation

and horses [46, 49, 50]. Most fractures, including comminuted ones, can heal and remodel adequately, without adversely affecting the functional recovery of the limb [48].

Bone plating is not advised in young animals, as there is little soft tissue covering and the bones are too soft for screw fixation. Nevertheless, in juvenile bones, LCPs can provide stable bone fixation with good prognosis in surgical repair of fractures [51]. In adult animals, DCP or LCP fixation provides rigid fixation of MC/MT fractures [52]. Usually, one plate fixed on dorsolateral surface is sufficient to provide rigid fixation. In heavy adult animals, double plating provides more stable fixation (Fig. 4.34). Additional external support along with plate fixation

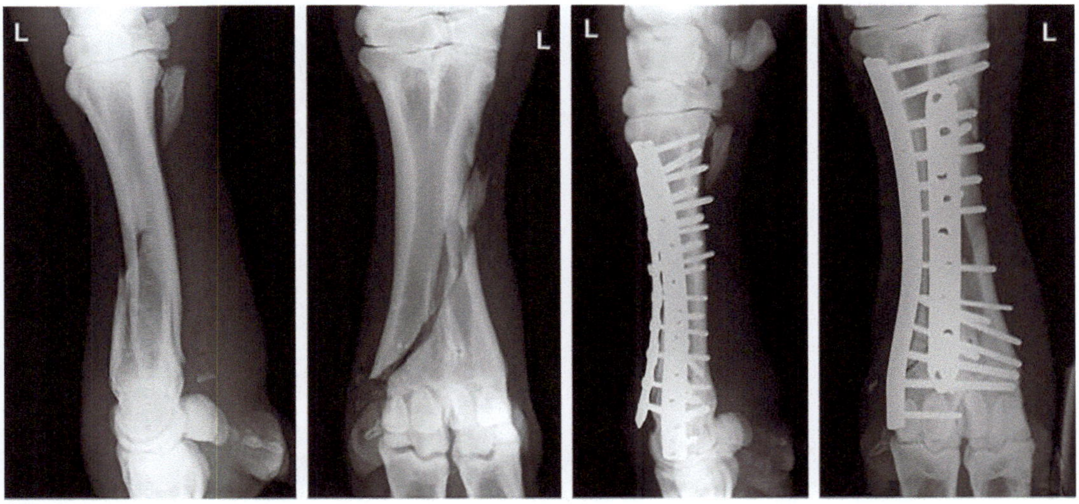


**Fig. 4.34** Left metacarpal bone with several fragments in an adult cow; A DCP was placed medially and an LCP was placed dorsally (Reproduced with permission from: Karl Nuss, Plates, Pins, and Interlocking Nails. Vet Clin Food Anim 30: 91–126, 2014)

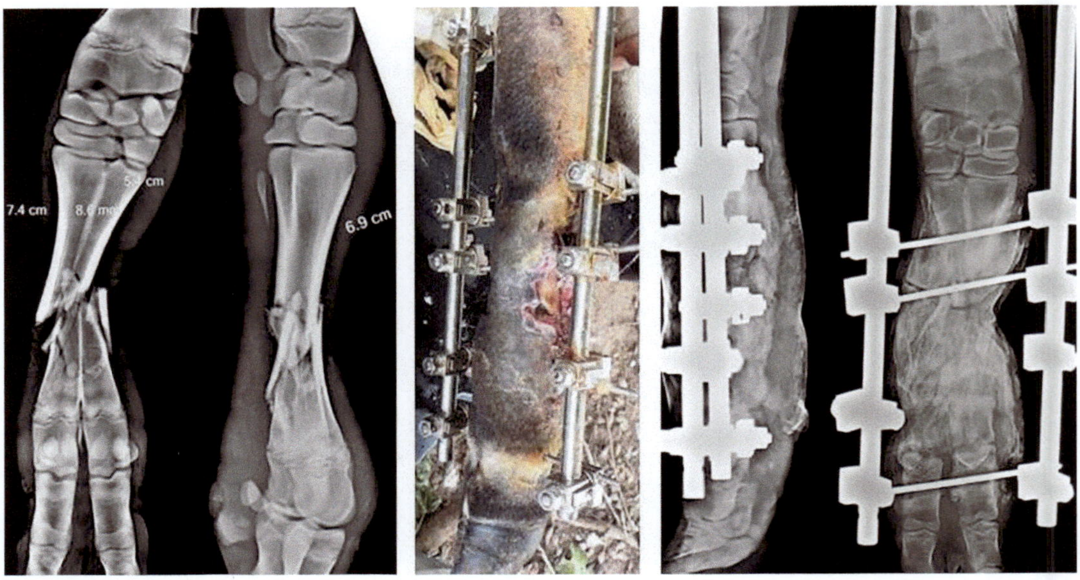


**Fig. 4.35** Open comminuted fracture of metacarpus in a cattle treated using transcarpal application of a bilateral linear fixator. Note staged destabilization, leading to bone healing with large external callus formation (Courtesy: Dr. Remala Sridhar, Tanuku, Andhra Pradesh, India)

may be provided for 3–4 weeks to protect the fracture site from direct weight-bearing loads. Prognosis of MC and MT fracture repair is usually favorable with good functional recovery.

As most of the fractures of MC and MT in large animals are open and infected, external skeletal fixation is more often used [4, 53]. As these bones are placed relatively straight along the long axis of the limb, transfixation pinning and bilateral linear fixation systems are very well suited (Fig. 4.35 and 4.36). Use of circular fixator, however, provides more stable fixation in heavy

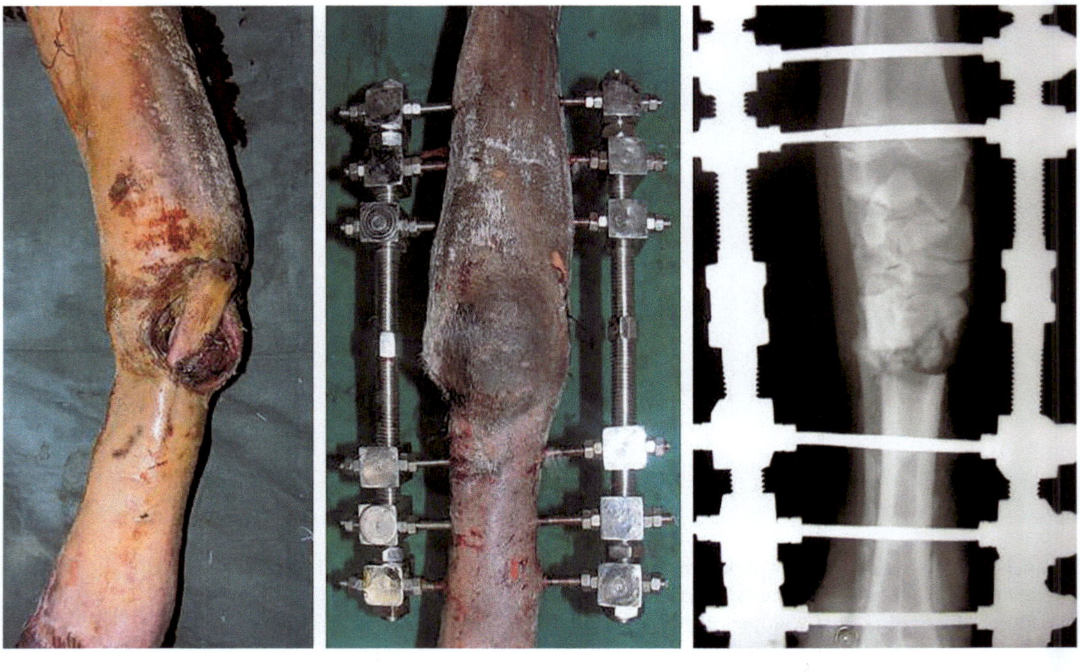

**Fig. 4.36** Transcarpal application of novel bilateral linear fixator for proximal metacarpal fracture fixation in cattle

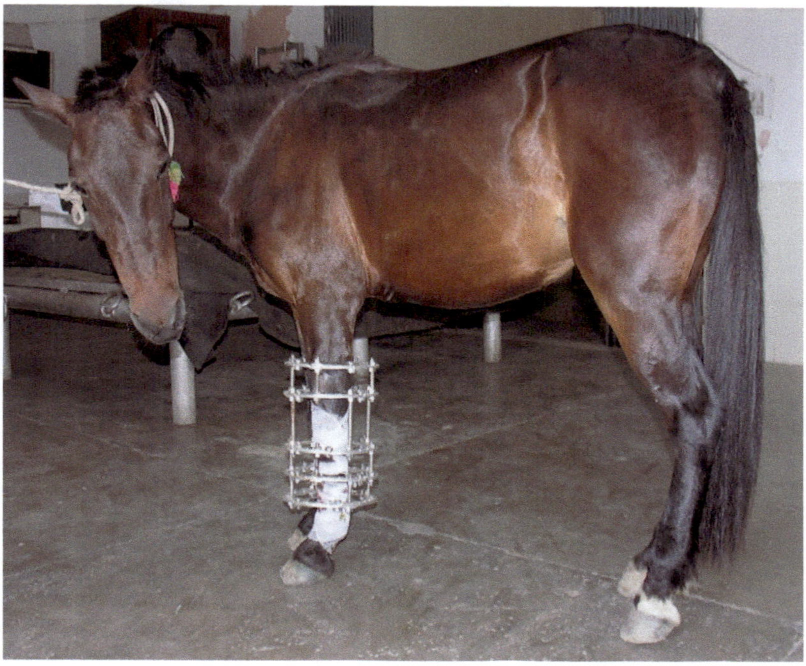

**Fig. 4.37** Use of circular external fixator in metacarpal fracture repair in a horse

animals (Fig. 4.37). ESF is all the more useful in cases where the fracture is near the joint (at one end of the bone) needing transarticular fixation. Proximal MC fractures can be treated using either linear or circular fixator [23, 54]. However, in proximal MT, fractures only circular fixators are recommended, as in angularly placed tibia, linear fixators cannot provide stability (Fig. 4.38).

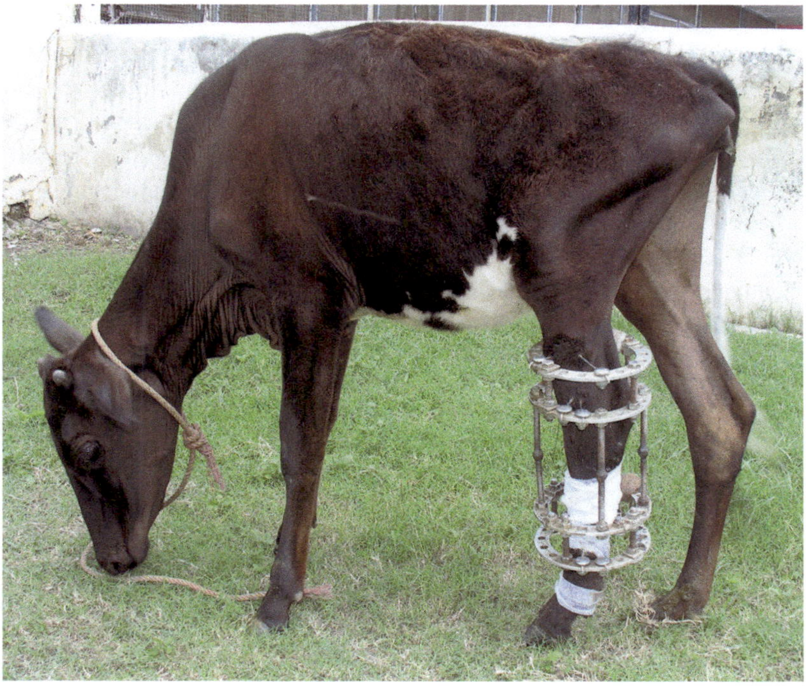

**Fig. 4.38** Transtarsal application of CEF in proximal metatarsal fracture in a calf

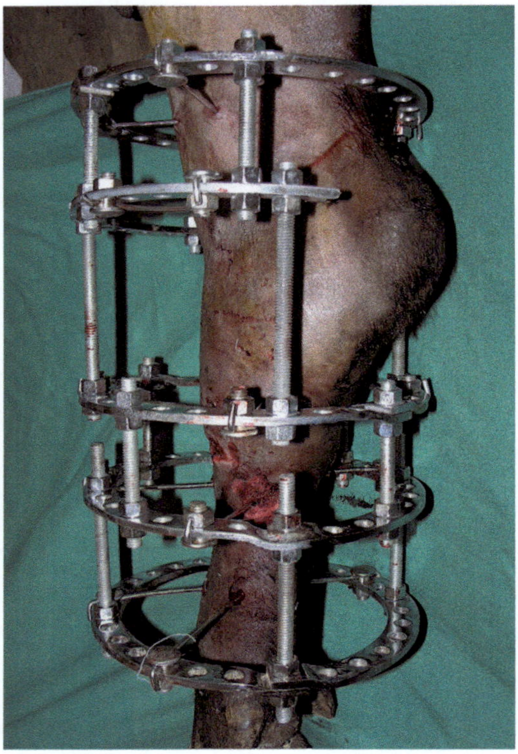

**Fig. 4.39** Use of incomplete rings in transtarsal application of CEF

Fixation near the tarsal joint requires use of incomplete rings to avoid injury to Achilles tendon or tuber calcis (Fig. 4.39). As MC and MT are straight bones, most fractures can be rigidly immobilized, and usually, even severely infected open fractures can heal normally with good functional recovery of the limb. However, in cases where the bone is severely crushed along the whole length of bone, even conventional ESF techniques may fail to yield desired results. In such cases, modified walking cast, which can immobilize the joints, and the fractured bone can be shielded from load bearing, may be attempted (Fig. 4.40). In young animals (weighing <100 kg), open fractures may be better managed with epoxy-pin external skeletal fixation [26] (Fig. 4.41).

Fracture/luxation of the phalanges is often seen in large ruminants. The distal phalanx (medial/lateral claw) is most often involved. In such cases, the affected claw may be trimmed, and if severely necrosed, it may be amputated completely and bandaged. Closed fractures of the proximal and middle phalanges are best immobilized with a plaster cast/fiberglass cast. The cast should completely encase the foot and extend proximally up to the level of carpus or tarsus. The incorporation of a metallic walking bar within the cast prevents direct loading of the injured site during weight bearing. Open fractures/luxations with evidence of infection can be treated by surgical removal of the loose necrotic tissues and by application of an ESF (Figs. 4.42 and 4.43).

## 4.6 Fractures of Pelvis

Pelvic fractures usually occur in mature adult animals, and the wing of ilium is the most common site in large ruminants [4]. In foals, fractures involving the tuber coxae, tuber ischii, acetabulum, and shaft of the ilium are common. Fractures involving multiple pelvic bones are usually seen as a result of an automobile accident. Pelvic fractures in equines are often caused due to trauma related to athletic activities. Separation of the pubic symphysis is often seen due to dystocia and subsequent obstetrical manipulations.

Fractures of the ilium are easy to diagnose on physical examination. The attachment of the *tensor fascia lata* and *obliquus abdominis internus* muscles results in ventral displacement of the fractured ilium, leading to "knocked down hip." The rectal examination is useful to evaluate the internal symmetry of the pelvic cavity. Fractures involving the acetabulum often cause severe pain and non-weight-bearing lameness. In case of multiple fractures of the pelvis, the animal is generally recumbent and unable to stand. Digital radiography will aid in confirmatory diagnosis; however, often, it is difficult to obtain desired images; hence, combination of nuclear scintigraphy and ultrasonography can be used especially in equines.

Due to heavy surrounding musculature, the pelvis is difficult to approach surgically, especially in heavy adult animals. Conservatively, pelvic fracture can be treated by stall confinement for 8–12 weeks. The prognosis following a pelvic

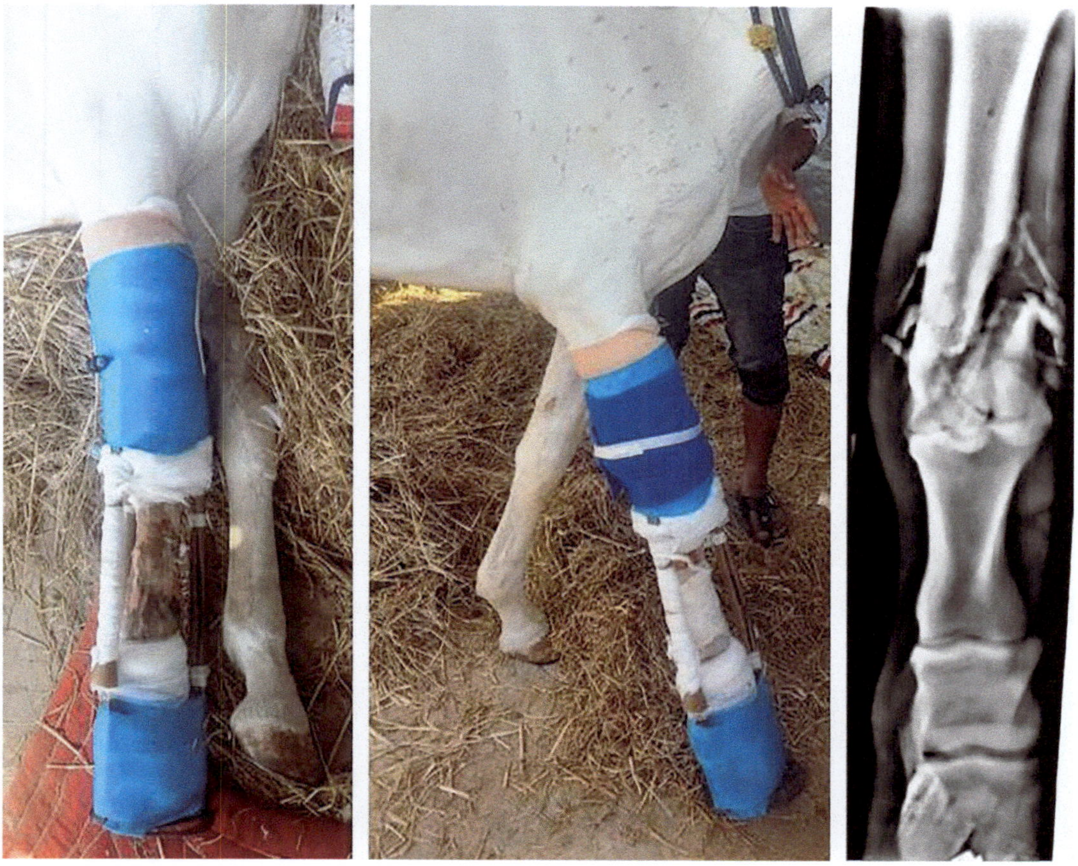

**Fig. 4.40** Modified walking cast used to stabilize a case of open comminuted fracture of metacarpus in a horse. Both the joints above and below are immobilized with fiberglass cast interconnected with strong steel side rods fixed to a circular foot rest and a ring at carpal region to transmit the load by shielding the fracture site. The wound site is kept open for drainage and dressing. Good functional recovery achieved. (Courtesy: Col. RV Dhumal, Navi Mumbai, India)

fracture depends on its location, and ilial fractures usually heal well. However, deformity of the pelvic cavity (due to large callus formation or otherwise) may affect the breeding value of the animal, often leading to dystocia during subsequent pregnancies. The prognosis is generally poor in cases of multiple pelvic fractures, especially when the acetabulum is involved (leads to osteoarthritis) and the obturator nerve is injured.

## 4.7 Fractures of Mandible

Mandibular fractures are relatively uncommon in bovines, but they are the most frequently recorded fractures of the head region in cattle as well as camels [4]. The fractures are commonly located at the interdental space, the molar region, and the mandibular symphysis. Animals less than 1 year old are more commonly affected. In neonates, the most common cause of mandibular fractures is trauma during obstetrical manipulation, due to excessive force applied to mandibular loop attached to the lower jaw to correct a malposition of fetus. Fractures may also occur when an animal slips or falls striking the head on a hard object. In camels, mandibular fractures usually occur due to infighting during breeding season or due to a solid blow by a hard object.

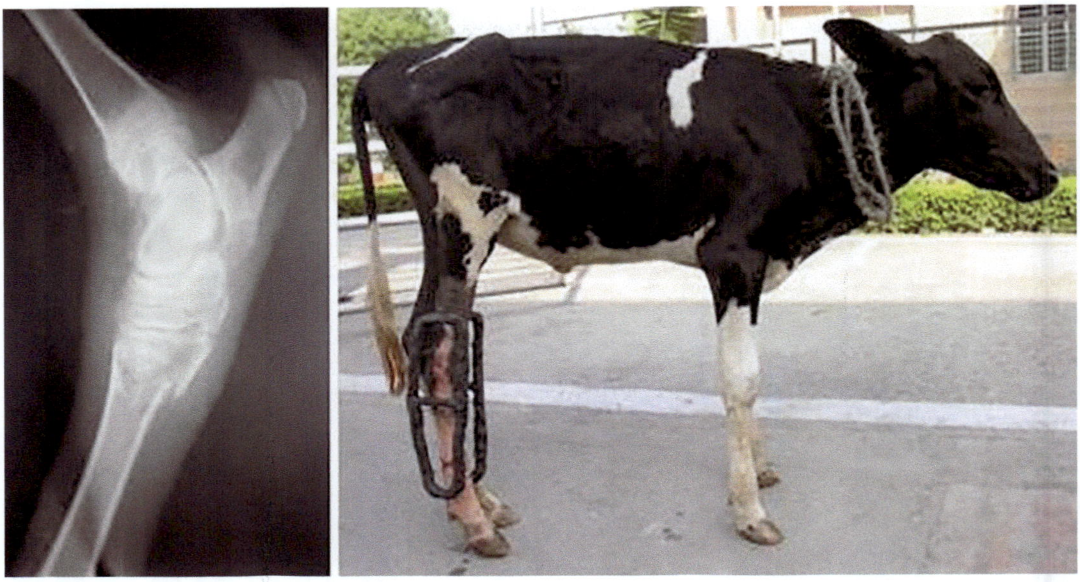

**Fig. 4.41** Epoxy-pin ESF applied transtarsally for repair of proximal metatarsal open fracture in a calf

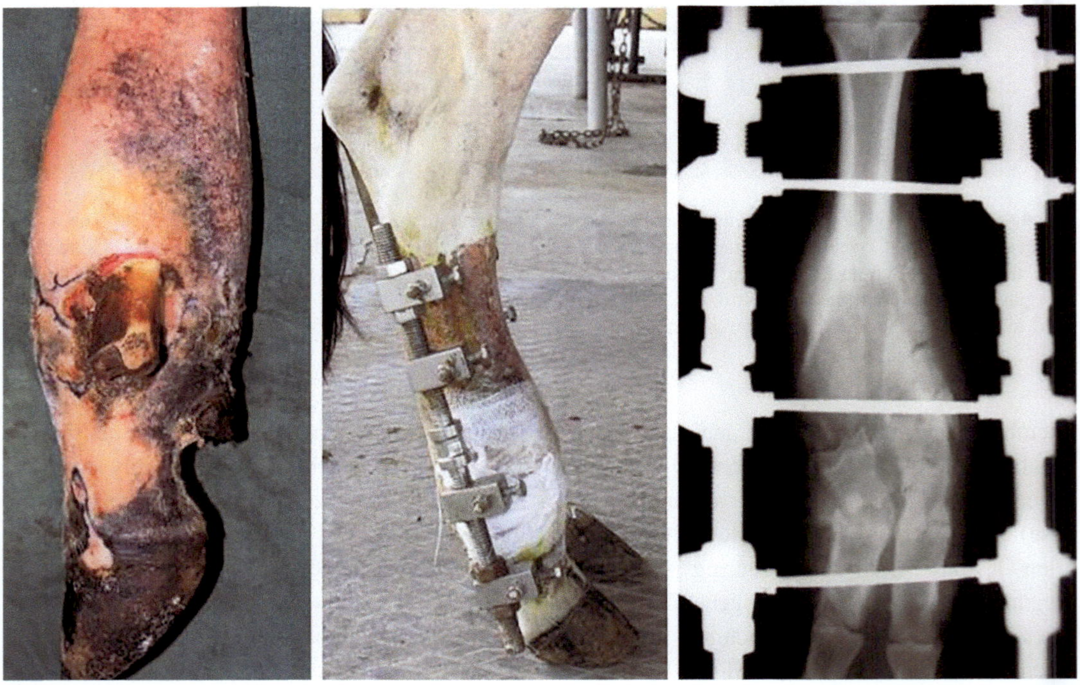

**Fig. 4.42** Open fracture at distal end of metatarsus treated using linear ESF

In neonates, the fractures are mostly open and located rostral to the premolars, and in cattle over 1 year of age, fractures are often seen in the molar region. Very rarely adult cattle and horses sustain fractures caudal to the interdental region. Fractures of the vertical ramus are rare due to protection from the masseter and pterygoid muscles. Fractures are frequently seen in both

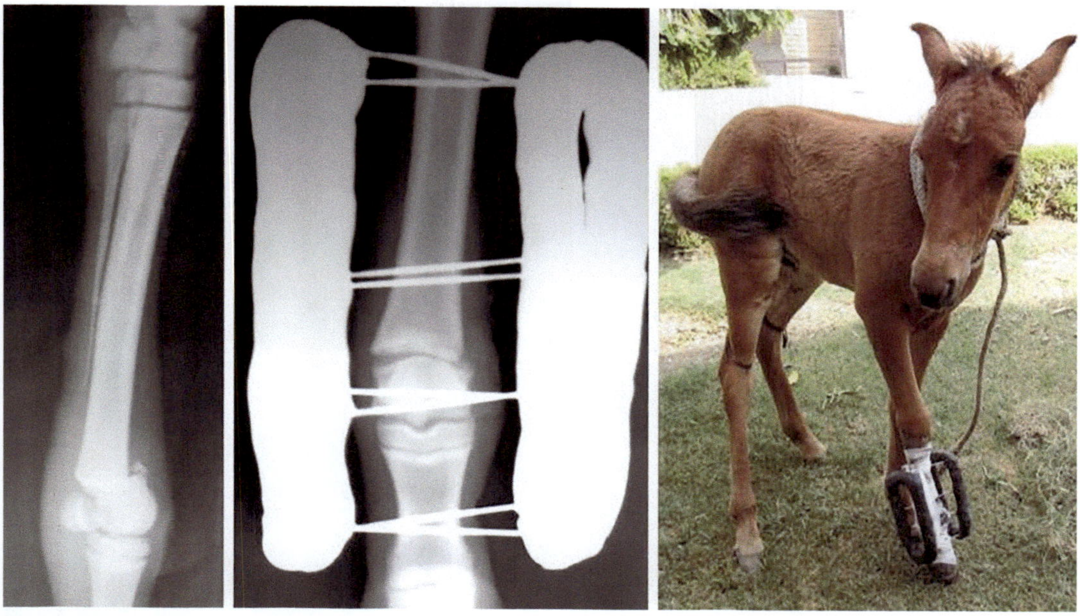

**Fig. 4.43** Epoxy-pin fixation for distal metaphyseal fracture of metacarpus in a foal

mandibles, but in mature cattle, unilateral mandibular fractures are often encountered. Open fractures are more common than closed fractures.

Mandibular fractures exhibit clinical signs of downward hanging of the rostral fractured fragment, protrusion of the tongue, drooling of saliva, and malaligned teeth, and in many cases, variable size of open wound may be visible with protruding fractured bone ends. The oral wound is generally filled with food materials, with the animal exhibiting difficulty in prehension and mastication. Mandibular fracture can easily be diagnosed by physical examination, and radiography is needed only to determine the configuration and extent of fracture [4].

The conservative treatment of mandibular fractures in cattle generally does not result in favorable outcome, as there will be difficulty in chewing and mastication. Rostral mandibular fractures in calves have been successfully treated using external coaptation [55]. The surgical fixation of mandibular fractures can provide sufficient stability of broken segments allowing painless mastication and rumination until fracture healing. Due to difficulty in accessing the fracture site and persistent tongue and jaw motions, general anesthesia is always preferred for surgical fixation of mandibular fractures. Treatment should include debridement, lavage, and suturing of gum lacerations, in addition to fixation of fractured bone.

In young calves, mandibular fractures can be repaired either by using a modified Kirschner-Ehmer apparatus, bilateral intramedullary pins, or cerclage wires (Fig. 4.44). Internal fixation generally provides satisfactory results, due to good speed of healing in young animals and the relative technical ease of exposure and stabilization. However, pins have a tendency to migrate or become loose before fracture healing. Intraosseous implants may often damage tooth roots. Intraoral PMMA splint positioned on the tension surface of the mandible has been reported to have less disadvantages and provide stable fixation.

In mature cattle, conservative treatment can be attempted if there is a unilateral nondisplaced fracture of the mandible. However, constant movement and infiltration of saliva and food into fractured dental alveoli may result in delayed healing. Interdental wiring and cross pinning techniques have been reported to provide adequate fixation in simple fractures [56–59]. Bone plating (DCP/LCP) of the ventrolateral aspect of the mandibule provides a stable reduction [60–62]. The ramus can be exposed by giving an

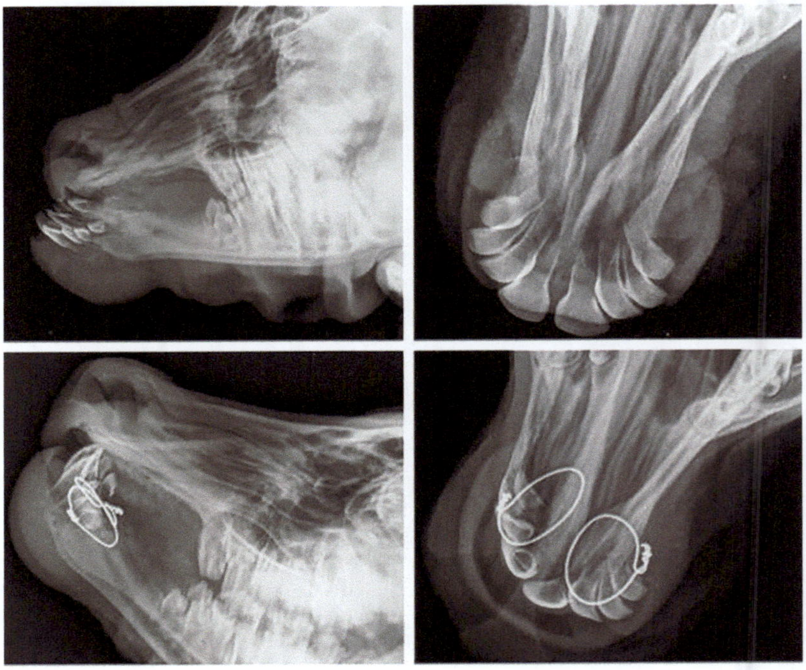

**Fig. 4.44** Interdental wiring for repair mandibular fracture in a cattle

incision directly over its ventrolateral aspect, by protecting the parotid duct, artery, and vein. The screws are placed on the lower side of horizontal ramus to avoid damage to the teeth roots. A bone plate can be applied similarly on the other side in case of a bilateral fracture. Use of type I and II external fixators have been used successfully in adult animals [63, 64] (Fig. 4.45). Acrylic/epoxy-pin ESF can also be used, as it has the advantage of ease of application and better contouring to the

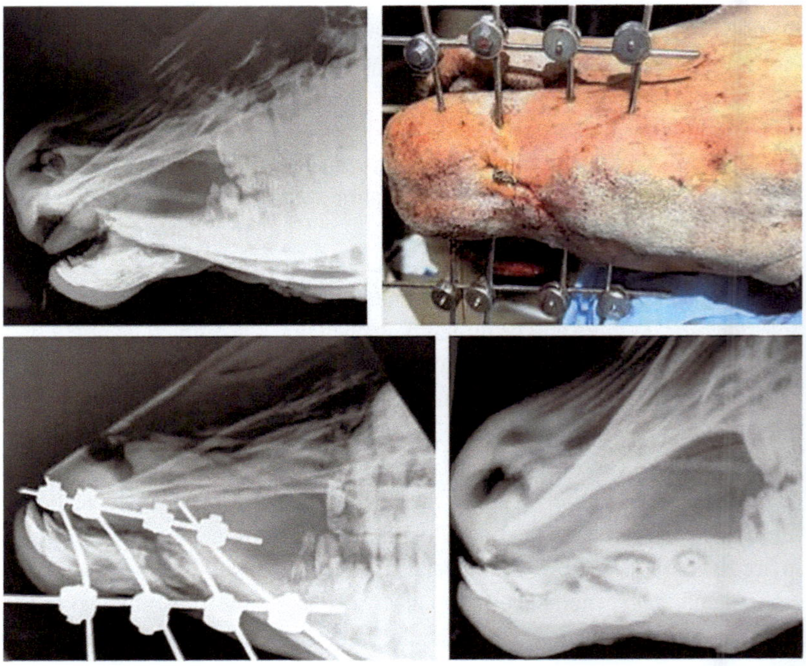

**Fig. 4.45** Type II ESF used for repair of mandibular fracture in cattle (Courtesy: Dr. Sachin Vende and Dr. Sandip Pawar, Veterinary Polyclinic, Nashik, Maharashtra, India)

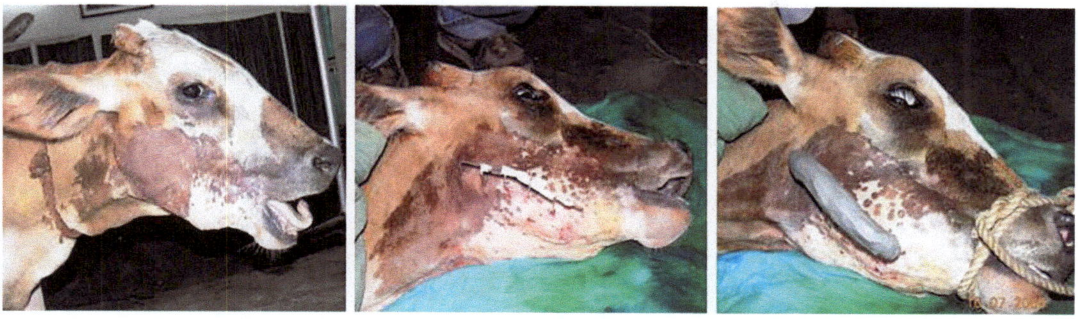

**Fig. 4.46** Epoxy-pin ESF for repair of bilateral mandibular fracture in cattle

fractured bone [65] (Fig. 4.46). An AO/ASIF pinless external fixator was found to provide stable fixation of unilateral mandibular fractures in cattle and horses [66, 67]. The major benefits of this technique are ease of application and least surgical trauma without causing any injury to the tooth roots.

Different treatment methods have been described for fixation of symphyseal fractures, such as fixation of an external fixator, application of Steinmann pins or clamps, lag screw fixation, and fixation of cerclage wires by fastening and securing between the teeth externally. Use of an external fixator for treatment of mandibular fractures has the limitations of accidental injury to the tooth roots and possible pin tract infections. Use of external clamps in place of Steinmann pins can prevent damage to tooth roots and possible infection. Lag screw fixation also has the potential to damage the tooth roots and harbor infection, especially in open infected fractures.

An external fixation technique using a cerclage wires anchored to the incisors has been described for fixation of open infected mandibular symphyseal fractures [68, 69]. The technique includes placing the cerclage wire loops (1.5 mm wires) around the base of each incisor from the inner (lingual) side to outer/external (labial) side, and the free end of the wire is secured along by inserting through each wire loop on the external side (Fig. 4.47). Lastly, each wire loop (also the wire ends) is tightened gently between the teeth alternatively till the symphyseal gap disappear and the fracture is secured. If applied correctly, cerclage wires can provide stable fixation leading to good bone healing as the fracture site is devoid of any implant. As the cerclage wires do not pierce the bone, injury to the tooth roots is prevented.

Postoperative care in mandibular fracture repair consists of a course of antibiotic therapy, with regular removal of food material trapped at the fracture site and along the internal fixation device and lavage of the oral cavity with mild antiseptic solution [4]. The animal should be fed a soft liquid diet for the initial 2–3 weeks. Results of surgical fixation of mandibular fractures in bovines and equines are generally successful, particularly with more rostral fractures. The primary complications are related to management of concurrent problems such as nutritional deficiency, septicemia, and osteomyelitis, which should be a concern in therapy of bovine open mandibular fractures, despite the relative resistance to infection in wounds of the oral cavity.

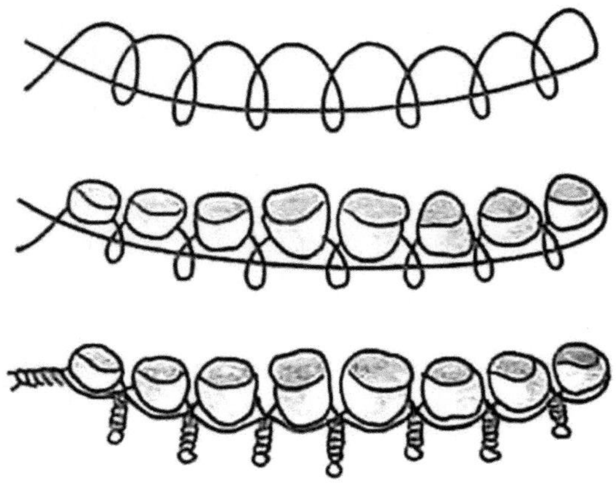

**Fig. 4.47** Schematic presentation of cerclage wires anchored externally to the teeth to immobilize mandibular symphyseal fracture

## Chapter 4: Sample Questions

### Q. No. 1: Mark the correct answer

1. In diaphyseal fracture of humerus, double plating is done on the following surfaces
   (a) laterally and medially (b) laterally and caudally (c) cranially and laterally (d) cranially and medially
2. In young lightweight animals, open infected fractures of metacarpus/metatarsus can be better managed using
   (a) cast application (b) modified Thomas splint (c) bone plating (d) epoxy-pin ESF
3. For tibial fractures in heavy animals, which of the following technique provides most rigid fixation
   (a) standard full limb cast (b) hanging limb pin cast (c) walking limb cast (d) transfixation pin and cast
4. Preferred technique for the management of distal femoral fractures in young animals is
   (a) bone plating (b) interlocking nailing (c) multiple cross pinning (d) external skeletal fixation
5. Compound fracture of radius/ulna in large heavy animals can be best managed with
   (a) IM pinning (b) plaster cast (c) bone plating (d) external fixator

### Q. No. 2: State true or false

1. Fracture of scapula is uncommon in large animals.
2. Stack pinning or cross IM pinning generally provides stable fixation of humerus fractures leading to good healing in young large ruminants.
3. Radius-ulna are well suited for external fixation as the bones are fairly straight and surrounded by little soft tissues.
4. As the fore limb is straight, bilateral linear fixators generally provide good fixation of open fractures of the radius-ulna.
5. The lateral surface of the distal tibia is devoid of much soft tissue coverage; hence, most often, distal tibial fractures get open on the lateral surface.
6. A nail can be placed in the medullary cavity without damaging the articulating surface of the stifle joint through the cranio-lateral surface of proximal tibia.
7. For trans-tarsal applications, linear ESF system is better than circular ESF system.
8. The fractures of metacarpus and metatarsus are the common in large animals.
9. Cerclage wire anchored to the incisors can provide good stability of symphyseal fracture of the mandible without penetrating the medullary cavity and causing damage to the tooth roots.

### Q. No. 3: Fill up the blanks

1. The humeral diaphysis is surgically exposed by retracting the ______________________ muscle caudally and the ______________________ muscle cranially, and the distal humerus is approached by cranial retraction of ______________________ and caudal retraction of ______________________ muscle.
2. For plate osteosynthesis, the radius is either approached through the ______________________ approach, which provides easier access to the bone, or the ______________________ approach, which allows adequate soft tissue covering of the plate.

3. In femoral diaphyseal fractures, double plate fixation can be achieved by fixing one on the ____________________ and another on the ______________________ surface to provide greater stability.
4. In supracondylar femoral fractures, interlocking nail could be introduced by normograde technique through the ________ ____________________________ to provide better anchorage in the small distal segment.
5. Cast application is difficult in tibia due to __________________________________-____, ______________________________ and ______________ and ______________________.
6. Due to angular placement of bone, open tibial fractures can be better treated using ______ ____________ ESF than ___________ _________ ESF systems.
7. ______________________________________ is the most common site of pelvic fracture in adult ruminants.

**Q. No. 4: Write short note on the following**

1. Multiple cross pin fixation in supracondylar femoral fractures
2. Metacarpal and metatarsal fractures
3. Interlocking nailing in bovine tibia
4. Plate osteosynthesis in radius-ulna
5. Mandibular fracture repair using cerclage wiring
6. Open fracture repair in radius vs. tibia using an ESF
7. Hanging limb pin cast for tibial fracture management

## References


1. Auer, J.A., and A. Furst. 2015. Fractures of the scapula. *Equine Veterinary Education* 29 (4): 184. https://doi.org/10.1111/eve.12496.
2. Ferguson, J.D. 1997. Surgical conditions of the proximal limb. In *Lamenesss in cattle*, ed. P.R. Greenough, 3rd ed., 252–276. Philadelphia: W.B. Saunders Company.
3. Tulleners, E P. 1986. Management of bovine orthopedic problems. Part 1. Fractures. *Compendium on Continuing Education for the Practicing Veterinarian* 8: S69–S80.
4. Singh, A.P., G.R. Singh, H.P. Aithal, and P. Singh. 2020. Section D – fractures, chapter on the musculoskeletal system. In *Ruminant surgery: A textbook of the surgical diseases of cattle, buffaloes, camels, sheep and goats*, ed. J. Singh, S. Singh, and R.P.S. Tyagi, 2nd ed. New Delhi: CBS Publishers and Distributers.
5. Rakestraw, P.C. 1996. Fractures of the humerus. *The Veterinary Clinics of North America. Food Animal Practice* 12: 153–168.
6. St. Jean, G., and B.L. Hull. 1987. Conservative treatment of humeral fracture in a heifer. *The Canadian Veterinary Journal* 28: 704–706.
7. Markel, M.D., D.M. Nunamaker, J.D. Wheat, and A.E. Sams. 1988. In vitro comparison of three fixation methods for humeral fracture repair in adult horses. *American Journal of Veterinary Research* 49: 586–593.
8. Rakestraw, P.C., A.J. Nixon, R.E. Kaderly, and N.G. Ducharme. 1991. Cranial approach to the humerus for repair of fractures in horses and cattle. *Veterinary Surgery* 20: 1–8.
9. Ramakumar, V., G.R. Singh, and S.C. Datt. 1976. Use of Kuntschner nail in spiral fracture of humerus in a buffalo heifer-a case report. *The Indian Veterinary Journal* 53: 64–65.
10. Nuss, K. 2014. Plates, pins and interlocking nails. *Veterinary Clinics of North America: Food Animal Practice* 30: 91–126.
11. Gamper, S., A. Steiner, K. Nuss, S. Ohlerth, A. Furst, J. Ferguson, J. Auer, and C. Lischer. 2006. Clinical evaluation of the CRIF 4.5/5.5 system for long-bone fracture repair in cattle. *Veterinary Surgery* 35: 361–368.
12. Yamagishi, N., B. Devkota, and M. Takahashi. 2014. Outpatient treatment for humeral fractures in five calves. *The Journal of Veterinary Medical Science* 76: 1519–1522.
13. Aithal, H.P., and G.R. Singh. 1999. A survey of bone fractures in cattle, sheep and goats. *The Indian Veterinary Journal* 76: 636–639.
14. Gangl, M., Grulke, S., Serteyn, D. And Touati, K. 2006. Retrospective study of 99 cases of bone fractures in cattle treated by external coaptation or confinement. The Veterinary Record 158: 264–268
15. Lozier, J.W., A.J. Niehaus, A. Muir, and J. Lakritz. 2018. Short- and long-term success of transfixation pin casts used to stabilize long bone fractures in ruminants. *The Canadian Veterinary Journal* 59: 635–641.
16. Trostle, S.S. 2004. Internal fixation. In *Farm animal surgery*, ed. D.L. Fubini and G. Ducharme, 290–315. St Louis (MO): Saunders.
17. Auer, J., A. Steiner, U. Iselin, and C. Lischer. 1993. Internal fixation of long bone fractures in farm animals. *Veterinary and Comparative Orthopaedics and Traumatology* 6: 36–41.
18. Trostle, S., D. Wilson, P. Hanson, and C.E. Brown. 1995. Management of radial fracture in an adult bull.

*Journal of the American Veterinary Medical Association* 206: 1917–1919.
19. Ahmad, R.A. 2013. Development and evaluation of designer locking plates for fixation of tibial and radial fractures in large ruminants. PhD thesis submitted to Deemed University, Indian Veterinary Research Institute, Izatnagar- 243 122 (UP), India.
20. Hague, B.A., R.N. Hooper, A.J. Roussel, T.S. Taylor, and J.P. Watkins. 1997. Tension band plating of an olecranon fracture in a bull. *Journal of the American Veterinary Medical Association* 211: 757–758.
21. Aithal, H.P. 2015. Management of fractures. In *A handbook on field veterinary surgery*, ed. M.M.S. Zama, H.P. Aithal, and A.M. Pawde, 145–154. New Delhi: Published by Astral.
22. Aithal, H.P., Amarpal, P. Kinjavdekar, A.M. Pawde, K. Pratap, P. Kumar, D.K. Sinha, and H.C. Setia. 2009. A novel bilateral linear external skeletal fixation device for treatment of long bone fractures in large animals: A report of 12 clinical cases. 33rd Congress of ISVS held at Veterinary college, GADVASU, Ludhiana (Punjab), 11–13 Nov. 2009, Abst: OR-1.
23. Aithal, H.P., Amarpal, P. Kinjavdekar, A.M. Pawde, G.R. Singh, M. Hoque, S.K. Maiti, and H.C. Setia. 2007. Management of fractures near carpal joint of two calves by transarticular fixation with a circular external fixator. *The Veterinary Record* 161: 193–198.
24. Aithal, H.P., G.R. Singh, P. Kinjavdekar, Amarpal, M. Hoque, S.K. Maiti, A.M. Pawed, and H.C. Setia. 2007. Hybrid construct of linear and circular external skeletal fixation devices for fixation of long bone osteotomies in large ruminants. *The Indian Journal of Animal Sciences* 77: 1083–1090.
25. Singh, G.R., H.P. Aithal, Amarpal, P. Kinjavdekar, S.K. Maiti, M. Hoque, A.M. Pawde, and H.C. Joshi. 2007. Evaluation of two dynamic axial fixators for large ruminants. *Veterinary Surgery* 36: 88–97.
26. Aithal, H.P., P. Kinjavdekar, Pawde Amarpal, and A. M., Zama, M.M.S., Prasoon Dubey, Rohit Kumar, Tyagi S.K. and Madhu, D.N. 2019. Epoxy-pin external skeletal fixation for management of open bone fractures in calves and foals: a review of 32 cases. *Veterinary and Comparative Orthopaedics and Traumatology* 32: 257–268.
27. Nuss, K., A. Spiess, M. Feist, and R. Köstlin. 2011. Treatment of long bone fractures in 125 newborn calves. A retrospective study. *Tierärztliche Praxis. Ausgabe G, Grosstiere/Nutztiere* 39: 15–26.
28. McCann, M.E., and R.J. Hunt. 1993. Conservative management of femoral diaphyseal fractures in four foals. *The Cornell Veterinarian* 83: 125–132.
29. Nichols, S., D.E. Anderson, M.D. Miesner, and K.D. Newman. 2010. Femoral diaphyseal fractures in cattle: 26 cases (1994-2005). *Australian Veterinary Journal* 88: 39–44.
30. Bellon, J., and P.Y. Mulon. 2011. Use of a novel intramedullary nail for femoral fracture repair in calves: 25 cases (2008–2009). *Journal of the American Veterinary Medical Association* 238: 1490–1496.
31. Madhu, D.N. 2015. Development and evaluation of interlocking nail and tubular locking plate for management of femur fracture in large ruminants. PhD thesis submitted to Deemed University, Indian Veterinary Research Institute, Izatnagar- 243 122 (UP), India.
32. Denny, H.R., B. Sridhar, B.M. Weaver, and A. Waterman. 1988. The management of bovine fractures: a review of 59 cases. *The Veterinary Record* 123: 289–295.
33. Ashworth, C., M.J. Boero, G.J. Baker, and J. Huhn. 1990. Repair of distal femoral fractures in calves using a 90° blade plate. Scientific meeting abstracts - ACVS. *Veterinary Surgery* 19: 56.
34. Singh, A.P., K.K. Mirakhur, and J.M. Nigam. 1983. A study on the incidence and anatomical location of fractures in canine, caprine, bovine, equine and camel. *Indian Journal of Veterinary Surgery* 4: 61–66.
35. Ramakumar, V., M. Manohar, and R.P.S. Tyagi. 1973. Hanging pin cast for oblique fracture of tibia in a cow-A disadvantage. *The Indian Veterinary Journal* 50: 114.
36. Adams, S.B., and J.F. Fessler. 1983. Treatment of radial, ulnar and tibial fractures in cattle, using a modified Thomas splint cast combination. *Journal of the American Veterinary Medical Association* 183: 430–433.
37. Anderson, D.E., and St. Jean, G. 2008. Management of fractures in field settings. *The Veterinary Clinics of North America. Food Animal Practice* 24: 567–582.
38. Vijaykumar, D.S., J.M. Nigham, A.P. Singh, et al. 1984. Experimental studies on fracture repair of the tibia in the bovine. *Journal of Veterinary Orthopedics* 3: 6–12.
39. Bhat, S.A., H.P. Aithal, P. Kinjavdekar, Amarpal, M.M.S. Zama, P.C. Gope, A.M. Pawde, R.A. Ahmad, and M.B. Gugjoo. 2014. An in vitro biomechanical investigation of an intramedullary interlocking nail system developed for buffalo tibia. *Veterinary and Comparative Orthopaedics and Traumatology* 27: 36–44.
40. Ahmad, R.A., H.P. Aithal, D.N. Madhu, Amarpal, P. Kinjavdekar, and A.M. Pawde. 2017. Use of locking plate in combination with dynamic compression plate for repair of tibial fracture in a young horse. *Iranian Journal of Veterinary Research* 18: 138–141.
41. Ahmad, R.A., H.P. Aithal, Amarpal, P. Kinjavdekar, P.C. Gope, and D.N. Madhu. 2021. Biomechanical properties of a novel locking compression plate to stabilize oblique tibial osteotomies in buffaloes. *Veterinary Surgery* 50: 444–454.
42. Aithal, H.P., Amarpal, P. Kinjavdekar, A.M. Pawde, G.R. Singh, and H.C. Setia. 2010. Management of tibial fractures using a circular external fixator in two calves. *Veterinary Surgery* 39: 621–626.
43. Aithal, H.P., G.R. Singh, M. Hoque, S.K. Maiti, P. Kinjavdekar, Amarpal, A.M. Pawde, and H.C. Setia. 2004. The use of circular external skeletal fixation device for the management of long bone

osteotomies in large ruminants: an experimental study. *Journal of Veterinary Medicine* A51: 284–293.
44. Shah, M.A., Rohit Kumar, P. Kinjavdekar, Amarpal, H.P. Aithal, Mohammad Arif Basha, and Asif Majid. 2022. The use of circular and hybrid external skeletal fixation systems to repair open tibial fractures in large ruminants: a report of six clinical cases. *Veterinary Research Communications* 46: 563–575.
45. Singh, G.R., H.P. Aithal, R.K. Saxena, P. Kinjavdekar, Amarpal, M. Hoque, S.K. Maiti, A.M. Pawde, and H.C. Joshi. 2007. In-vitro biomechanical properties of linear, circular and hybrid external skeletal fixation devices developed for use in large ruminants. *Veterinary Surgery* 36: 80–87.
46. Mulon, P.Y. 2017. Fractures of the metatarsal/metacarpal. In *Farm animal surgery*, ed. S.L. Fubini and N.G. Ducharme, 2nd ed., 416. S. Louis: Elsevier.
47. Koestlin, R., K. Nuss, and E. Elma. 1990. Metacarpal and metatarsal fractures in cattle. Treatment and results. *Tierärztliche Praxis* 18: 131–144.
48. Tulleners, E.P. 1986. Metacarpal and metatarsal fractures in dairy cattle-33 cases (1979-1985). *Journal of the American Veterinary Medical Association* 189: 463–468.
49. Lescun, T.B., S.R. McClure, M.P. Ward, C. Downs, D.A. Wilson, S.B. Adams, J.F. Hawkins, and E.L. Reinertson. 2007. Evaluation of transfixation casting for treatment of third metacarpal, third metatarsal, and phalangeal fractures in horses: 37 cases (1994–2004) *Journal of the American Veterinary Medical Association* 230 (9): 1340–1349.
50. Mulon, P.Y. 2017. External fixation. In *Farm animal surgery*, ed. S.L. Fubini and N.G. Ducharme, 2nd ed., 400–405. St. Louis: Elsevier.
51. Belge, A., I Akin, A. Gulaydin, and M.F. Yazici. 2016. The treatment of distal metacarpus fracture with locking compression plate in calves. *Turkish Journal of Veterinary and Animal Sciences* 40: 234–242.
52. Gillespie, A. 2018. Internal fixation of a comminuted metacarpal fracture in a bull. *Veterinary Record Case Reports*. https://doi.org/10.1136/vetreccr-2018-000630.
53. Dubey, P., H.P. Aithal, P. Kinjavdekar, Amarpal, P.C. Gope, D.N. Madhu, Rohit Kumar, T.B. Sivanarayanan, A.M. Pawde, and M.M.S. Zama. 2021. A comparative in vitro biomechanical investigation of a novel bilateral linear fixator vs. circular and multiplanar epoxy-pin external fixation systems using a fracture model in buffalo metacarpal bone. *World Journal of Surgery and Surgical Research* 4: 1331.
54. Bilgili, H., B. Kurum, and O. Captug. 2008. Use of a circular external skeletal fixator to treat comminuted metacarpal and tibial fractures in six calves. *The Veterinary Record* 163: 683–687.
55. Taguchi, K., and K. Hyakutake. 2012. External coaptation of rostral mandibular fractures in calves. *The Veterinary Record* 170: 598. https://doi.org/10.1136/vr.100606.
56. Nuss, K., R. Kostlin, E. Elma, and U. Matis. 1991. Mandibular fractures in cattle-treatment and results. *Tierärztliche Praxis* 19: 27–33.
57. Ramakumar, V., B. Prasad, J. Singh, and R.N. Kohli. 1981. Cross-pinning for repair of bilateral mandibular fracture in a bullock. *Modern Veterinary Practice* 62: 317.
58. Rizk, A., and M. Hamed. 2018. The use of cerclage wire for surgical repair of unilateral rostral mandibular fracture in horses. *Iranian Journal of Veterinary Research* 19: 123–127.
59. Trent, A.M., and J.G. Ferguson. 1985. Bovine mandibular fractures. *The Canadian Veterinary Journal* 26: 396–399.
60. Kuemmerle, J.M., M.A. Kummer, J.A. Auer, D. Nitzl, and A.E. Fürst. 2009. Locking compression plate osteosynthesis of complicated mandibular fractures in six horses. *Veterinary and Comparative Orthopaedics and Traumatology* 22: 54–58.
61. Murch, K.M. 1980. Repair of bovine and equine mandibular fractures. *The Canadian Veterinary Journal* 21: 69–73.
62. Wilson, D.G., A.M. Trent, and W.H. Crawford. 1990. A surgical approach to the ramus of the mandible in cattle and horses. Case reports of a bull and a horse. *Veterinary Surgery* 19: 191–195.
63. Belsito, K.A., and A.T. Fischer. 2001. External skeletal fixation in the management of equine mandibular fractures: 16 cases (1988–1998). *Equine Veterinary Journal* 33: 176–183.
64. Turek, B., O. Drewnowska, and M. Kaplan. 2019. External unilateral fixator of own design for the treatment of selected mandibular fractures in horses. *Applied Sciences* 9 (13): 2624. https://doi.org/10.3390/app9132624.
65. Colahan, P.T., and J.R. Pascoe. 1983. Stabilization of equine and bovine mandibular and maxilar fractures, using an acrylic splint. *Journal of the American Veterinary Medical Association* 182: 1117–1119.
66. Haralambus, R.M.A., C. Werren, W. Brehm, and C. Tessier. 2010. Use of a pinless external fixator for unilateral mandibular fracture repair in nine equids. *Veterinary Surgery* 39: 761–764.
67. Lischer, C.J., E. Fluri, B. Kaser-Hotz, R. Bettschart-Wolfensberger, and J.A. Auer. 1997. Pinless external fixation of mandible fractures in cattle. *Veterinary Surgery* 26: 14–19.
68. Rasekh, M., D. Devaux, J. Becker, and A. Steiner. 2011. Surgical fixation of symphyseal fracture of the mandible in a cow using cerclage wire. *The Veterinary Record* 169: 252. https://doi.org/10.1136/vr.d4303. Epub 2011 Aug 10.
69. Yaygingul, R., N. Kilic, and B. Kibar. 2018. Surgical treatment of a mandibular symphyseal fracture in a calf using a continuous wire-loop technique: a case report. *Veterinary Medicine* 63: 248–250.

# 5 Fractures in Young, Osteoporotic, and Avian Bones

**Learning Objectives**

You will be able to understand the following after reading this chapter:

- Principles of fracture fixation in young animals; open reduction and internal fixation, fractures involving the growth plate
- Principles and techniques of fracture management in osteopenic/osteoporotic bones.
- Management of fractures in avian bones

**Summary**

- The bone cortices in young animals are considerably thinner; hence, immature bone is highly susceptible to implant failure by pin migration or screw pullout.
- Fracture or trauma to the open growth plate in immature animals may arrest or alter the longitudinal growth of the bone leading to varied degrees of shortening and deformity of the limb.
- Fracture healing in young growing bones is rapid with abundant callus formation.
- The ideal form of internal fixation for bone fractures in young animals is smooth K-wires placed perpendicular to the epiphyseal plate; cross IM pinning using small K-wires is the method of choice in fractures near the stifle or elbow joints.
- In young animals, relatively small diameter Steinmann pins or K-wires are advised for IM fixation, as the greater portion of medullary cavity is filled with cancellous bone allowing better anchorage of pins than in adult animals.
- Locking compression plate developed using titanium alloy is light weight and hence may prove ideal for plate osteosynthesis in juvenile long bones.
- In hyperparathyroidism condition, the parathyroid gland produces excessive amounts of parathyroid hormone in response to reduced blood calcium level, leading to drainage of minerals from the bones ensuing in osteopenia.
- Osteopenic bones in young animals are elastic and have thin cortices and show mostly folding fractures, whereas osteoporotic bones in adult animals are brittle leading to comminution of bone.
- IM pin fixation provides favorable results in young animals, and plate osteosynthesis may prove better in adult animals with osteoporosis. Treatment of fractures in osteoporotic bones

(continued)


H. P. Aithal et al., *Textbook of Veterinary Orthopaedic Surgery*,
https://doi.org/10.1007/978-981-99-2575-9_5

should also include the treatment of primary cause of osteopenia.

- Birds have hollow pneumatic bones containing large air-filled medullary canals; hence, it is very important not to allow fluid to enter the proximal fracture segment during surgery, as it may result in aspiration pneumonia or/and asphyxiation.
- IM pinning is the most common type of internal fixation used in birds; instead of stainless steel pins, absorbable and lightweight pins developed from other materials such as polydioxanone have been used to stabilize fractures. When compared, healing usually occurs relatively faster in avian bones than mammalian bones.

## 5.1 Fractures in Young Animals

Young or immature animals are those animals having open growth plate, and based on the species and breed of the animal, the age may vary from 5 to18 months. Long bone fractures are frequently encountered in young dogs and cats [1] as well as calves and foals [2] and are more frequently observed in proximal bones of the limb such as femur, humerus, tibia-fibula, and radius-ulna. In large ruminants, femoral and humeral fractures are more common in young calves than in adults. In growing animals, fractures at or near the growth plate are often seen due to the presence of weak unmineralized cartilage (Fig. 5.1a, b).

As most of the bone growth occurs during the early growing period, the structural and material characteristics of immature bones in growing animals are markedly distinct from that of adult animals [3, 4]. Young bones have lesser strength, stiffness, yield stress, and elastic modulus. Immature bones generally have more collagen fibers and less mineral content and have vast blood circulation; hence, the fracture type and pattern of healing differ. Young bones, however, are more resilient and therefore can withstand greater deformation before getting fractured. The periosteum is thick and highly vascular but loosely attached and hence can easily strip when subjected to trauma. Additionally, the bone

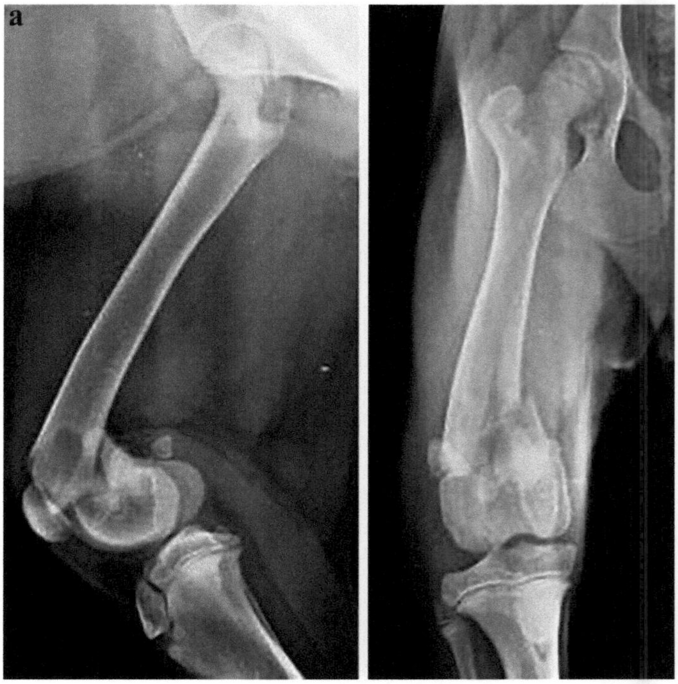


**Fig. 5.1** (**a**) Fracture at distal metaphysis of femur involving the growth plate, a common location of fracture in young animals. (**b**) Fracture involving the proximal metaphysis and physis of tibia in a young calf

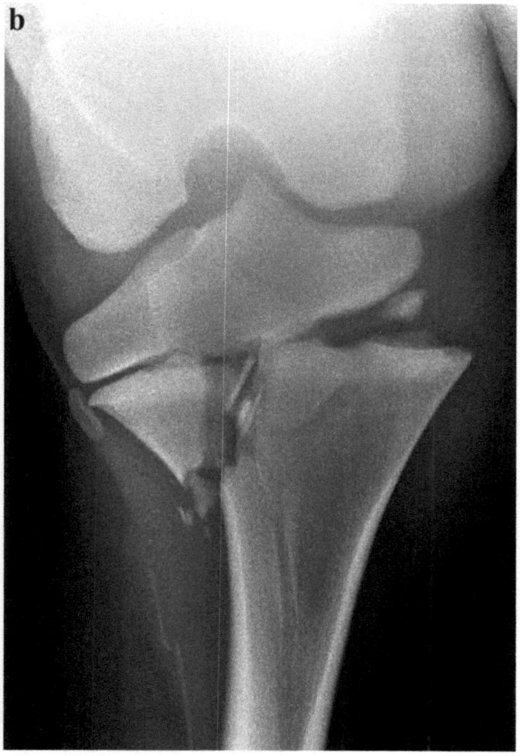

Fig. 5.1 (continued)

cortices are substantially thinner in young animals in comparison to adults [5]. Consequently, implant failure in terms of pin migration or screw pullout is more common in immature bones. As the growth plate is open in immature animals, any injury to the growth plate may halt or modify the longitudinal growth of the long bone leading to varied degrees of shortening and deformity of the limb. Fracture healing, however, is rapid in young growing bones with abundant callus formation. All these factors should be taken into consideration while treating fractures in young animals.

Incomplete or greenstick fractures of the diaphysis are more frequent, especially in small animals [1]. The animal may be presented with or without any history of trauma and may show signs of lameness with partial weight bearing. As the cortex is not completely broken, there will not be any crepitus, but the local swelling and pain would be evident. Diagnosis can be confirmed by radiographic examination. Incomplete fractures generally respond well to closed reduction and conservative treatment. Fractures below the elbow and stifle can be treated using any one of the external fixation techniques. The splint or cast should be of lightweight (like fiberglass cast), and the joints are fixed in normal angulations (should not be hyper extended) to prevent the occurrence of fracture disease (Fig. 5.2). Incomplete fractures of femur and humerus may require internal fixation to provide stability against bending. This can easily be achieved by normograde fixation of IM Steinmann pin by close method in femur, humerus, and tibia (Figs. 5.3 and 5.4). As there is no displacement of bone segments, angular deviation at the fracture site can be corrected by external manipulation, and the bone can be straightened easily. Diaphyseal fractures in young animals heal quickly with minimal complications like shortening and angulation. The splint/cast should be removed as early as possible (within 2–3 weeks) to prevent any joint stiffness and fracture disease [5]. The stabilization of the knee in young animals, albeit for short duration, can result in joint stiffness due to development of adhesions and quadriceps contracture, affecting limb function. This complication can be prevented by early mobilization of the joint. Similarly, IM pin should be removed within 2–3 weeks (may be after clinical union of bone) so that the pin does not get trapped within the fast-growing long bone.

### 5.1.1 Open Reduction and Internal Fixation

Open reduction and internal fixation of fracture in young animals are indicated only when there is complete fracture of long bones possibly leading to shortening of limb and rotational deformity, fractures involving growth plates, and those resulting in congruency of articular surface. Principles of internal fixation in immature bone include gentle tissue handling (during the surgical approach and fracture reduction), early reduction and fixation of fracture post-trauma (to avoid difficulty in fracture reduction due to callus formation), and use of minimum implant (both is size and number) for a shortest period of time [5–8].

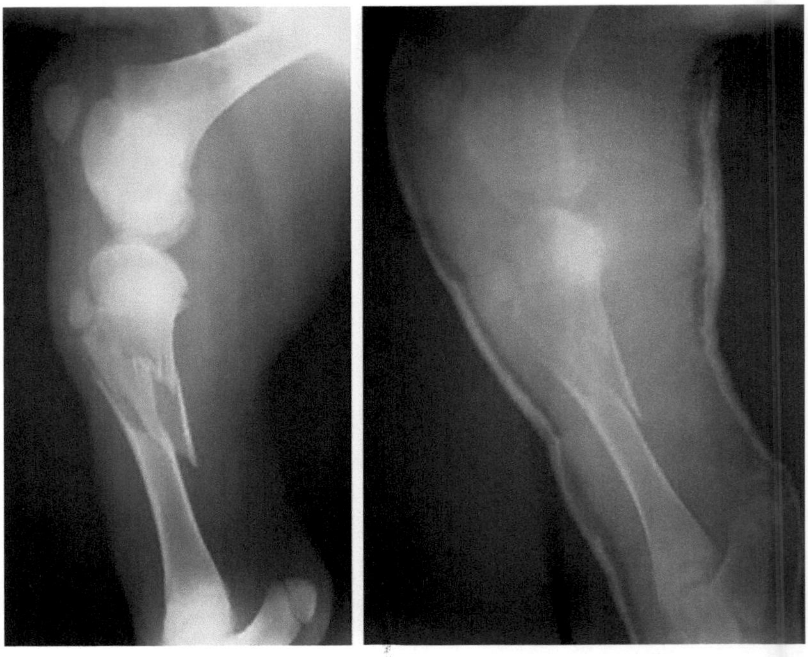

**Fig. 5.2** Proximal tibial fracture in a young calf immobilized with fiberglass cast

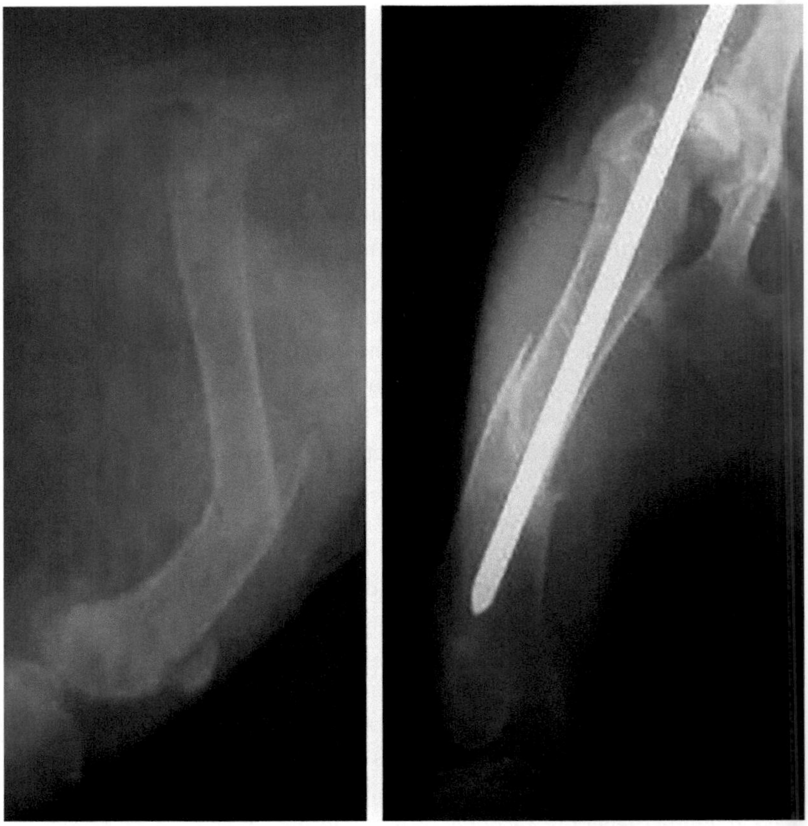

**Fig. 5.3** Greenstick fracture of femur in a dog treated with normograde IM pinning by close method. As there was no displacement of bone segments, fracture can be easily reduced by close method and IM pin fixed

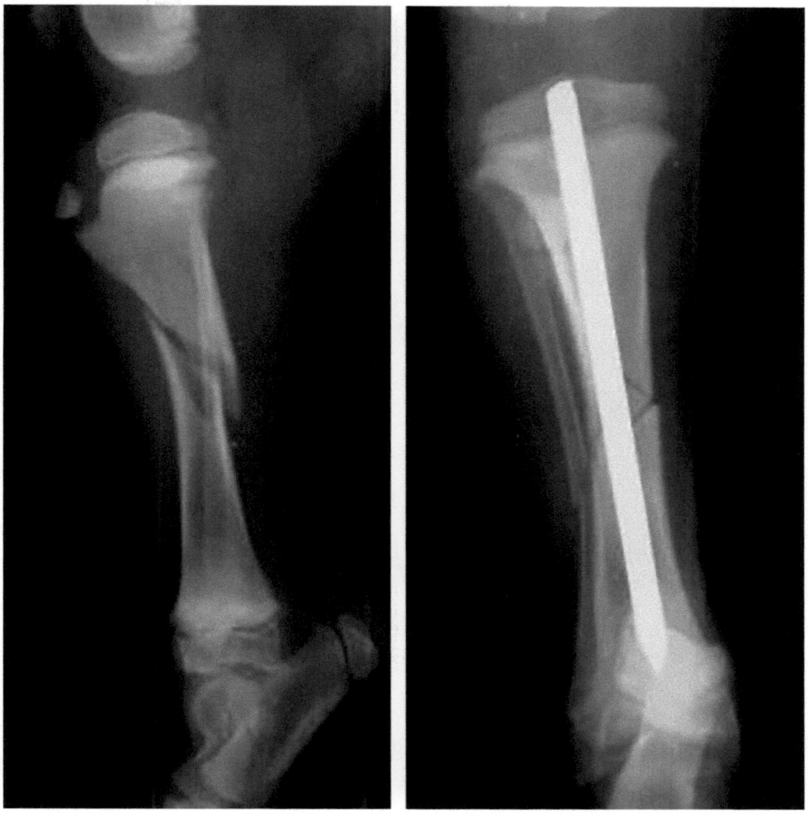

**Fig. 5.4** Spiral fracture of tibia in a young dog stabilized with IM pin fixation by close method. Note the fibula was intact, keeping the fractured segments in alignment with minimal displacement

Surgical fixation of long bone fractures in growing animals has several concerns. During open reduction, the fracture site should only be minimally disturbed by careful handling, and the bone segments are reduced by separating of the soft tissues with little manipulation and when possible using the fingers without the use of hard instruments. Rough handling during reduction may cause further cracks in the thin and fragile bony cortex. If the fracture is of a few days old, one should be very careful while breaking the adhesions and callus. During the internal fixation trans-physes, damage to the growth plates should be minimal. Generally, smooth pins are least traumatic, while threaded pins, rush pins, or plate and screws may cause major growth plate damage, leading to growth disturbances.

Intramedullary pin fixation can be used in young growing animals to obtain satisfactory fixation of diaphyseal fracture of long bones [9, 10]. But one should remember that often the presence of large medullary cavity due to very thin bony cortices may cause difficulty in achieving stable fixation with single IM pin, as the use of a very large pin may cause material property mismatch between the implant and bone leading to fixation failure. However, in young animals, as the greater percentage of medullary cavity is filled with cancellous bone than in adult animals, it allows fixation of relatively small diameter pins. Hence, it is always advised to use relatively small diameter Steinmann pin during IM fixation, or when required two or more smaller pins, or K-wires can be used to achieve rotational stability. Reaming of medullary cavity should not be practiced, and classic IM nailing through the trochanteric fossa may cause severe structural changes in the femoral head and neck, such as small disfigured femoral head, short and thin femoral neck, increased angulation between the femoral neck and shaft, and subluxation of coxofemoral joint [11] (Fig. 5.5). Similarly, the use of cerclage wires should be avoided in young

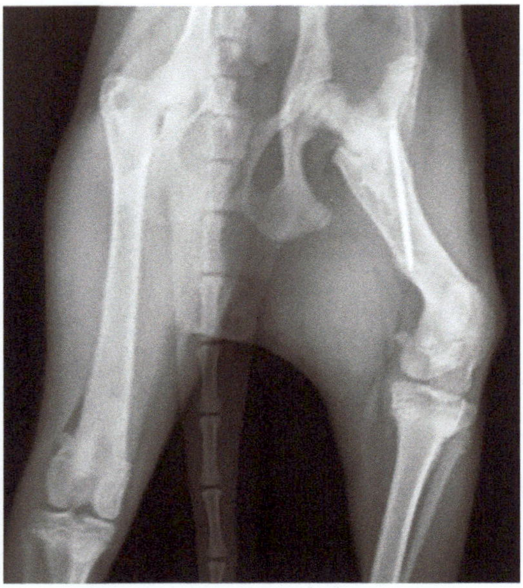

**Fig. 5.5** Deformation of proximal femur with shortening of the bone subsequent to IM pin fixation of proximal femoral fracture in a young dog

bones, as it may hinder the widening of cortex and may get trapped within the large periosteal callus. Instead, absorbable suture materials such as PGA can be used to secure the bone fragments by circling around the bone and tightening (Fig. 5.6). With IM pin fixation using least traumatic technique, the fracture healing and functional recovery are generally good in young dogs/cats and calves/foals (Fig. 5.7). Lightweight tubular interlocking nail could be effective to provide stable fixation in young large animals [12]. Due to faster healing in growing animals, maintenance of fixation for even 15–20 days will suffice to achieve clinical fracture union. IM pin/nail should be removed as soon as the clinical union is achieved (2–4 weeks) to avoid complications of pin migration and trapping of pin/nail within the medullary cavity (Fig. 5.8).

As IM nailing and ESF techniques have drawbacks in young animals, plate fixation has become popular for treating fractures in long bones such as femur, where external fixation technique cannot be used. However, technique of anatomical reduction and rigid internal fixation using standard bone plate during the early growth

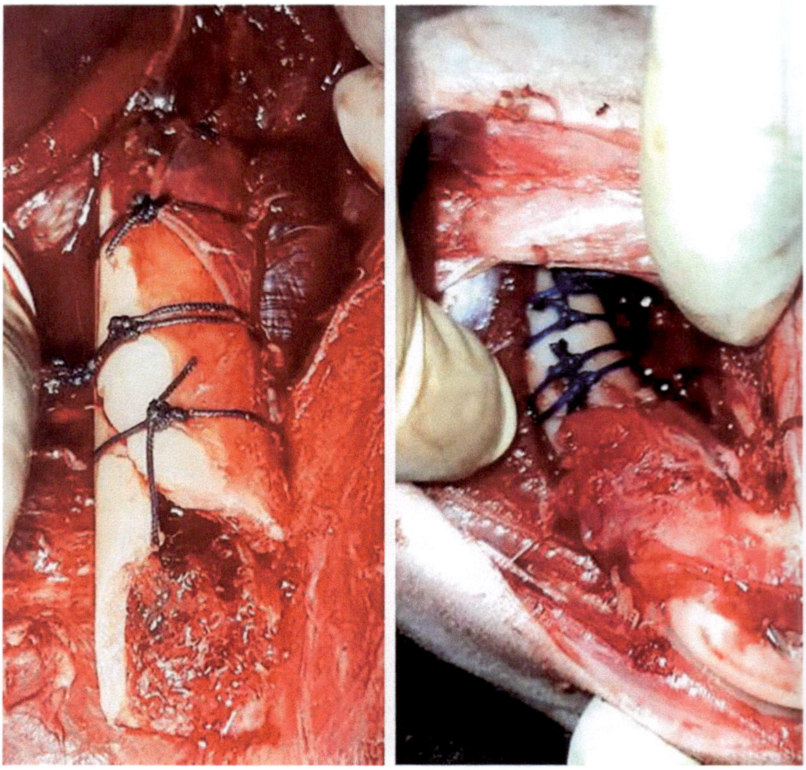

**Fig. 5.6** Use of absorbable sutures (instead of orthopedic wires) for stabilization of fracture fragments in young bones

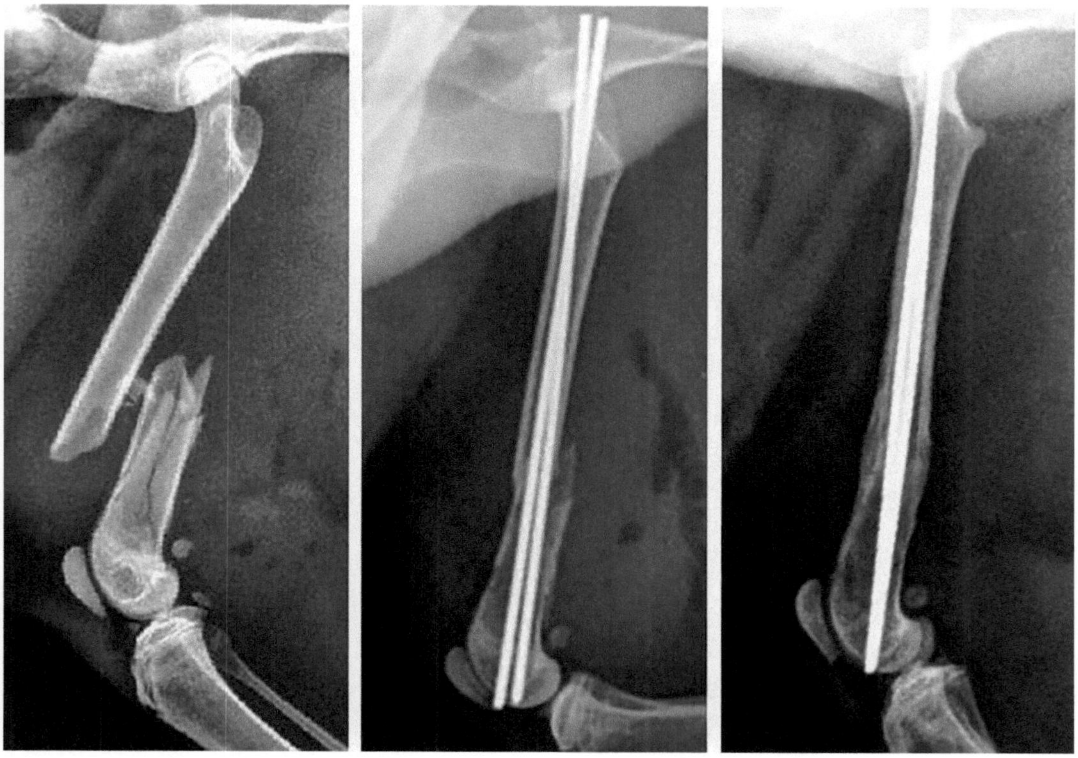

**Fig. 5.7** Comminuted fracture of distal femur in a young cat stabilized with cross IM pinning along with absorbable sutures used in cerclage fashion. Note that the bone fragments were well retained in position leading to good bone healing

period may lead to catastrophic implant failure via screw pullout. This has led to more biological semirigid plate [13] or elastic plate osteosynthesis technique, where veterinary cuttable plates (VCP) are applied in the form of bridge plating (fixation of a long plate with only a few screws) [7, 14]. In this technique, fracture segments are reduced by indirect method by applying traction on the distal bone segment using forceps, without precise anatomical reduction. The optimum length plate (by cutting the extra length) is positioned along the bone, and two screws each are fixed in the most proximal and most distal holes without tapping and taking care not to insert the screws along/across the growth plate. The adjacent screws are placed in diverging planes to increase pullout resistance. VCP permits controlled micromovement at the site of fracture promoting early callus formation and healing. The middle part of plate without screws should be long enough (>3 empty screw holes) to decrease the stress concentration effect of a single empty hole and to increase the overall strength of the repaired bone-plate composite, thereby limiting the chances of implant failure. The minimally invasive percutaneous plate osteosynthesis technique can further reduce postoperative morbidity. This approach eliminates exposure of the fracture site, preserves the fracture hematoma, and minimizes injury to the soft tissues, thus promoting biological healing and early use of the fractured limb. More recently, developed locking compression plate (LCP) using titanium alloy, which is lightweight, may prove ideal for plate osteosynthesis in juvenile long bones, as it will virtually eliminate the chances of fixation failure through screw pullout. The LCP fixation could be more effective in young calves and foals [15].

To overcome the limitations of plate and screw fixation in young growing bones via reduced purchase of screws in thin cortex and screw pullout, tubular plates (with different diameter and length)

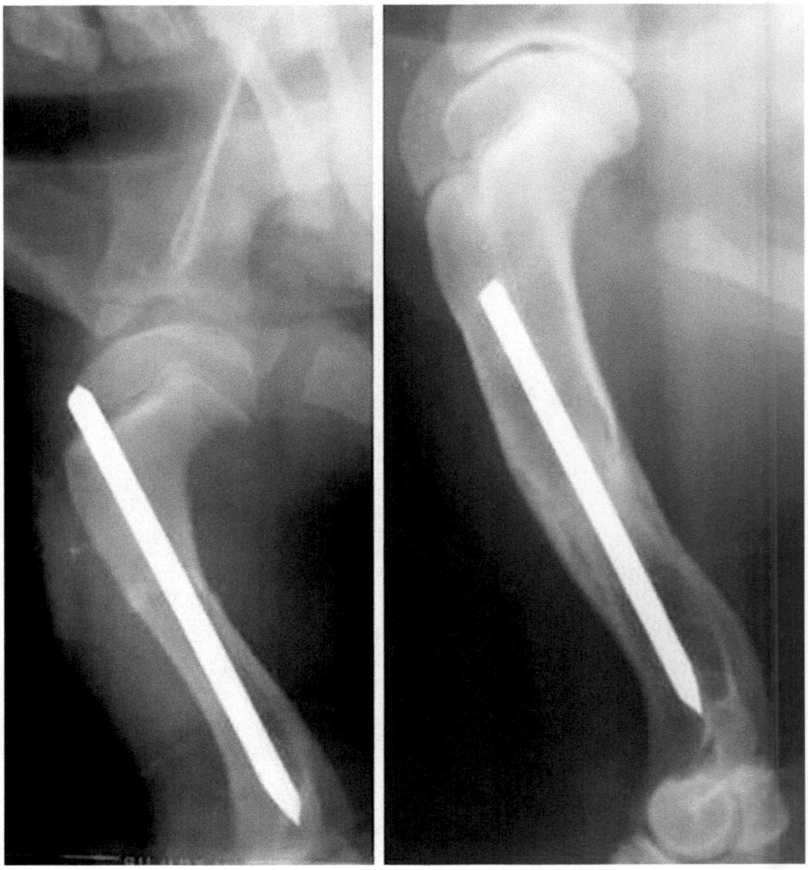

**Fig. 5.8** IM pinning of humeral fracture in a young dog. Note that the delay in removal of pin resulted in trapping of the pin within the medullary cavity due to rapid growth of the bone

that are fixed without screws can be used. The tubular plate (which is thinner and lighter in weight than standard plates and has small holes along the borders) is cut to proper length before placing and securing along a tubular long bone such as femur. After exposing the bone and reducing the fracture, the plate is placed on the craniolateral surface of femur by sliding underneath the muscle. The plate is then fixed and secured with the bone using interrupted sutures using either stainless steel cerclage wires or synthetic absorbable sutures (PGA is better than a SS wire), which are passed through the small holes present along the edges of the plate and taken around the bone. Although tubular plate may provide adequate fixation in lightweight animals, the plate when applied alone may not resist the bending load. Hence, it may be used along with a small IM pin (filling up to 30% of medullary diameter) to provide stable fixation (Fig. 5.9). A small diameter Steinmann pin is first passed into the medullary cavity to align the bone segments, and subsequently, the tubular plate is fixed. When IM pin can resist bending, the tubular plate can counteract rotational force. This “combi-fix” can thus provide stable fixation in young thin bones, without causing further damage to the fragile cortex.

External skeletal fixation is another technique, which can be employed in selected cases of long bone fractures in young growing animals. However, thin soft cortex reduces the pullout strength of fixation pins in unilateral configurations, making them less stable. In certain cases and if the fracture is open, bilateral, multiplanar fixations systems that employ small diameter pins can be used. Lightweight acrylic/epoxy-pin fixation may be particularly useful in such cases and can be applied by closed method without

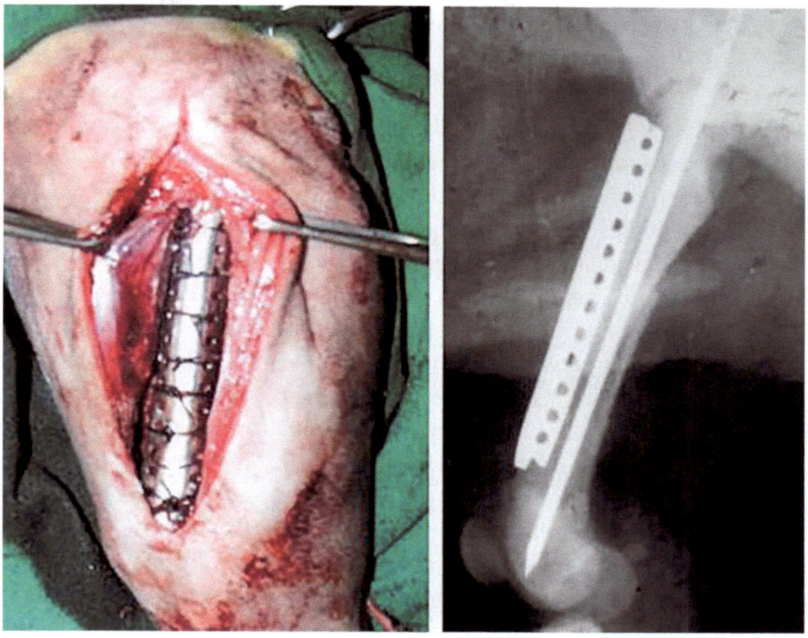

**Fig. 5.9** Use of tubular plate for fixation of femoral fracture in a dog

open reduction, or with semi-open method (in open fractures) (Fig. 5.10).

Postoperatively, the movement of the animal should be restricted; however, limited weight bearing on the limb along with range of joint motion is advised soon after surgical fixation. Physical activities such as leash walking, trotting, and swimming should be encouraged as early as possible, which are beneficial to achieve early healing and return to function. However, high impact activities such as running and jumping should be avoided. Supplementation of vitamin D and calcium will definitely help promote healing in growing animals. The plate and screws should be removed as early as possible (3–4 weeks) post-fixation.

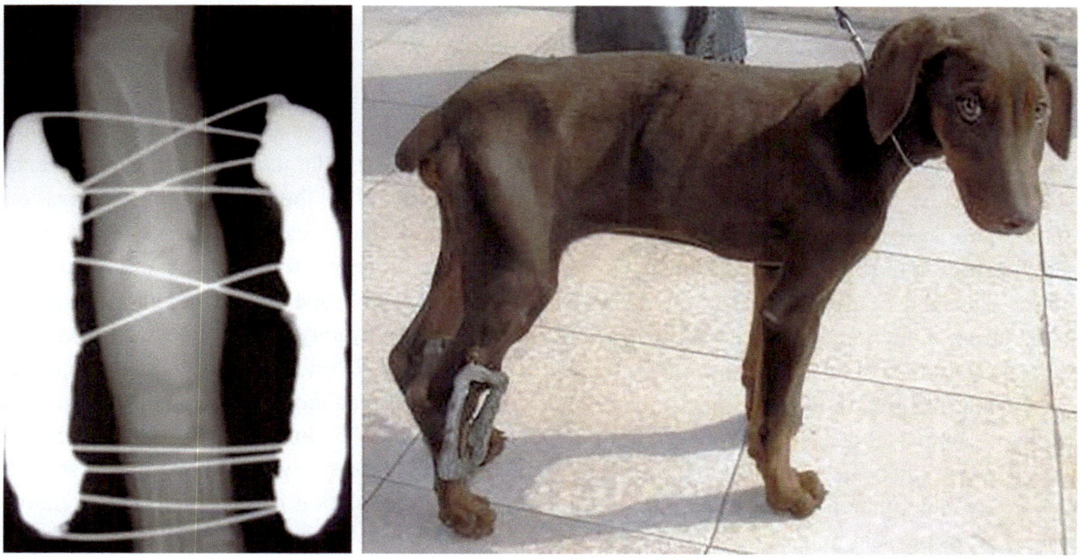

**Fig. 5.10** Treatment of open tibial fracture in a young dog with epoxy-pin ESF

### 5.1.2 Fractures Involving the Growth Plate

Growth plate injuries are frequently encountered in young growing animals, especially in dogs [16]. Injuries can occur at the growth plate at traction epiphyses (origin/insertion of major muscles, such as tibial tuberosity, greater trochanter, olecranon process, etc.), which do not significantly alter the future growth of long bones, whereas injuries at pressure epiphyses, that is, at the end of long bones, normally result in stunted growth of long bones, often accompanied with angular deformities (common at the distal radius-ulna).

Diagnosis of epiphyseal plate injury or fracture is often difficult, since there may be minimal or no displacement of bone segments. Pain, swelling, and distortion at the end of a long bone near the joint in a young growing animal may indicate an injury or fracture of the growth plate. Radiographic examination should be carefully done to observe for the thickness and uniformity of the physeal plate and deflection of the epiphysis from the shaft. Comparison with the contralateral normal limb physis will help diagnose any changes in the injured physis. Crushing injuries are challenging to detect, especially if bilateral, as there is no displacement of the epiphysis with perfect alignment.

Epiphyseal plate fractures should be reduced within 24 h following injury with careful handling and manipulation. Closed reduction (fluoroscopic-assisted) and percutaneous fixation of pins are advised when possible [17, 18]. Regardless of the method (closed or open), care is necessary while reducing epiphyseal fractures as the bone is delicate and it may get further damaged. Sharp instruments should not be used during reduction and alignment of fracture segments, as they may injure the physeal cells responsible for growth. Type I and II injuries in immature animals if they are old (present for more than 10 days) can be better managed by corrective osteotomy rather than forcible reduction, to avoid more serious physeal injury.

If type I and II fractures can be adequately reduced by closed method and alignment maintained, external fixation can be done using casts or coaptation splints; if not, internal fixation should be considered. The ideal method of internal fixation in young animals is placement of small, smooth pins (K-wires) across the physeal plate (Fig. 5.11). Cross pinning or cross IM pinning using K-wires is the method of choice, especially in fractures near the stifle or elbow joints [7, 9]. Threaded implants should not be used across the growth plate to avoid injury. Hence, in open physeal injuries, devices such as threaded pins, screws, tension band wires, or plates should not be used bridging the growth plate. In case they are used, they need to be removed as early as possible after fracture union, since prolonged presence of these devices may lead to closure of the epiphyseal plate and angular deformities. The custom-made “arrow pins” have been shown to provide adequate stability and resistance to rotational and axial forces in supracondylar femoral fractures in young dogs and cats [19]. ESF using small diameter pins (circular) spanning the injured site could also be used to provide stable fixation, which may allow correction of angular deformities even after bone fixation or during the course of healing. Irrespective of the technique used, in fractures involving the articular surface, anatomical reduction of fractured bone and rigid fixation are necessary to restore the joint function [5].

Subsequent to repair of growth plate injury, the animal should be examined periodically up to healing. Articular cartilage defect can heal satisfactorily after the removal of the fixation pin [20]. Regular examination of the animal should continue even after bone union for 2–3 months or until the closure of growth plate to ensure that deformity does not occur. In general, types 1, II, or III fractures heal quicker (in about half the time) than those involving the metaphysis (types IV and V). Similarly, most types I, II, and III injuries if properly and immediately treated and blood circulation is preserved have a favorable prognosis. Types IV, V, and VI injuries are more likely to cause varied degrees of growth plate closure regardless of the treatment method

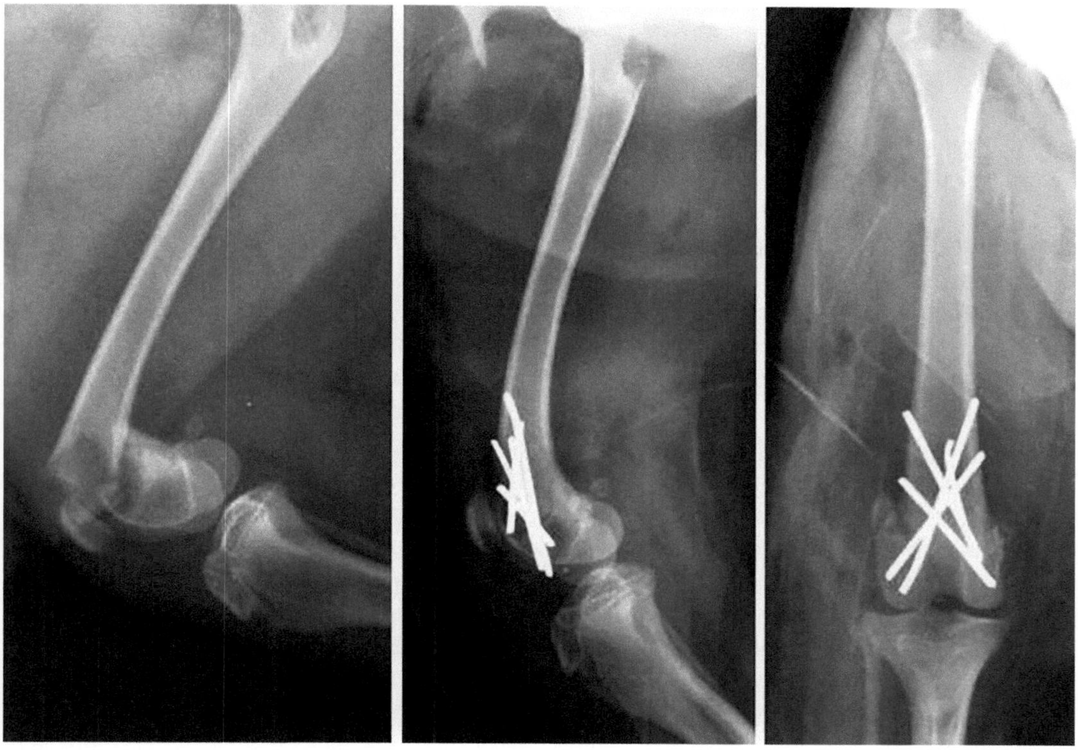

**Fig. 5.11** Use of multiple small K-wires (cross pins) for fixation of supracondylar femoral fracture in a young dog (Courtesy: Dr Tarunbir Singh, GADVASU, Ludhiana, India)

followed. The extent of shortening or deformity is normally proportional to the extent of physeal injury and the existing growth potential while trauma. In dogs, the injuries involving the distal radial and ulnar growth plates and the proximal femoral (capital) growth plate generally have a guarded prognosis.

## 5.2 Fractures in Osteopenic/Osteoporotic Bones

Osteopenia refers to the loss of bone density due to either the loss of minerals or the failure of mineralization. Primary osteoporosis, which affects millions of people throughout the world, does not seem to occur in animals, but osteoporosis marked by perceptible loss of bone (atrophy of bone) can affect animals as well. There is a reduction in the organic and inorganic matter of bone in equal proportion (bone is normal). Osteoporosis is known to occur because of disparity between bone formation and bone resorption; the bone formation is either unable to match with normal bone resorption, or bone resorption exceeds bone formation. Osteoporosis thus causes osteopenia due to the loss of minerals in the bone matrix, characterized by reduction in the number of bony trabeculae and cortical thinning. Thus, the affected bones can become weak, porous, and fragile and have increased risk of fractures; weak bones can break during a simple jump or fall from a height [21–23].

The diseases essentially affecting either organic or inorganic matrix can cause generalized osteoporosis. Deficiency of ascorbic acid (scurvy) can result in defective formation and maintenance of intracellular substances in the mesenchymal cells and osteoblasts. Insufficient availability of protein or copper may lead to decreased bone formation. Similarly, variations in estrogen, adrenal, thyroid, and pituitary hormone levels can also lead to decreased bone formation and thus induce osteoporosis. Metabolic disorders involving mineral metabolism like fibrous osteodystrophy (hyperparathyroidism) (excessive osteoclastic resorption) and rickets or osteomalacia (failure in the mineralization of the organic matrix) may also cause osteoporosis [24–26]. In hyperparathyroidism condition, the parathyroid gland produces excessive amounts of parathormone in response to reduced blood calcium level, which can drain minerals from the bones, leading to reduced bone density or osteopenia (Figs. 5.12 and 5.13). Nutritional secondary hyperparathyroidism is a very common condition due to the imbalance in the dietary calcium and phosphorus, which causes osteopenia in growing animals (common in dogs) [21, 27]. Other conditions, which can cause osteopenia, are long-term kidney diseases/failure, diabetes mellitus, neoplasia, and hyperadrenocorticism.

Disuse osteoporosis is a condition caused primarily due to prolonged immobilization leading to loss of bone density in one or more bones, or all the bones in the body. Reduction in bone density is attributed to lack of normal stress. In veterinary practice, it is normally seen in the bony cortex underneath a rigid bone plate or in the limb bones immobilized by an external cast for a prolonged period. Often, this may also result from paralysis. The osteoporosis occurs due to diminished blood flow to the bone as a result of decreased muscular activity surrounding the bone.

Osteopetrosis is a congenital or inherited abnormality of developing skeleton in man and animals, which is rare but can also lead to osteoporosis. The development and maturation of cartilage cells in the growth plate, matrix, and primary trabecular bone are normal, leading to relatively normal length and shape of bone. But there is interruption in the remaining cycle of endochondral ossification, including maturation, resorption, and replacement of immature bone, remodeling and formation of new bony cortex. The accumulation and persistence of calcified cartilage core, osteoid, or immature bone in the medullary cavity may lead to unusually dense bone.

Development of osteopenia/osteoporosis is a gradual process, which may take long time. Very often, it is difficult to diagnose osteoporosis in the initial period; hence, many times it is detected accidentally when a radiographic examination is done for other conditions like fracture. Radiographically, the affected bones may look more radiolucent than normal. Secondary osteoporosis may be diagnosed by clinical and radiographic signs, along with the signs of the primary disease. A primary disease condition should be diagnosed based on laboratory findings.

In veterinary practice, osteopenia is common in young growing animals, and osteopenic/osteoporotic bones in young animals will show thin cortices, which are elastic causing mostly incomplete/folding fractures, whereas osteoporotic bones in adult animals may be brittle, leading to comminution of bone segments. All the fracture fixation techniques/principles described in preceding text for young animals are applicable in osteopenic/osteoporotic bones as well. However, results with IM pin fixation are more favorable in young animals, and plate osteosynthesis may prove better in adult animals with osteoporosis (Figs. 5.14, 5.15, and 5.16). Use of proper application of the basic principles of fracture fixation and the advanced implant designs and fixation techniques can provide stable bone fixation and allow early weight-bearing resulting in normal fracture healing even in osteoporotic patients [28, 29].

Bone healing is determined by mechanical and biological factors, which are affected by age and osteoporosis. Although a fracture can heal normally in an osteoporotic animal, fracture healing is delayed as regards to callus mineralization and strength. The incidence of fracture malunions and nonunions is more common, especially in older patients. This is mostly attributed to implant loosening, due to unstable fixation in the weak and fragile bone. Pin loosening may also occur due to thermal and mechanical damage caused while inserting the pin and fibrous tissue formation at the pin-bone interface. The type of implant material may also determine the fixation strength. Pins coated with titanium have shown a higher osteointegration than stainless steel pins. Use of

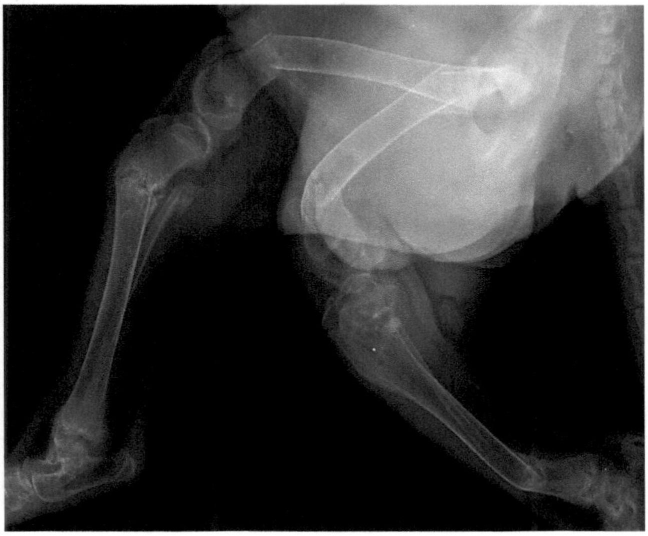

**Fig. 5.12** Multiple fractures in femur and tibia bones in a young dog affected with severe osteopenia due to nutritional secondary hyperparathyroidism. Note paper-thin cortices of long bones

anti-osteoporotic drugs has also been shown to improve implant fixation. Bisphosphonates such as alendronate and the selective estrogen receptor modulators (SERM) like raloxifene are the most popular antiresorptive drugs used for the prevention and treatment of osteoporosis in humans, and both are equally effective in the prevention of osteoporotic fracture [30, 31]. Bisphosphonates are known to selectively get integrated into osteoclasts and hamper with their biological activity to inhibit bone resorption. The studies have demonstrated that biphosphonates can

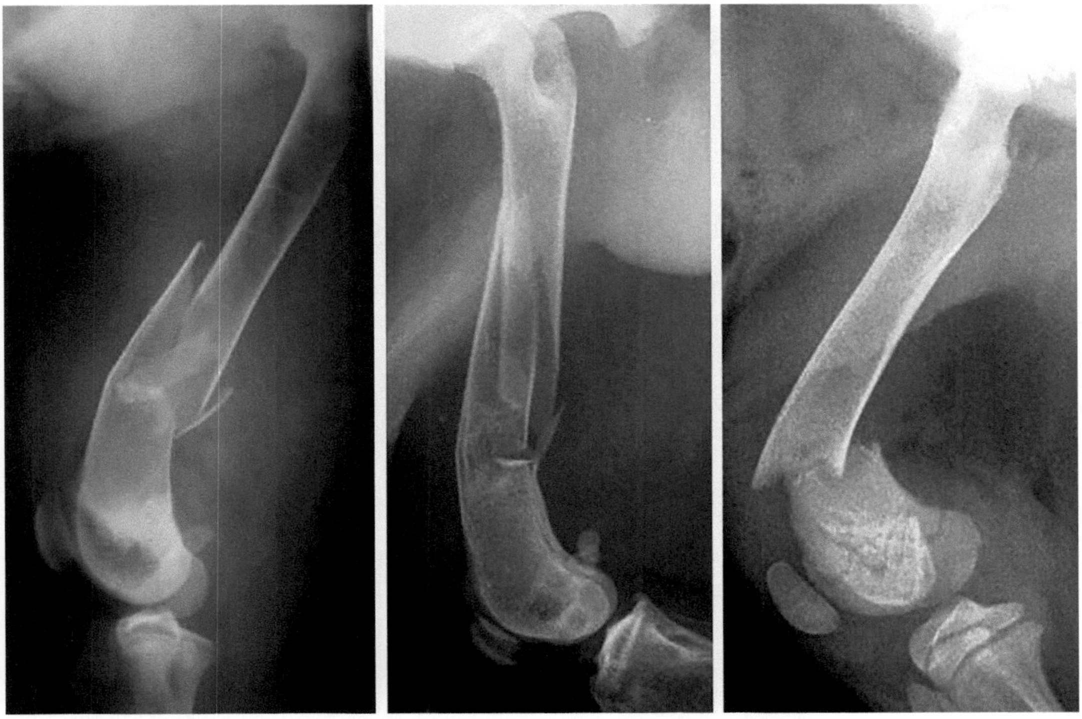

**Fig. 5.13** Fractures in femur bones affected with osteopenia. Note very thin bony cortices

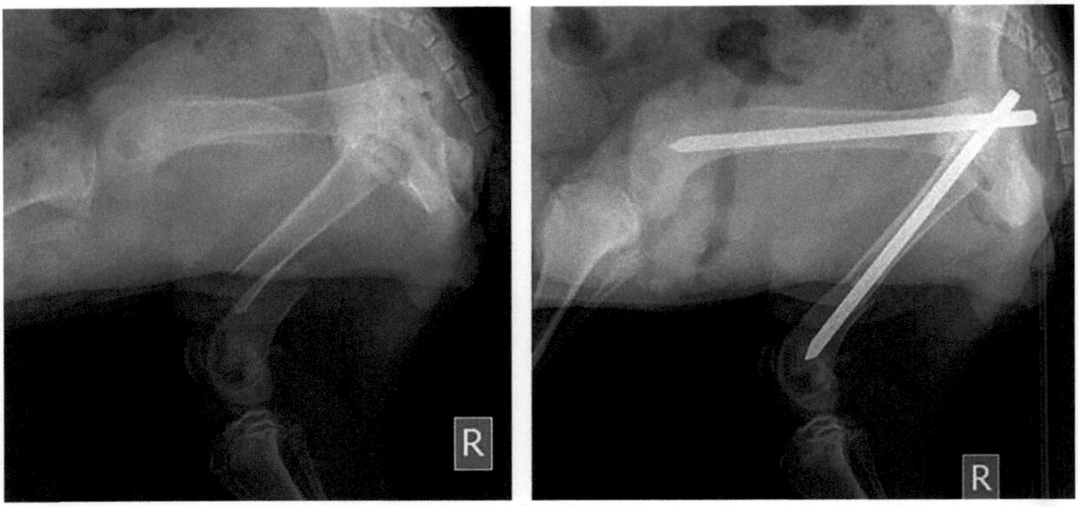


**Fig. 5.14** Bilateral fractures of osteopenic femur bones stabilized with IM pinning

enhance early fixation strength in both cortical and cancellous bones. Other studies have shown that alendronate can also improve fixation stability by inhibiting bone resorption at the bone-screw interface. Alendronate is known to initiate active bone remodeling around the implant, thereby providing stable bone-screw fixation and preventing pin loosening and infection. Anabolic agents have also been proved effective to treat osteoporosis and hence are expected to improve

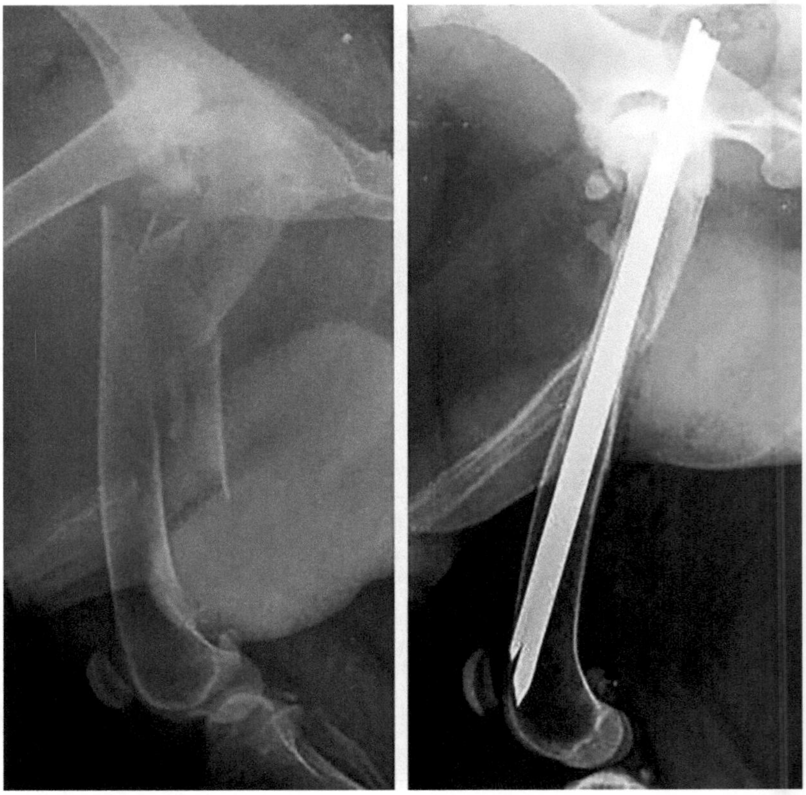

**Fig. 5.15** Comminuted fracture of osteoporotic femur bone stabilized with stack pinning along with absorbable sutures

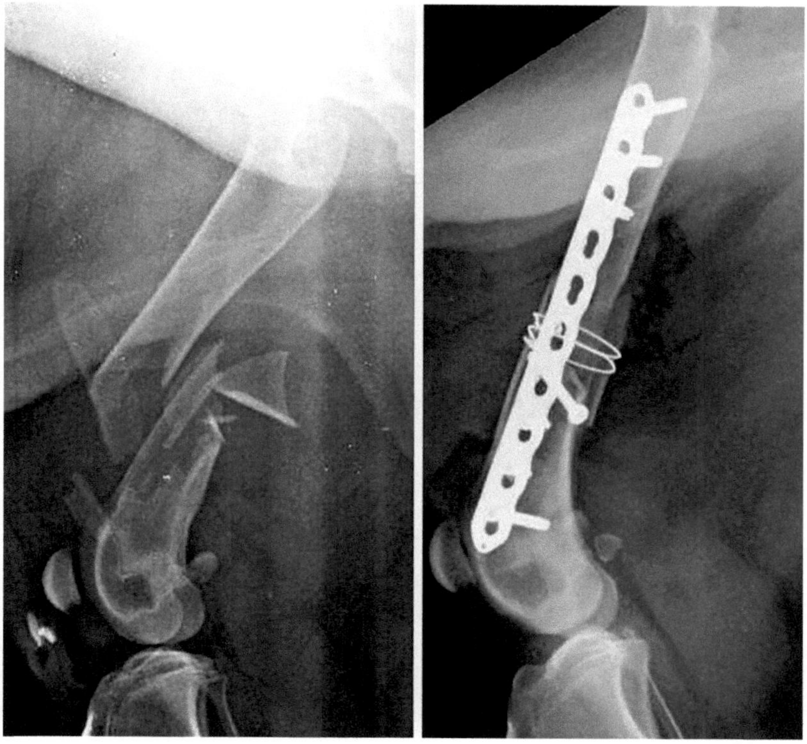

**Fig. 5.16** Severely comminuted fracture of osteoporotic femur bone in a dog stabilized with lag screw, cerclage wires and LCP with locking head screws

fracture healing in osteoporotic bones. Nandrolone decanoate, an anabolic steroid, has been shown to increase the bone mass in growing rabbits with osteopenic bones [32]. Similarly, in growing dogs with osteopenic bone diseases, among different drugs like Nandrolone, Raloxifene, Alendronate, and TGF-β, Nandrolone was found to be the most effective drug to enhance bone mineralization [33]. Calcitonin has been shown to inhibit the bone resorption stimulated by PTH and increase bone mass by transiently inhibiting osteoclastic activity, and it has been used to treat conditions like osteoporosis and rickets in animals and man [34, 35].

Treatment of fractures in osteopenic/osteoporotic bones should also include the treatment of primary disease condition. The dogs suffering from prolonged osteoporosis may experience pain, which can be severe at times. Administration of analgesics can help relieving the pain and keep the dogs active and help manage the disease condition, as they should get regular exercise to prevent further deterioration in the condition. Another approach to treat a dog with osteoporosis is by trying to restore some of the lost bone density. There are certain supplements designed to facilitate bone growth, which can be given to juvenile dogs. Calcium is an important element in the diet, which promotes bone growth. Other nutrients such as vitamin D and omega-3 fatty acids are also important. Collagen supplements such as fish collagen can help restore bone density and maintain the strength of joints, tendons, and bones in osteoporotic dogs.

## 5.3 Fractures in Avian Bones

The main principles of fracture treatment in avian species are not very different from mammals. Most of the fracture fixation techniques used in humans or animals can be employed in birds as well; however, certain anatomical differences in avian species must be taken into account before contemplating to treat a fracture [36].

Hollow pneumatic bones in birds make their body lightweight and facilitate them to fly. Several bones such as pelvis, humerus, and femur contain large air-filled medullary canals, which are involved in respiration during flight. Fracture of a pneumatic bone many a time leads to subcutaneous emphysema, but normally, it gets resolved on its own. The bones of birds are thin containing more calcium than mammalian bone and hence are relatively more brittle. Fractures at distal part of leg below the tibiotarsus and proximal humerus often become open and comminuted due to very less soft tissue covering [36].

### 5.3.1 Methods of Fracture Repair

There are similarities between avian and mammalian bone growth and fracture healing, but in birds, the fractures must be properly reduced, stabilized, and immobilized, ensuring adequate blood supply to the bone fragments for optimal healing [37]. A method used for fracture repair in birds depends on several factors, namely, the pattern and location of the injury, the age and weight of the bird, and also most importantly the functional utility of the bird after treatment. Wild birds should be able to fly and catch prey normally once released after treatment; breeder birds must have enough limb function for successful breeding; however, in pet birds, even salvage procedures like limb amputation can be done to save their life [38]. In pneumatic bones, it is important not to allow fluid to get into the fractured bone segments during surgery, as it may lead to aspiration pneumonia and asphyxiation. Fractures of the wing also require extra care not to damage the periosteum during surgical fixation, as feather follicles attached to the periosteum may get damaged.

External coaptation using bandages, splints, or slings often works well, especially for tibiotarsal fractures and joint luxations in small birds, where internal fixation is not advised or impossible [39–41]. Manual restraint can be used most often during application of splints, if the bones need not be manipulated extensively. In small birds, simple tape bandage can be used to immobilize fractures of tibiotarsus, whereas in larger birds, lightweight splints made of wood, aluminum, or any other material may be incorporated into the splint to provide additional support (Fig. 5.17). Immobilization of the wing in its natural resting location can bring the bone segments in proper alignment. However, while covering a splint and bandage to the body to immobilize the wings, it is taken care not to interfere with natural respiration or hinder crop function. In pet birds, application of splints in places acceptive to external coaptation often provides stable fixation of fracture. However, splint application may cause improper alignment and shortening of the bone, ankylosis of the joint, and tendon contracture or entrapment within the callus.

Internal fixation will provide proper anatomic alignment and functional recovery [36]. As general anesthesia is required, the patient must be stabilized and well hydrated so that they can withstand the surgical fixation. Intramedullary pinning is the most common type of internal fixation used (Fig. 5.18) [42]. Use of cerclage and hemicerclage wires along with the IM pin can help to resist rotational and shear forces. Metaphyseal fractures may be stabilized effectively using cross pins. Pins developed using

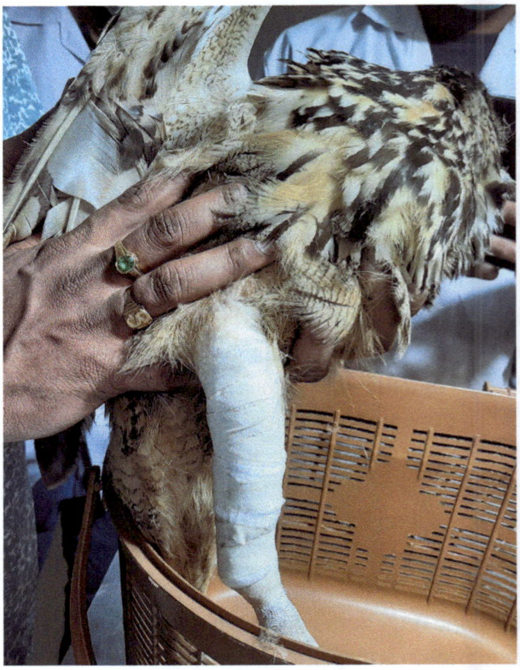

**Fig. 5.17** Splint-bandage application for immobilization of fracture fragments in an Eagle

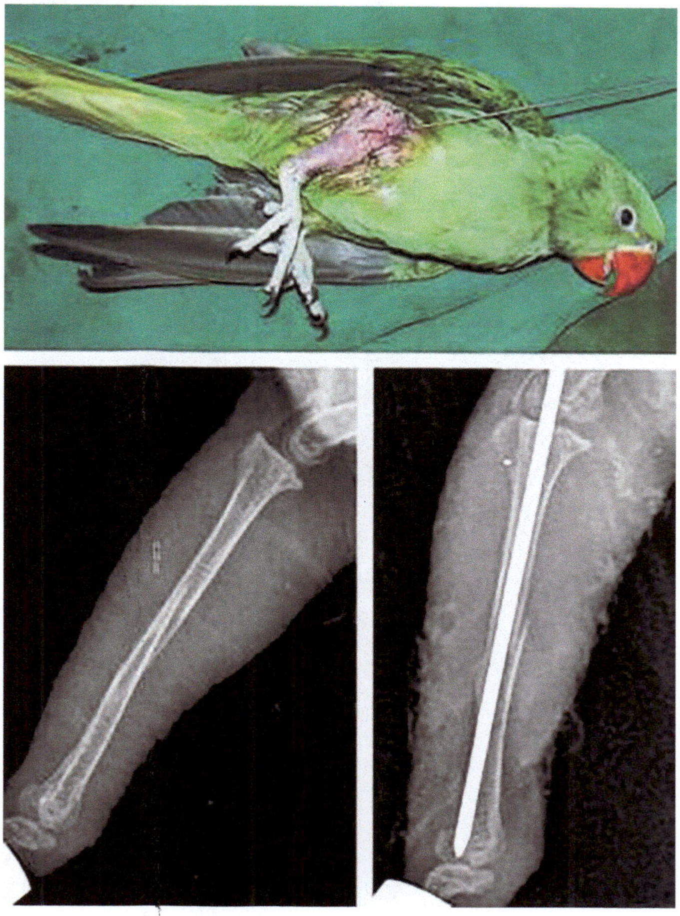

**Fig. 5.18** Intramedullary pinning for fixation of tibiotarsal bone fracture in a parrot

absorbable materials such as Polydioxanone (PDS), which are lightweight, has also been used to immobilize fractures in birds. However, PDS is not as rigid and stable as stainless steel, and therefore, PDS pin fixation should be supplemented with some external support. PDS pins are generally inserted by shuttle technique. In this technique, a small hole is drilled at the center of the rod using a small K-wire or hypodemic needle, and a suture material is inserted through the hole. The PDS rod is first inserted into the longer segment of the fractured bone by retrograde technique. The other bone segment is then aligned with the opposite end of the rod (by toggling), which is then pushed into the shorter segment by pulling the suture. To achieve rotational stability, polymethylmethacrylate (PMMA) bone cement can be used under strict aseptic conditions to fill the medullary cavity. Bone plates can also be used in birds, especially in larger flighted birds. PMMA may be used to improve screw purchase in the bone. Alternatively, locking compression plate/reconstruction plate may be used (Fig. 5.19), and plates developed using lightweight titanium alloy is ideal for use in birds.

External skeletal fixation such as K-E splint has been used for fracture repair in birds. Birds tolerate ESF devices well and return to early function without affecting the joint motion [43]. Small PVC or latex pipes or drinking straws can be used as connecting rods by filling with PMMA or dental acrylic cement. Epoxy putty can also be used as an external fixator component, either for attaching the fixation pins with steel connecting bars or constructing the epoxy-pin connecting bar by incorporating the bent fixation pins within (Figs. 5.20 and 5.21). IM pin used to

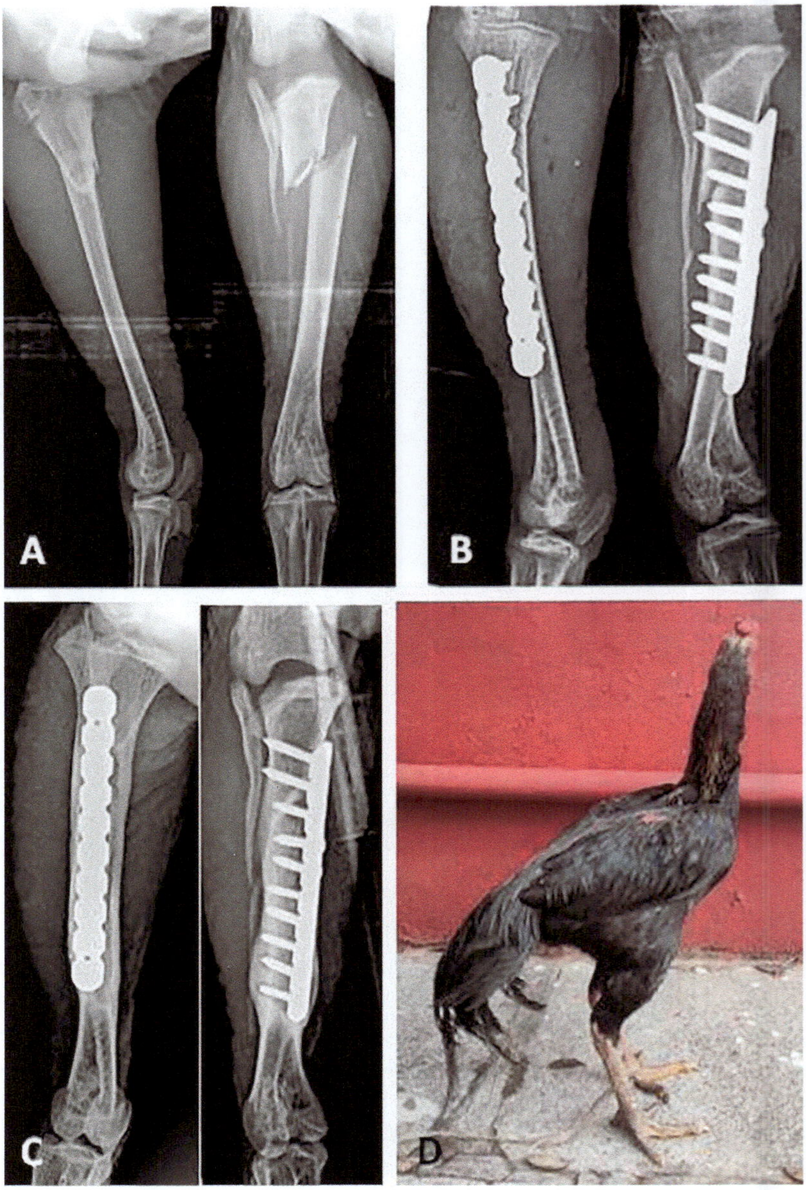


**Fig. 5.19** Use of locking reconstruction plate for the repair of tibiotarsal bone: Complete short oblique metaphyseal fracture of tibiotarsus (**a**), postoperative radiograph (day 0) showing the use stainless steel locking reconstruction plate to stabilize the fracture (**b**), radiograph made on day 60 shows complete bone union (**c**), good weight bearing and use of limb on day 60 (**d**) (Courtesy: Dr Pallavi and Dr Dilipkumar D, Veterinary College, Bidar, Karnataka, India)

immobilize the fracture can be bent and joined with the connecting bar of an ESF to provide further rotational stability [44]. Application of ESF device at an early date post-injury can prevent muscle atrophy, maintain the proper bone length, and help early return to full functional flight. ESF can also be used for repair of joint luxations.

Fractures of mandibles can be treated by the use of K-wires, or acrylic or mesh splints. However, management of avian mandibular fractures is difficult, and complications such as infection, necrosis, and nonunion are common.

Perioperatively, an analgesic anti-inflammatory drug should be given routinely. In case of severe pain, opioids such as morphine or hydrocodone may be given, and in case of moderate pain, butorphanol can been administered. It is also important to begin physical therapy at the earliest after fracture repair to preserve/regain the range of joint motion and enable the bird to be released into the wild as soon as possible.

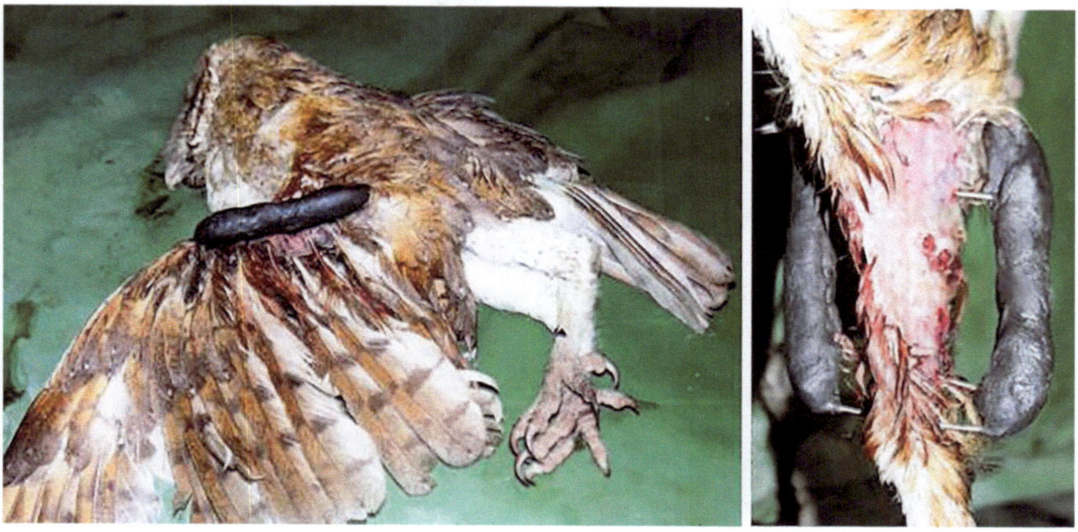

**Fig. 5.20** Epoxy-pin fixation for repair of wing bone in an owl

Like mammalian bone, avian bone can heal either by primary or secondary healing; nevertheless, majority of fractures in birds heal by secondary healing by external callus formation, generally due to the presence of fracture gaps and instability at the fracture site [36]. When compared, healing usually occurs relatively faster in avian bones than mammalian bones. Callus may not be visible radiographically for 3–6 weeks; however, a simple midshaft fracture of a long bone such as tibiotarsal fracture may be clinically stable within 2–3 weeks; by then, it is advised to remove the fixation device if needed. Complications such as nonunion and osteomyelitis can arise in birds also and are treated with the same principles as in mammals. Birds having osteomyelitis generally show increased white blood cell count but may not show generalized systemic signs and are treated by administering specific antibiotic. Nonunions can be treated by

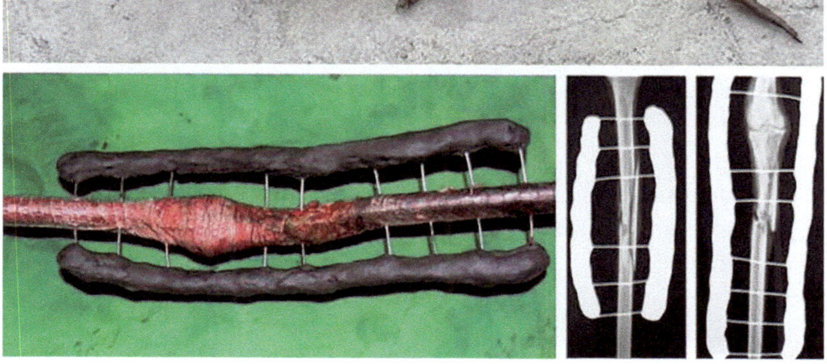

**Fig. 5.21** Epoxy-pin fixation for bilateral tibiotarsal bone fractures in a crane

providing rigid and stable fixation along with autografts.

## Chapter 5: Sample Questions

### Q. No. 1: Mark the correct answer

1. Which of the following is not true with respect to young bones as compared to adult bones
(a) contain more collagen fibers and less minerals (b) have thin cortices (c) have more blood supply (d) are less resilient
2. The splint or cast in young animals should be
(a) light weight (b) the joints are fixed in normal angulations (c) removed as early as possible after bone healing (d) all are true
3. The implant that is least traumatic to the growth plate
(a) smooth pins (b) threaded pins (c) rush pins (d) plate and screws
4. Preferred technique of fixation for diaphyseal fractures in juvenile animals, which cannot be immobilized by external fixation is
(a) IM nailing (b) bone plating (c) ESF technique (d) none of these
5. Decreased bone formation in osteoporotic animals may be associated with deficiency of
(a) protein (b) copper (c) ascorbic acid (d) all of the above

### Q. No. 2: State True or False

1. Fracture or trauma to the growth plate in immature animals can arrest the longitudinal growth of bone leading to shortening and deformity of the limb.
2. Incomplete or greenstick fractures of the diaphysis are more common in adult bone.
3. In young and osteoporotic bones, it is always advised to use relatively large diameter intramedullary pins to achieve greater stability.
4. Types IV, V, and VI physeal injuries are more likely to result in varied degrees of epiphyseal plate closure regardless of the treatment method used.
5. Alendronate can help achieve good bone-screw fixation and prevent the pin loosening.
6. The bones of birds are thin and contain less calcium than mammalian bone.

### Q. No. 3: Fill up the blanks

1. The most common cause of failure of bone plating in young and osteoporotic bones is ________________.
2. Use of cerclage wire should be avoided in young bones, as it may ________________ ________________ and ________________ ________________.
3. Failure in the mineralization of the organic matrix of the bone is called as ________________.
4. Nutritional secondary hyperparathyroidism is commonly caused due to the imbalance in the dietary minerals, namely, ________________ and ________________.
5. Loss of bone density caused due to prolonged immobilization of the bone is called ________________.
6. The condition causing accumulation of calcified cartilage cores, osteoid, and primitive bone in the medullary cavities resulting in abnormally dense bone is known as ________________.
7. Usually, internal fixation with ________________ gives favorable results in young animals, and ________________ is better in adult animals with osteoporosis.
8. In pneumatic bones, entry of fluid into the proximal fracture segment may cause ________________ and ________________.
9. ________________ is the most common type of internal fixation used in birds.

### Q. No. 4: Write short note on the following

1. Structural difference between mammalian and avian bones
2. Internal fixation in young animals
3. Management of fractures involving the growth plate

4. Treatment of fractures in osteoporotic bones
5. Fracture treatment in avian bones

## References


1. Kumar, K., I.V. Mogha, H.P. Aithal, P. Kinjavdekar, Amarpal, G.R. Singh, A.M. Pawde, and R.B. Kushwaha. 2007. Occurrence and pattern of long bone fractures in growing dogs with normal and osteopenic bones. *Journal of Veterinary Medicine A* 54: 484–490.
2. Singh, A.P., G.R. Singh, H.P. Aithal, and P. Singh. 2020. Section D – fractures, chapter on the musculoskeletal system. In *Ruminant surgery: A textbook of the surgical diseases of cattle, buffaloes, camels, sheep and goats*, ed. J. Singh, S. Singh, and R.P.S. Tyagi, 2nd ed. New Delhi: CBS Publishers and Distributers.
3. Torzilli, P.A., K. Takebe, A.H. Burstein, and K.G. Heiple. 1981. Structural properties of immature canine bone. *Journal of Biomechanical Engineering* 103: 232–238.
4. Torzilli, P.A., K. Takebe, A.H. Burstein, J.M. Zika, and K.G. Heiple. 1982. The material properties of immature bone. *Journal of Biomechanical Engineering* 104: 12–20.
5. DeCamp, C.E., S.A. Johnston, L.M. Déjardin, and S.L. Schaefer. 2016. Fractures in growing animals. In *Brinker, Piermattei and Flo's handbook of small animal orthopedics and fracture repair*, 5th ed., 781–790. St. Louis, MO: Elsevier.
6. Bush, D. 2011. Management and treatment of fractures in immature animals. Vet Times September 26, 2011. https://www.vettimes.co.uk
7. Perry, K., and S. Woods. 2018. Fracture management in growing animals. Companion. *Animal* 23 (3): 120. https://doi.org/10.12968/COAN.2018.23.3.120.
8. Stubbs, W.P. 2013. Fracture management in skeletally immature dogs. Proceedings of NAVC conference 2013 small animal and exotics
9. Howard, P.E. 1991. Principles of intramedullary pin and wire fixation. *Seminars in Veterinary Medicine and Surgery (Small Animal)* 6 (1): 52–67.
10. St-Jean, G., R.M. DeBowes, B.L. Hull, and P.D. Constable. 1992. Intramedullary pinning of femoral diaphyseal fractures in neonatal calves: 12 cases (1980–1990). *Journal of the American Veterinary Medical Association* 200: 1372–1376.
11. Black, A., and S. Withrow. 1979. Changes in the proximal femur and coxofemoral joint following intramedullary pinning of diaphyseal fractures in young dogs. *Veterinary Surgery* 8: 19–24.
12. Trostle, S., D. Wilson, R. Dueland, and M.D. Markel. 1995. In vitro biomechanical comparison of solid and tubular interlocking nails in neonatal bovine femurs. *Veterinary Surgery* 24: 235–243.
13. Kumar, K., I.V. Mogha, H.P. Aithal, Amarpal, P. Kinjavdekar G.R. Singh, A.M. Pawde, and V.P. Varshney. 2007. Management of osteopenic bone fractures in growing dogs using semi-rigid bone plates. *The Indian Journal of Animal Sciences* 77: 1091–1098.
14. Cabassu, J. 2001. Elastic plate osteosynthesis of femoral shaft fractures in young dogs. *Veterinary and Comparative Orthopaedics and Traumatology* 14: 40–45.
15. Hoerdemann, M., Gedet, P., Ferguson, S.J., Sauter-Louis, C. And Nuss, K. 2012. In-vitro comparison of LC-DCP and LCP-constructs in the femur of newborn calves - a pilot study. BMC Veterinary Research 8: 139
16. Newton, C.D., and D.M. Nunamaker. 1985. Pediatric fractures. In *Textbook of small animal orthopaedics*, ed. C.D. Newton and D.M. Nunamaker, 461–466. Philadelphia: J.B. Lippincott.
17. Boekhout-Ta, C.L., S.E. Kim, A.R. Cross, R. Evans, and A. Pozzi. 2017. Closed reduction and fluoroscopic-assisted percutaneous pinning of 42 physeal fractures in 37 dogs and 4 cats. *Veterinary Surgery* 46: 103–110.
18. Cook, J.L., J.L. Tomlinson, and A.L. Reed. 1999. Fluoroscopically guided closed reduction and internal fixation of fractures of the lateral portion of the humeral condyle: prospective clinical study of the technique and results in ten dogs. *Veterinary Surgery* 28: 315–321.
19. Rathnadiwakara, R., D. de Silva, and H. Wijekoon. 2020. Treatment of supracondylar femoral fractures in young cats and dogs using "arrow pin" technique. *Journal of Veterinary Medicine and Animal Sciences* 3 (1): 1017.
20. Aithal, H.P., G.R. Singh, and A.K. Sharma. 1999a. Healing of articular cartilage following intra-articular pin fixation in dogs. *The Indian Journal of Animal Sciences* 69: 46–48.
21. Aithal, H.P., G.R. Singh, Amarpal, P. Kinjavdekar, and H.C. Setia. 1999b. Fractures secondary to nutritional bone disease in dogs: A review of 38 cases. *Journal of Veterinary Medicine* A46: 483–487.
22. Kumar, K., I.V. Mogha, H.P. Aithal, Amarpal, P. Kinjavdekar, G.R. Singh, A.M. Pawde, and H.C. Setia. 2009. Determinants of bone mass, density and growth in growing dogs with normal and osteopenic bones. *Veterinary Research Communications* 33: 57–66.
23. Tanaka, S. 2019. Molecular understanding of pharmacological treatment of osteoporosis. *EFORT Open Review* 4 (4): 158. https://doi.org/10.1302/2058-5241.4.180018.
24. Bennett, D. 1976. Nutrition and bone disease in the dog and cat. *The Veterinary Record* 98: 313–320.
25. Campbell, J.R., and I.R. Griffiths. 1984. Bone and muscles. In *Canine medicine and therapeutics*, ed. E.A. Chandler, J.B. Sutton, and D.J. Thompson, 2nd ed., 138–166. Oxford: Blackwell.

26. Jubb, K.V.F., P.C. Kennedy, and N. Palmer. 1995. *Pathology of domestic animals*. 3rd ed, 34–50. New York: Academic Press.
27. Kushwaha, R.B., H.P. Aithal, Amarpal, P. Kinjavdekar, A.M. Pawde, G.R. Singh, V.P. Varshney, and H.C. Setia. 2011. Therapeutic management of hyperparathyroidism in growing dogs. *The Indian Veterinary Journal* 88: 79–82.
28. Giannoudis, P.V., and E. Schneider. 2006. Principles of fixation of osteoporotic fractures. *Journal of Bone and Joint Surgery* 88-B: 1272–1278.
29. Hollensteiner, M., S. Sandriesser, E. Bliven, C. von Rüden, and P. Augat. 2019. Biomechanics of osteoporotic fracture fixation. *Current Osteoporosis Reports* 17 (6): 363–374.
30. Gatti, D., and A. Fassio. 2019. Pharmacological management of osteoporosis in postmenopausal women: the current state of the art. *Journal of Population Therapeutics and Clinical Pharmacology* 26 (4): e19. https://doi.org/10.15586/jptcp.v26i4.646.
31. Kim, Y., Y. Tian, J. Yang, V. Huser, P. Jin, C.G. Lambert, H. Park, S.C. You, R.W. Park, P.R. Rijnbeek, M. Van Zandt, C. Reich, R. Vashisht, Y. Wu, J. Duke, G. Hripcsak, D. Madigan, N.H. Shah, P.B. Ryan, M.J. Schuemie, and M.A. Suchard. 2020. Comparative safety and effectiveness of alendronate versus raloxifene in women with osteoporosis. *Scientific Reports* 10: 11115. (2020). https://doi.org/10.1038/s41598-020-68037-8.
32. Aithal, H.P., P. Kinjavdekar, Amarpal, A.M. Pawde, G.R. Singh, A.K. Pattanaik, V.P. Varshney, T.K. Goswami, and H.C. Setia. 2009. Effects of Nandrolone and TGF-β1 in growing rabbits with osteopenia induced by over-supplementation of calcium and vitamin D3. *Veterinary Research Communications* 33: 331–343.
33. Parti, M., H.P. Aithal, Amarpal, P. Kinjavdekar, A.M. Pawde, G.R. Singh, T.K. Goswami, and H.C. Setia. 2008. Evaluation of certain antiresorptive drugs in growing dogs affected with osteopenic bone diseases (rickets, NSH). *The Indian Journal of Animal Sciences* 78: 1333–1337.
34. Copp, D.H. 1994. Calcitonin: discovery, development and clinical application. *Clinical and Investigative Medicine* 17: 268–277.
35. Ladelnet, A. 1999. Rickets and osteoporosis in puppies and kittens, and the therapeutic use of calcitonin. *Animal-de-compagnie* 14: 469–497.
36. Wissman, M.A. 2006. Avian orthopaedics. www.exoticpetvet.net
37. Tully, T.N., Jr. 2002. Basic avian bone growth and healing. *The Veterinary Clinics of North America. Exotic Animal Practice* 5 (1): 23–30.
38. Madhu, D.N., S.W. Monsang, H.P. Aithal, Amarpal, A.M. Pawde, P. Kinjavedkar, and M.M.S. Zama. 2013. Unilateral wing amputation for the management of humerus fracture in a black kite (*Milvus migrans*). *Advances in Animal and Veterinary Sciences* 1 (2S): 24–25.
39. Duerr, R. 2010. Splinting avian fractures. Duerr Splinting Manual, 2nd edn. https://theiwrc.org
40. Singh, J., D.N. Madhu, Rohit Kumar, and H.P. Aithal. 2013. External coaptation for elbow joint luxation in a rock pigeon (*Columba livia intermedia*). *Indian Wildlife Year Book* 10: 80–81.
41. Wright, L., C. Mans, G. Olsen, and G. Doss. 2018. Retrospective evaluation of tibiotarsal fractures treated with tape splints in birds: 86 cases (2006–2015). *Journal of Avian Medicine and Surgery* 32: 205–209.
42. Hoque, M., H.P. Aithal, and S.K. Maiti. 2001. Hypodermic needle for intramedullary fixation of femoral fracture in a stork. *Wild Life Information Bulletin* 8: 12–13.
43. MacCoy, D.M. 1992. Treatment of fractures in avian species. *The Veterinary Clinics of North America. Small Animal Practice* 22 (1): 225–238.
44. Aithal, H.P., J. Singh, P. Kinjavdekar, and Amarpal. 2012. Epoxy-pin fixation for management of tarsometarsus fracture in a Sarus crane. *Intas Polivet* 13: 469–472.

# Open Fractures

# 6

**Learning Objectives**

You will be able to understand the following after reading this chapter:

- Classification of open fractures
- Infection of soft tissues and bone and their treatment
- Management of soft tissue injuries and wound closure in open fractures
- Stabilization of open fractures
- Postoperative care of open fractures

**Summary**

- Primary goals of open fracture management are to prevent/control the infection by providing drainage and suitable antibiotic therapy, protect the surrounding soft tissues, and provide stable fixation to achieve early bone union and functional recovery.
- Fractures that are adequately stabilized, either with internal or external fixation, can heal despite bacterial infection; however, unstable fixation with the presence of loose bone fragment/implant may perpetuate infection.
- Animals with open fractures should be treated aggressively with a broad-spectrum antibiotic, which should be continued until the wound is completely healed.
- The closure of wound in open fractures can be considered at different time intervals; small puncture wounds can be sutured immediately, and larger clean lacerated wounds with little contamination and infection may also be closed primarily after thorough flushing and debridement, but heavily traumatized and contaminated wounds should not be closed immediately.
- Osteomyelitis may be characterized by aggressive, irregular and purposeless periosteal and endosteal bone formation, the presence of radiodense bone fragments surrounded by radiolucent areas, and increased soft tissue density and swelling at injured site.
- Any fixation technique used in open fractures should be minimally invasive and should not lead to further damage to the surrounding soft tissues, allowing biological healing. Open fractures below the stifle and elbow may be treated using a suitable external skeletal fixator, whereas fractures in femur or humerus may be treated using bone plate (DCP/LCP) and screws fixation.

(continued)





H. P. Aithal et al., *Textbook of Veterinary Orthopaedic Surgery*,
https://doi.org/10.1007/978-981-99-2575-9_6

- A cancellous autograft can be used in contaminated or infected fractures to promote biological healing without concerns of rejection or sequestration; however, its survival depends on adequate vascularization.

Open fractures are frequently encountered in both small and large animal practice, specifically in the distal bones of the limb due to minimal coverage of soft tissues [1, 2]. The management of open fractures continues to be challenging for the veterinary surgeons, despite better understanding of fracture biology and improvement in the surgical techniques in recent years. As the protective skin covering is damaged, the chances for bacterial infection, osteomyelitis, and nonunion are higher in open fractures than in closed fractures. Open fractures with extensive soft tissue injury and severe comminution of bone segments pose greater difficulty in treatment, especially in large animals [2, 3]. However, timely and appropriate management of these injuries can help reduce infection, leading to favorable outcomes. This can be achieved by proper understanding of fracture type and classification, pathogenesis of infection, and principles of biological fixation. Each case is treated differently, some with open wound management using external fixation initially with delayed definitive fixation, and others with immediate debridement, primary closure, and rigid fixation with either internal fixation or external skeletal fixation. The decision on selection of fracture fixation is mostly determined by the degree of soft tissue trauma, which also guides the early management [4]. Primary objectives of open fracture management include the prevention or control of infection by providing drainage and suitable antibiotic therapy and protection of surrounding soft tissues and providing stable fixation to achieve early bony union and restoration of function [2, 5–9].

## 6.1 Classification of Open Fractures

The purpose of open fracture classification system is to help decision-making on treatment options. The classification systems mostly take into consideration the extent of skeletal and surrounding soft tissue injury and infection. There are several methods of classification of open fractures [5, 8, 9], yet the most commonly used method in animal practice is: Grade I (or first degree): fractures with a tiny puncture in the skin at or near the fracture site, wherein the fractured bone may or may not be seen protruding through the wound and soft tissue injury is minimal (Fig. 6.1); Grade II (or second degree): fractures with a varying sizes of skin wounds along with the minimally comminuted fractures, soft tissue damage is relatively more with some degree of contamination; and Grade III (or third degree): fractures with severe comminution of bone, with or without bone loss, and extensive soft tissue damage and contamination. Such fractures are typically caused by high energy trauma like automobile accidents or gunshot injuries [10].

The infection rate in Grade I and Grade II fractures is generally less, and the prognosis is usually favorable if stable fixation is provided. However, grade III fractures are most difficult to treat, and complications such as infection, implant failure, delayed union, and nonunion are increasingly common. In severe cases, amputation of the limb may be considered carefully based not only on the extent of fracture injury but also on the emotional and social factors. The outcome of the treatment much depends on how the patient is taken care of by the animal owner.

## 6.2 Soft Tissue Infection, Osteomyelitis, and Antibiotic Therapy

Soft tissue injury with vascular compromise and contamination predispose the open fracture site

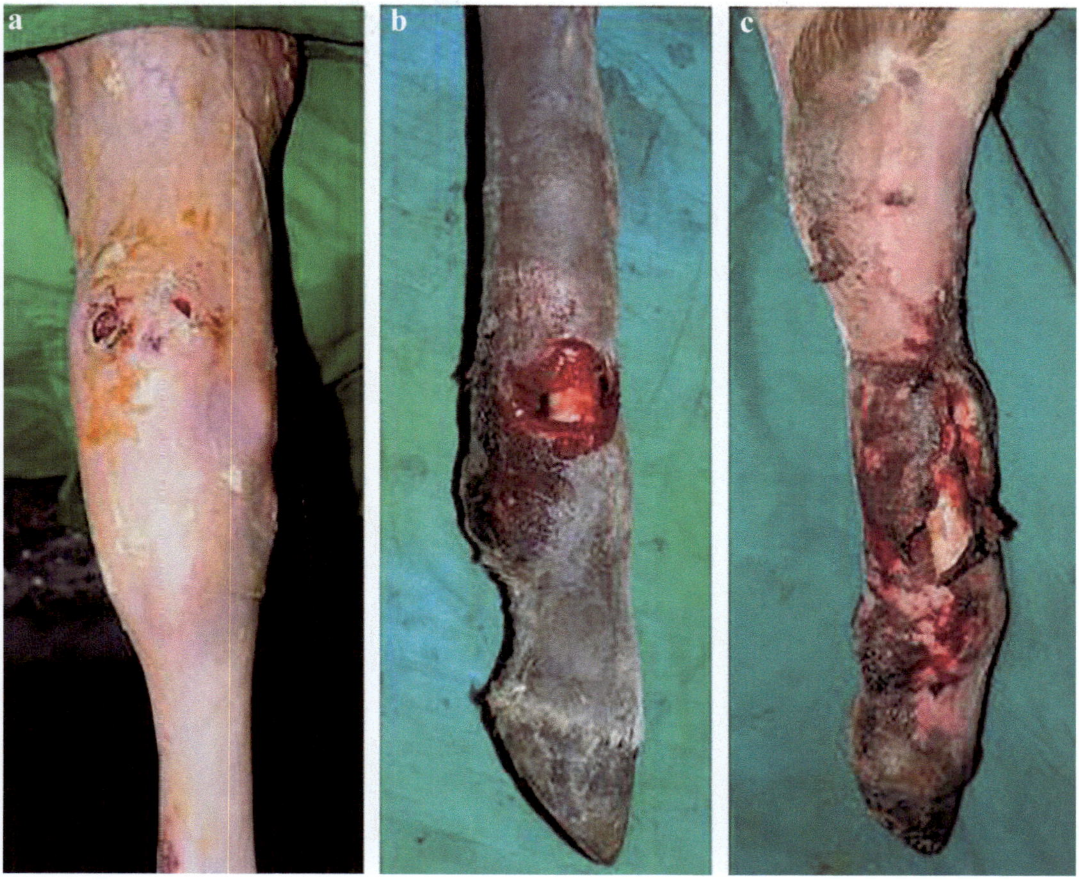


**Fig. 6.1** Broad classification of open fractures: Grade I (**a**), Grade II (**b**), and Grade III (**c**)

for infection. Soft tissue infection can be controlled with regular drainage of exudate, dressing and antibiotic therapy [6, 9]. Spread of infection from the surrounding injured soft tissue to the fractured bone can lead to osteomyelitis (Fig. 6.2). Infections get established when the revascularization to the fracture site is compromised by the presence of avascular bone or soft tissues along with bacterial contamination. Unstable fracture fixation, the presence of loose bone pieces, and loose implants will provide a conducive environment for development of osteomyelitis [11]. Rigid immobilization using stable internal or external skeletal fixation may allow fractures to heal, despite bacterial infection [2, 12]; nonetheless, unstable fixation by internal implants may perpetuate infection. Further, rigid immobilization with external skeletal fixation (ESF) will allow drainage and dressing of open wound and thus facilitate treatment of infection, and osteomyelitis is rarely seen with ESF of open contaminated fractures.

All open fractures ought to be considered as contaminated and managed accordingly [10]. The method of treatment may be chosen based on the fracture pattern and also the risk of infection. To minimize the risk of infection, animals with open fractures must be administered with a broad spectrum antibiotic as soon as possible (within 3 h of trauma). As Grade I and II fractures are more frequently tend to get infected with gram-positive bacteria, a first-generation cephalosporin is usually advised. Grade III fractures often get contaminated with gram-positive and gram-negative organisms; hence, a broad spectrum antibiotic should be employed. In the case of soil-contaminated wounds, an antibiotic that is also effective against anaerobic bacteria such as *Clostridia* should be used. Antibiotic therapy should be started before surgery and

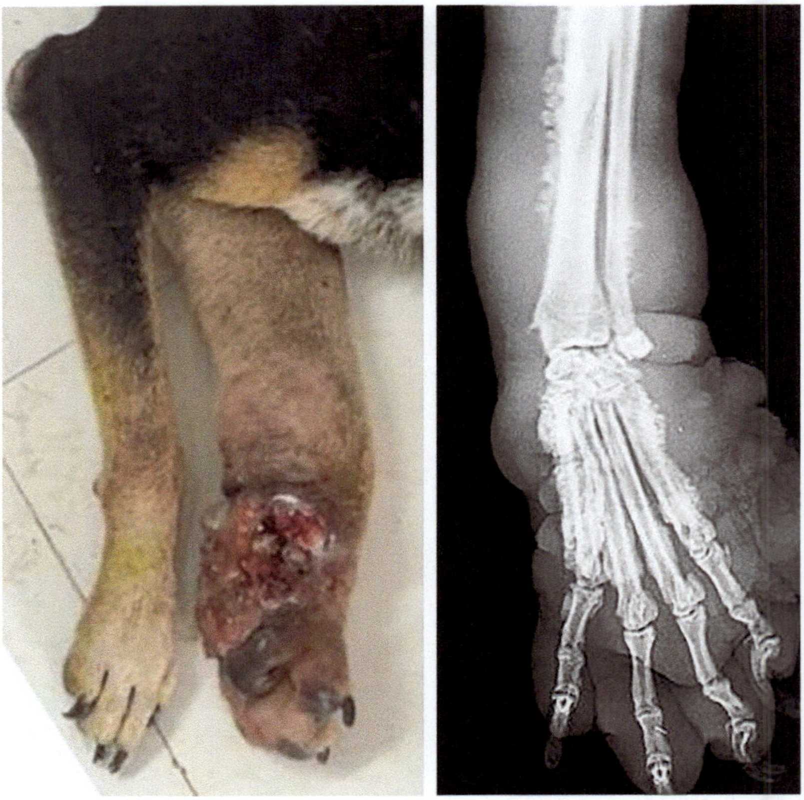

**Fig. 6.2** Spread of infection from a chronic soft tissue wound to the surrounding bone (Courtesy: Dr. Snehal Pundkar, Mumbai, India)

continued during the course of surgery and early in the postoperative period [6, 13]. In principle, the antibiotic therapy should be given until the wound is completely closed or healed. Initially, the therapy may be given for 3–5 days; if wound infection or osteomyelitis occurs or persists for longer period, specific antibiotic should be administered based on the culture and sensitivity test of samples (swabs) collected from the infected area. In patients with confirmed infections or osteomyelitis, prolonged antibiotic administration is advised for 6–8 weeks. Local antibiotic therapy should be considered when extensive contamination is present. The antibiotic powder or liquid may be sprayed over the open wound, or it may be administered in the form of "antibiotic beads" (constructs formed with antibiotic powder and polymethylmethacrylate cement for sustained release) along with systemic administration, to control the infection in severely contaminated open fractures.

Animals with contaminated wounds should also be given tetanus toxoid, which is more critical in horses. Toxoid should be administered as early as possible after the trauma as it will take about 15–20 days to obtain desired antibody level in the blood.

## 6.3 Management of Soft Tissue Injuries and Wound Closure

The most crucial part in the management of open fractures is the early intervention, including flushing, washing, and debridement of the injured site [6, 8–10, 14]. The timing of intervention may vary depending on several factors such as patient's physiological status, surgeon's availability, etc. However, an animal with open fracture should undergo initial debridement as early as possible, which should include removing any devitalized tissues and free bone pieces at the injured site under appropriate analgesia. After the initial assessment and stabilization of the traumatized animal, the hair around the wound is clipped and the skin scrubbed with the animal under sedation. The wound is carefully but thoroughly cleansed using sterile normal saline, lactated Ringers or a 0.5–1.0% chlorhexidine solution, and the necrotic tissues and debris are trimmed and removed. Severely comminuted fractures with tissue necrosis due to vascular compromise and severe fecal or soil contamination require special attention. The vascularity of the affected tissues should be assessed carefully. Along with debridement, it is crucial to irrigate the open wound liberally to remove the contaminating debris and to decrease the potentially infective bacterial loads. An antibiotic agent added to the irrigating solution will help contain infection.

The wound closure can be done at different time intervals, that is, immediately when the animal is brought for treatment, as early as possible (within 3 days) or delayed (beyond 3 days). Immediate primary closure or earlier closure may be performed in cases having no or minimal contamination and vascular insufficiency and where it is possible to approximate the skin without tension (Fig. 6.3). Traditionally, it has been advised to delay the closure if gross contamination of the wound is suspected with possible chances of clostridial infections and gangrene. However, studies have shown that early closure of wounds results in reduced infection rates and complications and early fracture healing. Small puncture wounds need not be sutured and may be covered with nonadherent dressings. Larger, cleanly lacerated skin wounds with little contamination and infection (Grade I and II fractures) may be closed primarily following careful flushing and debridement. In case there is any suspicion about the safety of primary closure, it is better to wait for few more days until second debridement is done and decide accordingly. Heavily traumatized or contaminated wounds should not be closed immediately and are cleaned and covered with gauze sponges soaked with antiseptic solutions and bandaged. Initially, the bandage should be changed daily, until there is minimal exudation; subsequently, the duration may be increased. The unsutured wound may be allowed to heal by second intention. Often, problems such as abscess formation and wound dehiscence may occur after premature closure of a wound. In such cases, the wound edges are freshened or re-opened to provide drainage for the exudate. Regular flushing and dressing of the wound may lead to early healing.

Contaminated and infected open fractures should be thoroughly lavaged and drained and temporarily fixed with an external support until the final surgical fixation [8, 9, 14]. In fractures below the elbow or stifle, a full limb splint and bandage is applied preoperatively, which will help cover the wound and prevent more contamination, protect the soft tissues from further trauma and provide temporary fracture stabilization allowing comfort to the patient. The dressing and the splint should be kept intact until the patient is taken to the surgical room for definitive fracture fixation in cases of early fracture stabilization. If fracture fixation is delayed, the splint and bandage should be regularly removed for wound dressing and reapplied. Wounds over the joints are thoroughly cleaned and wrapped with a bandage along with the spica splint used to immobilize the fracture. An elastic bandage may be applied to compress the injured tissues gently to prevent or reduce inflammatory swelling.

## 6.4 Treatment of Open Fractures

Early stabilization of open fractures has several benefits. It helps to protect the soft tissues from further getting injured by the free movement of fracture segments, maintains bone reduction and alignment, improves circulation at the fracture site (decrease infection), and assists in quick functional recovery of fractured limb. While selecting a fracture fixation technique, both mechanical and biological condition of the fracture should be considered. Mechanically, weak severely comminuted fractures cannot withstand the load of weight bearing, and hence, the bone fixation should be rigid and stable by use of implants that can buttress the fracture site and resist the load of weight bearing during the period of bone healing. Similarly, open fractures with severe soft tissue damage (Grade III) do not have a conducive biological environment for normal healing. Therefore, any fixation technique used should be

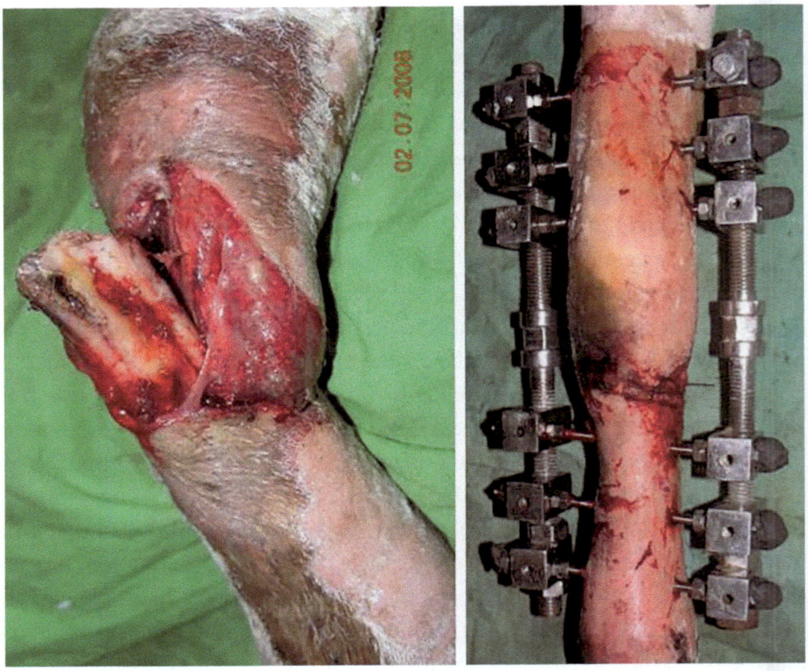


**Fig. 6.3** Open metacarpal fracture in cattle with relatively clean lacerated skin, treated by primary closure of skin and ESF

minimally invasive and should not cause any further damage to the surrounding soft tissues, allowing biological healing. Old age, poor general health, additional limb injuries, and preexisting diseases are some other factors, which may adversely affect the biological environment. Uncooperative patients and owners can further complicate the postoperative management.

In Grade I and II open fractures, there is minimal comminution of bone and less soft tissue damage and contamination; hence, the selection of fracture fixation technique depends mainly on the species and nature of animal patient and location and type of fracture, irrespective of open wound. Any stable internal fixation technique can be used, including interlocking nails or plates and screws [2, 12]. Fractures below the stifle and elbow may be suitably treated using either internal fixation or external skeletal fixators, whereas open fractures in femur or humerus may be treated by fixation of bone plate and screws (DCP/LCP). Stable fixation leads to early healing, and the implants may be removed early. Less rigid fixation using IM Steinmann pins should be avoided. Use of cerclage wire should also be avoided, which, unless properly fixed, harbors infection at the fracture site.

In Grade III open fractures, minimally invasive biological osteosynthesis technique, which will minimally disturb the fracture site biology, should be used. Surgical debridement should also be limited only to accessible superficial necrotic tissues. Generally, the wounds are not sutured to allow drainage. It is also possible that after thorough flushing and debridement of heavily traumatized and contaminated wounds, the wound edges may be partially closed using simple interrupted sutures, taking care not to exert undue tension at the wound edges (to avoid interference with wound healing) (Fig. 6.4). If not possible, the skin edges need not be apposed, only brought closer. This technique of partial closure of skin edges will not only allow drainage but also help reduce the wound gap and cover the fracture site with soft tissues and hence will promote early vascularization and healing. Deep tissue infections are treated by keeping drainage and daily lavage of the wound until the exudates cease to exist. The implant used for fixation of bone should help bridge the comminuted fracture (fracture gap) and sufficiently strong to resist bending or breakage. Hence, closed reduction and minimally invasive external skeletal fixation is optimal for Grade III open fractures of the radius,

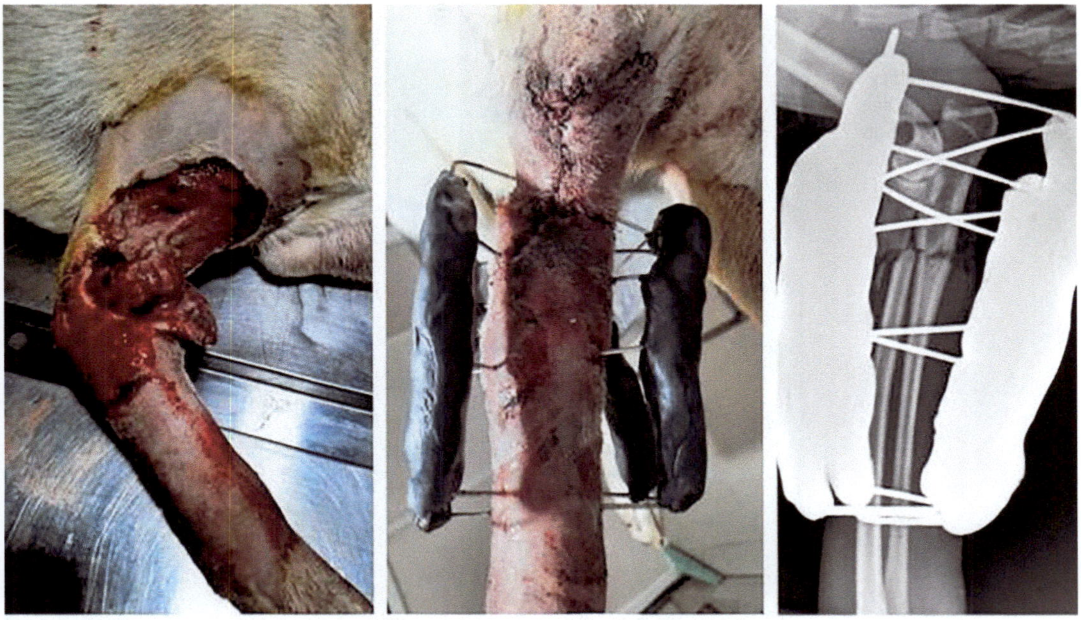

**Fig. 6.4** In a case of open fracture of radius-ulna (Grade III), traumatized and contaminated wound was thoroughly flushed and debrided, before partially closing the wound edges using simple interrupted sutures. This would allow drainage and also reduce the wound gap and cover the fracture site with soft tissues, and hence would promote early bone healing

tibia, metacarpus, and metatarsus in both small and large animals [15–18]. In large animals, open fractures of digits can also be managed successfully using transarticular fixation of external fixators. In angularly placed tibia or hock region, multiplanar or circular fixators are preferred. In small animals including calves and foals (weighing up to about 100 kg), epoxy-pin fixation may be preferred, as it is very versatile and can be applied to any type of fracture and can provide stable fixation and economical too [19–22] (Fig. 6.5). In Grade III open comminuted fractures of the humerus or femur, minimally invasive internal fixation techniques such as bridging plate can be employed without disturbing the bone segments at the fracture site. The technique of bridging plate osteosynthesis is easy to apply with minimum time and leads to early healing even in open fracture environment.

In certain cases of open fractures, where the soft tissue infection persists or osteomyelitis develops, replacement of one technique with another may be needed. An ESF may be replaced with a rigid internal fixation like intramedullary nail or plate and screw fixation, or otherwise. Replacement of one technique with another may require additional time and antibiotic treatment before refixation.

In open fractures with severe comminution, it is advised to preserve the large bone fragments in place, especially those with soft tissue attachments. Only free bone fragments, which may predispose for sequestra formation, should be removed. Similarly, dead or necrosed bone ends need not be removed and if removed may lead to or increase the fracture gap. After thorough flushing of the open wound and the bone ends, the "dead bone" may be left in place, which can help bridge the fracture gap and may act as osteoinducer (formation of new bone) before getting detached from the healthy bone (Fig. 6.6). It is, however, more unlikely that the dead bone gets incorporated during the healing process. During the course of healing, the dead bone may get detached, and the free moving dead bone piece can be removed using a bone rongeur during routine dressing of open wound. Rigidly immobilized open fracture at times can heal

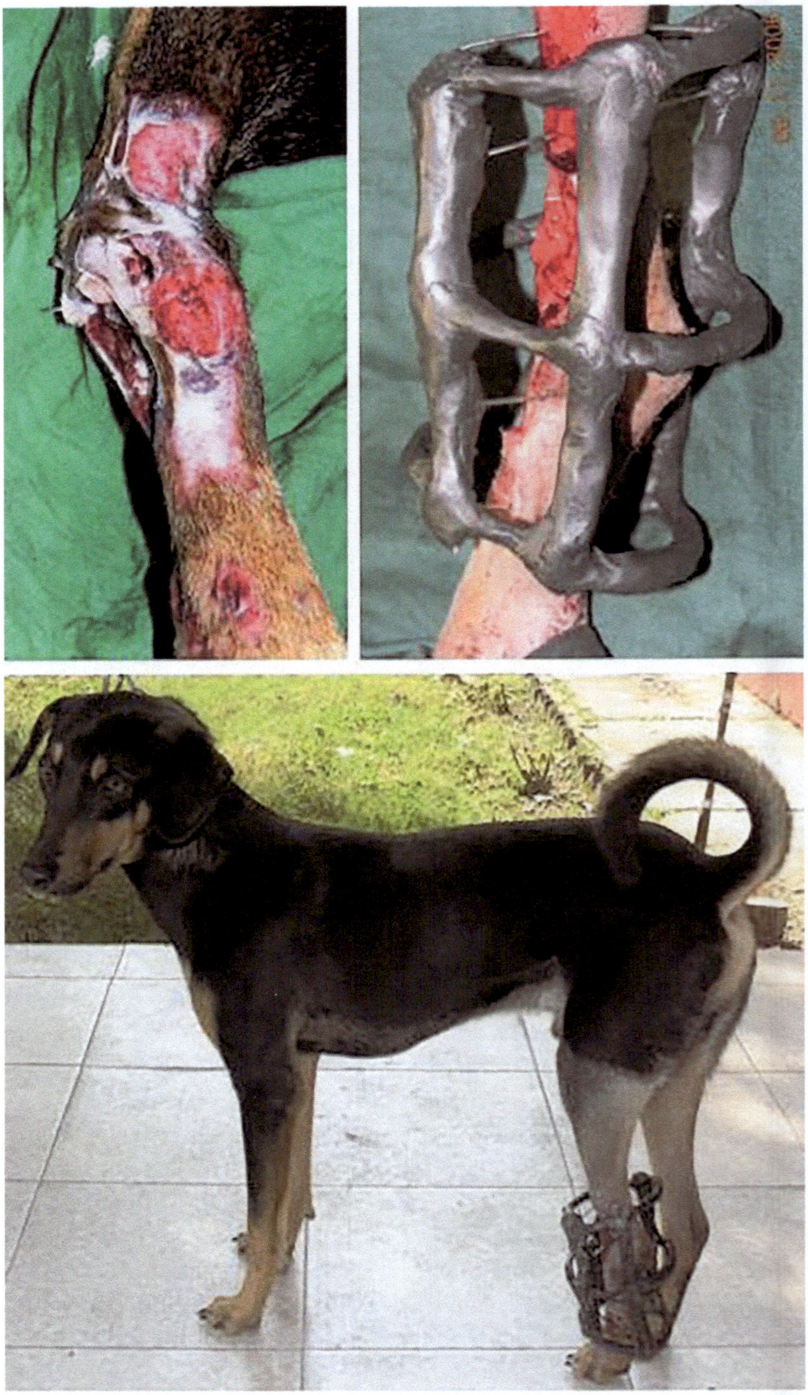

**Fig. 6.5** Grade III open fracture-luxation of tarsus in a dog treated with epoxy-pin circular ESF, which provided stable fixation leading to early weight bearing on the affected limb

even with fracture gap (Fig. 6.7). A cancellous bone autograft may also be used in contaminated or infected fractures to promote bone healing without apprehension of rejection or sequestration. The bone graft incorporation, however, depends on adequate fixation stability and soft tissue viability and vascularization; hence, it should be used only when adequate soft tissue coverage in ensured in a rigidly fixed fracture. In cases where there is severe soft tissue damage and

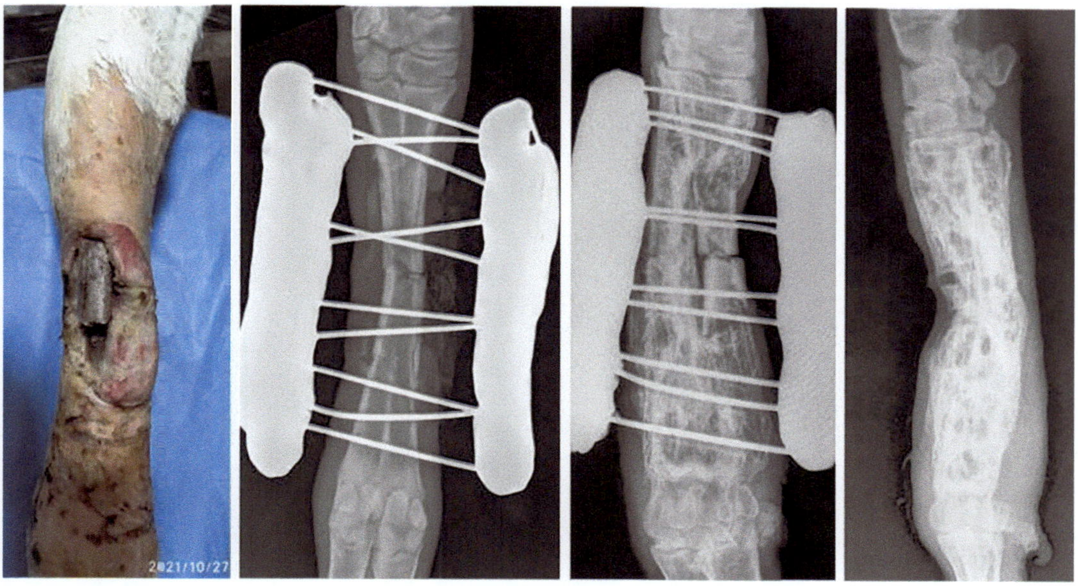


**Fig. 6.6** The "dead bone" induced new bone before getting detached at the site of pin insertion, leading to fracture healing (Epoxy-pin ESF in open fracture of metacarpus in a calf)

infection, it is better to first stabilize the fracture and treat the open wound until healthy granulation tissue is formed before going for bone grafting.

## 6.5 Postoperative Care of Open Fractures

Postoperative care and management of open fractures include everything needed after routine fracture fixation in a normal animal. Regular flushing and dressing of open wound is essential along with administration of broad spectrum antibiotics [8, 10, 23]. Deep tissue infections are treated by keeping drainage tubes and regularly lavaging the wound until the discharge recedes. In ESF, regular cleaning and dressing of the pin-skin interfaces is needed as it has been observed that pin tract infections are often more with open fracture fixations. If infection persists for longer period, culture and sensitivity test of the discharge or exudate should be done, and antibiotic regimen should be changed accordingly. Normally, within first few weeks, newly formed granulation tissue emerges on the wound surface. In certain cases with severe tissue trauma, debriding of necrosed tissue may be needed, which can be undertaken during regular dressing. In cases where devascularized bone (either attached with or detached from the major bone segment) is detected in the wound, it is required to remove the exposed bone so as to allow complete covering of granulation tissue. The wound will ultimately heal by contraction and fibrous tissue (scar) formation. If needed, skin graft may be used to cover the healing granulation tissue.

Postoperatively, radiographs are taken at regular intervals to evaluate fracture reduction and alignment, position of the implants, and bone healing. Care must be taken while interpreting and differentiating the radiographic signs of healing bone and signs of osteomyelitis in open comminuted fractures. Increased soft tissue density may be visible in both cases. In general, fractures stabilized with rigid internal fixation will heal with endosteal callus, and healing is usually delayed. In open fractures treated with an ESF, external callus may also be evident. There is gradual increase in the radiographic density between the bone ends, leading to bridging callus. In open fractures with exposed bone ends

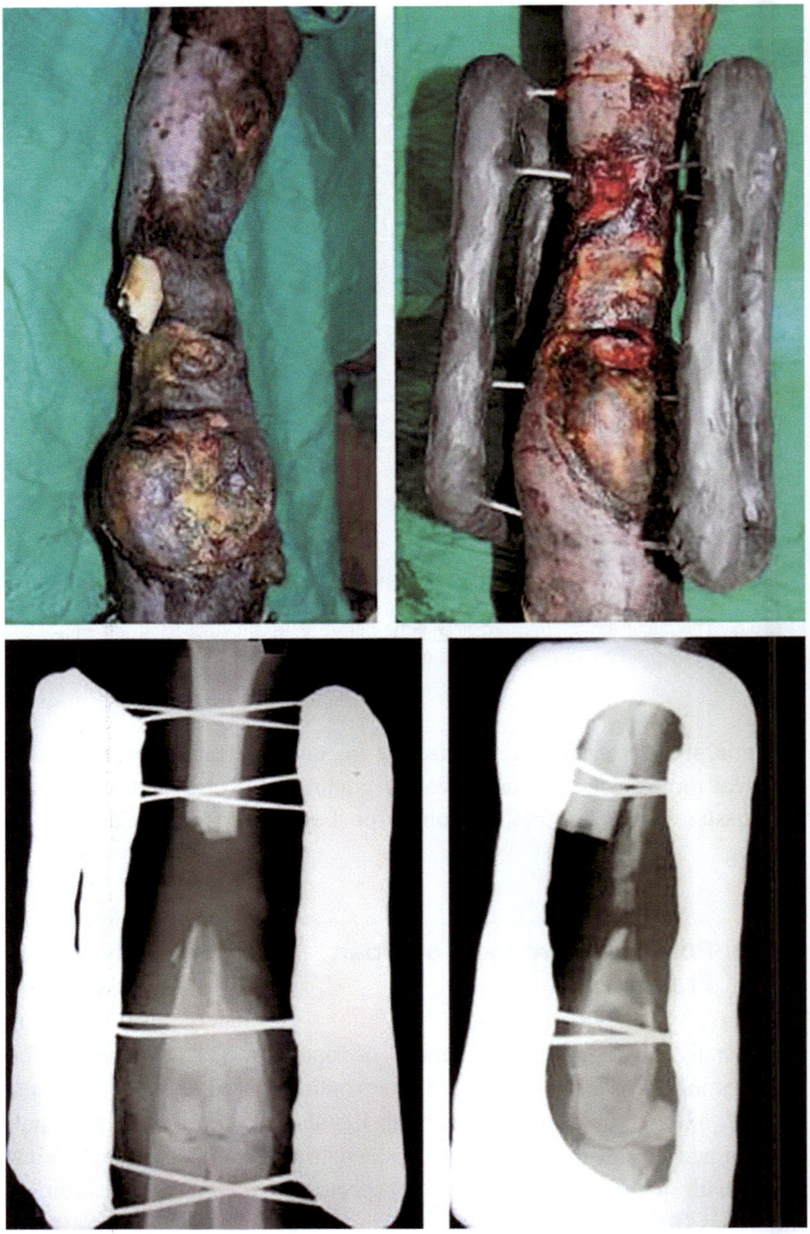

**Fig. 6.7** Severely comminuted fracture of metatarsal bone with bone loss (>25 mm) immobilized with epoxy-pin fixation. Note the presence of fracture gap and induction of new bone at the fracture site

and loss of soft tissues, new bone formation (periosteal callus) is generally seen on the outer surface of far cortex, which is covered with soft tissues. On the outer surface of the exposed bone, there will not be any callus reaction. During the course of healing, increased periosteal callus reaction may also be seen around the junction between the healthy and dead bone (with a radiolucent line at the junction indicating separation of necrosed bone from the healthy part) and also at the level of pin-bone interfaces. Radiolucency may be visible along the pin tracts. Increased radiolucency along the pin tracts and increased periosteal reaction at the pin-bone interfaces may indicate the presence or persistence of infection. Radiographic evidences of osteomyelitis include intense but irregular and purposeless new bone formation along the periosteal and endosteal surfaces, the presence of dense bone fragment enclosed by a radiolucent zone (sequestrum), and increased soft tissue density and swelling at injured site. Clinically, an animal with osteomyelitis may exhibit swelling, lameness, and drainage from the fracture site in the form of a fistulous tract.

If ostoemyelitis occurs in a fracture with stable fixation with implants in position and there is no formation of sequestrum, long-term treatment should be done with suitable antibiotics. Osteomyelitis concurrent with loose implants or sequestered bone fragments may lead to nonunion, which has to be managed by removing the affected implants and bone fragments surgically. In such cases, the fracture site should be thoroughly flushed with a sterile solution containing a broad-spectrum antibiotic, and the bone ends should be freshened (using bone rongeurs) before stabilizing them using an alternate technique. Re-fixation of fracture can be done either immediately or later, along with bone grafts and long-term antibiotic therapy.

In open fractures, it is advised to remove the implants soon after the bone healing, to avert possible long-term complications. After removal of implants, the fracture site may be temporarily stabilized using splints and bandages for a few days. With an ESF, the pin tracts are flushed with antiseptic solutions before splinting. In general, by adhering to the principles such as providing proper drainage, preserving of soft tissues, stable bone fixation, specific antibiotic therapy, and proper postoperative care will help better management of open fractures, in both small and large animals.

## Chapter 6: Sample Questions

### Q. No. 1: Mark the correct answer

1. Open fracture with a small puncture wound with or without protrusion of the fractured bone and with minimal soft tissue injury can be classified as
   (a) Grade I (b) Grade II (c) Grade III (d) Grade IV
2. Severely comminuted fractures with soft tissue injuries can be ideally stabilized using
   (a) interlocking nail (b) external skeletal fixation (c) bone plate and screws (d) none of these
3. The bone graft which can be safely used in contaminated/infected fractures to promote biological healing
   (a) cancellous autograft (b) cortical autograft (c) cancellous allograft (d) cortical allograft
4. Aggressive, irregular, and purposeless periosteal and endosteal bone formation is characteristic of
   (a) normal bone healing (b) delayed union (c) nonunion (d) osteomyelitis
5. The important factor contributing to onset of infection at fracture site is
   (a) compromised vascularity (b) soft tissue injury (c) unstable fracture fixation (d) all of the above

### Q. No. 2: State true or false

1. The chances for bacterial infection, osteomyelitis, and nonunion is higher in open fractures than in closed fractures.
2. Fractures that are adequately stabilized, either with internal implants or external fixators, can heal despite bacterial infection.
3. Heavily traumatized or contaminated wounds should be closed immediately to prevent further contamination.
4. Severely comminuted fractures with soft tissue injury should be treated using minimally invasive technique which can also provide rigid bone fixation.
5. In open fractures with comminution, it is advised to preserve the large bone fragments in place, especially those with soft tissue attachments.
6. Open fractures treated with an ESF generally heal with endosteal callus.

### Q. No. 3: Fill up the blanks

1. Open fractures are more frequently seen at the distal extremities of the limbs due to _______ ______________________________.

2. The classification of open fracture is done based on the ___________________________ _____ and _______________________________ ____________________.
3. _________________________________ refers to infection of bone and marrow.
4. Primary objectives of open fracture management are the ___________________________ ___, _______________________________ ____, and ___________________________________ ________.
5. During the course of healing, increased periosteal callus reaction around the junction between the healthy and dead bone with a radiolucent line at the junction may indicate ___________________________________ ____________________.
6. Increased radiolucency along the pin tracts and increased periosteal reaction at the pin-bone interfaces may indicate __________________ ______________________________.
7. Osteomyelitis associated with loose implants or sequestered bone fragments may be treated surgically by ___________________________ _____________________________ and ___ ___________________________________ ______________________________.

**Q. No. 4: Write short note on the following**

1. Classification of open fractures
2. Closure of open wounds with fractures
3. Clinical and radiographic signs of osteomyelitis
4. Treatment of soft tissue and bone infection

## References


1. Kumar, P., H.P. Aithal, P. Kinjavdekar, Amarpal, A.M. Pawde, K. Pratap, and G.S. Bisht. 2013. The occurrence and pattern of simple and compound fractures in limb bones in different domestic animals: A retrospective study of 989 cases. *Indian Journal of Veterinary Research* 34: 35–40.
2. Nixon, A.J., J.A. Auer, and J.P. Watkins. 2020. Principles of fracture fixation (chapter 9). In *Equine fracture repair*, ed. A.J. Nixon, 2nd ed. Hoboken, NJ: John Wiley and Sons.
3. Adams, S.B. 1985. The role of external fixation and emergency fracture management in bovine orthopedics. *The Veterinary Clinics of North America. Food Animal Practice* 1: 109–129.
4. Patzakis, M.J., and J. Wilkins. 1989. Factors influencing infection rate in open fracture wounds. *Clinical Orthopaedics and Related Research* 243: 36–40.
5. Bright, S. 2016. Open fractures. In: BSAVA Manual of Canine and Feline Fracture Repair and Management Chapter 12. 106–111.
6. Cross, W.W., and M.F. Swiontkowski. 2008. Treatment principles in the management of open fractures. *Indian Journal of Orthopaedics* 42 (4): 377–386.
7. Johnson, A.L. 1999. Management of open fractures in dogs and cats. *Waltham Focus* 9 (4): 11–17.
8. Johnson. K.A. 2012. How to manage an open fracture. BSAVA Congress, 11–15 April 2012. Birmingham, U.K. URL: https://www.vin.com/doc/?id=5328297
9. Perry, K.L. 2016. Open fractures- emergency treatment and management. 41st World Small Animal Veterinary Association Congress Proceedings Sept 27-30, Cartagena, Colombia. https://www.vin.com
10. Nunamaker, D.M. 1985. Open fractures and gunshot injuries: section one- management of open fractures. In *Textbook of small animal orthopaedics*, ed. C.D. Newton and D.M. Nunamaker, 481–485. Philadelphia: J.B. Lippincott.
11. Hoque, M., G.R. Singh, and H.P. Aithal. 1998. Post-traumatic osteomyelitis in animals: A retrospective analysis. *Indian Journal of Veterinary Research* 7: 53–57.
12. Buehler, M., M.A. Jackson, and A. Furst. 2011. Successful reduction and internal fixation of an open tibial fracture in an adult Icelandic horse. *Pferdeheilkunde* 27 (6): 681–686.
13. Gosselin, R.A., I. Roberts, and W.J. Gillespie. 2004. Antibiotics for preventing infection in open limb fractures. *Cochrane Database of Systematic Reviews* 2004 (1): CD003764.
14. Crowley, D.J., N.K. Kanakaris, and P.V. Giannoudis. 2007. Irrigation of the wounds in open fractures. *Journal of Bone and Joint Surgery. British Volume (London)* 89B: 580–585.
15. Aithal, H.P., Amarpal, P. Kinjavdekar, A.M. Pawde, G.R. Singh, M. Hoque, S.K. Maiti, and H.C. Setia. 2007. Management of fractures near carpal joint of two calves by transarticular fixation with a circular external fixator. *The Veterinary Record* 161: 193–198.
16. Dubey, P., H.P. Aithal, P. Kinjavdekar, Amarpal, P.C. Gope, D.N. Madhu, Rohit Kumar, T.B. Sivanarayanan, A.M. Pawde, and M.M.S. Zama. 2021. A comparative in vitro biomechanical investigation of a novel bilateral linear fixator vs. circular and multiplanar epoxy-pin external fixation systems using a fracture model in buffalo metacarpal bone. *World Journal of Surgery and Surgical Research* 4: 1331.
17. Shah, M.A., Rohit Kumar, P. Kinjavdekar, Amarpal, H.P. Aithal, Mohammad Arif Basha, and Asif Majid.

2022. The use of circular and hybrid external skeletal fixation systems to repair open tibial fractures in large ruminants: a report of six clinical cases. *Veterinary Research Communications* 46: 563–575.

18. Singh, A.P., G.R. Singh, H.P. Aithal, and P. Singh. 2020. Section D – fractures, chapter on the musculo-skeletal system. In *Ruminant surgery: A textbook of the surgical diseases of cattle, buffaloes, camels, sheep and goats.*, ed. J. Singh, S. Singh, and R.P.S. Tyagi, 2nd ed. New Delhi: CBS Publishers and Distributers.
19. Aithal, H.P., P. Kinjavdekar, Amarpal, A.M. Pawde, Rohit Kumar, Rekha Pathak, P. Kumar, S.K. Tyagi, P. Dubey, and D.N. Madhu. 2019. Treatment of open bone fractures using epoxy-pin fixation in small ruminants: a review of 26 cases. *Rum Science* 8: 103–114.
20. Aithal, H.P., P. Kinjavdekar, Amarpal, A.M. Pawde, M.M.S. Zama, Prasoon Dubey, Rohit Kumar, S.K. Tyagi, and D.N. Madhu. 2019. Epoxy-pin external skeletal fixation for management of open bone fractures in calves and foals: a review of 32 cases. *Veterinary and Comparative Orthopaedics and Traumatology* 32: 257–268.
21. Kumar, P., H.P. Aithal, P. Kinjavdekar, Amarpal, A.M. Pawde, K. Pratap, Surbhi, and D.K. Sinha. 2012. Epoxy-pin external skeletal fixation for treatment of open fractures or dislocations in 36 dogs. *Indian Journal of Veterinary Surgery* 33: 128–132.
22. Tyagi, S.K., H.P. Aithal, P. Kinjavdekar, Amarpal, A.M. Pawde, and Abhishek Kumar Saxena. 2021. Acrylic and epoxy-pin external skeletal fixation systems for fracture management in dogs. *Indian Journal of Animal Research*. https://doi.org/10.18805/IJAR.B-4265.
23. Tillson, D.M. 1995. Open fracture management. *The Veterinary Clinics of North America. Small Animal Practice* 25 (5): 1093–1110.

# 7 Bone Grafts and Scaffolds in Fracture Repair

**Learning Objectives**

You will be able to understand the following after reading this chapter:

- Different functions of bone grafts/implants such as osteogenesis, osteoinduction, osteoconduction, and mechanical support
- Classification of bone grafts according to origin and composition
- Different techniques used for processing the bone grafts
- Process of bone graft incorporation
- Different bone substitutes like demineralized bone matrix, calcium phosphate synthetic substitutes, synthetic polymers
- Bone inducers- bone morphogenic protein, transforming growth factor-β, insulin-like growth factor, growth hormone
- Different types of stem cells and their therapeutic application in bone healing

**Summary**

- The bone grafts or implants when transplanted into the host tissue may perform four different types of functions, namely, osteogenesis, osteoinduction, osteoconduction, and mechanical support, depending on their nature and composition.
- Autograft, the bone harvested from one site to and transplanted another site within the same individual, is the most preferred graft because it is non-immunogenic and it does not carry the risk of disease transmission.
- Several methods of preservation have been found to reduce the immunogenicity of bone allografts and xenografts; the most common methods are deep freezing, ethylene oxide treatment, and decalcification.
- Demineralization removes most of the structural components of an allograft (decrease the immune response) but still preserves the osteoinductive proteins such as bone morphogenic proteins.
- Bone morphogenic proteins (BMPs) are osteoindutive substances, which can induce the differentiation of mesenchymal cells into chondrocytes and osteoblasts during embryogenesis, growth, adulthood, and healing.
- Tricalcium phosphate (TCP) and hydroxyapatite (HA) are resorbable

(continued)


H. P. Aithal et al., *Textbook of Veterinary Orthopaedic Surgery*,
https://doi.org/10.1007/978-981-99-2575-9_7

ceramics commonly used in bone reconstruction. HA is highly brittle and slowly resorbed, whereas TCP is less brittle and has a faster resorption rate; TCP and HA are combined to form a biphasic calcium phosphate composite, which is less brittle and has a faster resorption rate than pure HA.

- Stem cells are unspecialized cells having capacity of self-renewal by cell division (even after long periods of inactivity) to proliferate extensively (often indefinitely) and to differentiate into one or more cell/tissue types. Mesenchymal stem cells (stromal bone marrow stem cells), having the potential for in vitro expansion and osteogenic differentiation, are the most commonly used stem cells for therapeutic applications in bone repair.

A graft is a living tissue that is transplanted into the same individual or another individual to repair a defect. Bone graft is a bony tissue that is used to fill a defect in the bone. The main objective of the bone grafting is to repair the defects in the bone, but it can also be used to accelerate healing of the complex and nonhealing fractures [1–3]. The clinical situations for application of bone grafting in veterinary practice include comminuted fractures, segmental defects due to bone loss from surgical excision of a bony lesion (Fig. 7.1), and delayed unions and nonunions. In addition to the bone, a large number of nonviable materials may be used to facilitate bone healing in animals. A nonviable material put in a living system is defined as an implant. Implants used for orthopedic surgery may be composed of several organic or inorganic and natural or synthetic materials, which may include bone cement, processed cortical bone,

metal or ceramic material, etc. [4–7].

## 7.1 Functions of Bone Grafts or Implants

Depending on the nature and composition, the bone grafts or implants may perform four different types of functions, namely, osteogenesis, osteoinduction, osteoconduction, and mechanical support, when transplanted into the host tissue [8–10].

***Osteogenesis*:** Osteogenesis is the formation of new bone from the cells, namely, osteoblasts and mesenchymal stem cells, which are transferred to the recipient site with the graft. The osteogenesis occurs more frequently in fresh cancellous autografts than the cortical autografts because such grafts have a large surface area covered by quiescent lining cells, undifferentiated mesenchymal cells, or active osteoblasts and can be revascularized more rapidly due to their more porosity. Initiation of osteogenesis can occur as early as 5 days after transplantation, and it may continue up to 8 weeks after transplantation of the graft.

***Osteoinduction*:** Osteoinduction is the differentiation of undifferentiated mesenchymal cells into osteogenic cells (osteoblasts) under the influence of the environment and constituents of the bone matrix [11]. Mesenchymal cells can be stimulated to differentiate into chondroblasts and osteoblasts that proliferate and produce mineralized matrix under the influence of different factors like bone morphogenic proteins (BMPs), transforming growth factor beta, insulin-like growth factor, platelet-derived growth factor, tumor necrosis factor, prostaglandin E2, and several other cytokines [12, 13]. These factors supplied by the graft would help differentiation of progenitor mesenchymal cells into osteoblasts.

***Osteoconduction*:** Osteoconduction is the process of the passive ingrowth of new bone into the graft from the recipient bed [14]. The process includes the progression of blood capillaries, perivascular tissue, and mesenchymal cells from

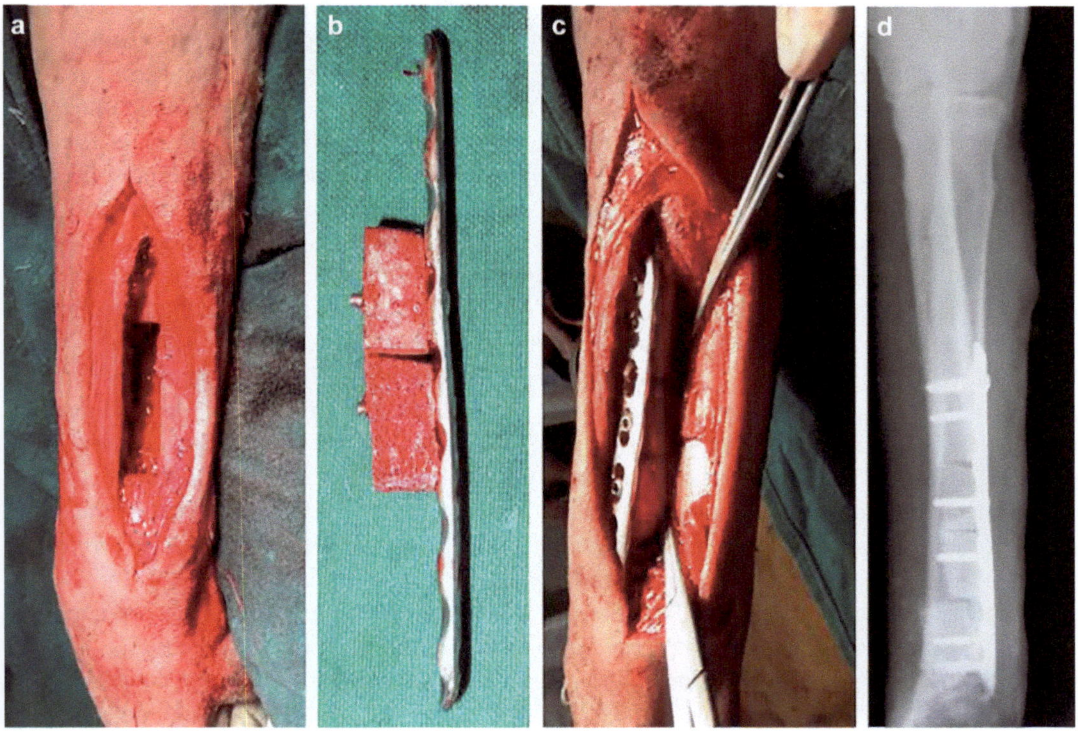


**Fig. 7.1** In a German shepherd dog with early stage of bone tumor at the distal diaphysis of ulna, the lesion site (including the surrounding normal bone) was resected (**a**), allogenic cortical bone grafts of same size was secured to a locking compression plate (**b**), fixation of graft along with plate at the defect site (**c**), and radiograph taken soon after bone fixation showing the defect site filled with bone graft (**d**)

the host bed into the scaffold. In this process, the new viable bone replaces the old necrotic bone, and it is called as creeping substitution. However, in autogenous cancellous bone graft, the new bone is formed directly over the existing necrotic trabeculae, which would be resorbed subsequent to the deposition of new bone.

***Mechanical support***: In addition to providing osteogenesis, osteoinduction, or osteoconduction, the grafts also provide mechanical support when used to fill large bony defects, particularly in weight-bearing structures. Cortical bone grafts or synthetic scaffolds are better than the cancellous grafts for providing mechanical support. Adequate mechanical support would require stabilization of these grafts adequately using suitable fracture fixation techniques such as compression plating.

## 7.2 Types of Bone Grafts

Bone grafts can be categorized according to their site of origin and their composition [15].

### 7.2.1 According to Origin

*Autografts*: If the bone is harvested from one site and transplanted to another site within the same individual, it is called as autograft [9]. Autografts are the most preferred grafts because they are readily accepted owing to their histocompatibility with the host's immune system. Further, they do not carry the risk of disease transmission. In addition to filling the gap, autografts provide the osteogenic cells and matrix proteins that can induce new bone formation and hasten bone healing. The use of autologous bone is supposed to be gold standard for fracture healing; however, their non-availability is the main limitation, and there is very little information about their clinical use in veterinary orthopedics.

*Allografts*: An allograft is the bone harvested from one individual and transplanted to another individual of the same species. Allografts may initiate significant host-graft reaction and also carry the risk of disease transmission on transplantation. However, their immunogenicity can be reduced by freezing, freeze-drying, autoclaving, or chemical treatment before transplantation. Allografts can provide instant mechanical support at the fracture site and may act as osteoinductive and osteoconductive material, but do not possess the osteogenic potential [16–18]. Inadequate availability of the autografts favors the use of allografts in clinical situations.

*Xenografts*: If the bone is harvested from an individual and transplanted to an individual of another species, it is called as xenograft. Xenografts may cause serious immunogenic reactions and carry the risk of disease transmission if not pretreated suitably. Xenogeneic bone can be used safely after tissue engineering, processing, and developing them into composite scaffolds by addition of osteogenic cells and growth factors. The composite scaffolds can provide mechanical support as well as the osteogenic environment. Nevertheless, xenografts are not routinely used in clinical practice [15].

### 7.2.2 According to Composition

According to their composition, the bone grafts may be categorized as cancellous, cortical, corticocancellous, composite, and osteochondral grafts [16, 18–20].

*Cancellous grafts*: They consist of highly cellular trabecular bone and thus enhance bone healing very rapidly but do not provide adequate mechanical strength or structural support [6, 7]. Cancellous grafts can be obtained from greater tubercle of the humerus, the tuber ischium and ilial body, and the medial condyle of the tibia. The subtrochanteric region and distal lateral femoral condyle have also been described as additional harvesting sites in dogs. Each site has very little available bone, and sometimes, the amount of the bone required for grafting may demand removal of tissue from more than one site. The wing of the ilium is the most common site for collection of bone graft because of easy approach. Harvesting of the autogenous cancellous graft involves a small incision over the donor site. A bone curette then can be used to collect the bone graft.

*Cortical grafts*: They consist of dense cortical bone and provide structural support and mechanical scaffolding for the ingrowth of new bone. Cortical grafts are usually allogeneic in origin and require adequate processing before transplantation. They are usually obtained from the cadaveric bone.

*Corticocancellous grafts*: They are a mixture of both cortical and cancellous bone.

*Composite grafts*: They are a combination of both fresh cancellous bone and preserved all implants.

*Osteochondral grafts*: They include articular cartilage as well as bone.

## 7.3 Processing of Bone Grafts

Bone contains different types of cells that are capable of inducing an immune response in the host. This response is most marked when fresh allogenic bone grafts are used. The immune response results in vascular compromise and ischemic damage. Therefore, this response can modulate the graft and implant revascularization as well as remodeling. Immunosuppression of the host animal may result in bony union of the host bone with an allograft. Matching histocompatibility antigens favorably affects the incorporation of fresh and frozen allografts. In unmatched grafts, preservation decreases the immunogenic properties of an allograft. Several methods of preservation have been reported to decrease the immunogenic properties of the allografts and xenografts. The common methods of preservation include decalcification, boiling, autoclaving, deep freezing, freeze-drying, lyophilization, irradiation, and ethylene-oxide treatment [21, 22]. The most common methods are deep freezing, ethylene oxide treatment, and decalcification. Deep freezing of allogenic bone can decrease the immune response, without much effect on the compressive, torsional, or bending strength of the bone. However, freeze-drying markedly decreases the torsional and bending strengths of the allograft. Decalcified bone grafts were found to be more successful than the inorganic grafts. Commercially produced cortical allografts are now available for veterinary use.

## 7.4 Process of Bone Graft Incorporation

The incorporation of the graft is dictated by the recipient site environment and viable cells in the fresh autograft. The cellular response is different to the cancellous graft and cortical graft, but initiation of their incorporation is the same. Initial environment for the new graft is provided by the blood clot and hematoma formation at the recipient site, which is followed by inflammatory response and invasion of the area by vascular granulation tissue. The vascular response in cancellous autografts is much more than cortical grafts, and the complete graft bed may be fully revascularized within a short period of 1 to 2 weeks. Cellular components of the graft, which are not reached by the vascular response, may die within 2 weeks. The osteoblasts provided by the recipient site or transplanted graft line the graft bone trabeculae and osteoid seam are laid around the dead bone. The osteoclasts then gradually resorb the entrapped dead bone. In the processed and stored cancellous allografts, the vascular response is less, and cellular reaction is slow as the transplanted cells are dead.

Revascularization of the cortical bone would be very slow and may take up to 2 months. The revascularization in cortical bone takes place through the existing old Haversian and Volkmann canals. Revascularization starts from periphery and gradually extends to inner parts, beginning the process of creeping substitution. Remodeling is more complete toward of the ends and the periphery of the graft than at the center of the graft. Repair of the bone completes with completion of remodeling activity.

The process of incorporation is different in cortical allografts than autografts. The allografts may induce inflammatory response, which would last for several weeks. The revascularization of allografts is considerably slower, and the new bone formation is lesser than autografts. Initially, there may be encapsulation of the allograft, which may be incorporated into the host tissue gradually.

## 7.5 Bone Substitutes

### 7.5.1 Demineralized Bone Matrix

Demineralized bone matrix (DBM) can be used as a substitute to bone graft in several situations as it could be made easily available and does not lead to comorbidity associated with autografts [23, 24]. It is prepared by demineralization of the bone tissue using chemical processing. Mineral components of the allogenic cortical bone are removed by extracting with an acid solution. Demineralization removes most of the structural components of an allograft but still preserves the osteoinductive proteins and makes them osteoconductive. DBM contains type-1 collagen, non-collagenous proteins, and growth factors such as bone morphogenic proteins (BMPs). Acid-resistant BMPs and other growth factors are potent inducers of bone formation even at extraskeletal sites. BMPs promote bone formation by inducing the transformation of perivascular mesenchymal cells to chondroblasts, which produce bone usually through endochondral ossification. DBMs have been shown to induce excellent bone formation in fracture healing in segmental defects.

### 7.5.2 Calcium Phosphate Synthetic Substitutes

Calcium phosphate synthetic substitutes are osteoconductive but can also be made osteoinductive by adding growth factors, BMPs, or other osteoinductive substances to produce a composite graft. However, they are brittle and do not have sufficient strength. As simple scaffolds, they provide osteoconductive matrix for bone formation by the host osteogenic cells with the effect of osteoinductive factors. Calcium phosphate substitutes are available in the form of ceramics, powders, and cements [25–27]. Ceramics are highly crystalline structures developed by sintering mineral salts at very high temperatures (>1000°C). The phosphate materials are relatively slowly incorporated than sulfate materials, and tricalcium phosphate is the most widely available resorbable ceramic. The structure and porosity of coralline tricalcium phosphate ceramic, formed by thermochemical treatment of coral with ammonium phosphate, is very similar to cancellous bone. A bioartificial composite bone graft consisting of beta-tricalcium phosphate and platelet-rich plasma has been used clinically [28, 29].

Synthetic hydroxyapatite is another ceramic bone substitute with osteoconductive property, and chemically, it is calcium phosphate crystals produced by a sintering process [30]. As hydroxyapatite is highly brittle, and in vivo resorption is very slow, and it is not commonly used alone. Therefore, it is combined with tricalcium phosphate to form a biphasic calcium phosphate composite, which is less brittle and has a faster resorption rate than simple hydroxyapatite.

Calcium phosphate "cement" can also be used as a bone substitute [31]. It is manufactured by dissolving the calcium by adding an aqueous solution, resulting in precipitation of calcium phosphate crystals and hardening of cement. The cement has the ability to fill the defects perfectly with higher compressive strength. However, it has the disadvantage of spilling beyond the boundaries of the fracture gap causing potential damage to the surrounding tissues and joints.

Over the past few years, a number of synthetic "grafts" have been introduced to the veterinary market and have found some favor with orthopedic surgeons although the data on their effectiveness is not extensive [27, 28, 32]. Particulate ceramic compound known as bioglass has been prepared by combining calcium oxide (CaO), sodium oxide (Na2O), silicon dioxide (SiO2), and phosphorus oxide (P2O5). A synthetic bone graft produced by the incorporation of P2O5-CaO glass within the hydroxyapatite matrix has been shown to have osteoinductive and osteoconductive properties in experimental studies and has also been used clinically [33].

### 7.5.3 Synthetic Polymers

Some of the synthetic polymers studied as bone substitutes are based on an ester polymer backbone, like poly L-lactic acid (PLA), poly glycolic acid (PGA), poly D, L-lactic acid-co-glycolic acid (PLGA), poly caprolactone, and poly propylene fumarate. They have the advantages of slow degradation and hydrophobicity allowing protein adsorption and cell adhesion, hence favored as scaffolds for cell transplantation in bone tissue engineering. Other degradable polymers used in bone regeneration are polyanhydrides, namely, poly methacrylated sebacic anhydride and poly methacrylated 1, 6-bis carboxyphenoxy hexane. Poly ethylene glycol (PEG), a nondegradable polymer, has been extensively used for manufacturing of hydrogels. It is a highly hydrophilic molecule and has great biocompatibility.

## 7.6 Bone Inducers

Bone inducers are different types of peptides and proteins that can be added as a component of composite scaffolds for bone regeneration [34–40]. Some of the important bone inducers are listed below.

### 7.6.1 Bone Morphogenic Protein (BMP)

The BMPs comprise a family of more than 12 related proteins that were originally identified by their presence in osteoinductive extracts of demineralized bone [41, 42]. They are the major active component in DBM. Their primary function is to induce the transformation of undifferentiated mesenchymal cells into chondrocytes and osteoblasts during different stages of life like embryogenesis, growth, adulthood, and bone healing [13, 43]. Recombinant technology has made available a large quantity of recombinant BMP for clinical application [44].

### 7.6.2 Transforming Growth Factor-β

TGF-β is a versatile growth factor that mediates several normal cellular physiological functions and tissue embryogenesis. The largest source of TGF-β in the body is the extracellular matrix of bone, followed by platelets. It controls proliferation and metabolic activity of skeletal mesenchymal precursor cells such as chondrocytes, osteoblasts, and osteoclasts and thus plays a significant role in directing tissue differentiation during fracture healing [45].

### 7.6.3 Insulin-like Growth Factor

Insulin-like growth factors IGF-I and growth hormone (GH) are known to have marked anabolic effects on bone [46]. IGF accelerates proliferation and increases the metabolic activity of osteoblasts that result in increased production of osteocalcin. The primary function of osteocalcin in bone is the regulation of bone maturation and the mineralization of bone matrix [12].

### 7.6.4 Growth Hormone

Growth hormone (GH) has an anabolic effect on bone metabolism and may act through an increased synthesis of IGF-1 in osteoblasts [46, 47].

## 7.7 Stem Cells

The stem cell research and application has attracted enormous interest in the recent past due to potential application of stem cells in various incurable diseases. Stem cells are primitive undifferentiated cells, which possess the capacity to proliferate extensively by cell division and differentiate into one or more cell or tissue types even after a prolonged period. There are many types of stem cells like embryonic stem cells and adult or tissue-specific stem cells that exist in various fetal and adult tissues. Some specialized adult cells can be transformed genetically to stem cell-like cells, termed as "induced pluripotent stem cells (iPSCs)" [12, 48, 49].

Adult stem cells, also known as tissue-specific stem cells, have been identified in many tissues and organs such as blood and blood vessels, bone marrow, skeletal muscle, skin, teeth, heart, liver, brain, gut, ovarian epithelium, uterine endothelium, Wharton's jelly, and testes [50]. They are believed to inhabit in a distinct area of each tissue, called a stem cell niche.

Bone marrow adult stem cells have been classified based on their differential potential as either hematopoietic or mesenchymal stem cells (MSC). Mesenchymal stem cells are often called as stromal stem cells, stromal bone marrow stem cells, or multipotent mesenchymal stromal cells (suggested by The International Society for Cellular Therapy). Mesenchymal stem cells are most commonly used stem cells for therapeutic applications [12, 49].

Conventionally, it is more rational to use autologous cultured stem cells than allogeneic cells, which could have the risk of immune rejection and disease transmission. However, the main drawback of using autologous mesenchymal stem cells in therapeutic applications is the long time required for their culture and expansion. Nevertheless, bone marrow-derived stem cells seem to possess certain degree of immune privilege that avoid allogenic rejection and minimal requirement of immunosuppressive drugs. Hypoimmunogenicity of MSCs is attributed to lack of major histocompatibility complex (MHC)-II and co-stimulatory molecule expression preventing T-cell responses (by modulating dendritic cells, and disrupting natural killer (NK) and CD8+, CD4+ T cell function) [51]. MSCs thus have a great prospect for therapeutic applications in a variety of medical conditions.

For therapeutic applications, stem cells can be administered through local delivery or by systemic infusion. Different mechanisms proposed by which MSCs repair tissue injury include: (a) creation of an environment for enhancing regeneration of endogenous cells, (b) trans-differentiation of stem cells into host tissue cells, or (c) cell fusion [12, 49].

Stimulation of new bone formation at the site of implantation of MSCs indicates that these cells either themselves act as osteogenic cells or stimulate the host bone to regenerate. MSCs having the potential for in vitro expansion and osteogenic differentiation are the most commonly used seed cells for bone regeneration. Clinical studies have indicated that the use of autologous MSCs in bone reconstruction produces strong osteogenic activity, but allogenic MSCs are the next best alternative. Experimental studies of bone defects have also revealed that allogenic MSCs are as effective as autogenic stem cells with little chances of immune reaction and rejection [51]. Segmental bone defects in canines have been treated with bone marrow-derived canine MSCs along with demineralized bone matrix and ceramic implants. Similarly, cultured goat bone marrow-derived MSCs have also been used along with scaffolds for reconstruction of segmental bone defect in goat tibia. Successful management of nonunion of radius-ulna in a cross bred dog has been reported with the use of composite scaffold made from implanting autologous adipose-derived stem cells (ADSCs) ($3.2 \times 10^7$ cells) on hydroxyapatite (HA) and chitosan (CH) fibers [52]. Nonunion in a dog has also been successfully treated by injecting bone marrow-derived MSCs ($2 \times 10^6$) locally (Fig. 7.2). Promising clinical results of stem cell therapy have also been recorded in spinal cord injuries in dogs [53] (Fig. 7.3).

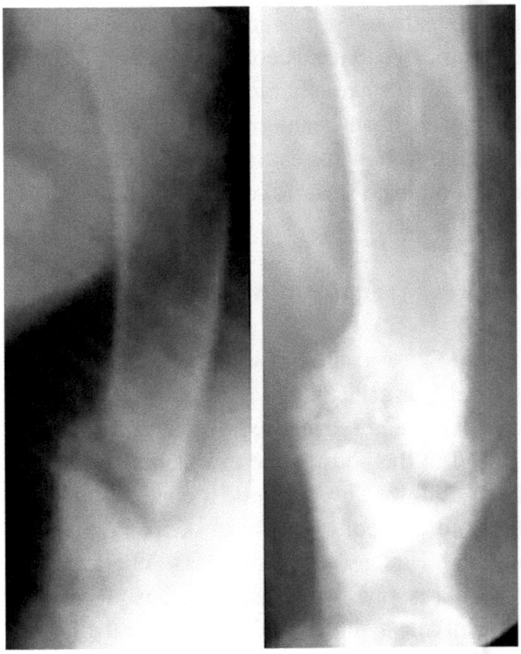

**Fig. 7.2** A nonunion fracture of distal humerus (**a**), 15 days after treatment with local injection of stem cell, local injection of $1 \times 10^6$ autogenic bone marrow derived mesenchymal stem cells, showing increased osseous density at the fracture site indicating healing

## Chapter 7: Sample Questions

**Q. No. 1: Mark the correct answer**

1. The process of differentiation of undifferentiated mesenchymal cells into bone is called as
   (a) osteoinduction (b) osteoconduction (c) osteogenesis (d) incorporation
2. A tissue sample that is taken from one individual and transplanted into another individual from the same species is called as
   (a) autograft (b) isograft (c) allograft (d) xenograft
3. Homograft is also know as
   (a) autograft (b) allograft (c) xenograft (d) isograft

**Q. No. 2: State true or false**

1. Hydroxy apatite ceramic can be used as a scaffold to fill the bone defect.
2. Osteoconduction is the process of differentiation of undifferentiated mesenchymal cells into bone cells.
3. Demineralization removes most of the structural components of an allograft but preserves the osteoinductive proteins and makes them osteoconductive.
4. Deep freezing of allogenic bone may markedly reduce the compressive, torsional, or bending strength, whereas freeze-drying may not affect

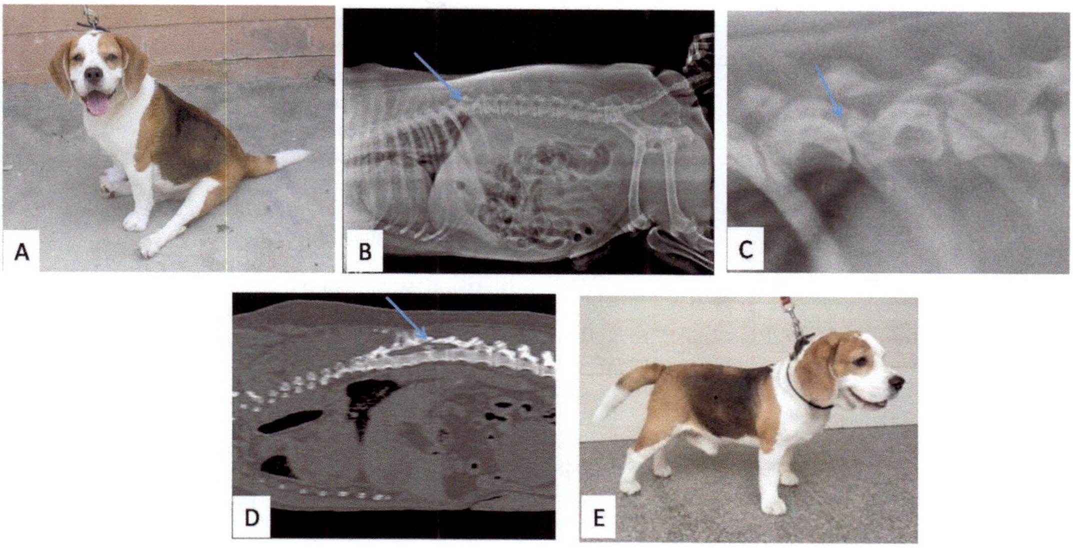

**Fig. 7.3** A 6-year-old male Beagle dog with sudden onset of paraplegia (**a**), lateral radiograph showing decreased intervertebral space at T12-T13 level (**b**), magnified view of the radiograph (**c**), CT image of the vertebral column showed Hensen type I disk protrusion (**d**), the animal showed complete recovery after 4 doses of intralesional administration of allogenic mesenchymal stem cell ($1 \times 10^6$ cell in 1 ml PBS) at 15 day interval (**e**)

the torsional and bending strengths of the bone.

5. Hydroxyapatite is less brittle and has a faster resorption rate than tricalcium phosphate.
6. Insulin-like growth factors are known to have marked anabolic effects on the bone.
7. MSCs are immune-privileged cells as they are hypoimmunogenic, due to lack of major histocompatibility complex (MHC)-II and co-stimulatory molecule expression.

## Q. No. 3: Fill up the blanks

1. The process of the passive ingrowth of new bone into the graft from the recipient bed is called ____________________.
2. A material that is taken from one individual and transplanted into another genetically identical individual is ____________________ ________.
3. The most common site for collection of bone autograft is the ____________________.
4. The synthetic polymers most commonly investigated for bone tissue engineering scaffold applications are ________________ ________________, ________________ ________________ and ________________ ________________.
5. The largest source of TGF-β, a multifunctional growth factor, in the body, is the ____________________ and ____________________.
6. Unspecialized cells having capacity of self-renewal by cell division and differentiate into one or more cell/tissue types are called as ____________________.
7. Bone marrow adult stem cells based on their differential potential can be grouped as ______ ________________ or ________________ ________________ stem cells, and the most commonly used stem cells for therapeutic applications are ________________ ________________.

## Q. No. 4: Write short note on the following

1. Differentiate between osteoinduction and osteoconduction
2. Types of bone grafts
3. Processing and preservation of bone grafts
4. Incorporation of bone grafts

5. Bone morphogenic proteins
6. Therapeutic application of stem cells in bone regeneration

## References


1. Johnson, A.L. 1991. Principles of bone grafting. *Seminars in Veterinary Medicine and Surgery (Small Animal)* 6 (1): 90–99.
2. Nunamaker, D.M., and F.W. Rhinelander. 1985. Bone grafting. In *Textbook of small animal orthopaedics*, ed. C.D. Newton and D.M. Nunamaker, 519–526. Philadelphia: J.B. Lippincott.
3. Stevenson, S. 1985. Bone grafting. In *Textbook of small animal surgery*, ed. D.H. Slatter, 2035–2048. Philadelphia: PA Saunders.
4. Nandi, S.K., S. Roy, P. Mukherjee, B. Kundu, D.K. De, and D. Basu. 2010. Orthopaedic applications of bone graft and graft substitutes: a review. *The Indian Journal of Medical Research* 132: 15–30.
5. Pinho, P.O., J.M. Campos, C. Mendonça, A.R. Caseiro, J.D. Santos, A.C. Maurício, and L.M. Atayde. 2017. Clinical application of macroporous ceramic to promote bone healing in veterinary clinical cases. In *Materials, technologies and clinical applications*, ed. F. Baino. London: IntechOpen. https://doi.org/10.5772/intechopen.70341. https://www.intechopen.com/books/5922.
6. Roberts, T.T., and A.J. Rosenbaum. 2012. Bone grafts, bone substitutes and orthobiologics: the bridge between basic science and clinical advancements in fracture healing. *Organogenesis* 8 (4): 114–124.
7. Wang, W., and K.W.K. Yeung. 2017. Bone grafts and biomaterials substitutes for bone defect repair: a review. *Bioactive Materials* 2 (4): 224–247.
8. Burchardt, H. 1983. The biology of bone graft repair. *Clinical Orthopaedics and Related Research* 174: 28–42.
9. Old, R.B., K. Sinibaldi, M. DeAngelis, S.G. Stoll, and H. Rosen. 1973. Autogenous cancellous bone grafting in small animals. *Journal of the American Animal Hospital Association* 9: 454–457.
10. Urist, M.R. 1972. Osteoinduction in undemineralized bone implants modified by chemical inhibitors of endogenous matrix enzymes. *Clinical Orthopaedics* 87: 132–137.
11. Wilson-Hench, J. 1987. Osteoinduction. In *Progress in biomedical engineering*, Definitions in biomaterials, ed. D.F. Williams, vol. 4, 29. Amsterdam: Elsevier.
12. Gugjoo, M.B., Amarpal, Ahmed Abdelbaset-Ismailc, H.P. Aithal, P. Kinjavdekar, A.M. Pawde, G. Sai Kumar, and G.T. Sharma. 2017. Mesenchymal stem cells with IGF-1 and TGF- β1 in laminin gel for osteochondral defects in rabbits. *Biomedicine & Pharmacotherapy* 93: 1165–1174.
13. Yu, D.A., J. Han, and B.S. Kim. 2012. Stimulation of chondrogenic differentiation of mesenchymal stem cells. *International Journal of Stem Cells* 5 (1): 16–22.
14. Cornell, C.N., and J.M. Lane. 1998. Current understanding of osteoconduction in bone regeneration. *Clinical Orthopaedics and Related Research* 355S: S267–S273.
15. Harasen, G. 2011. Stimulating bone growth in the small animal patient: grafts and beyond! *The Canadian Veterinary Journal* 52 (2): 199–200.
16. Henry, W.B., and P.L. Wadsworth. 1981. Diaphyseal allografts in the repair of long bone fractures. *Journal of the American Animal Hospital Association* 17: 525–534.
17. Roe, S.C., G.J. Pijanowski, and A.L. Johnson. 1988. Biomechanical properties of cortical bone allografts: effects of preparation and storage. *American Journal of Veterinary Research* 49: 873–877.
18. Sinibaldi, K.R. 1989. Evaluation of full cortical allografts in 25 dogs. *Journal of the American Veterinary Medical Association* 194: 1570–1577.
19. Alexander, J.W. 1983. Use of combination of cortical bone allografts and cancellous bone autografts to replace massive bone loss in fresh fractures and selected nonunions. *Journal of the American Animal Hospital Association* 19: 671–687.
20. Heiple, K.G., V.M. Goldberg, A.E. Powell, G.D. Bos, and J.M. Zika. 1987. Biology of cancellous bone grafts. *The Orthopedic Clinics of North America* 18: 179–185.
21. Kerwin, S.C., D.D. Lewis, A.D. Elkins, J. Oliver, R. Pechman, R.J. McCarthy, and G. Hosgood. 1996. Deep-frozen allogeneic cancellous bone grafts in 10 dogs: a case series. *Veterinary Surgery* 25: 18–28.
22. Schwarz, N., G. Schlag, M. Thurnher, J. Eschberger, H.P. Dinges, and H. Redl. 1991. Fresh autogeneic, frozen allogeneic, and decalcified allogeneic bone grafts in dogs. *Journal of Bone and Joint Surgery* B73 (5): 787–790.
23. Hoffer, M.J., D.J. Griffon, D.J. Schaeffer, A.L. Johnson, and M.W. Thomas. 2008. Clinical applications of demineralised bone matrix: a retrospective and case-matched study of seventy-five dogs. *Veterinary Surgery* 37 (7): 639–647.
24. Vertenten, G., F. Gasthuys, M. Cornelissen, and E. Schacht. 2010. Enhancing bone healing and regeneration: present and future perspectives in veterinary orthopaedics. *Veterinary and Comparative Orthopaedics and Traumatology* 23: 153–162.
25. Aithal, H.P., I.V. Mogha, and G.R. Singh. 1993. Clinical and radiological evaluation of bone grafts and ALCAP ceramic used in the treatment of bone defects in goats. *Indian Journal of Veterinary Surgery* 14: 16–20.
26. Aithal, H.P., I.V. Mogha, O.P. Paliwal, and G.R. Singh. 1992. Comparative histopathological evaluation of different bone grafts and ALCAP ceramics in goats. *Indian Journal of Veterinary Pathology* 16: 91–94.

27. Franch, J., C. Diaz-Bertrana, P. Lafuente, P. Fontecha, and I. Durall. 2006. Beta-tricalcium phosphate as a synthetic cancellous bone graft in veterinary orthopedics: a retrospective study of 13 clinical cases. *Veterinary and Comparative Orthopaedics and Traumatology* 19: 196–204.
28. Hauschild, G., H.-A. Merten, A. Bader, G. Uhr, A. Deivick, A. Meyer-Lindenberg, and M. Fehr. 2005. Bioartificial bone grafting: tarsal joint fusion in a dog using a bioartificial composite bone graft consisting of beta-tricalciumphosphate and platelet rich plasma-A case report. *Veterinary and Comparative Orthopaedics and Traumatology* 18 (1): 52–54.
29. Rabillard, M., J.-G. Grand, E. Dalibert, B. Fellah, O. Gauthier, and G. Niebauer. 2009. Effects of autologous platelet rich plasma gel and calcium phosphate biomaterials on bone healing in an ulnar ostectomy model in dogs. *Veterinary and Comparative Orthopaedics and Traumatology* 22 (6): 460–466.
30. Roy, D.M., and S.K. Linnehan. 1974. Hydroxyapatite formed from coral skeletal carbonate by hydrothermal exchange. *Nature* 247: 220–222.
31. Blokhuis, T.J., M.F. Termaat, F.C. den Boer, P. Patka, F.C. Bakker, and H.J. Haarman. 2000. Properties of calcium phosphate ceramics in relation to their in vivo behavior. *The Journal of Trauma* 48 (1): 179–186.
32. Wheeler, D.L., E.J. Eschbach, R.G. Hoellrich, M.J. Montfort, and D.L. Chamberland. 2000. Assessment of resorbable bioactive material for grafting of critical-size cancellous defects. *Journal of Orthopaedic Research* 18: 140–148.
33. Pinto, P.O., J.M. Campos, A.R. Caseiro, T. Pereira, J.D. Santos, L.M. Atayde, and A.C. Maurício. 2016. *Use of a macroporous glass-reinforced hydroxyapatite synthetic bone substitute in treatment of long-bone atrophic non-union fracture- two clinical cases in dogs*, 448–449. London: ESVOT.
34. Celeste, A.J., J.A. Iannazzi, R.C. Taylor, R.M. Hewick, V. Rosen, E.A. Wang, and J.M. Wozney. 1990. Identification of transforming growth factor β family members present in bone inductive protein purified from bovine bone. *Proceedings of the National Academy of Sciences of the United States of America* 87: 9843–9847.
35. Chang, S.C., B. Hoang, J.T. Thomas, S. Vukicevic, F.P. Luyten, N.J. Ryba, C.A. Kozak, A.H. Reddi, and M. Moos Jr. 1994. Cartilage-derived morphogenetic proteins. New members of the transforming growth factor-β super family predominantly expressed in long bones during human embryonic development. *The Journal of Biological Chemistry* 269: 28227–28234.
36. Chen, G., C. Deng, and Y.P. Li. 2012. TGF-β and BMP signalling in osteoblast differentiation and bone formation. *International Journal of Biological Sciences* 8: 272–288.
37. Horner, A., P. Kemp, C. Summers, S. Bord, N.J. Bishop, A.W. Kelsall, N. Coleman, and J.E. Compston. 1998. Expression and distribution of transforming growth factor-β isoforms and their signalling receptors in growing human bone. *Bone* 23: 95–102.
38. Klar, R.M., R. Duarte, T. Dix-Peek, and U. Ripamonti. 2014. The induction of bone formation by the recombinant human transforming growth factor- β3. *Biomaterials* 35: 2773–2788.
39. Klar, R.M. 2018. The induction of bone formation: the translation enigma. *Frontiers in Bioengineering and Biotechnology*, 07 June 2018. Sec. Tissue Engineering and Regenerative Medicine. https://doi.org/10.3389/fbioe.2018.00074.
40. Reddi, A.H. 2000. Role of bone morphogenetic proteins in skeletal tissue engineering of bone and cartilage: inductive signals, stem cells, and biomimetic biomaterials. *Tissue Engineering* 6: 351–359.
41. Jain, A.P., S. Pundir, and A. Sharma. 2013. Bone morphogenetic proteins: the anomalous molecules. *Journal of Indian Society of Periodontology* 17: 583–586.
42. Reddi, A.H. 2005. BMPs: from bone morphogenetic proteins to body morphogenetic proteins. *Cytokine & Growth Factor Reviews* 16: 249–250.
43. Scarfì, S. 2016. Use of bone morphogenetic proteins in mesenchymal stem cell stimulation of cartilage and bone repair. *World Journal of Stem Cells* 8 (1): 1–12.
44. Gupta, V., M. Sengupta, J. Prakash, and B.C. Tripathy. 2016. Production of recombinant pharmaceutical proteins. *Basic and Applied Aspects of Biotechnology*: 77–101. https://doi.org/10.1007/978-981-10-0875-7_4.
45. Wang, X., Y. Wang, W. Gou, Q. Lu, J. Peng, and S. Lu. 2013. Role of mesenchymal stem cells in bone regeneration and fracture repair: a review. *International Orthopaedics* 37 (12): 2491–2498.
46. Giustina, A., G. Mazziotti, and E. Canalis. 2008. Growth hormone, insulin-like growth factors, and the skeleton. *Endocrine Reviews* 29 (5): 535–559.
47. Gugjoo, M.B., Amarpal, Ahmed Abdelbaset-Ismail, H.P. Aithal, P. Kinjavdekar, G. Sai Kumar, and G.T. Sharma. 2020. Allogeneic mesenchymal stem cells and growth factors in gel scaffold repair osteochondral defect in rabbit. *Regenerative Medicine* 15: 1261. https://doi.org/10.2217/rme-2018-0138.
48. Gade, N.E., M.D. Pratheesh, A. Nath, P.K. Dubey, Amarpal, B. Sharma, G. Saikumar, and G.T. Sharma. 2013. Molecular and cellular characterization of buffalo bone marrow derived mesenchymal stem cells. *Reproduction in Domestic Animals* 48: 358e67.
49. Gugjoo, M.B., Amarpal, G.T. Sharma, P. Kinjavdekar, H.P. Aithal, and A.M. Pawde. 2016. Cartilage tissue engineering: role of mesenchymal stem cells along with growth factors and scaffolds. *The Indian Journal of Medical Research* 144 (3): 339–347.
50. Gugjoo, M.B.A., P. Kinjavdeka, H.P. Aithal, M. Matin Ansa, A.M. Pawde, and G.T. Sharma. 2015. Isolation, culturing and characterization of New Zealand white rabbit mesenchymal stem cells derived from bone marrow. *Asian Journal of Animal and Veterinary* 10 (10): 537–548.

51. Udehiya, R.K., Amarpal, H.P. Aithal, P. Kinjavdekar, A.M. Pawde, R. Singh, and G.T. Sharma. 2013. Comparison of autogenic and allogenic bone marrow derived mesenchymal stem cells for repair of segmental bone defects in rabbits. *Research in Veterinary Science* 94: 743–752.
52. Lee, H.B., Y.S. Chung, S.Y. Heo, and N.S. Kim. 2009. Augmentation of bone healing of nonunion fracture using stem cell based tissue engineering in a dog: a case report. *Veterinary Medicine* 54 (4): 198–203.
53. Sharun, K., R. Kumar, V. Chandra, A.C. Saxena, A.M. Pawde, P. Kinjavdekar, K. Dhama, Amarpal, and G.T. Sharma. 2021. Percutaneous transplantation of allogenic bone marrow-derived mesenchymal stem cells for the management of paraplegia secondary to Hansen type I intervertebral disc herniation in a Beagle dog. *Iranian Journal of Veterinary Research* 22 (2): 161–166.

# Complications of Fracture Fixation

# 8

**Learning Objectives**

You will be able to understand the following after reading this chapter:

- Etiology; clinical symptoms; radiographic diagnosis and treatment of delayed union, nonunion, and malunion of fracture; and fixation failure
- Diagnosis and management of soft tissue infection and osteomyelitis
- Prevention and treatment of fracture disease and supporting limb laminitis
- Complications associated with dislocation of joints


**Summary**

- Most complications in fracture fixation occur due to selection of improper method for fracture stabilization; thus, many of them can be avoided or minimized by appropriate selection and application of fracture fixation technique.
- Delayed union is a fracture, which fails to heal within a stipulated period of time that is normally required for healing for a particular location and type of fracture, whereas when fracture ends fail to unite with complete cessation of healing process, it is called a nonunion.
- Basic principles of treatment in osteomyelitis include establishment of drainage through debridement of infected and necrosed tissues; antibiotic therapy based on sensitivity test, providing stable fracture fixation by avoiding dead space and by using bone grafts; and quick removal of the implant after bone union.
- Quadriceps contracture, where vastus intermedius muscle forms a fibrotic scar with the femoral fracture bone callus resulting in an inability to flex or extend the stifle, is the most common and severe form of fracture disease seen in small animal patients.
- Support limb laminitis is more common in horses than cattle treated for fracture fixation as a horse tends to stand on contralateral normal limb all the time resting the injured limb, whereas cattle lie down more frequently giving rest to the affected limb.
- Complications involving dislocation of joints can be due to the inability to reduce the joint adequately, the inability to maintain the reduction, or to the loss of joint function following successful/unsuccessful/delayed attempts.





H. P. Aithal et al., *Textbook of Veterinary Orthopaedic Surgery*,
https://doi.org/10.1007/978-981-99-2575-9_8

Complications related to fracture and its fixation can be associated with initial trauma, fixation technique, or postoperative care following a fracture repair. Complications of fracture are mostly related to improper care and delayed treatment (Figs. 8.1 and 8.2). Most complications in fracture fixation occur due to selection of improper method for fracture stabilization [1–3]. Many of them thus can be avoided or minimized by selecting appropriate fracture fixation technique adopting standard method. The complications are often related to undersized or oversized implant (IM pin/bone plate), improper number of implants (pins/screws), malpositioning and poor contouring of implants (bone plate), and failure to use bone grafts/scaffolds when a gap is present at the fracture site. A thorough understanding of the principles of fracture fixation technique helps avoid most of the problems. At times, in spite of our best efforts, complications in bone healing are unavoidable, but their resolution may be aided by early diagnosis of the problem and initiating appropriate treatment. The common complications include (i) cast/splint sores (with external fixation), (ii) unsuccessful functional bone union (delayed union, nonunion, malunion, premature closure of growth plate, etc.), (iii) pin tract sepsis (with ESF) and osteomyelitis (more with internal fixation), (iv) fixation failure (bone-implant construct failure, which can occur due to defects with the implant, bone, or fixation of implant to the bone), (v) fracture disease (atrophy, stiffness, adhesions), (vi) contralateral/supporting limb laminitis (more common in equines), and (vii) nerve and vascular injuries leading to denervation and avascular necrosis.

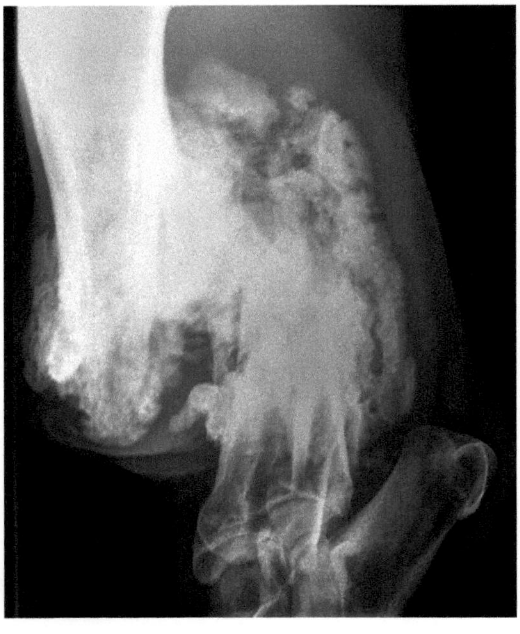

**Fig. 8.1** An untreated fracture of distal tibia in cattle, resulting in malunion

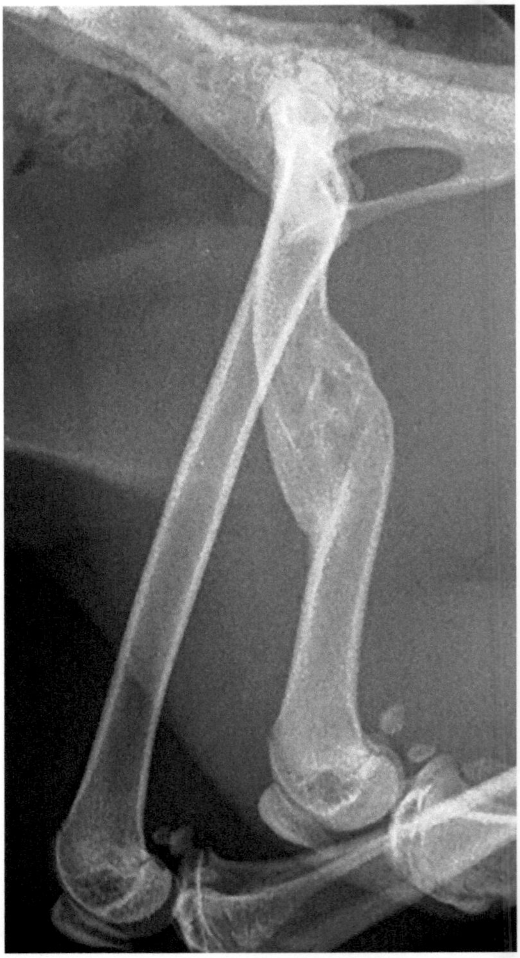

**Fig. 8.2** Malunion and shortening of femur in a dog due to delay in seeking treatment

The normal time period required for fracture healing may vary with animal's age, type and location of fracture, type of bone involved, severity of soft tissue injury, infection, nutritional status of the animal, and the presence of concomitant metabolic disease. Healing is faster in young growing animals and with increasing age and complexity of fracture healing delays. Further, with less rigid fixation (micromotion at the fracture site), healing is faster, and with more rigid fixation, healing is delayed. Under proper conditions, healing should progress normally leading to union between the fracture segments before the implant/fixation fails. Generally, it may take about 2–4 weeks in very young animals, 4–6 weeks in adult dogs and young calves/foals, and about 6–12 weeks in adult large animals, depending on the type of fixation used.

## 8.1 Delayed Union

When a fracture fails to heal within a stipulated period of time that is normally required for healing for a particular location and type of fracture, it is called as *delayed union* [4–6]. It is difficult to diagnose a delayed union, as one should know about what is "normal period" for a specific fracture to heal. Delayed union can be caused either by mechanical or biological factors, or both. Biological causes include periosteal damage, vascular compromise, and infection, whereas mechanical causes include excessive fracture gaps, soft tissue interposition between the fracture ends, and suboptimal fixation or fixation for an inadequate period of time. Old age, accompanied with corticosteroid administration and metabolic diseases (such as hyperadrenocorticism), can also delay the fracture healing. Some of the common findings related to delayed union are broken implants, radiolucency between the fracture ends and at bone-implant interface, pain on palpation of the fracture site, and persistent or escalating lameness (Fig. 8.3). In an uncertain biological or mechanical condition, immediate surgical intervention is needed to provide rigid immobilization [7, 8].

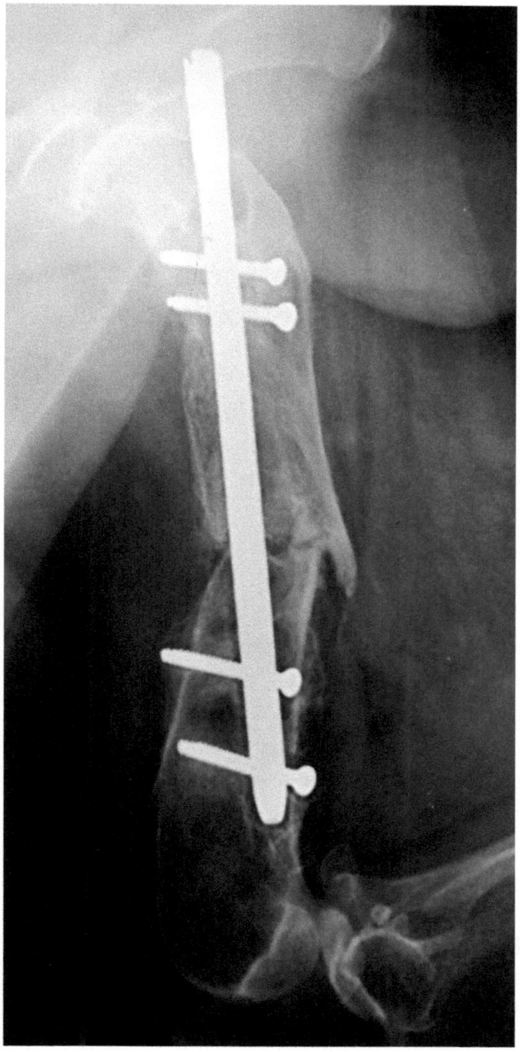

**Fig. 8.3** Delayed union of femur fracture treated with interlocking nail fixation in a dog. Callus reaction is visible at the fracture site, but purposeful bridging callus is not present. The reason for delayed union could be osteoporosis

## 8.2 Nonunion

In a *nonunion*, the fracture ends fail to unite with complete cessation of healing process, requiring surgical correction to achieve a functional bone union [4, 6, 8]. Distal radius/ulna and tibia are the common sites of nonunion [9]. Nonunion can be viable (hypertrophic, moderately hypertrophic, and oligotrophic) or nonviable (dystrophic, necrotic, defect, and atrophic). In viable nonunion, vascular supply and biological environment at the fracture site is adequate, but there is inadequate mechanical stability, whereas nonviable nonunion is distinguished by insufficient vascular and biological conditions. Besides impaired circulation, several other factors such as bone loss due to injury or surgical dissection, faulty fracture reduction (unsuitable implant), technical error during fracture fixation and devascularization of fracture segments during the surgical correction, infection, or instability may also contribute to nonunion. Common and variable clinical signs of a nonunion may include lameness (recent, continuous, or aggravated), instability and pain on palpation at the site or movement of the limb, and disuse atrophy and stiffness of muscles. Radiographically, sclerotic fracture ends with rounding of edges are characteristic, which differentiates it from a delayed union. A viable nonunion can be treated by dissecting the fibrous tissue between the fracture segments, freshening the sclerotic bone ends to open the medullary cavity, filling the fracture gap with a bone graft, and providing rigid and stable fixation (bone plating or external skeletal fixation), while in a nonviable nonunion, the focus of treatment should be on protecting the soft tissues and maintaining circulation in addition to providing a rigid fixation (Fig. 8.4). Use of bone inducers such as bone morphogenic protein can be beneficial to achieve a favorable outcome especially in nonviable nonunion cases.

## 8.3 Malunion

When fracture union occurs away from the normal anatomical alignment, that is, in an abnormal position, it is called *malunion* [4, 7, 10]. Inadequate fracture reduction, alignment, or fixation failure may lead to malunion (Fig. 8.5). Nonunion is common with inadequate bone reduction and alignment during the application of a cast or splint in large animals. Correction of malunion is required only when it leads to functional disability to the animal. Surgical correction includes osteotomies of the bone at the site of nonunion, realignment, and rigid fixation of fracture segments using a bone plate or external skeletal fixation.

## 8.4 Fixation Failure

Fixation failure or bone-implant construct failure can occur either due to failure of the fixation implant, that is, breaking of screws or bending of plate, or due to breaking of the bone (Fig. 8.6). But they are rarely primarily attributed to the implant alone, and in majority of cases, the cause is a technical error, including the selection of improper type of implant, use of inappropriate sized implants, improper placement of implants, and poor owner compliance [3, 10, 11]. Generally, fixation failure occurs in the early postoperative period; as the time since surgery increases, the possibility of fixation failure reduces. In large animal fracture fixation, there are every chances of fixation failure during recovery from anesthesia; hence, they need assistance while rising and lying down during recovery from anesthesia and also during the immediate post-fixation period [12]. Cattle are generally less prone to implant failure and refracture during recovery from anesthesia than horses, but risk is higher in internal fixation of humerus, femur, and tibial fractures.

Fixation failure can be diagnosed by evaluating orthogonal views of sequential follow-up radiographs taken after fracture fixation. Implant loosening or breakage can be diagnosed by assessing the relative position of the implant as compared to previous radiographs (Fig. 8.7). Reduced bone density or radiolucency adjoining to the implant may indicate implant loosening or infection. There can be loss of reduction and alignment of bone segments at the fracture site. In cases of fixation failure, surgical correction is advised, and rigid fixation may be provided by changing the fixator type (internal fixation to ESF or vice versa). If infection is evident, an ESF is preferred.

## 8.5 Soft Tissue Infection and Osteomyelitis

Infection of soft tissues and bone can occur during or following fracture fixation. Osteomyelitis, inflammation of bone marrow and cortex, is usually linked with open, contaminated fractures and internal fixation [13–17]. Although fungal, viral, and parasitic invasion of bone are known, osteomyelitis mainly implies to bacterial invasion, most commonly caused by *Staphylococcus* species. Infection develops either through

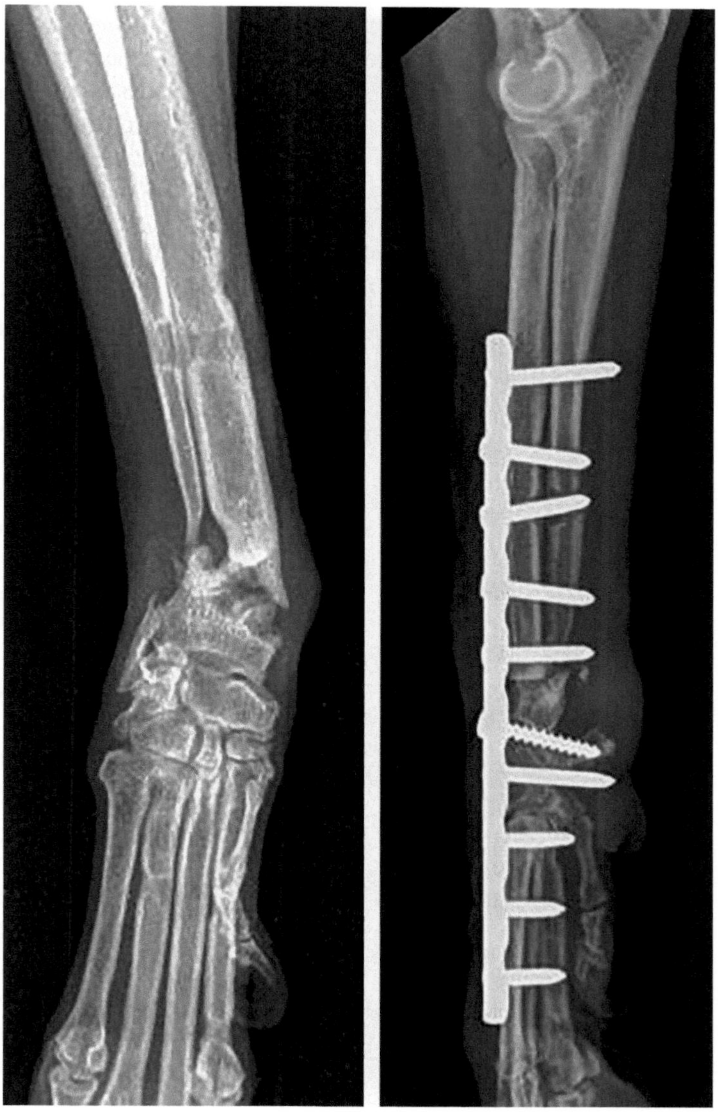

**Fig. 8.4** Nonunion of distal radius-ulna fracture treated with an ESF application in a dog. The fracture ends are rounded off with no union between the bone segments (**a**); treated by freshening of the fracture ends and transcarpal fixation with a LCP

hematogenous or exogenous routes. Exogenous route of infection is common in animals. Bacteria may be inoculated into an open wound either at the time of injury or during the surgical intervention. Tissue damage, presence of implant, lack of blood supply and mobility at the fracture site potentiates the proliferation of bacteria.

Clinical signs associated with an infection may comprise inflammatory swelling at the incision site, pain on palpation over the fracture site or implant, fistulous tracts discharging the exudates, and sudden onset or aggravation of lameness (Fig. 8.8). Drainage from the pin tracts is characteristic with ESF [12, 18–22]. Radiographically, soft tissue swelling adjacent to/surrounding the affected site is the early indication of infection/osteomyelitis. Excessive and irregular periosteal reaction and cortical lysis/radiolucency associated with implant/bone interface may be visible.

Infection can be prevented by the use of sterile surgical materials, following standard aseptic procedures, minimal tissue handling/damage, providing stable fracture fixation and judicious use of antibiotics. Management of osteomyelitis is often frustrating and unrewarding. Basic

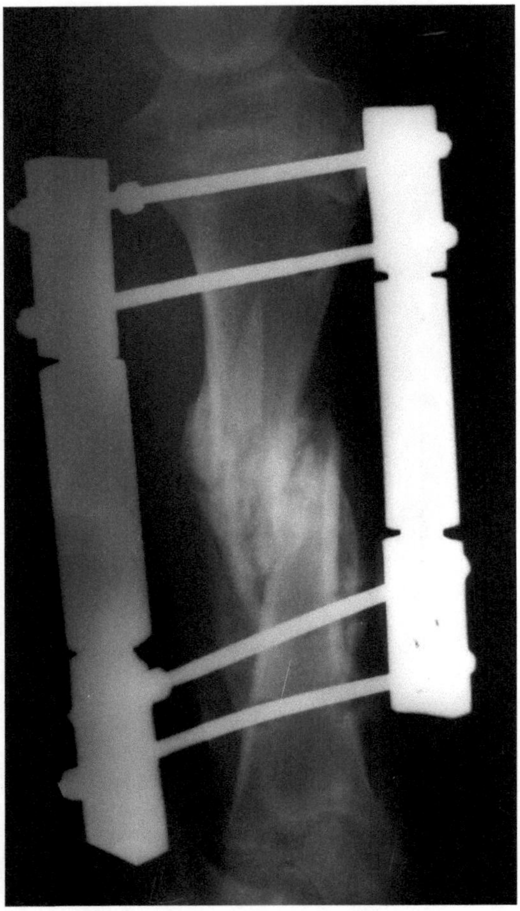

**Fig. 8.5** Malunion of tibial fracture in a calf stabilized with a bilateral ESF. Reduction and alignment of bone segments in angularly placed tibia is always difficult without ancillary fixation devices like cerclage wire or lag screws

principles of therapy include (i) establishment of drainage from the infected bone and tissues, (ii) antibiotic therapy based on sensitivity test, (iii) removal of the implant after bone union, and (iv) if instability persists, providing stable fracture fixation by avoiding dead space and by using bone grafts.

Infections accompanied with the surgical incision and surrounding soft tissues may not affect bone healing, and they can normally be treated with specific antimicrobial therapy. If the fixation is stable, a fracture can heal in spite of infection. And infections associated with the fixation implant or/and the bone are more troublesome. Typically, a bacterial biofilm develops around the implant offering resistance to antimicrobial drugs. Hence, to treat the infection, it is advised to remove the implant as soon as the bone healing is complete. It is also important to remove any avascular bone/sequestra that may exist at the site of infection. Prolonged systemic administration (at least for 6–8 weeks) of specific antibiotic based on culture and sensitivity tests is essential. It is also advised to make serial radiographic evaluation every 15–30 days until all the signs of infection are resolved and bone heals completely. Prognosis is usually favorable in most cases except where there is significant involvement/loss of tissues and if the infection involves the implant, which then needs to be removed for the complete resolution of infection.

## 8.6 Fracture Disease

Fracture disease is a complication of fracture repair characterized by muscle atrophy, joint stiffness, osteopenia, and articular cartilage degeneration, etc. attributed mainly to disuse of the affected limb [23, 24]. Quadricep contracture is the most common and serious form of fracture disease recorded in dogs and cats after femoral fracture repair (Fig. 8.9). It is particularly of great concern in patients where the fractured limb is immobilized in extension for a prolonged period using an external coaptation. Hence, it is important to monitor the quadricep muscles regularly (at 2–4 week intervals) during the post-fixation period by palpating the muscle for firmness or contracture and for range of joint motion (using a goniometer; normal angles: flexion $<45°$, extension about 160°), especially in young animals. The risk of fracture disease reduces as the bone heals and limb usage improves. This complication can be prevented or minimized by following atraumatic surgical procedure, rigid immobilization using internal fixation, early ambulation, and passive exercise and other physiotherapy techniques. In large animal practice also, fracture disease is common subsequent to prolonged cast immobilization [25, 26]. Hence, it is advised to remove the cast as quickly as the

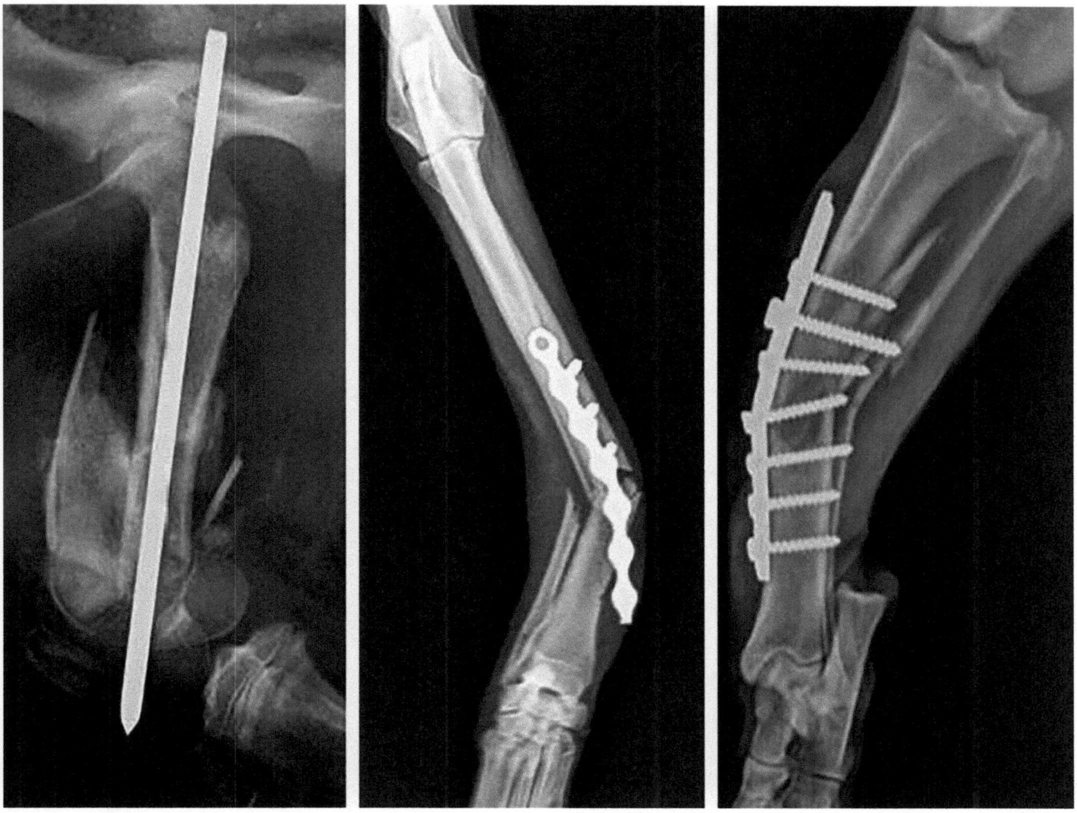

**Fig. 8.6** Fixation failure in a femur fracture treated with IM pin (**a**), and radius-ulna fracture (**b**) and tibial fracture (**c**) treated with bone plating techniques (see bending of plates at fracture site)

bone heals to prevent/minimize the development of fracture disease condition.

## 8.7 Supporting Limb Laminitis

Hyperextension of fetlock and digits and laminitis of support limb are common complications in large animals treated for limb fractures (Fig. 8.10). Support limb laminitis is relatively more often seen in horses than cattle, especially in those cases managed with cast application [26, 27]. This complication is more commonly seen in heavy animals and in cases with longer duration of casting. Mechanical overload (when one of the limbs has to carry much more weight than normal) results in weakening and tearing of the sensitive laminae, the interlocking Velcro-like tissues that secure the hoof wall with the third phalanx. This causes further overloading and tearing of the remaining laminae, leading to dropping or rotation of the third phalanx within the hoof. Inflammatory swelling in the injured laminae further deteriorates the blood flow badly required to nourish the broken tissues.

The success lies in preventing the development of laminitis, as it is a lot more difficult to manage once it begins. Laminitis can be prevented if diagnosed early and treated aggressively. If the vascular supply to the foot is cut off for many days, the hoof capsule sloughs off. When a horse keeps standing all the time on one limb and constantly loading the laminae (protecting and resting the injured limb), it is at a greater risk of developing laminitis. Supporting limb laminitis is rare in cattle because they lie down more frequently than horses. However, in inadequate fixation and complications during

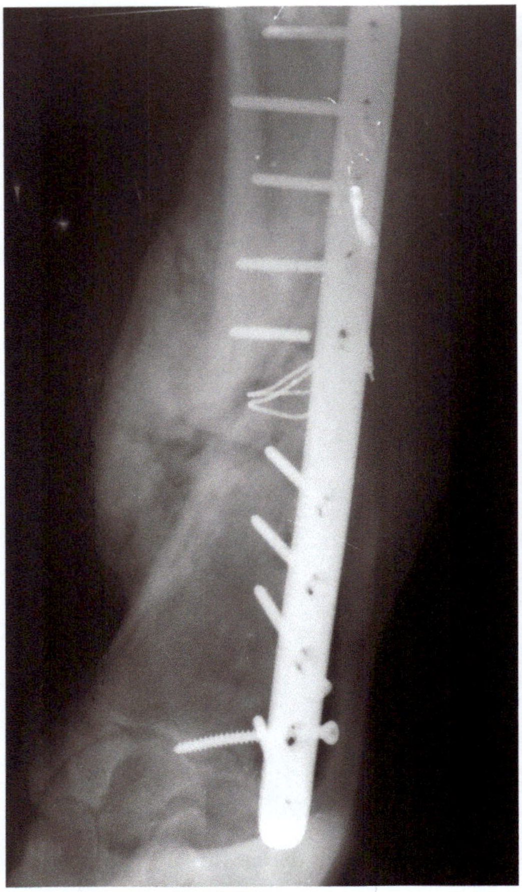

**Fig. 8.7** Screw loosening and breakage leading to fracture instability in a case of tibial fracture repair by plate osteosynthesis in cattle. However, the fracture segments are in alignment and healing occurred with a large periosteal callus

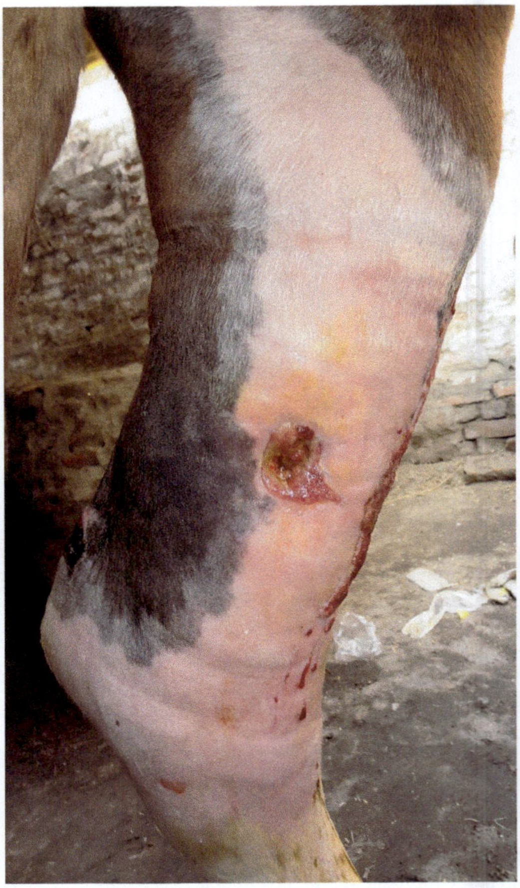

**Fig. 8.8** Fistulous tract draining the exudates on the medial surface of tibia indicating soft tissue infection in a horse treated for tibial fracture by bone plating

fracture healing, varus/valgus deformity of the contralateral limb may occur.

To prevent supporting limb laminitis, it is desirable to give a mechanical support to the weight-bearing foot to maintain the vascular supply to the laminae during full loading. This can be accomplished by (1) making the horse prefer standing with a P3 palmar angle of 20° by elevating the heels and moving back the functional breakover point and (2) giving arch support by placing a support device immediately after injury. Specialized ambulatory slings are now available, which can be used to prevent overloading of legs. It permits the horse to bear some weight on the legs without allowing overloading on any one leg. It also enables the horse to move around, graze, and thus improve its mindset.

Application of a shoe that can reduce tension on the deep digital flexor tendon is advised to preserve the blood flow to the dorsal laminae. A tenotomy of the deep digital flexor tendon may be considered when other approaches fail, or when the shoe does not work, or when the coffin bone has sunk below the circumflex blood vessels. Ablation/removal of the entire detached hoof wall and application of pin cast (cast built around pins in the cannon bone to hold the horse's weight, leading to floating foot) may give good results. During a severe limb injury, the immediate priority must be protecting the good foot, without waiting until the problem appears. This

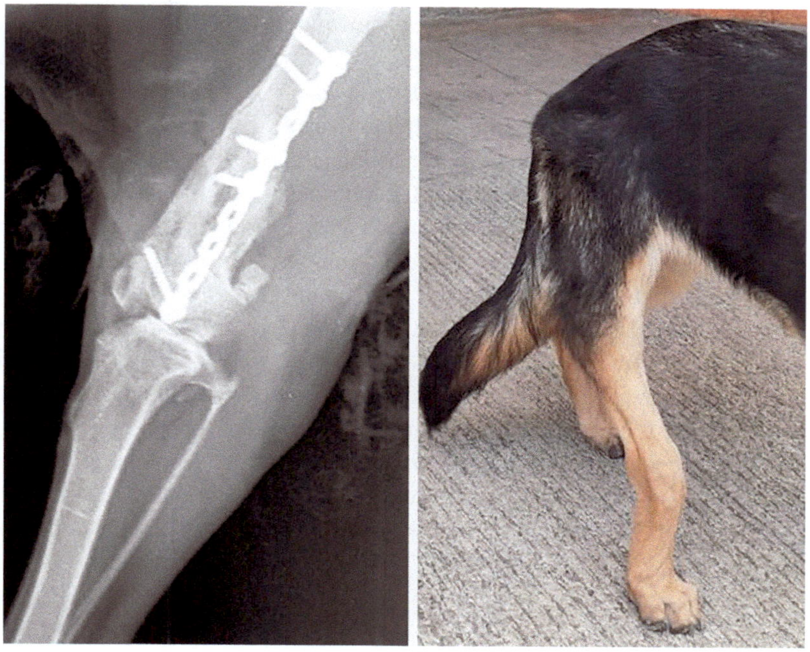

**Fig. 8.9** Severe quadriceps contracture and other signs of fracture disease following bone plate fixation of distal femoral fracture in a dog

can be done by applying either a splint-bandage or a cast. In catastrophic injury, amputation of the limb is a better option, and the horse can be put on prosthesis to maintain the limb length and protect the stump.

Postoperatively, it is important to treat acute pain and inflammation by administering higher doses of nonsteroidal anti-inflammatory drugs. Phenylbutazone, flunixin meglumine, or Banamine are the most often used NSAIDs. Early intravenous administration of lidocaine has been found beneficial by decreasing leukocytes and endothelium activation of

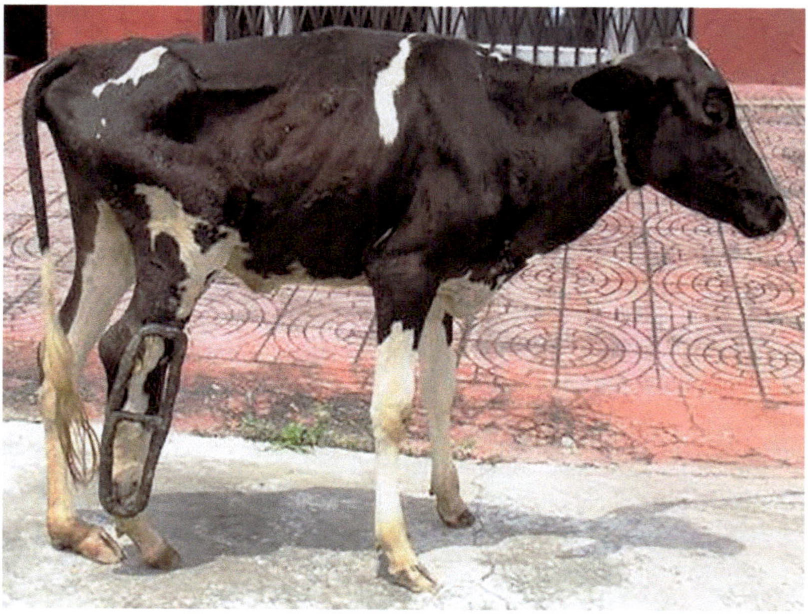

**Fig. 8.10** Hyperextension of fetlock in contralateral limb (left) in a calf treated for right metatarsal fracture using epoxy-pin ESF. Contralateral normal limb is subjected to more load due to non-weight bearing or reduced weight bearing on the treated limb leading to the deformity

neutrophils. Acepromazine has been shown to increase the blood flow to the hoof.

The prognosis is very good in unilateral cases provided that the limb injured initially has healed almost completely when the supporting limb laminitis aggravates to cause lameness. If supporting limb lameness persists for weeks, an aggressive approach should be adopted, and if stable enough, the injured limb should be used as the support limb for the next few days. Supporting limb laminitis in hind limbs is generally less severe than that of fore limbs as hind limbs bear relatively less body weight. It has also been seen that the fillies will acquire contralateral limb laminitis more speedily (3–4 weeks) as compared to colts (5–8 weeks), suggesting possible effect of hormones.

## Chapter 8: Sample Questions

### Q. No. 1: Mark the correct answer

1. Most common site of nonunion in dogs is
   (a) distal femur, (b) proximal tibia, (c) distal radius/ulna, (d) distal tibia
2. Cessation of reparative processes of healing without bony union is called as
   (a) delayed union (b) nonunion (c) malunion (d) osteomyelitis
3. Which of the following is not true with regard to laminitis
   (a) is the inflammation of laminae and papillae inside the hoof (b) caused by increased feeding of fermentable carbohydrates (c) not related to inheritance (d) characterized by lameness accompanied by systemic illness
4. Disuse of the affected limb can lead to
   (a) muscle atrophy (b) joint stiffness (c) osteopenia (d) all the above

### Q. No. 2: State true or false

1. Most of the complications in fracture fixation occur due to selection of improper method for fracture stabilization.
2. Hematogenous route of infection is more common in osteomyelitis.
3. Radiographically, sclerotic fracture ends with rounding of fracture ends is characteristic of nonunion.
4. Implant failure is primarily attributed to the implant alone, and rarely, it is caused due to technical error.
5. In large animal fracture fixation, there are every chances of fixation failure during recovery from anesthesia.
6. The risk of fracture disease decreases as the fracture heals and limb usage improves.
7. Long duration of immobilization of limb and higher bodyweight increase the likelihood of developing laminitis.
8. Contralateral limb laminitis is more common in cattle than horses.
9. Contralateral hind limb laminitis has a poor prognosis than front limb laminitis, as the hind limbs bear more weight.
10. Open reduction of joint luxation is less difficult in fresh cases than in delayed cases.
11. In large animals, hip dislocation is very difficult to reduce and retain either by closed or by open method.

### Q. No. 3: Fill up the blanks

1. Delayed union is usually caused either by ______________________ or ______________________ factors.
2. A nonunion that has an adequate blood supply and biologic environment but lacks sufficient mechanical stability is called ______________________, while a nonunion with avascular and biologically inactive environment is termed as ______________________.
3. Basic principles of therapy in osteomyelitis include providing ______________________, ______________________-______, and ______________________ ______________.
4. Postoperative complication associated with the fracture or its repair such as muscle atrophy and joint stiffness is generally referred as ______________________.
5. ______________________-__________ is the most common and severe

form of fracture disease seen in animal patients.

**Q. No. 4: Write short note on the following**

1. Radiographic features of osteomyelitis and osteosarcoma
2. Difference between delayed union and nonunion
3. Fracture disease
4. Supporting limb laminitis

## References


1. Olmstead, M.L. 1991. Complications of fractures repaired with plates and screws. The Veterinary Clinics of North America. *Small Animal Practice* 21 (4): 669–686.
2. Singh, A.P., K.N.M. Nayar, I.S. Chandna, S.K. Chawla, and J.M. Nigam. 1984. Postoperative complications associated with fracture repair in long bones in bovine, equine and ovine. *Indian Journal of Veterinary Surgery* 5: 47.
3. Smith, G.I. 2014. *Complications of fracture repair.* World Small Animal Veterinary Association World Congress Proceedings. https://www.vin.com/doc/id7054691.
4. Kaderly, R.E. 1993. Delayed union, non-union and malunion. In *Textbook of small animal surgery*, ed. D.H. Slatter, vol. 2, 1676–1685. Philadelphia: W.B. Saunders.
5. Piermattei, D.L., and G.L. Flo. 1997. *Handbook of small animal orthopaedics and fracture repair*, 68–95. Philadelphia: W.B. Saunders.
6. Robins, G.M. 1998. Delayed union and nonunion. In *Manual of internal fixation in small animals*, ed. W.O. Brinker, M.L. Olmstead, G. Summer-Smith, and W.D. Prieur, vol. 2, 227–239. Berlin: Springer Verlag.
7. Jackson, L.C., and P.D. Pacchiana. 2004. Common complications of fracture repair. *Clinical Techniques in Small Animal Practice* 19 (3): 168–179.
8. Lincoln, J.D. 1992. Treatment of open, delayed union, non-union fractures with external skeletal fixation. The Veterinary Clinics of North America. *Small Animal Practice* 22: 195–209.
9. Vaughan, L.C. 1964. A clinical study of non-union fractures in the dog. *The Journal of Small Animal Practice* 5: 173–177.
10. McLaughlin, R. 1999. Internal fixation. *The Veterinary Clinics of North America. Small Animal Practice* 29 (5): 1097–1115.
11. Nuss, K. 2014. Plates, pins, and interlocking nails. *Veterinary Clinics of North America: Food Animal Practice* 30: 91–126.
12. Aithal, H.P., G.R. Singh, M. Hoque, S.K. Maiti, P. Kinjavdekar, Amarpal, A.M. Pawde, and H.C. Setia. 2004. The use of circular external skeletal fixation device for the management of long bone osteotomies in large ruminants: an experimental study. *Journal of Veterinary Medicine.* A51: 284–293.
13. Caywood, D.D., L.J. Wallace, and T.D. Braden. 1978. Osteomyelitis in the dog: a review of 67 cases. *Journal of the American Veterinary Medical Association* 172: 943–946.
14. Gieling, F., S. Peters, C. Erichsen, R. Geoff Richards, S. Zeiter, and T. Fintan Moriarty. 2019. Bacterial osteomyelitis in veterinary orthopaedics: pathophysiology, clinical presentation and advances in treatment across multiple species. *Veterinary Journal* 250: 4454.
15. Griffon, D. 2016. Osteomyelitis. In *Complications in small animal surgery*, ed. D. Griffon and A. Hamaide, 28–33. Hoboken, NJ: John Wiley & Sons.
16. Herron, M.R. 1993. Osteomyelitis. In *Disease mechanisms in small animal surgery*, ed. M.J. Bojrab, 692–728. Philadelphia: Lea and Febiger.
17. Hoque, M., G.R. Singh, and H.P. Aithal. 1998. Post-traumatic osteomyelitis in animals: a retrospective analysis. *Indian Journal of Veterinary Research* 7: 53–57.
18. Aithal, H.P., P. AmarpalKinjavdekar, A.M. Pawde, G.R. Singh, and H.C. Setia. 2010. Management of tibial fractures using a circular external fixator in two calves. *Veterinary Surgery* 39: 621–626.
19. Egger, E.L. 1991. Complications of external fixation: a problem-oriented approach. The Veterinary Clinics of North America. *Small Animal Practice* 21 (4): 705–733.
20. Hararri, J. 1992. Complications of external skeletal fixation. The Veterinary Clinics of North America. *Small Animal Practice* 22: 99–107.
21. Rovesti, G.L. 2016. Complications in external skeletal fixation. In *Complications in small animal surgery*, ed. D. Griffon and A. Hamaide, 704–713. Hoboken, NJ: John Wiley & Sons.
22. Shah, M.A., Rohit Kumar, P. Kinjavdekar, Amarpal, H.P. Aithal, Mohammad Arif Basha, and Asif Majid. 2022. The use of circular and hybrid external skeletal fixation systems to repair open tibial fractures in large ruminants: a report of six clinical cases. *Veterinary Research Communications* 46 (2): 563–575. https://doi.org/10.1007/s11259-022-09884-w.
23. Johnson, A.L., and C.E. DeCamp. 1999. External skeletal fixation: linear fixation. The Veterinary Clinics of North America. *Small Animal Practice* 29: 1135–1151.
24. Millis, D. 2016. Quadriceps contracture. In *Complications in small animal surgery*, ed. D. Griffon and A. Hamaide, 692–696. John Wiley & Sons.
25. Gangl, M., S. Grulke, D. Serteyn, and K. Touati. 2006. Retrospective study of 99 cases of bone fractures in

cattle treated by external coaptation or confinement. *The Veterinary Record* 158: 264–268.

26. Lozier, J.W., A.J. Niehaus, A. Muir, and J. Lakritz. 2018. Short- and long-term success of transfixation pin casts used to stabilize long bone fractures in ruminants. *The Canadian Veterinary Journal* 59 (6): 635–641.

27. Virjin, J.E., L.R. Goodrich, G.M. Baxter, and S. Rao. 2011. Incidence of support limb laminitis in horses treated with half limb, full limb or transfixation pin casts: A retrospective study of 113 horses (2000–2009). *Equine Veterinary Journal. Supplement* 40: 7–11.

# Metabolic Bone Diseases

# 9

**Learning Objectives**
You will be able to understand the following after reading this chapter:

- The causes, clinical signs, diagnosis, and management of important metabolic bone diseases such as nutritional secondary hyperparathyroidism, rickets, hypertrophic osteodystrophy, osteochondrosis/osteochondritis dissecans, retained cartilage core, metaphyseal chondrodysplasia, and hip dysplasia
- Prevention and control of bone disorders

**Summary**

- Calcium homeostasis depends on dietary contents of calcium, phosphorus, and vitamin D and also on endogenous hormones such as parathyroid hormone, calcitonin, and vitamin D; hence, any imbalance of dietary mineral contents or disturbed endogenous hormone levels and/or normal metabolic activity may lead to a variety of skeletal disorders in growing animals.
- Nutritional secondary hyperparathyroidism, the most frequently recorded bone disease in dogs, is induced by nutritional imbalances, mainly calcium deficiency or excessive phosphorus intake, which stimulates the release of parathyroid hormone from the parathyroid glands leading to drainage of minerals from bone.
- Rickets is a disease occurring in young animals due to deficiency of vitamin D, characterized by widening of growth plate of long bones, mushrooming, or cupping of the enlarged metaphyses often leading to bone deformities.
- Hypertrophic osteodystrophy primarily affects the young, rapidly growing large breeds, and mostly appears in 3–4 months of age. Clinical signs include swelling and pain in long bone metaphyses, lameness, and refusal to bear weight on the affected limbs. Radiographically, a radiolucent zone in the metaphysis parallel to the physeal plate is most evident in the distal radius and ulna.
- Osteochondrosis is an abnormal development of the cartilage, characterized by a radiolucent area within the subchondral bone, flattening of the articular surface, presence of joint mice,

(continued)


H. P. Aithal et al., *Textbook of Veterinary Orthopaedic Surgery*,
https://doi.org/10.1007/978-981-99-2575-9_9

subchondral bone sclerosis, and in advanced cases degenerative changes in the joint.
- Hip dysplasia is associated with abnormal structure and laxity of the coxofemoral joint, leading to osteoarthritis in chronic cases. It can be surgically treated by palliative methods (before the development of osteoarthritis) such as juvenile pubic symphysiodesis, triple pelvic osteotomy and trochanteric wedge osteotomy of femur, or salvage procedures (after the development of osteoarthritis) such as total hip replacement or femoral head and neck excision.
- The incidence of developmental skeletal disorders can be reduced by providing balanced diet, especially in the early stage of life. Further, early diagnosis and treatment can minimize the extent of damage/deformity.

The bone growth is regulated by several factors involving the interaction of various body minerals, hormones, and nutritional elements (detailed in Chapter 1B). The role of minerals, especially of calcium and phosphorus, is very important and crucial during the period of bone growth as they are essential structural components of the skeleton. In addition to dietary contents of calcium, phosphorus, and vitamin D, calcium homeostasis also depends on endogenous hormones, especially parathyroid hormone (PTH), calcitonin (CT), and vitamin D. Any imbalance in the mineral contents in the diet of growing animals or disturbance in the endogenous hormone levels and/or normal metabolic activity can cause different skeletal deformities/disorders. Such skeletal abnormalities are more often seen in small growing animals. Some of the common abnormalities are nutritional secondary hyperparathyroidism, rickets and hypertrophic osteodystrophy, and hip dysplasia [1, 2].

## 9.1 Nutritional Secondary Hyperparathyroidism

Nutritional secondary hyperparathyroidism (NSH) is the most common bone disease, often reported in dogs fed with meat or meat products without bone. The condition can also occur in cats, certain nonhuman primates and laboratory animals in addition to other livestock. NSH is also called as osteodystrophy fibrosa, osteogenesis imperfecta, nutritional osteoporosis, juvenile osteoporosis, osteitis fibrosa, or all meat syndrome [3–6].

NSH can be recorded in any small or large breed of dogs and cats, and it is frequently seen in young large breed growing dogs having greater calcium requirements. The basic underlying cause of the disease is the prolonged mineral imbalance in the diet, mostly deficiency of calcium or excess of phosphorus, which can stimulate the release of parathyroid hormone (PTH) from the parathyroid glands. Hypocalcemia can occur due to inadequate dietary calcium (less availability of calcium in meat, cereal, grains, and fruits), or ineffective absorption of calcium from the intestines. Also in conditions such as rickets and osteomalacia, calcium deficiency can stimulate increased PTH secretion leading to hyperparathyroidism. And excess of dietary phosphorus and various other factors, which can lead to hypocalcemia (lack of vitamin A and D, renal and thyroid disease, and dietary magnesium, phytate, and fluorine, etc.), may also cause secondary hyperparathyroidism.

In young growing dogs, the initial clinical sign of NSH is lameness, which can be mild to severe (Fig. 9.1). Palpation of bones can exhibit pain. Often, folding or compression fractures can be seen in long bones and vertebrae, due to difference in the physical characteristics and composition of bone. Enlarged metaphyses of long bones and costo-chondral junctions of ribs and abnormal development of teeth are also often noticed. Deterioration in the general body condition and paresis or paralysis due to vertebral compression are other signs, which can be noticed.

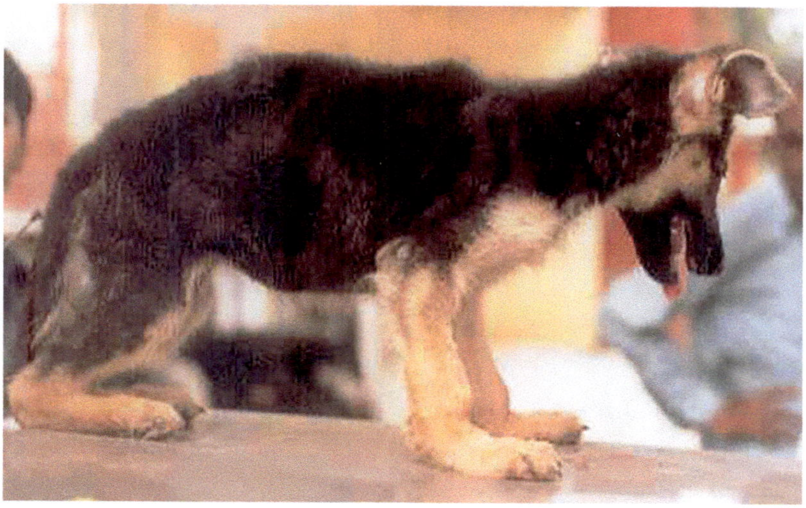

**Fig. 9.1** A German shepherd dog suffering from nutritional secondary hyperparathyroidism shows emaciation and severe hyperextension of hock and knee joints

Calcium and phosphorus levels in the blood are usually maintained in the normal range, due to normal homeostatic mechanism. However, phosphorus and alkaline phosphatase levels in the serum tend to increase. Urinary excretion of phosphorus increase and calcium excretion decrease due to the action of PTH on kidneys. Renal function parameters such as urea nitrogen and creatinine levels in the blood usually remain within normal range.

Radiographically, generalized decrease in density and thinning of bony cortices, with normal physeal plate, are characteristics of NSH. The area adjoining to the physeal plate may show increased bone density suggesting preferential mineralization. Metaphyses may broaden to give a "saucer" effect contrary to "cupping" effect seen in rickets (Fig. 9.2). These radiographic findings are more appreciable at the distal radius and ulna.

Treatment of NSH includes termination of feeding of diet with mineral imbalance, such as whole meat diet, and feeding of balanced diet supplemented with calcium and phosphorus in appropriate ratio [7]. The dogs may be fed with bones (large bones for chewing or finely chopped) and milk and milk products as they are rich sources of calcium. To combat severe muscle pain, a combination of selenium and tocopherols (0.1 ml/kg body weight) can be administered intramuscularly every week.

Supplementation of 265 mg calcium and 220 mg phosphorus/kg body weight per day to adult dogs and twice a day to immature dogs is advised. It has been recommended that diet fed to dogs should have a Ca:P ratio of 1.2:1.0 to 2.0:1. The calcitonin hormone, which has an action opposite to parathormone and facilitates deposition of calcium in the bone, has been used for the treatment of NSH. Anabolic steroid *Nandrolone Decanoate* has shown to increase the bone mineral density and thickness in osteopenic bones [8]. Homeopathic drugs such as *Calcarea phosphorica* and *Symphytum 30* have also been shown to increase the mineral density of long bones both in experimental animals and in clinical applications. Antiresorptive drugs like *Alendronate* and *Raloxifene* did not show consistent results in experimental animals. It is possible to treat osteopenia and reverse the pathological changes in the bone associated with NSH if treatment is initiated in early stage.

## 9.2 Rickets

Rickets is a disease condition occurring in young animals, showing defective mineralization in bone including at the cartilaginous area of the growth plate [9]. Failure of mineralization of proliferating cartilage at the growth plate results in thickening of the physis, often leading to deformity and bowing due to weight-bearing loads. Osteomalacia is a condition similar to rickets occurring in adult animals, characterized by

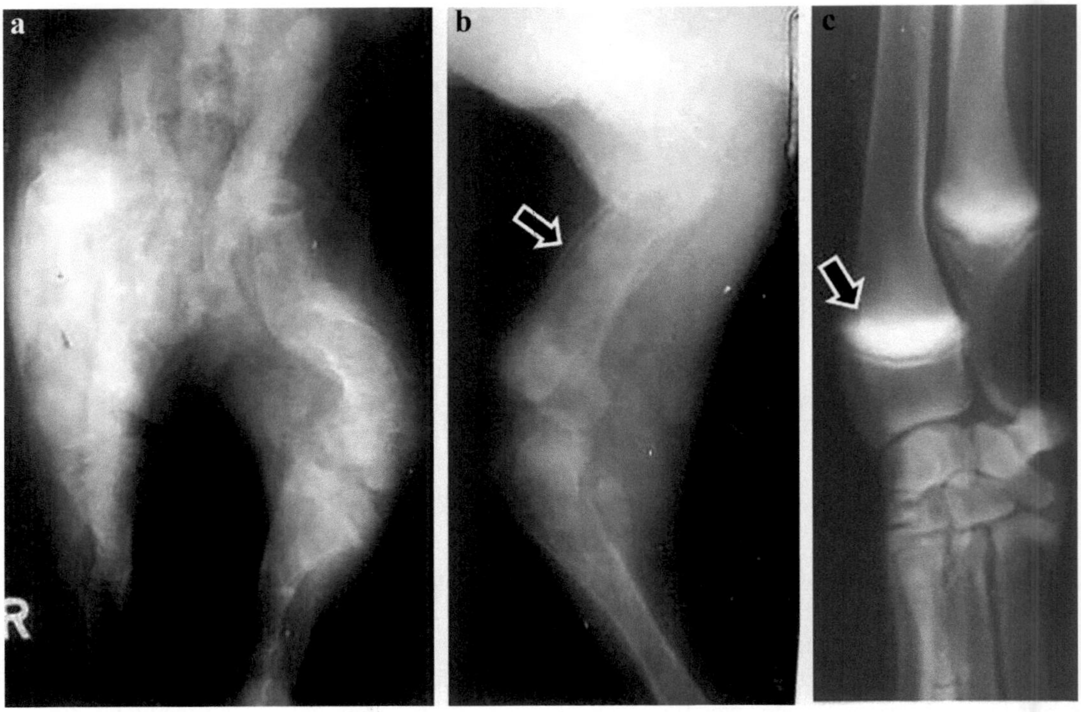


**Fig. 9.2** Radiographs of dogs affected with secondary hyperparathyroidism show generalized thinning of bone cortices with multiple fractures (**a**), double cortical lines (arrow) (**b**), and area adjoining to the physeal plate showing increased bone density (**c**)

poor mineralization of newly laid down osteoid during the normal remodeling process resulting in accumulation of excessive unmineralized osteoid on trabecular surfaces (no growth plate changes, as adult animals do not have growth plates).

Vitamin D (cholecalciferol) deficiency due to inadequate intake or diminished endogenous production is the primary cause of rickets [10–12]. Most commonly, a diet deficient in both bioavailable calcium and vitamin D causes rickets in growing pups. Phosphorus or vitamin D deficiency (or inadequate sunlight) or inborn error in vitamin D metabolism could also cause rickets. Experimentally, feeding of diet low in calcium, phosphorus, or both calcium and phosphorus has shown to induce rickets. Similarly, feeding of diets deficient in vitamin D to young animals, which are housed indoors without exposure to sunlight (ultraviolet radiation) developed rickets. Whereas feeding of diets with insufficient vitamin D, adequate calcium and phosphorus did not induce rickets in growing animals. Nutritional deficiencies and/or poor exposure to sunlight have been shown to induce rickets in different domestic animals such as swine, cattle, sheep, and birds, but horses are generally less susceptible. In human beings, rickets also results from gastric abnormalities, biliary disease, and enteric absorption defects. Animals with chronic glomerular renal disease can also develop rickets and osteopenia due to renal secondary hyperparathyroidism (detailed in Chapter 1).

Pups are normally presented with a "bow legged" condition of the forelimb (Fig. 9.3) followed by pathological fractures [13]. Enlarged joints, enlarged metaphyseal regions of the bones (including costo-chondral junctions), pliable limb bones, and dropped pasterns resulting in flat footed or plantigrade appearance are other signs. Occasionally, "cow hock" conditions of the hind limbs and very rarely knock-knee with outward rotation of the paw regions and deformity of the pelvic girdle are also observed. Other signs like listlessness, severe muscle weakness,

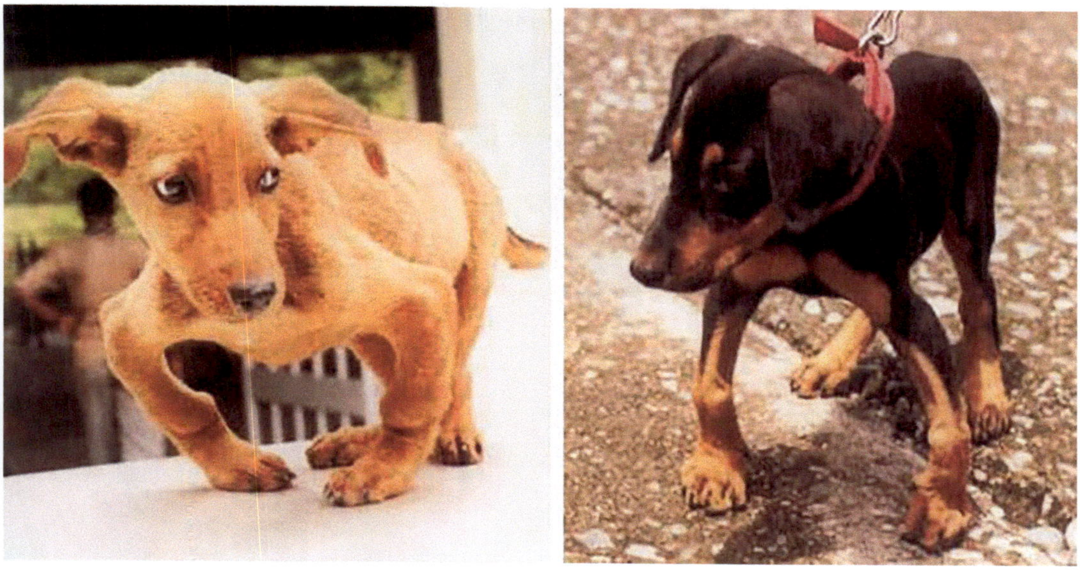

**Fig. 9.3** Pups affected with rickets show emaciation, bow legged condition (genu varum) of forelegs with enlarged metaphyseal regions of long bones

lameness, and lateral bowing of the ante-brachii can also be seen. Sometimes, pups may show hyperextended carpus (palmagrade stance) and tarsus (plantigrade stance). Pathological fractures, lordosis, and abnormal eruption of permanent teeth are also seen frequently. Clinical manifestations of rickets in human beings include generalized symptoms like intense muscle hypotonia, weakness, and disturbance in growth along with reduced bone density, skeletal malformation, and vulnerability to fractures.

Radiographically, poorly mineralized and extremely thin cortices may be seen indicating generalized osteopenia. The diaphyses of all long bones have their cortices with cancellous bone of normal density as seen in the medullary cavity and metaphyses. Grossly epiphyseal line (growth plate) is thickened or widened with "mushrooming" or "cupping" of the enlarged metaphyses often resulting in bone defects (Fig. 9.4). Epiphyses and metaphyses are enlarged, compressed and laterally displaced. Widened epiphyseal growth plate (unmineralized cartilage) often extends into the metaphyses giving an appearance of "islands" of radiolucent patches. Although these changes can be seen in any long bone, they are more prominent at distal ulna and radius. The costo-chondral junctions are generally two to three folds larger in diameter than the ribs.

The 25(OH) vitamin D concentration in rachitic pups may remain below the reference range. Hypomagnesemia and hyperparathyroidism are also reported occasionally. Decrease in Hb content, packed cell volume, total erythrocyte count, and leukocytosis are reported in cases of rickets. Blood protein, calcium, phosphorus, and zinc levels may decrease, whereas serum alkaline phosphatase and transaminase activities may increase in cases of rickets. Serum sodium and potassium levels may be normal, while serum magnesium, copper, and iron may decline. An increase of Ca:P ratio (>2) may indicate rickets. Measured basal plasma CT concentration in rickets cases may range from 12–80 ng/L, and there may be an 8–20 times increase after infusion of calcium bolus (1 and 2.5 mg/kg body weight).

In cases of rickets, it is advised to get exposure to early morning sunlight for synthesis of vitamin D. Further, it is also recommended to maintain adequate intake of vitamin D in the diet, which is about 20 and 7 IU/kg body weight for growth and maintenance, respectively. However, oversupplementation of vitamin D should be

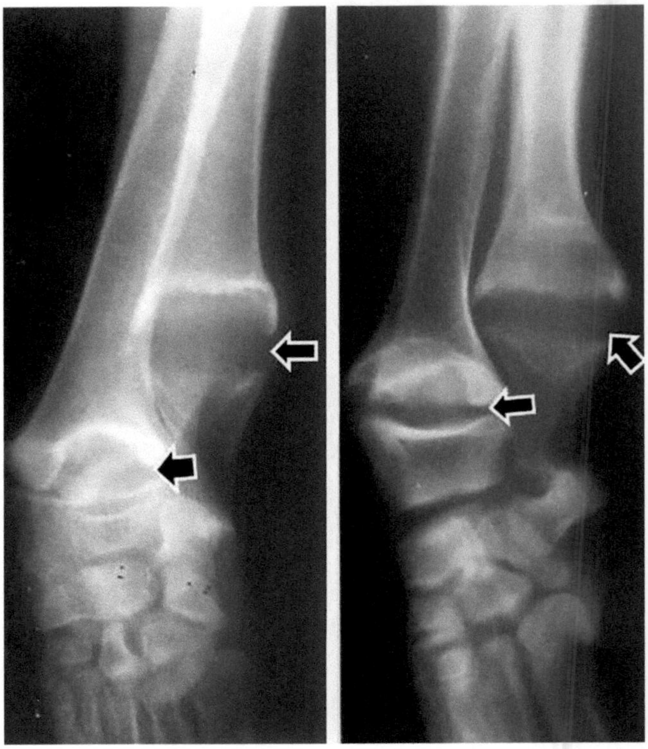

**Fig. 9.4** Radiographs of pups affected with rickets show poorly mineralized thin cortices, and the growth plates of long bones thickened (widened) with "mushrooming" (cupping) of the enlarged metaphyses (arrows)

avoided as it can produce a deficient and defective matrix, which can be vulnerable to even minor trauma. Excessive intake of vitamin D may also cause anorexia, nausea, fatigue, renal damage, soft tissue calcification, hypercalcemia, diarrhea, dehydration, and even death. It is also recommended to feed a diet rich in calcium such as bones, milk, and milk products, and it is ensured that dietary Ca and P are adequate and in their correct ratio.

Treatment with homeopathic drugs, *Calcarea phosphorica* and *Symphytum 30,* has been shown to improve the conditions of rachitic lesions in long bones. In cases of angular limb deformities, cast or splint and bandage could be applied to keep the limb in extended position and to prevent further angulation. However, the cast or splint should be changed after every 2 weeks to prevent any injury to the bony prominences of the fast growing animals. Severe angular deformities may require surgical correction.

## 9.3 Hypertrophic Osteodystrophy

Collett and Morell in 1935 first reported Hypertrophic Osteodystrophy (HOD) in veterinary literature. The disease hypertrophic osteodystrophy has been previously called by various names such as Moller-Barlowsche Krankheit beim Hund, Barlow's disease, Skeletal scurvy, hypertrophic osteodystrophy associated with disturbances of vitamin C synthesis, and Osteodystrophy II. Metaphyseal osteopathy (MO) is a better term for hypertrophic osteodystrophy, since the hypertrophy does not always develop and lesions are always seen at metaphysis. Bruyere (1972) has described hypertrophic osteodystrophy and skeletal scurvy as separate diseases and suggested that the former often accompanied the latter. Carlson in 1967 introduced the term idiopathic osteodystrophy.

HOD primarily affects the young, rapidly growing large and giant breed dogs such as Great Dane, Irish Wolfhound, St. Bernard, Borzoi, Boxer, Dalmatian, Irish setter, Weimaraner,

German Short Haired Pointer, Doberman Pinscher, German shepherd, Labrador Retriever, Collie, Greyhound, Bassett hound, and Terriers [14–17].

Vitamin C deficiency was thought to be the primary etiological factor for HOD [18]. Other causes speculated include oversupplementation of minerals and vitamins including vitamin D in the diet. Detection of Canine Distemper virus RNA in the bone cells suggested a role of this virus in etiopathogenesis of MO in dogs. *E. coli* bacteraemia has been detected in a 6-month-old Great Dane having HOD to suggest a possible role of this bacterium in causing the disease.

The clinical signs of the disease generally start in 3–4 months of age in most animals, which may include variable extent of lameness, swelling, and pain on palpation of the affected metaphyses of long bones, along with generalized symptoms like weight loss, anorexia, and pyrexia [19–21]. Metaphyses of all long bones could be affected including metacarpals, mandible and maxilla, scapula, ilium, and costochondral junctions of the ribs; however, metaphyses of long bones distal to the elbow and stifle (radius-ulna and tibia) are most commonly affected. Clinical signs generally subside in a few days, and later, it may recur after many days. Hemorrhage may often be seen at various locations, more prominently in gingivae.

In the early stages of the disease, radiographic changes may be visible in the metaphyseal region of long bones. A radiolucent band parallel to the growth plate is most evident in the distal radius and ulna, and sometimes, a radiodense line may be visible adjacent to the growth plate (Fig. 9.5). Soft tissues swelling may be seen around the metaphyses. These radiographic changes are normally bilateral. In later stages, irregular periosteal new bone formation and enlargement of metaphyses may be observed in some of the affected animals.

Hematological changes during the acute stage of the disease are nonspecific, which may include neutrophilia, lymphopenia, and monocytosis suggesting inflammation and stress. Low level of ascorbic acid has been recorded in the blood and urine of some of the affected animals, but it was not consistent.

Complete rest and withdrawal of dietary supplementation of excessive vitamins and minerals may improve the condition in HOD-affected animals. Vitamin C therapy usually does not provide favorable response, although some researchers have found good outcome in some cases. Supplementation of minerals and vitamin D must be avoided as they might hasten the rate of dystrophic calcification and reduce bone remodeling. Anti-rachitic therapy has been found to worsen the condition.

## 9.4 Osteochondrosis

Osteochondrosis (OC) is an abnormal development of the joint cartilage, often seen in human beings and animals most commonly pigs, horses, cattle, dogs, and cats. OC syndrome is considered to be a biochemical disease, which occurs due to disturbance in the endochondral ossification resulting in severe lameness and skeletal deformities [22, 23]. Osteochondritis dissecans (OCD) is the manifestation of osteochondrosis, wherein a piece of articular cartilage detaches. Growing dogs of large and giant breeds are predisposed mostly. Incidence is higher in rapidly growing male than female dogs. Shoulder joint is most commonly affected, but it can also be seen in other joints such as elbow, hip, and stifle.

The etiology of OC is poorly understood. Feeding of excess energy, protein, calcium, and phosphorus and rapid skeletal growth due to the overnutrition are reported to be the common causes of OC. By experimentally feeding excess of energy, protein, calcium, phosphorus, and vitamin D, OC could be induced in Great Dane pups. By increasing only the calcium content of the diet, also the occurrence and severity of OC could be increased. High calcium intake (independent of the Ca:P ratio) is an important determinant of disturbance in endochondral ossification. Rapid skeletal growth and an overloading of the growing skeleton due to increasing muscle mass and body weight produce biochemical forces on forming joint surface,

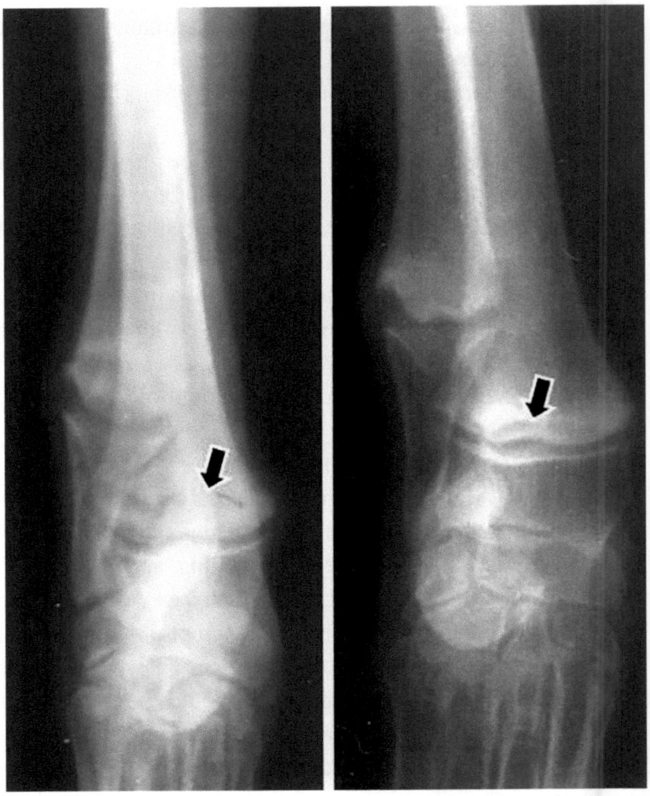

**Fig. 9.5** Radiographs of distal radius-ulna in a dog affected with hypertrophic osteodystrophy show radiolucent band parallel to the growth plate (arrows) along with a radiodense line adjacent to the growth plate

while they are still structurally weak, causing OC. Some have suggested involvement of genetic factors in the origin of OC.

Clinical signs are usually exhibited between 5 and 10 months of age, and males are about three times more frequently affected than females. Sudden onset of lameness is the early sign of the disease. Initially, lameness may be slight to moderate, and it typically decreases after rest and increases after exercise. In majority of dogs, the lameness may increase over a period of 3–4 weeks. The dogs may show abducted stance. Hyperextension or flexion of the affected part may elicit the signs of pain. Muscle atrophy might be marked over the affected area, particularly in chronic cases.

Radiographically, a radiolucent area within the subchondral bone or a flattening of the articular surface is seen. A joint mice or calcified cartilage fragment might be visible. Subchondral bone sclerosis might be present, although it is difficult to identify in most cases. In advanced cases, degenerative changes can be seen in and around the joint. OC has also been reported in vertebral body, and pathological signs include short-ended vertebral body, deformity and erosion of the end plate, reduction in the intervertebral space, and osteophytosis.

Haemato-biochemical changes include a significant increase in plasma total protein and creatinine concentrations. High blood serum phosphorus and normal calcium concentrations and low Ca:P ratio may be evident.

Conservative treatment of OC is controversial, and regardless of the method used, in most of the cases, lameness persists, and secondary complications such as osteoarthritis may develop. Conventional treatment may include a combination of rest (movement restriction), restriction of body weight, and management of pain using either steroidal or nonsteroidal anti-inflammatory drugs, nutraceuticals and polysulfated glycosamino-glycans. More recently, laser therapy and administration of platelet-rich plasma have also been included in conservative treatment regime to help alleviate progressive arthritis.

Even though this conservative treatment may not help to treat the primary condition by itself, it has been recommended in the postoperative period to augment the outcome of surgical treatment.

Surgical treatment is often the method of choice for OC to avert worsening of joint degradation. During surgery, the flap of unhealthy cartilage along with the surrounding abnormal cartilage tissue is trimmed with a curette and retrieved. Multiple holes are then drilled in the lesion bed, with a 1–2 mm drill bit or a small K-wire, deep into the subchondral bone to promote blood circulation, which will promote the migration of pluripotent stem cells into the articular defect site and restore the defect by the formation of fibrocartilage. The residual tissue debris including the cartilage particles are then flushed out by joint lavage. Surgery significantly diminishes the rapidity of onset of chronic secondary degenerative joint disease. Surgical treatment can be undertaken either by conventional method or by arthroscopic procedure, which is minimally invasive and allows better visualization of intra-articular structures with less disruption of the periarticular soft tissues leading to less postoperative pain and morbidity. Arthroscopic surgery has the advantage especially when multiple joints are involved.

Following surgical treatment, the dogs should be restricted to leash confinement for at least 4 weeks. Subsequently, controlled activity may be gradually increased over the period of time. Medical treatment described earlier should be continued. The response of OCD to surgical intervention (standard arthrotomy or arthroscopic surgery) is usually favorable with normal functional recovery of the affected dogs, except in long-standing cases with severe degenerative arthritic changes. A good to excellent prognosis is expected in more than 90% of cases when surgical treatment is coupled with suitable medical therapy postoperatively.

## 9.5 Retained Cartilage Core

Retention of cartilage core occurs due to abnormalities in the process of endochondral ossification of the growth plate of long bones, often leading to bone deformities [24–26]. In this condition, the hypertrophic chondrocytes at the growth plate fail to mature and mineralize the surrounding matrix leading to aggregation of cartilage cells in columns extending deep into the metaphysis. It is thought to be a developmental bone disease, and disturbance in the mineral and vitamin metabolism could also lead to retention of cartilage core. It is more common in young, large, and giant breed dogs. It can occur in any long bone, but distal ulna is most often involved causing antebrachial deformities.

Common clinical signs include varied degrees of lameness, lateral deviation of the foot (carpus valgus) ,and retarded bone growth. Usually, it is a bilateral condition affecting both forelimbs similarly. Cartilage retention in the distal ulnar growth plate leads to retarded growth and relative shortening of ulna (compared to radius) causing cranial bowing of radius, lateral rotation (valgus) of paw, and subluxation of elbow and carpal joints.

Radiographically, an inverted radiolucent column in the form of a cone can be seen extending from the distal growth plate proximally deep into the metaphyseal region (Fig. 9.6). Widening of growth plate may or may not be seen. Metaphyses of other long bones may also show irregular densities, which may persist even after maturity.

Any growth abnormality/angular deformity arising from the retention of cartilage core may be corrected surgically as per the case, depending on the time of detection and growth potential of the bone (detailed in Chapter 10).

## 9.6 Metaphyseal Chondrodysplasia

Metaphyseal chondrodysplasia is a cluster of abnormalities affecting predominantly the metaphyses of long bones with typically normal epiphyses, and skull, and trunk bones [27].

The mode of inheritance is compatible with a simple autosomal recessive trait [28]. The condition is believed to be caused due to exceptionally rapid ossification of the metaphyseal cortex of long bones in animals fed with the diet having

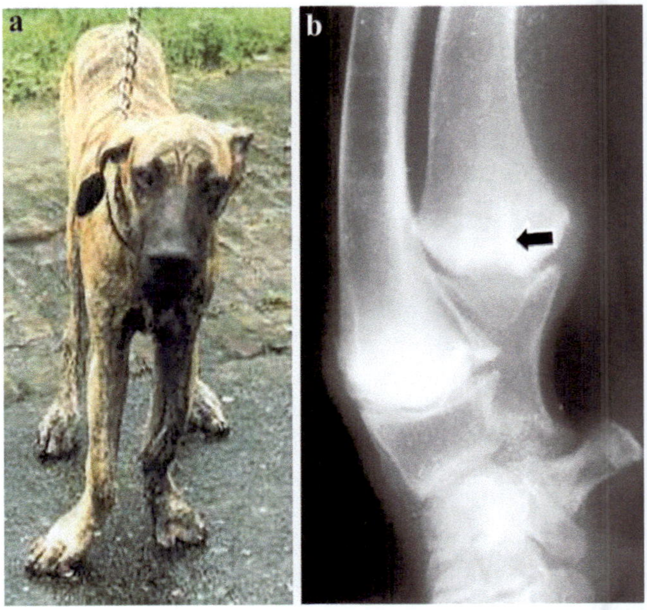


**Fig. 9.6** A dog having retention of cartilage core shows carpus valgus (**a**) and radiograph of distal radius-ulna shows an inverted radiolucent column (cone) extending from the distal growth plate proximally into the metaphysis (**b**)

mineral imbalance (Ca:P ratio) giving rise to the syndrome of metaphyseal dysplasia or retention of cartilage.

Clinically, the affected dogs show lameness and enlarged distal metaphysis with no pain. Radiographically, triangular metaphyseal radiolucency is observed, which is usually most obvious in the distal ulna [29] (Fig. 9.7). Other signs include flaring of the metaphyses of all long bones and the costo-chondral junction of ribs. Vertebral bodies may look short and less radiodense and have a beak like appendage on the caudal extremity. Histologically, the growth plate may reveal disorderly arranged chondrocyte columns and quantitative changes in the chondrocytes at proliferative zone.

## 9.7 Panosteitis

Panosteitis is an idiopathic bone disease of young, rapidly growing, large breed dogs [30]. It is also referred to as juvenile osteomyelitis, eosinophilic panosteitis, enostosis, endosteal proliferation of new bone, and eopan. The disease is evidenced by acute, recurrent shifting lameness in the limb with variable extent of pain on palpation of the diaphysis of long bones.

The dogs in the age group of 6–18 months are more commonly affected. Larger breeds of dogs such as German shepherds, Great Danes, St. Bernards, Golden Retrievers, Basset Hounds, Dobermanns, Labrador Retrievers, and Rottweilers are frequently involved and are known genetically predisposed to the condition. Males are more commonly affected (about 70%) than females. Humerus is most commonly affected, and other bones such as ulna, radius, femur, and tibia can also be involved, with the symptoms generally starting in the forelimbs.

The cause of panosteitis is obscure [31, 32]. Apart from genetic predisposition, several other factors such as stress, impaired metabolism, infection, or an autoimmune cause might also play an important role. It has been suggested that rapid weight gain and high-protein diet are involved in the pathogenesis of the disease. Oversupplementation of minerals, as well as excess calcium in particular, may predispose to the condition. Blood analysis might show an elevated white blood cell count, indicating the possibility of an infection; nevertheless, no specific bacteria could be cultured or isolated from the affected animals, and hence, viral etiology is suspected. It has been postulated that an excessive buildup of protein may cause intraosseous edema,

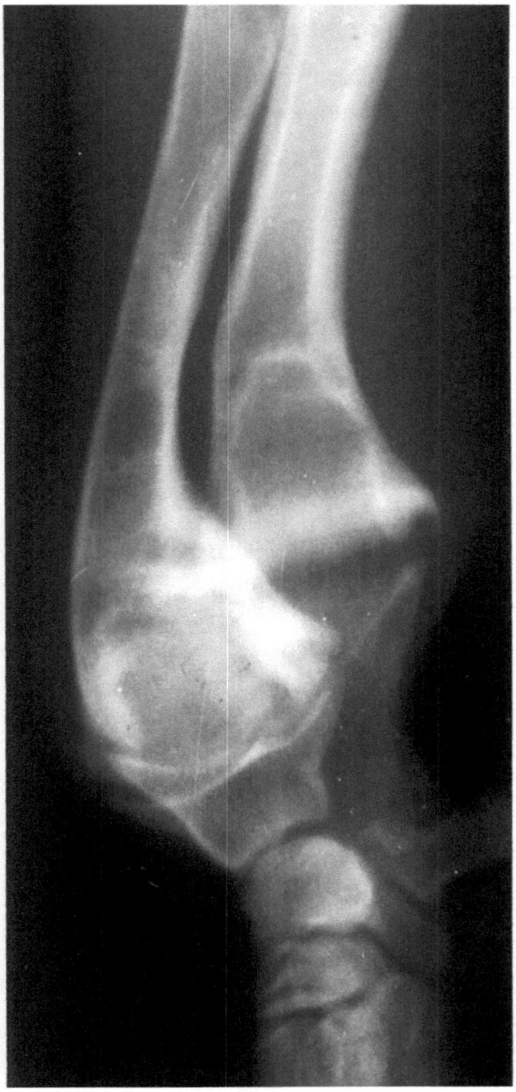

**Fig. 9.7** Radiograph of distal radius-ulna in a case of metaphyseal chondrodysplasia showing a large triangular radiolucent area in the metaphyseal region

leading to an increased intramedullary pressure and constriction of blood vessels. Subsequent osseous ischemia may cause hypoxia, acidosis, and disruption of biochemical processes resulting in local inflammation. Increased intramedullary pressure and stimulation of pain receptors in the periosteum may cause pain. Extreme physical activity is likely to aggravate the condition by increasing metabolism.

Panosteitis can be diagnosed based on the clinical signs and radiographic findings [33, 34]. The clinical signs of panosteitis may vary, and the animals may experience moderate to severe pain in one or more long bones of the limb. Intermittent and "shifting leg" lameness is characteristic of the disease. The pain can last for a few days to weeks, and it may relapse even after a month or two. Fever, pain upon palpation of limb, loss of appetite, weight loss, lethargy, and reluctance to exercise can be other symptoms of the disease.

In the initial days of lameness (for about 10 days), the radiographs may not show any evidence of the disease. Subsequently, radiographs of the affected long bones may reveal an increased medullary cavity density and an aggravated trabecular pattern around the nutrient foramen. As the disease progresses, there may be further mottling and increased opacity in the medullary cavity along with cortical and periosteal thickening (Fig. 9.8).

Panosteitis is a self-limiting condition, and the symptoms may get resolved within a few days or weeks without any treatment. Treatment is done only to alleviate the pain and inflammation so as to make the dog comfortable. This can be achieved by administering analgesics and anti-inflammatory drugs, such as NSAIDs (like meloxicam and carprofen) and non-narcotic opiates (like tramadol). Steroids may be given in more acute and severe cases to reduce inflammation. It is also advised to limit the physical activity during the period of treatment to prevent worsening of the condition. Generally, the symptoms resolve mostly around the age of 18 months; however, it may often persist even up to 5 years of age. The prognosis is always favorable.

Panosteitis can be prevented by giving careful attention to nutrition. Large breed dogs should be fed lower concentration of protein and fat to maintain "optimum" growth. Calcium should not be provided in excess. Vitamin C and Omega 3 supplements may be given, and the animals should be restricted to moderate exercise only. Due to heritability of the disease, the affected dogs and their parents should not be used for breeding, and they may be spayed and neutered to prevent genetic transmission.

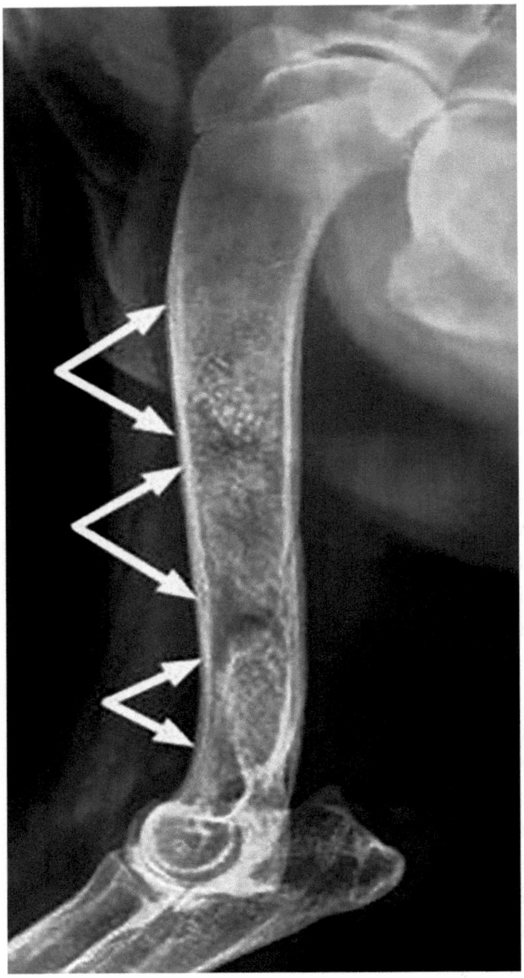

**Fig. 9.8** Radiograph of humerus showing increased medullary cavity density with trabecular pattern indicating panosteitis (Source: Praveen Kumar et al., Radiographic diagnosis of congenital and developmental orthopedic diseases in 50 dogs, Indian J. Vet. Surg. 35 (2): 116–120, 1014)

Panosteitis is basically a disease condition affecting dogs, and its occurrence in other pet or domestic animals is extremely rare. But suspected cases of panosteitis have been reported in horses, cattle, and a camel [34–36]. These animals had clinical signs characteristic to dogs such as juvenile onset, shifting leg lameness, and pain on palpation of the long bones. The radiographic findings also matched with that of dogs. Clinical improvement was seen with symptomatic treatment in most cases.

## 9.8 Hip Dysplasia

Hip dysplasia is one of the most common skeletal conditions affecting dogs, but cats may also get affected. It is characterized by abnormal structure of hip joint associated with a laxity of the muscles, connective tissues, and ligaments supporting the joint, leading to subluxation of hip or coxofemoral joint. Subluxation creates abnormal wear and erosion and severe structural changes in the articular surfaces of the joint leading to osteoarthritis and pain, resulting in varied clinical signs [37–40].

Hip dysplasia is generally bilateral and may also affect only right or left hip joint. Both male and female dogs are equally affected. It is predominantly a disease of large and giant breeds of dogs. Labrador Retrievers, Rottweilers, Great Danes, Golden Retrievers, and Saint Bernards are most frequently affected, whereas Greyhound is rarely affected. On the other hand, small breed dogs are rarely affected, and they seldom exhibit clinical signs of hip dysplasia.

Early clinical signs of hip dysplasia like pain and discomfort during or after exercise may be observed in young puppies aged about 5 months. The signs of discomfort may aggravate gradually as age advances. The clinical condition may become apparent in many animals below 1 year of age; however, in some cases, the symptoms may not be seen before the middle or later years of life. Clinical signs generally depend on the extent of joint laxity, inflammation, and duration of the condition; in early stages, they are mostly related to joint laxity, whereas in later stages, they are due to degenerative changes in the joint [41].

The affected dogs may show decreased activity, lameness, and gait abnormality. Hind limb lameness may be first noticed early in the morning, which can be irregular or continual and often can get aggravated after exercise. The animals generally avoid complete extension or flexion of the hind limbs. They may be reluctant to do normal day to day activities, such as rising, running, jumping, or climbing stairs. They often run with a "bunny hopping" gait. Gradually, the range of hip joint motion decreases with atrophy and loss of thigh muscle mass. The shoulder muscles may get enlarged due to extra load of weight bearing on the forelegs. Back legs look unnaturally close together with narrow stance in the hind limbs. With progression of the disease, the condition of dogs may get worsen with generalized weakness and loss of muscle tone needing assistance even to get up and move around.

Both genetic and environmental factors influence the development and progression of hip dysplasia. Researchers have found genetic susceptibility for hip looseness or laxity. The amount of calories and the period of life when they were consumed will determine whether a genetically susceptible dog will eventually develop hip dysplasia. The severity of the condition may increase in obese animals. Rapid growth during the young age (3–10 months) may also contribute to development of hip dysplasia. Feeding a diet with mineral imbalance (including calcium and phosphorus) can also have deleterious effects on the normal evolution of the hip joint predisposing to hip dysplasia. Overexercise at a young age may also predispose to hip dysplasia in dogs that are genetically predisposed to the disease; however, normal exercise can generally help maintain good muscle mass and thus reduce the incidence of hip dysplasia.

Hip dysplasia in canines can be diagnosed based on the clinical signs of osteoarthritis (pain and lameness), physical examination, and radiographic evaluation [42]. Clinical examination may exhibit loosening in the joint, and pain may be elicited through extension and flexion of the hind limb. The most popular and widely used radiographic technique for the diagnosis of hip dysplasia is the standard ventrodorsal hip extended view. Ventrodorsal radiographic view is made with the dog positioned in dorsal recumbency and the femur bones held stretched and parallel to each other with the stifle joints rotated internally (Fig. 9.9). The aim is to get a radiograph with symmetrical pelvis, parallel femurs, and patella centered on the distal femoral metaphysis. Radiographs should be assessed for both the primary laxity and secondary degenerative changes of hip joints.

Radiographically, formation of solitary bone osteophytes on the caudal part of the femoral neck may be visualized as an opaque line directed distally. There may be varied degrees of sclerosis of the subchondral bone of the femoral head and acetabulum. Femoral head may lose its spheroid shape and become flattened along its articular surface (Fig. 9.10). The femoral neck may become thickened and the surface of the neck irregular owing to formation of osteophytes. The acetabulum loses its cup-like shape and may become shallow. A variable degree of coxofemoral subluxation may be evident, and in distinct cases of arthritis, degenerative changes in the joint can be easily visible on the radiographs.

For more objective evaluation of the hip joint laxity, different methods have been used. The Norberg angle (NA) measured in degrees is the angle formed by a line drawn between the centers of the femoral heads and another line drawn from the center of the femoral head to the craniolateral margin of the acetabular rim (Fig. 9.11). This helps to quantify the position of the femoral head with respect to the acetabulum [43, 44]. Although normal NA may differ among different breeds of dogs, generally an angle of 105° or more is considered normal. There are three different scoring systems used worldwide to quantify the radiographic changes in canine hip dysplasia [45]. Federation Cynologique Internationale (FCI) system is followed in more than 80 nations located in most European countries, South America, Russia, and Asia; Orthopedic Foundation for Animals (OFA) scoring system is exclusively used in the United States and Canada, while British Veterinary Association/Kennel Club (BVA/KC) system is followed in Britain, Ireland, Australia, and New Zealand.

In FCI system, hip joint is described in five grades: A, no sign of hip dysplasia: the femoral head and the acetabulum may be congruent, and the craniolateral acetabular rim may appear sharp, slightly rounded, and in excellent hip joints, it may encircle the femoral head in caudolateral direction, and the joint space is narrow and even, and the NA is about 105°; B, near normal hip joint: the femoral head and acetabulum are

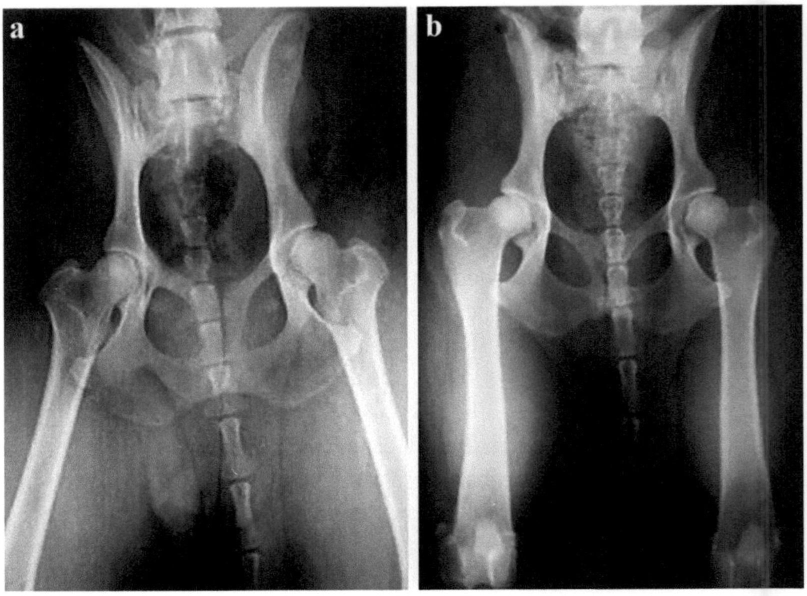


**Fig. 9.9** Diagnosis of hip dysplasia is made by ventrodorsal radiographic view with the dog positioned in dorsal recumbency and the femur bones held stretched and parallel to each other with the stifle joints rotated internally; (**a**) incorrect position and (**b**) correct position

slightly incongruent, and the NA is about 105° or the femoral head, and the acetabulum are congruent, and the NA is less than 105°; C, mild hip dysplasia: the femoral head and acetabulum are incongruent, and the NA is about 100, and/or there is slight flattening of the craniolateral acetabular rim with mild signs of osteoarthrosis on the cranial, caudal, or dorsal acetabular edge or on the femoral head and neck; D, moderate hip dysplasia: obvious incongruity between the femoral head and the acetabulum with subluxation, the NA is more than 90°, with flattening of the craniolateral rim and/or osteoarthritic signs; and E, severe hip dysplasia: with marked dysplastic changes such as luxation or distinct subluxation, the NA is less than 90°, with obvious flattening of the cranial acetabular ridge, deformation of the femoral head (mushroom shaped, flattening), or other signs of osteoarthrosis.

Medical management of hip dysplasia is mostly palliative; goal is to reduce pain, thereby improving the limb function and slowing the progress of degenerative changes in the hip joint [46–48]. It has three main approaches including nutritional, exercise and physical therapy, and administration of drugs. Administration of anti-inflammatory and analgesic drugs, providing suitable diet with supplements and regular exercises, may help to reduce the progression of degenerative arthritis; however, the joint laxity and the bony changes cannot be reversed or changed markedly. Exercise can help the dog to maintain proper weight and muscle building, in addition to preserve acceptable range of joint motion and limit wear and tear of joints. Massage and physical therapy may be considered for relaxing stiff muscles and promoting the range of joint movement. Several nonsteroidal anti-inflammatory drugs such as carprofen, etodolac, deracoxib, and meloxicam and corticosteroids have been used in dogs with hip dysplasia. For the management of osteoarthritis, compounds such as glucosamine and chondroitin, polysulfated glycosaminoglycan, and Omega-3 fatty acids have also been used extensively (detailed in Chapter 12). The present therapeutic approach to treat osteoarthritis is to prevent or delay the structural changes in the joint and hence to improve the limb function. In recent years, one such approach has been regenerative medicine using mesenchymal stem cells (MSC) and plasma-rich growth factor (PRGF) or platelet-rich plasma (PRP) [49, 50]. The findings with the use of MSCs and PRGF were not conclusive; however, their treatment has resulted in significant improvement in terms of pain reduction and improvement in limb function at least during the initial few months of treatment, indicating that

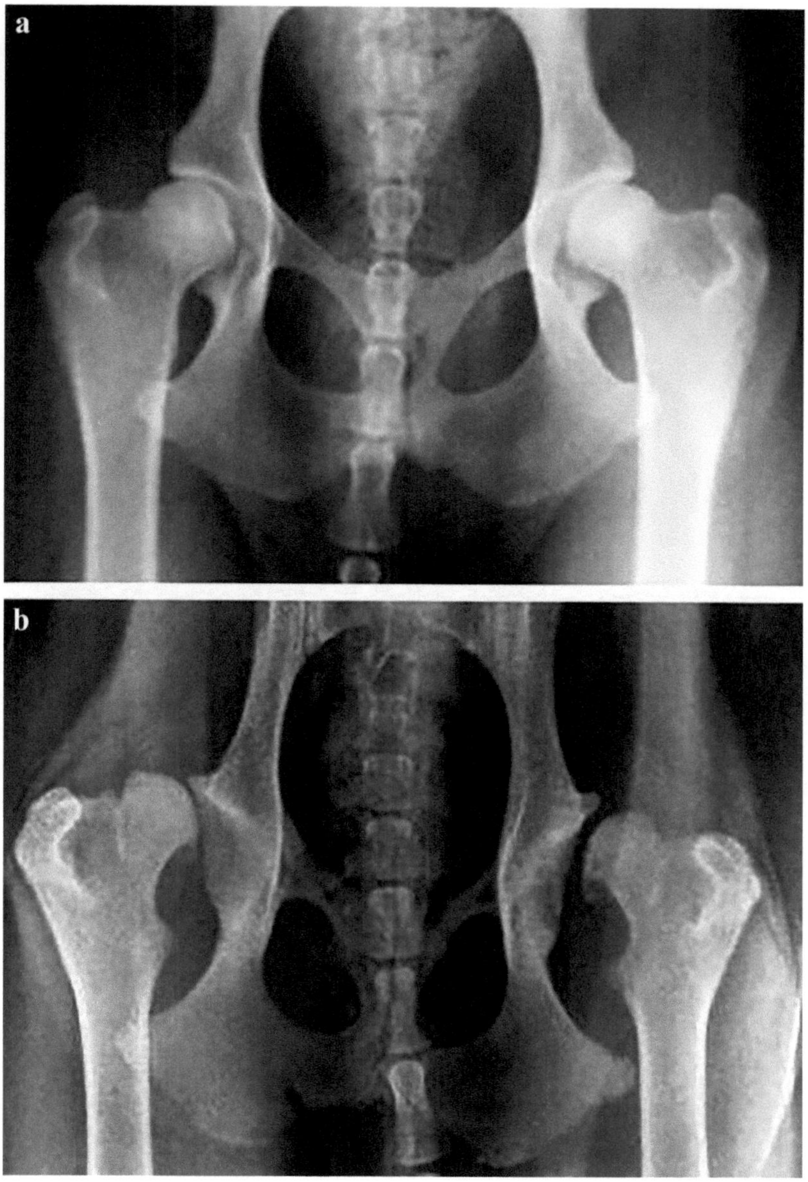

**Fig. 9.10** Radiographs of a normal hip (**a**) and a dysplastic hip (**b**) showing different signs of hip dysplasia such as sclerosis of the subchondral bone of the femoral head and acetabulum, flattening of femoral head, shallow acetabulum, osteophyte formation, and subluxation of coxo-femoral joints

stem cell-based therapy could become an effective alternate therapy for osteoarthritis in cases of canine hip dysplasia.

The surgical treatment of hip dysplasia includes palliative, prophylactic, and salvage procedures [51, 52]. Palliative procedures comprise pectineal myectomy/myotomy and hip denervation. ***Pectineal myectomy*** (resection of pectineus tendon) can reduce the ascending force striking the femoral head into the acetabulum and thus release tension on the joint capsule and the muscle, resulting in pain relief and better coverage of femoral head within the acetabulum [53]. However, the pain relief is mostly transient, and it does not ameliorate the joint instability. ***Denervation of the hip joint*** capsule is another palliative procedure used to treat hip dysplasia since many years. The rationale is the craniolateral capsule of the canine hip joint is highly innervated with pain receptors; hence, craniolateral denervation results in pain relief and make the animal comfortable. The technique

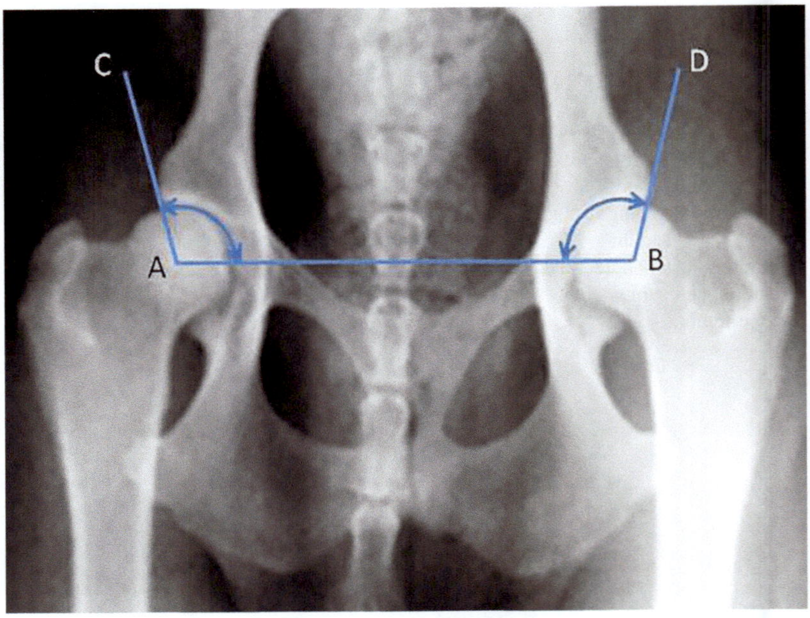


**Fig. 9.11** Measurement of the Norberg angle for diagnosis of hip dysplasia by measuring the angle (in degrees) formed by a line drawn between the centers of the femoral heads (A-B) and another line drawn from the center of the femoral head to the craniolateral margin of the acetabular rim (A-C and B-D)

includes deperiostation of acetabular rim resulting in denervation of cranial branches of gluteus nerve (on craniolateral aspect) and some sciatic nerve (on caudolateral aspect) branches. The craniolateral acetabulum is approached through a standard incision made in the cranial region of greater trochanter extending toward the iliac crest. Biceps femoris, gluteus medius, and tensor fascia lata muscles are diverged to expose the ilium. Denervation is achieved by debriding and scraping the periosteum from cranial surface of ilium, the craniodorsal joint capsule extending around the insertions of rectus femoris and deep gluteus muscles. The technique results in alleviation of pain and clinical improvement within a few days of surgery without the need for pain medications; however, the arthritic lesions caused by dysplasia and its progression cannot be changed. Due to decreased pain and increased activity, the pelvic and femoral muscles are expected to strengthen leading to improvement in the stability of dysplastic hip joint. As the technique is simple and minimally invasive, hip denervation can be a good option for management of hip dysplasia, especially in older and severely sick patients.

Prophylactic surgical procedures such as pubic symphysiodesis and corrective pelvic osteotomy are done in skeletally immature dogs not showing osteoarthritis signs, wherein the goal is to prevent the development of degenerative arthritis secondary to hip joint laxity.

***Juvenile public symphysiodesis*** is a minimally invasive technique, wherein the hyaline cartilage of the pubic symphysis is heated electrosurgically to induce necrosis of the germinal chondrocytes [54, 55]. It brings about premature closure of the pubic symphysis in immature dogs leading to shortening of the pubic ramus, thereby restricting the circumferential growth of the ventral segment of the pelvic canal while the dorsal segment continues to grow normally. With progression of growth, the acetabulum rotates ventrolaterally along the axial direction causing increased coverage of femoral head. The resulting changes in the angle and improvements in the articulation of the hip joint avert the possible development of osteoarthritis. The results are encouraging if the procedure is done in animals aged less than 20 weeks and before the development of arthritic signs.

***Corrective pelvic osteotomy*** is also a prophylactic surgical procedure aimed at minimizing the joint laxity and improving joint congruence through realignment the hip joint. Triple pelvic osteotomy technique is usually used in young dogs aged less than 10 months, having severe hip laxity without showing signs of joint damage. In this procedure, the pelvic bones are surgically incised (osteotomies of the pubis, ischium, and ilium) to achieve axial rotation and lateralization of the acetabulum; thereby, the femoral head and acetabulum are realigned (rotated) to provide greater dorsal coverage of the femoral head within the acetabular cavity [55–58]. The transverse osteotomy of the ilium is then stabilized with a pelvic osteotomy plate. Consequently, the extent of the force acting on the load-bearing parts of the acetabular rim and the femoral head is reduced, and the contact area is increased, thus improving the joint congruence during movement. The surgical correction can be performed on both sides simultaneously but more often done with a gap about 4–6 weeks. This surgical procedure is difficult and more invasive, but successful clinical outcome has occurred despite the development of osteoarthritis in some studies. Common complications are implant failure, acetabular fracture, sciatic nerve injury, infection, and pelvic canal narrowing.

***Intertrochanteric varus osteotomy*** of femur, another prophylactic technique used in human beings, has also been used and found beneficial to reduce subluxation and improve the acetabular coverage of the femoral head and hip congruency in canines [59, 60]. This technique can be considered for treatment of hip dysplasia in dogs with radiological signs of joint incongruence. In this technique, a femoral wedge osteotomy is performed proximal to the lesser trochanter (Fig. 9.12). The osteotomized segments are then reduced and stabilized using a bone plate, which results in decrease in the angle of inclination and anteversion, and push the proximal femoral segment into the acetabular cavity.

Total hip arthroplasty and femoral head and neck excision are salvage procedures used to restore the function of the leg.

***Total hip replacement*** may be the treatment of choice in chronic hip dysplasia cases having degenerative arthritic changes in dogs and cats [61]. In this procedure, the damaged joint is surgically resected, and it is replaced with a synthetic joint or prosthesis (Fig. 9.13). Total hip replacement implants normally include three components: acetabular cup (for implantation in the pelvis), femoral stem with a neck (for implantation inside the femur), and femoral head (for placement on the neck over the stem). All the implants are manufactured using the same specifications used for human applications. There are only a few implant manufacturers for veterinary applications; BioMedtrix (Whippany, New Jersey) is one such manufacturer of total hip replacement implants. Different techniques of cementless and cemented hip implant fixation have been described [62–68]. Cementless implants, used in medium and large dogs, are technically superior, as it can be stable instantly and become more stable with bone ingrowth (osteointegration) during the first 4–6 weeks of implantation. Cemented implants can also provide stable fixation and are mostly used in small dogs and cats. Postoperatively, the animals are confined to a small room and restricted to leash walk for 5–6 weeks. They are not allowed to run, jump, play, and climb stairs during the period. Subsequently, they may be allowed to go for walk two to four times a day for the next 30 days. Physical therapy specifically designed for the animal is carried out during the period. Normal activity is usually allowed within 2–3 months after surgery based on radiographic evaluation. Some of the complications of this surgery may include luxation or loosening of implant, fracture of femur shaft, infection, and sciatic nerve injury. The complications are generally less, and the surgery can be highly successful if performed by an experienced surgical team. The total hip replacement can alleviate the joint pain and restore the normal function of the joint at the earliest, and it is the most effective, successful and permanent treatment available. However, the procedure is quite expensive, the joint prosthesis is not readily available commercially, and there are only a few veterinary surgeons who can perform the procedure routinely.

***Femoral head and neck excision*** is a technique wherein the head and neck of femur bone is surgically resected and allowed to form a fibrous pseudo-joint [69–71]. It will help alleviate pain and permit normal activity, even though the range of joint motion and stability are compromised.

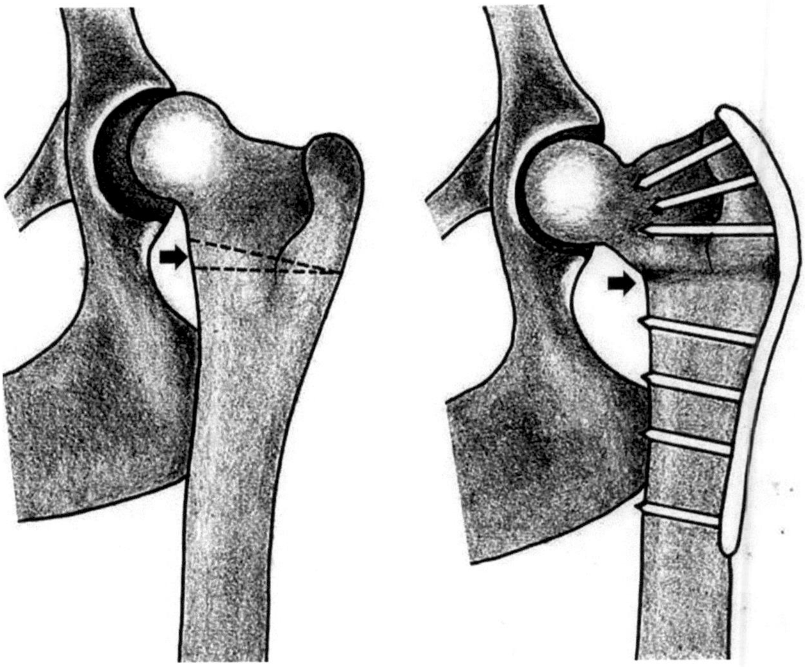

**Fig. 9.12** Intertrochanteric varus osteotomy, a prophylactic technique for hip dysplasia, wherein a femoral wedge osteotomy is performed proximal to the lesser trochanter and stabilized using a bone plate, to reduce the angle of inclination and anteversion, and to push the proximal femoral segment into the acetabular cavity

This procedure should be considered as a last option, and salvage procedure in cases with severe degenerative arthritis of hip joint and total hip replacement is not practicable [72]. The outcomes are better in lightweight animals.

The animal is restrained in lateral recumbency with the affected side held upward. A curvilinear incision is started slightly distal to the sacrococcygeal spine and extended distally up to the proximal third of the femoral shaft with its center just cranial to the greater trochanter. The subcutaneous tissues are incised to expose the underlying fascia and muscles. The fascia lata is incised just cranial to the greater trochanter, and the incision is extended distally between the tensor fascia lata and the biceps femoris muscles. Proximally, the incision is extended along the cranial margin of the superficial gluteal muscle, and the cranial margin of the middle gluteal is lifted dorsally to reveal the deep gluteal muscle tendon, which is stiff, bright, and shiny. After placing a stay suture, a partial tenotomy is done in the deep gluteal tendon, and the cut end is retracted proximally. The underlying vastus lateralis is separated by dissection to access the femur neck (Fig. 9.14).

Alternatively, the biceps femoris muscle is reflected caudally, and tensor fascia lata is reflected cranially to expose superficial gluteal muscle and its insertion on the greater trochanter. The superficial gluteal muscle is dissected from surrounding fascia at its tendon of insertion and reflected dorsally. The trochanter is then cut from the lateral surface with an osteotome or a saw so that the insertion of middle gluteal muscle remains attached to the resected trochanter. This approach will give better exposure of the joint capsule.

The hip joint is then extended or flexed and rotated internally or externally by manipulating the limb to exactly locate and palpate the femoral head and neck. Once affirmed, a linear incision is made in the dorsal joint capsule extending from the dorsal acetabular rim, across the femoral head and neck after placing stay sutures in the dorsal and ventral margins of the incised joint capsule. Then the joint capsule incision is extended circumferentially to separate the femoral neck. The junction of the femoral neck and proximal femoral shaft is visualized by elevating the origin of vastus lateralis muscle using a periosteal elevator. By retracting the joint capsule cranially and

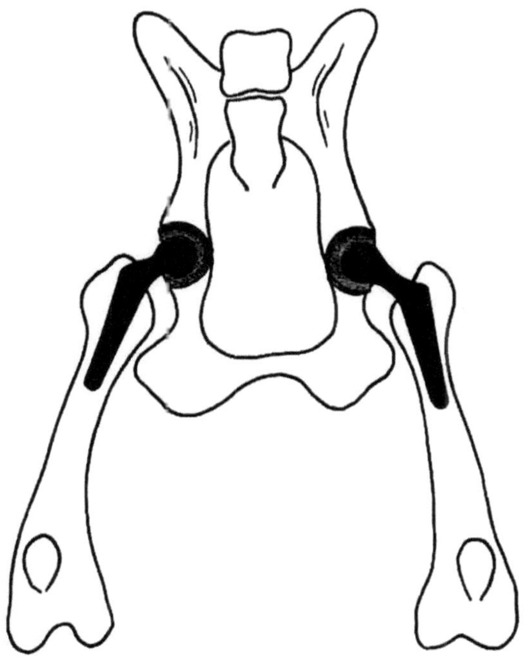

**Fig. 9.13** Schematic representation of bilateral total hip replacement with prosthesis

caudally using a retractor, a small curved scissor/sharp instrument is inserted between the femur head and the acetabulum to transect the round ligament. The limb is then externally rotated by about 90° (until the patella is pointed upwardly) to further expose the femoral head and neck and any soft tissue attachments if any are separated. A curved artery forceps may be inserted below the femoral neck to further exteriorize the femoral neck and head and allow better access for ostectomy.

Femoral head and neck excision is performed by preserving the lesser trochanter, which can be palpated along the caudomedial margin of the femoral neck (Fig. 9.15). Ostectomy procedure can be performed from distal to proximal direction using a saw, osteotome, and mallet. Experienced surgeons may sometime prefer an electric saw (reciprocating or oscillating) for excision of femoral head and neck. In any case, care should be taken to resect complete femoral neck and head without damaging the surrounding soft tissues. Incomplete removal may occur due to inadequate retraction of soft tissues, improper positioning and exposure of the femur neck, or inadequate external rotation. Once osteotomy is completed, ligamentous and capsular attachments are transected to allow excision of the femoral head and neck.

The limb is externally rotated, and the ostectomy surface of the proximal femur is palpated for any sharp edges or spurs using the index finger, and by using a rasp, the surface is smoothened, if required. A soft tissue layer is interposed between the ostectomy surface and the acetabulum to help improve the patient limb use and comfort. The incised edges of the joint capsule are identified with the help of previously placed stay sutures and are apposed by suturing. Effort should be made to close the transected capsule as much as possible, and if there is inadequate capsular tissue to accomplish apposition, the partially tenotomized deep gluteal tendon can be sutured at the ventral region. If trochanteric osteotomy was performed, the greater trochanter is reattached after proper positioning of femur, using small K-wires or cancellous screws.

Following the femoral head and neck excision, a false joint (pseudoarthrosis) develops due to scar tissue formation. Though movement should be restricted for a few days or 1–2 weeks (especially in heavy animals), early limb use is encouraged through passive physical therapy (warm compresses, massage, and passive range of motion) and active therapy (slow leash walks). Proper exercise, balanced nutrition, and physiotherapy modalities should be followed to maintain desirable body weight and maintain the hip joint congruence. The dogs may be provided with orthopedic foam beds, which can help distribute weight evenly and reduce pressure on joints. The dogs should not be allowed to go up and down the stairs. In addition, slightly warmer room temperature may be maintained. Prognosis is usually favorable with satisfactory functional recovery in more than 90% cases. Complications such as shortening of the operated limb, restricted range of joint motion, chronic lameness, disuse atrophy, recurrence of pain due to bony contact, and osteomyelitis due to breach in asepsis may occur occasionally. It could lead to severe functional deficits in large breed dogs [73].

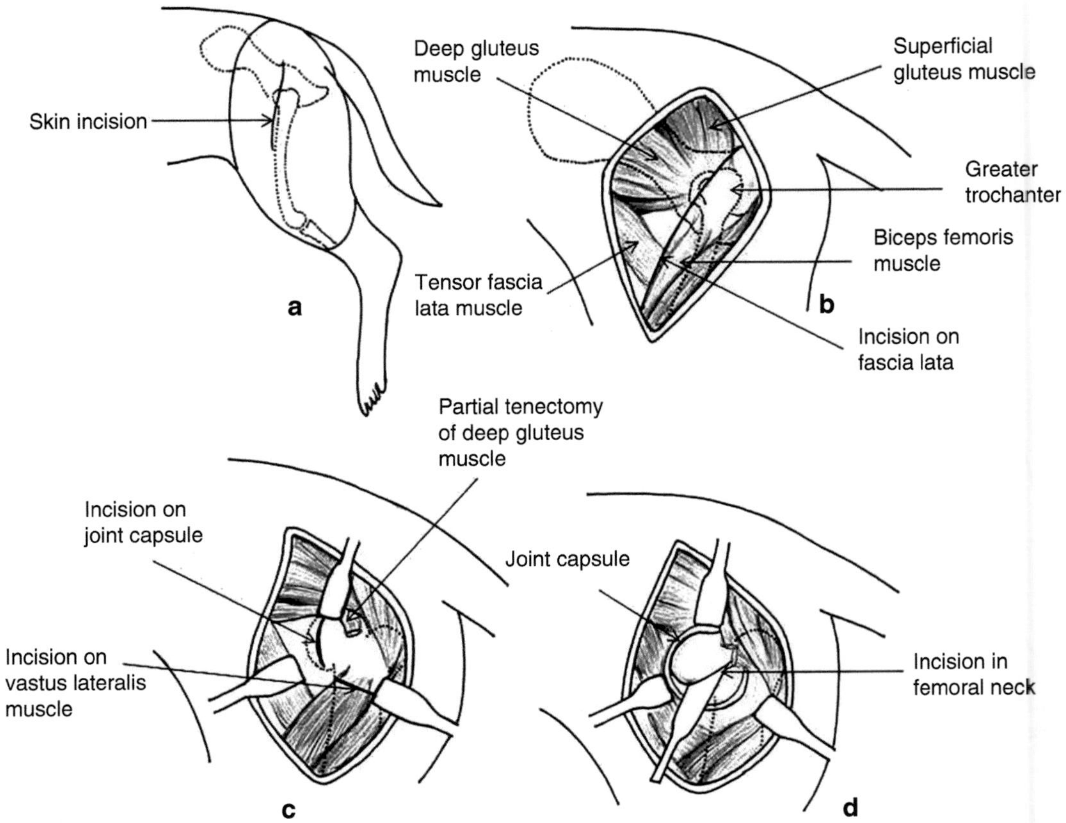


**Fig. 9.14** Schematic presentation of surgical approach to femoral head and neck ostectomy

Another technique of ***femoral neck lengthening*** and dorsal acetabular rim arthroplasty has been described recently to treat severe hip luxation in dog [74]. This treatment provided adequate femoral head coverage, and the dog could maintain full joint function over 7 years without any complication and with better functional recovery as compared to femoral head and neck ostectomy.

It is always difficult to cure hip dysplasia once set in; only the progression to degenerative joint disease can be delayed or reduced using different treatment options. Canine hip dysplasia can be prevented only by selective breeding; the affected dogs should not be used for breeding.

Hip dysplasia is also a relatively frequent congenital disease of cattle worldwide [75–80]. Similar to dogs, it is essentially an abnormality of the acetabulum leading to degenerative changes in the coxo-femoral joint. The shallow acetabular cavity (lower depth) is a characteristic feature that can help to distinguish hip dysplasia from an acquired osteoarthritis, or traumatic luxation. Further, in hip dysplasia, the malformation of the acetabulum is generally bilateral, even if the severity may vary. Young beef bulls of Aberdeen Angus, Charolais, Galloway, and Hereford breeds in the United Kingdom, North America, and Australia are more predisposed. Clinical signs are related to secondary osteoarthritis, which may include stiffness, hindlimb muscular atrophy, lameness, and reluctance to walk. Physical examination of the hip and rectal examination can help diagnose the condition; radiography will help in confirmatory diagnosis. Treatment is usually avoided, and severely affected cattle are often culled at a young age. Degenerative arthritis of the coxofemoral joint characterized by erosion of cartilage, deposition of new bone, and luxation of the joint and lameness, considered to be due to

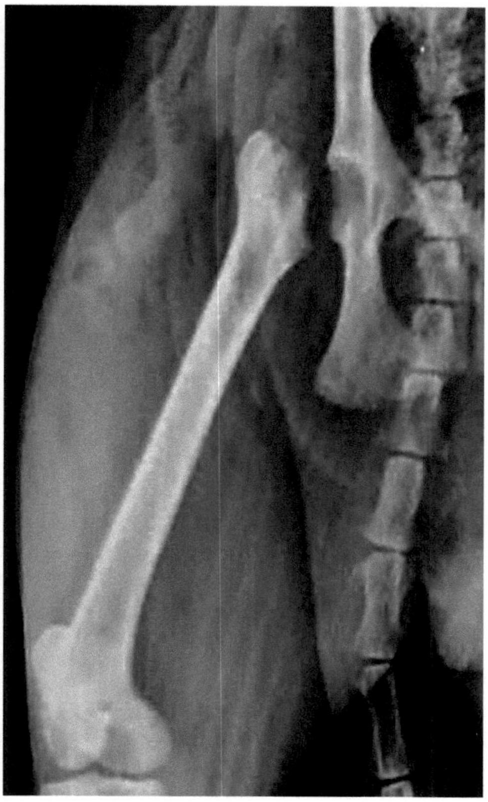

**Fig. 9.15** Radiograph of the hip joint made after femoral head and neck ostectomy

inherited hip dysplasia, has also been reported in foals [81].

## 9.9 Prevention and Control of Bone Disorders

The dog keeping is on rise in India. Along with indigenous or nondescript breeds of dogs, the craze for a pedigreed breed is increasing day by day. However, most of the pets are not fed with a balanced diet and are usually fed with kitchen leftover. The use of commercial dog feeds is in its infancy. Hence, the occurrence of nutritional and metabolic bone diseases has increased in recent years, as high as up to 30%.

Staples for dogs like meat and corn consist of adequate phosphorus but are deficient in calcium. Meat (skeletal muscle) contains about 0.02% calcium and 0.4% phosphorus on dry basis (meat byproducts including bones, however, are balanced diet). Corn (maize) may contain 0.03% calcium and 0.3% phosphorus; hence, both need to be supplemented with additional calcium. Similarly, milling byproducts such as wheat bran are deficient in calcium.

The recommended dietary contents of calcium and phosphorus are 1.1% and 0.9% for dogs, whereas, vitamin D requirement is 500 IU/kg body weight. In other words, dogs require 242 mg/kg body weight of calcium per day for maintenance and about 484 mg/kg per day for growth. Providing balanced diet, especially in the early period of life, may help reduce the incidence of skeletal disorders. However, some of these diseases appear to have genetic predisposition, though it is yet to be confirmed. Hence, it is advised not to breed the dogs affected with bone disorders.

Early diagnosis and treatment can reduce the extent of deformity or damage. Once detected, the imbalanced diet (like whole meat) should be discontinued, and a nutritionally balanced diet (supplemented with calcium and phosphorus) must be provided. Milk and milk products, which are natural sources of Ca and P, may be supplemented. The dog may be provided with chewing bones to supplement minerals. The affected animal may be housed in non-slippery floor, and for the first few weeks, it should be confined and activity restricted.

## Chapter 9: Sample Questions

**Q. No. 1: Mark the correct answer**

1. Failure of mineralization at the physeal cartilage resulting in thickening of the physis is characteristic of
   (a) nutritional secondary hyperparathyroidism (b) rickets (c) hypertrophic osteodystrophy (d) osteochondrosis
2. The onset of clinical signs of osteodystrophy occurs generally at
   (a) 3–4 months of age (b) 4–6 months of age (c) 6–12 months of age (d) above 12 months

3. Osteochondritis dissecans, a manifestation of osteochondrosis, most commonly affects the
   (a) hip joint (b) shoulder joint (c) elbow joint (d) stifle joint
4. The bone disease characterized by medullary fibrosis as well as both endosteal and subperiosteal new bone deposition is
   (a) panosteitis (b) osteodystrophy (c) osteopathy (d) osteomyelitis
5. Calcium homeostasis also depends upon endogenous hormones, namely,
   (a) Parathyroid hormone (b) calcitonin (c) vitamin D (d) all of the above

**Q. No. 2: State true or false**

1. Deficiency of phosphorus in the diet generally leads to secondary hyperparathyroidism.
2. PTH acts on the kidneys to increase urinary phosphorus excretion and decrease calcium loss in the urine.
3. Homeopathic drugs, *Calcarea phosphorica* and *Symphytum 30*, can improve the conditions of rachitic lesions in long bones of dogs.
4. Hip dysplasia is commonly first detected in dogs after 1 year of age.
5. Deficiency of vitamin C can cause hypertrophic osteodystrophy.

**Q. No. 3: Fill up the blanks**

1. An area of increased radio-density in the metaphyses of long bones adjacent to the growth plates is characteristic of ____________________________________________.
2. Grossly thickened radiolucent growth plate with "cupping" of the enlarged metaphysis is characteristic of ______________________________.
3. Retention of cartilage core leading to deformity of limbs is most commonly recorded at ____________________________________________.
4. Early signs of hip dysplasia are related to ______________________________, whereas in the later stage, the signs are related to ____________________________________________.
5. Juvenile pubic symphysiodesis is a surgical technique used to treat ______________________________.

**Q. No. 4: Write short note on the following**

1. Causes of Nutritional Secondary Hyperparathyroidism
2. Clinical and radiographic signs of rickets
3. Surgical treatment of Osteochondritis Dissecans
4. Causes of hip dysplasia

## References


1. Kumar, P., B.M. Yadav, S. Jangra, P. Chaudhary, and P. Jakhar. 2014. Radiographic diagnosis of congenital and developmental orthopaedic diseases in 50 dogs. *Indian Journal of Veterinary Surgery* 35 (2): 116–120.
2. Kushwaha, R.B., H.P. Aithal, P. Kinjavdekar, Amarpal, and K. Kumar. 2012. Incidence of skeletal diseases affecting long bones in growing dogs - A radiographic survey. *Intas Polivet* 13: 337–344.
3. Bennett, D. 1976. Nutrition and bone disease in the dog and cat. *The Veterinary Record* 98: 313–321.
4. Mendoza, F.J., R.E. Toribio, and A.P. Ecija. 2017. Nutritional secondary hyperparathyroidism in equids: overview and new insights. *Equine Veterinary Education* 29 (10): 558–563.
5. Merkle, C. 1976. Osteodystrophia fibrosa due to nutrition in the adult cat. *Tierärztliche Praxis* 4 (1): 77–84.
6. Tomsa, K., T. Glaus, B. Hauser, M. Flückiger, P. Arnold, G. Wess, and C. Reusch. 1999. Nutritional secondary hyperparathyroidism in six cats. *The Journal of Small Animal Practice* 40 (11): 533–539.
7. Kushwaha, R.B., H.P. Aithal, Amarpal, P. Kinjavdekar, A.M. Pawde, G.R. Singh, V.P. Varshney, and H.C. Setia. 2011. Therapeutic management of hyperpara-thyroidism in growing dogs. *The Indian Veterinary Journal* 88: 79–82.
8. Parti, M., H.P. Aithal, Amarpal, P. Kinjavdekar, A.M. Pawde, G.R. Singh, T.K. Goswami, and H.C. Setia. 2008. Evaluation of certain antiresorptive drugs in growing dogs affected with osteopenic bone diseases (rickets, NSH). *The Indian Journal of Animal Sciences* 78: 1333–1337.
9. Kushwaha, R.B., and H.P. Aithal. 2005. Rickets in a non-descript dog: A case report. *Intas Polivet* 6: 91–94.
10. Dittmer, K.E., and K.G. Thompson. 2011. Vitamin D metabolism and rickets in domestic animals: A review. *Veterinary Pathology* 48 (2): 389–407.
11. Elizabeth, W.U. 2018. The pathology of vitamin D deficiency in domestic animals: an evolutionary and comparative overview. *International Journal of Paleopathology* 23: 100–109.

12. Papadopoulou, A., E. Gole, and P. Nicolaidou. 2013. Hereditary rickets. How genetic alterations explain the biochemical and clinical phenotypes. *Endocrine, Metabolic & Immune Disorders Drug Targets* 13: 324–334.
13. Kushwaha, R.B., H.P. Aithal, Amarpal, P. Kinjavdekar, A.M. Pawde, G.R. Singh, V.P. Varshney, and A.K. Pattanaik. 2009. Studies on incidence, and clinical, radiographic and haematobiochemical profiles of growing dogs affected with rickets and their response to calcium-vitamin-D3 therapy. *Indian Journal of Veterinary Surgery* 30: 93–97.
14. Grondalen, J. 1976. Metaphyseal osteopathy (hypertrophic osteodystrophy) in growing dogs: a clinical study. *The Journal of Small Animal Practice* 17: 721–735.
15. Lenehan, T.M., and A.W. Fetter. 1985. Hypertrophic osteodystrophy In *Textbook of small animal orthopedics*, ed. C.D. Newton and D.M. Nunamaker, 597–601. Philadelphia: J.B. Lippincott.
16. Watson, A.D.J., R.C. Blair, B.R. Farrow, J.D. Baird, and H.L. Cooper. 1973. Hypertrophic osteodystrophy in the dog. Case report. *Australian Veterinary Journal* 49: 433–439.
17. Woodard, J.C. 1982. Canine hypertrophic osteodystrophy, a study of the spontaneous disease in littermates. *Veterinary Pathology* 19: 337–354.
18. Meier, H., S.T. Clark, G.B. Schnelle, and D.H. Will. 1957. Hypertrophic osteodystrophy associated with disturbance of vitamin C synthesis in dogs. *Journal of the American Veterinary Medical Association* 130: 483–491.
19. Bellah, J.R. 1993. Hypertrophic osteopathy. In *Disease mechanisms in small animal surgery*, ed. M.J. Bojrab, 858–864. Philadelphia: Lea & Febiger.
20. Kushwaha, R.B., H.P. Aithal, Amarpal, P. Kinjavdekar, A.M. Pawde, and G.R. Singh. 2005. Hypertrophic osteodystrophy in growing dogs: a clinical study. *Indian Journal of Veterinary Surgery* 26: 21–24.
21. Safra, N., E.G. Johnson, L. Lit, O. Foreman, Z.T. Wolf, M. Aguilar, N. Karmi, C.J. Finno, and D.L. Bannasch. 2013. Clinical manifestations, response to treatment, and clinical outcome for Weimaraners with hypertrophic osteodystrophy: 53 cases (2009–2011). *Journal of the American Veterinary Medical Association* 242 (9): 1260–1266.
22. Johnson, K.A. 1981. Retardation of endochondral ossification at the distal ulnar growth plate in dogs. *Australian Veterinary Journal* 57: 474–478.
23. Ytrehus, B., C.S. Carlson, and S. Ekman. 2007. Etiology and pathogenesis of osteochondrosis. *Veterinary Pathology* 44 (4): 429–448.
24. Altunatmaz, K., M. Saroglu, and O. Guzel. 2006. Retained endochondral ossification of the distal ulnar growth plate in dogs. *Medycyna Weterynaryjna* 62 (1): 40–42.
25. Kushwaha, R.B., H.P. Aithal, Amarpal, P. Kinjavdekar, G.R. Singh, A.M. Pawde, V.P. Varshney, and H.C. Setia. 2006. Clinical, radiographical and haematobiochemical changes in growing dogs with retained cartilage core. *The Indian Journal of Animal Sciences* 76: 886–890.
26. Piermatei, D.L., and G.L. Flo. 1997. Retained cartilage cores in the distal ulnar physis. In *Brinker, Piermatei and Flo's handbook of small animal orthopedics and fracture repair*, ed. D.L. Piermatei and G.L. Flo, 697–698. Philadelphia: W.B. Saunders.
27. Bingel, S.A., and R.D. Sande. 1994. Chondrodysplasia in five great Pyrenees. *Journal of the American Veterinary Medical Association* 205: 845–848.
28. Kyöstilä, K., A.K. Lappalainen, and H. Lohi. 2013. Canine chondrodysplasia caused by a truncating mutation in collagen-binding integrin alpha subunit 10. *PLoS One* 8 (9): e75621.
29. Breur, G.J., C.A. Zerbe, R.F. Slocombe, G.A. Padgett, and T.D. Braden. 1989. Clinical, radiographic, pathologic, and genetic features of osteochondrodysplasia in Scottish deerhounds. *Journal of the American Veterinary Medical Association* 195: 606–612.
30. Lenehan, T.M., D.C. VanSickle, and D.N. Biery. 1985. Canine panosteitis. In *Textbook of small animal orthopaedics*, ed. C.D. Newton and D.M. Nunamaker, 591–596. Philadelphia, Pennsylvania: J.B. Lippincott.
31. Schawalder, P., H.U. Andres, K. Jutzi, C. Stoupis, and C. Bösch. 2002. Canine panosteitis: an idiopathic bone disease investigated in the light of a new hypothesis concerning pathogenesis. Part 1: clinical and diagnostic aspects. *Schweizer Archiv für Tierheilkunde* 144 (3): 115–130.
32. Schawalder, P., K. Jutzi, H.U. Andres, and J. Blum. 2002. Canine panosteitis- an idiopathic bone disease investigated in the light of a new hypothesis concerning pathogenesis. Part two: Biochemical aspects and investigations. *Schweizer Archiv für Tierheilkunde* 144 (4): 163–173.
33. Böhning, R.H., Jr., P.F. Suter, R.B. Hohn, and J. Marshall. 1970. Clinical and radiologic survey of canine panosteitis. *Journal of the American Veterinary Medical Association* 156: 870–883.
34. O'Neill, H.D., and B.M. Bladon. 2011. Retrospective study of scintigraphic and radiological findings in 21 cases of enostosis-like lesions in horses. *The Veterinary Record* 168: 326–329.
35. Levine, D.G., J.J. Smith, D.W. Richardson, and V. Brown. 2007. Suspected panosteitis in a camel. *Journal of the American Veterinary Medical Association* 231 (3): 437–441.
36. Sato, R., T. Ito, T. Suganuma, Y. Une, T. Kudo, H. Kayanuma, E. Kanai, T. Suzuki, H. Ochiai, N. Enomoto, S. Itoh, K. Onda, and Y. Wada. 2015. Suspected panosteitis in a crossbred calf. *The Canadian Veterinary Journal* 56 (5): 463–465.
37. King, M.D. 2017. Etiopathogenesis of canine hip dysplasia, prevalence and genetics. *The Veterinary Clinics*

of North America. *Small Animal Practice* 47 (4): 753–767.
38. Lust, G. 1997. An overview of the pathogenesis of canine hip dysplasia. *Journal of the American Veterinary Medical Association* 210: 1443–1445.
39. Todhunter, R.J., and G. Lust. 2003. Hip dysplasia: pathogenesis. In *Textbook of small animal surgery*, ed. E.D. Slatter. Philadelphia: P.A. Saunders.
40. Zhang, Z.W., L. Zhu, J. Sandler, S.S. Friedenberg, J. Egelhoff, A.J. Williams, N.L. Dykes, W. Hornbuckle, U. Krotscheck, N.S. Moise, G. Lust, and R.J. Todhunter. 2009. Estimation of heritabilities, genetic correlations, and breeding values of four traits that collectively define hip dysplasia in dogs. *American Journal of Veterinary Research* 70: 483–492.
41. Fry, T.R., and D.M. Clark. 1992. Canine hip dysplasia: clinical signs and physical diagnosis. *The Veterinary Clinics of North America. Small Animal Practice* 22: 551–558.
42. Ginja, M.M.D., A.M. Silvestre, J.M. Gonzalo-Orden, and A.J. Ferreira. 2010. Diagnosis, genetic control and preventive management of canine hip dysplasia: a review. *Veterinary Journal* 184: 269–276.
43. Comhaire, F.H., A.C.C. Criel, C.A.A. Dassy, P.G.J. Guévar, and F.R. Snaps. 2009. Precision, reproducibility, and clinical usefulness of measuring the Norberg angle by means of computerized image analysis. *American Journal of Veterinary Research* 70: 228–235.
44. Culp, W.T., A.S. Kapatkin, T.P. Gregor, M.Y. Powers, P.J. McKelvie, and G.K. Smith. 2006. Evaluation of the Norberg angle threshold: a comparison of Norberg angle and distraction index as measures of coxofemoral degenerative joint disease susceptibility in seven breeds of dogs. *Veterinary Surgery* 35: 453–459.
45. Saunders, J., and B. Broeckx. 2017. Radiographic methods for diagnosis of hip dysplasia World Small Animal Veterinary Association Congress Proceedings, 2017. https://www.vin.com
46. Barr, A.R.S., H.R. Benny, and C. Gibbs. 1987. Clinical hip dysplasia in growing dogs: the long-term results of conservative management. *The Journal of Small Animal Practice* 28: 243–252.
47. Farrell, M., D.N. Clements, D. Mellor, T. Gemmill, S.P. Clarke, J.L. Arnott, D. Bennett, and S. Carmichael. 2007. Retrospective evaluation of the long-term outcome of non-surgical management of 74 dogs with clinical hip dysplasia. *The Veterinary Record* 160: 506–511.
48. Kirkby, K.A., and D.D. Lewis. 2012. Canine hip dysplasia: reviewing the evidence for nonsurgical management. *Veterinary Surgery* 41: 2–9.
49. Cuervo, B., M. Rubio, J. Sopena, J.M. Dominguez, J. Vilar, M. Morales, R. Cugat, and J.M. Carrillo. 2014. Hip osteoarthritis in dogs: a randomized study using mesenchymal stem cells from adipose tissue and plasma rich in growth factors. *International Journal of Molecular Sciences* 15: 13437–13460.
50. Vilar, J.M., M. Batista, M. Morales, A. Santana, B. Cuervo, M. Rubio, R. Cugat, J. Sopena, and J.M. Carrillo. 2014. Assessment of the effect of intraarticular injection of autologous adipose-derived mesenchymal stem cells in osteoarthritic dogs using a double blinded force platform analysis. *BMC Veterinary Research* 10: 143.
51. Bergh, M.S., and S.C. Budsberg. 2014. A systematic review of the literature describing the efficacy of surgical treatments for canine hip dysplasia. *Veterinary Surgery* 43: 501–506.
52. Schachner, E., and M. Lopez. 2015. Diagnosis, prevention, and management of canine hip dysplasia. *Veterinary Medicine: Research and Reports* 6: 181–192.
53. Wallace, L.J. 1992. Pectineus tendon surgery for the management of canine hip dysplasia. *The Veterinary Clinics of North America. Small Animal Practice* 22: 607–621.
54. Dueland, R.T., W.M. Adams, A.J. Patricelli, K.A. Linn, and P.M. Crump. 2010. Canine hip dysplasia treated by juvenile pubic symphysiodesis. Part I: two year results of computed tomography and distraction index. *Veterinary and Comparative Orthopaedics and Traumatology* 23: 306–317.
55. Manley, P.A., W.M. Adams, K.C. Danielson, R.T. Dueland, and K.A. Linn. 2007. Long-term outcome of juvenile pubic symphysiodesis and triple pelvic osteotomy in dogs with hip dysplasia. *Journal of the American Veterinary Medical Association* 230: 206–210.
56. Borostyankoi, F., R.L. Rooks, C.N. Kobluk, A.L. Reed, and E.T. Littledike. 2003. Results of single-session bilateral triple pelvic osteotomy with an eight-hole iliac bone plate in dogs: 95 cases (1996-1999). *Journal of the American Veterinary Medical Association* 222: 54–59.
57. Rose, S.A., K.A. Bruecker, S.W. Petersen, and N. Uddin. 2012. Use of locking plate and screws for triple pelvic osteotomy. *Veterinary Surgery* 41: 114–120.
58. Slocum, B., and T. Devine. 1986. Pelvic osteotomy technique for axial rotation of the acetabular segment in dogs. *Journal of the American Animal Hospital Association* 22: 331–338.
59. Pinna, S., E. Pizzuti, and F. Carli. 2013. Effects of intertrochanteric varus osteotomy on Norberg angle and percent coverage of the femoral head in displastic dogs. *Journal of Veterinary Science* 14 (2): 185–191.
60. Prieur, W.D. 1987. Intertrochanteric osteotomy in the dog: theoretical consideration and operative technique. *The Journal of Small Animal Practice* 28 (1): 3–20.
61. Allen, M.J. 2012. Advances in total joint replacement in small animals. *The Journal of Small Animal Practice* 53: 495–506.
62. DeSandre-Robinson, D.M., S.E. Kim, J.N. Peck, J.D. Coggeshall, G. Tremolada, and A. Pozzi. 2015. Effect of dorsal acetabular rim loss on stability of the

Zurich cementless total hip acetabular cup in dogs. *Veterinary Surgery* 44: 195–199.

63. Fitzpatrick, N., A.Y. Law, M.B. Bielecki, and S. Girling. 2014. Cementless total hip replacement in 20 juveniles using BFX™ arthroplasty. *Veterinary Surgery* 43: 715–725.
64. Gemmill, T.J., J. Pink, A. Renwick, B. Oxley, C. Downes, S. Roch, and W.M. McKee. 2010. Hybrid cemented/cementless total hip replacement in dogs: seventy-eight consecutive joint replacements. *Veterinary Surgery* 40: 621–630.
65. Heo, S.Y., J.W. Seol, and H.B. Lee. 2015. Total hip replacement in two dogs with unsuccessful femoral head ostectomy. *Journal of Veterinary Science* 16: 131–134.
66. Hummel, D. 2017. Zurich cementless total hip replacement. *The Veterinary Clinics of North America. Small Animal Practice* 47: 917–934.
67. Montgomery, M.L., S.E. Kim, J. Dyce, and A. Pozzi. 2015. The effect of dorsal rim loss on the initial stability of the BioMedtrix cementless acetabular cup. *BMC Veterinary Research* 11: 68.
68. Morshed, S., K.J. Bozic, M.D. Ries, H. Malchau, and J.M. Colford. 2007. Comparison of cemented and uncemented fixation in total hip replacement. *Acta Orthopaedica* 78: 315–326.
69. Lippincott, C.L. 1987. Excision arthroplasty of the femoral head and neck. *The Veterinary Clinics of North America. Small Animal Practice* 17 (4): 857–871.
70. Lippincott, C.L. 1992. Femoral head and neck excision in the management of canine hip dysplasia. *The Veterinary Clinics of North America. Small Animal Practice* 22 (3): 721–737.
71. Rawson, E.A., M.G. Aronsohn, and R.L. Burk. 2005. Simultaneous bilateral femoral head and neck ostectomy for the treatment of canine hip dysplasia. *Journal of the American Animal Hospital Association* 41 (3): 166–170.
72. Harper, T.A.M. 2017. Femoral head and neck excision. *The Veterinary Clinics of North America. Small Animal Practice* 47 (4): 885–897.
73. Ober, C., C. Pestean, L. Bel, M. Taulescu, J. Milgram, A. Todor, R. Ungur, M. Lesu, and L. Oana. 2018. Use of clinical and computed tomography findings to assess long-term unsatisfactory outcome after femoral head and neck ostectomy in four large breed dogs. *Acta Veterinaria Scandinavica* 60: 28. (2018). https://doi.org/10.1186/s13028-018-0382-8.
74. Petazzoni, M., and M. Dallago. 2019. Canine femoral neck lengthening combined with darthroplasty to manage severe canine juvenile hip dysplasia: a case report. *Veterinary and Comparative Orthopaedics and Traumatology Open* 2 (2). https://doi.org/10.1055/s-0039-1694036.
75. Agerholm, J., and A. Basse. 1993. Hip dysplasia in a nine-month-old male Jersey calf. *The Veterinary Record* 133: 273.
76. Carnahan, D.L., M.M. Guffy, C.M. Hibbs, H.W. Leipold, and K. Huston. 1968. Hip dysplasia in Hereford cattle. *Journal of the American Veterinary Medical Association* 152 (8): 1150–1157.
77. Howlett, C. 1972. Inherited degenerative arthropathy of the hip in young beef bulls. *Australian Veterinary Journal* 48: 562–563.
78. Mann, S., A. Blutke, A. Brühschwein, and M. Feist. 2011. A case of congenital unilateral hip dysplasia in a newborn calf. *Schweizer Archiv für Tierheilkunde* 153 (10): 457–461.
79. Vlierbergen, B.V., K. Chiers, M. Hoegaerts, D. Everaert, and R. Ducatelle. 2007. Hip dysplasia – like lesions in a Belgian blue cow. *The Veterinary Record* 160 (26): 910–912.
80. Weaver, A. 1978. Hip dysplasia in beef cattle. *The Veterinary Record* 102: 54–55.
81. Speirs, V.C., and R. Wrigley. 1979. A case of bilateral hip dysplasia in a foal. *Equine Veterinary Journal* 11 (3): 202–204.

# Antebrachial Bone Deformities

# 10

**Learning Objectives**
You will be able to understand the following after reading this chapter:

- Causes, clinical signs, and radiographic diagnosis of different forelimb deformities such as closure of distal ulnar growth plate, closure of distal radial growth plate, closure of proximal radial physis, and closure of both growth plates – distal radius and ulna
- Different methods of surgical treatment, postoperative care, management, and prognosis of antebrachial deformities

**Summary**

- Limb deformities are most common in the canine antebrachium; as the distal ulnar physis has to grow much faster than the distal radius to keep pace with it, any disparity in growth between the twin bones can predispose this area to growth abnormalities.
- Antebrachial limb deformities are more common in large giant breed dogs; the most common causes are fractures of the radius-ulna or metabolic diseases such as hypertrophic osteodystrophy and cartilage retention.
- The principles of treatment in limb deformities are to prevent, reduce, and/or correct the angular deformity, preserve the joint congruity, and maintain the bone length, in young growing animals. The aim should be to cut the slow-growing bone to allow the other bone to grow uninterrupted. In older dogs (after the closure of growth plate), the deformity is corrected by osteotomy/ostectomy procedure performed at the area of greatest curvature, and the bone is rigidly fixed using a bone plate/an ESF.

Angular limb deformity is a relatively common orthopedic condition encountered in dogs, more commonly in chondrodystrophic breeds [1–7]. Angular deformity has also been reported in other domestic animals such as horses. It may result in impaired limb function due to painful range of motion and dysfunction of the limb joints, ineffective locomotion from misaligned joints, or limb shortening. Although angular limb deformity may occur in any limb, in veterinary practice, the most common location is in the antebrachium. The twin bones, the radius and the ulna, which are strongly connected via


H. P. Aithal et al., *Textbook of Veterinary Orthopaedic Surgery*,
https://doi.org/10.1007/978-981-99-2575-9_10

the interosseous ligament, must grow simultaneously and proportionately for normal development of the antebrachium, failure of which is a common cause of development of angular limb deformities.

The longitudinal growth of the ulnar diaphysis occurs almost exclusively from the distal physis (about 85% of growth in length), while the proximal physis contributes only about 15%. Similarly, the distal radial physis contributes for about 70% of the growth and the proximal physis for 30% growth. This disproportionate growth of the radius and the ulna and their respective ends predisposes the antebrachium to growth abnormalities. Further, the conical shape and superficial location of the distal ulnar physis make it more vulnerable to injury [7–9]. The most common causes for antebrachial deformities are damage to the radius-ulna or diseases like cartilage retention and hypertrophic osteodystrophy [10]. Often even minor trauma, which may not be detected at the time of injury, would cause disruption of the distal ulnar physis. The deformity will be generally apparent in about two weeks time after the trauma. The retention of cartilage is most commonly seen at the distal physis of the ulna in giant breeds of dogs, which may slow down or completely arrest the physeal growth. In large breed dogs with long limb bones, foreleg deformities are more common, and the dogs with short limb tend to develop more severe abnormalities of joint alignment. Age of the animal at the time of injury or premature closure of growth plates would determine the extent of the deformity. In developmental abnormalities of elbow alignment, the lameness slowly progresses in one or both forelimbs, which may be exaggerated after exercise. Lameness is primarily due to abnormalities in the joint alignment and resultant arthritis.

Regardless of the affected growth plate, the principles of treatment are to (i) prevent, reduce, and/or correct the angular deformity, (ii) preserve the joint congruity, and (iii) maintain the bone length. Conservative treatment such as application of splint and bandage can be used to manage certain cases of slight antebrachial deformity with little or no growth potential left in the animal, and the joint is minimally subluxated [11]. In very young animals with a large growth potential remaining, the conservative treatment should be avoided as it can worsen the joint subluxation and deformity. In general, conservative treatment may help to reduce further worsening of the condition, but it is ineffective at correcting the limb deformity.

The method of surgical treatment depends on the animal's age, expected continued growth potential of the bones, severity of carpal valgus/rotational deformity, and the extent of bone shortening. In young, 3–4-month-old animals with significant potential of growth, the aim is to section the slow-growing bone so as to permit the uninterrupted growth of the other bone. If there is mild deformity, it can get corrected on its own; and if the deformity is more severe, it may be corrected when noted or when the bone growth stops. Such release osteotomies are least traumatic and can promote compensatory growth in young growing animals. Periosteal stripping is another technique, which can help to "release" the thick periosteum "restricting" the longitudinal growth of the bone in young animals. This technique is more popular in horses but can be performed in dogs having significant angular deformity without severe rotational deformity and joint subluxation [11]. Stapling is another corrective surgical procedure performed to restrict the longitudinal growth of one bony physis/part of the physis allowing the other bony physis/part of the physis to grow in young animals with minimal or partial premature closure of growth plate [11, 12]. The stapled animals should be carefully monitored for the correction of deformity, and the staple should be removed as early as possible to avoid complete cessation of growth plate.

In older dogs (>6–7 months), the deformity is corrected by osteotomy/ostectomy (usually wedge/dome osteotomy) procedure performed at the area of greatest curvature, and the bone is rigidly fixed [13, 14]. The plane of the carpal and elbow joints is kept parallel while determining the angle of the wedge to be removed by considering all the three planes of deformity – cranial bowing, angular, and rotational deformity – while planning the corrections [11, 15]. Traditionally these osteotomy techniques were planned from radiographic studies using orthogonal views. However, in recent years, three-dimensional images obtained from the CT scan have been used to provide more accurate measurements of the complex geometries and plan for bone resection [16–18]. Different stabilization techniques have been described for bone fixation after osteotomy for correction of angular deformities, such as external coaptation, bone plates and screws, linear fixation systems and circular and hybrid external fixators [19–30]. If an ESF is chosen for fixation, the transfixation pins may be placed parallel to the respective joint surfaces on both sides of the osteotomy and are later secured parallel to each other in the fixator to align the joint surfaces. With an ESF, adjustments can be made even after bone fixation, which cannot be done when using a plate. A circular or hybrid ESF has greater scope for maneuverability while correcting the rotational/angular deformations than a linear ESF.

The distal ulnar or distal/proximal radial closure can cause incongruity of the elbow joint. Osteotomy of the affected bone and allowing continuous weight bearing is usually sufficient to realign the elbow joint. Often when the humeroulnar joint luxation is severe, active realignment with circular ESF-facilitated bone transport (distraction osteosynthesis) may be indicated. Bone transport refers to the surgical technique of cutting the shortened bone and fixing it with external fixator system for its progressive and gradual lengthening to achieve normal bone length.

## 10.1 Closure of Distal Ulnar Growth Plate

The distal ulnar growth plate closure is the most common form of growth disturbance of the canine antebrachium and mostly occurs following a trauma or metabolic abnormality [4, 5, 7, 9, 25, 31]. Due to the conical shape of distal ulnar physis, the forces concentrate and compress at the site making it more susceptible to injuries. Closure or retardation of growth of ulnar physis results in the deformation of the distal radius and carpus because the radius continues to grow around the stationary ulna. In long standing cases, the carpus rotates internally and may bend caudally. Most often there will be marked outward deviation of the carpus or foot but the elbow may be spared; however, concurrent subluxation of the elbow is accompanied with severe pain.

Surgical treatment for the distal ulnar premature closure in young growing dogs includes removal of a section of the ulna (ostectomy) at the level of greatest deformity in the radius bone, which will help relieve the pressure on the radius. A sufficiently large (2–4 cm) gap should be created in the ulna, so that it will not bridge before the cessation of radial physeal growth (Fig. 10.1). The periosteum should be removed/excised completely especially along the radius, and fat may be grafted between the bone ends to prevent premature healing of the defect [32]. If healing occurs before growth ceases, a second osteotomy may be needed. If severe angular deformity is present at the time of osteotomy, it can be corrected by taking care to protect the continued growth of the distal radial physis. If the deformity is of mild nature, it would be better to wait until growth of the bone ceases to make final correction. In adult dogs, a single correction can be made by making the osteotomy (wedge/dome) at the point of greatest deformity in the radius including ulna (Figs. 10.2 and 10.3). In case there is concurrent subluxation of the elbow, then a second osteotomy should be made in the proximal ulna to relieve pressure. The osteotomized bone is fixed using an ESF, preferably a circular fixator to allow corrections/bone lengthening at a later date. In adult mature animals, during the final correction, which do not require limb lengthening, even an epoxy-pin fixation may prove successful.

## 10.2 Closure of Distal Radial Growth Plate

Although premature closure of distal ulnar physis is more common, deformities can also occur due

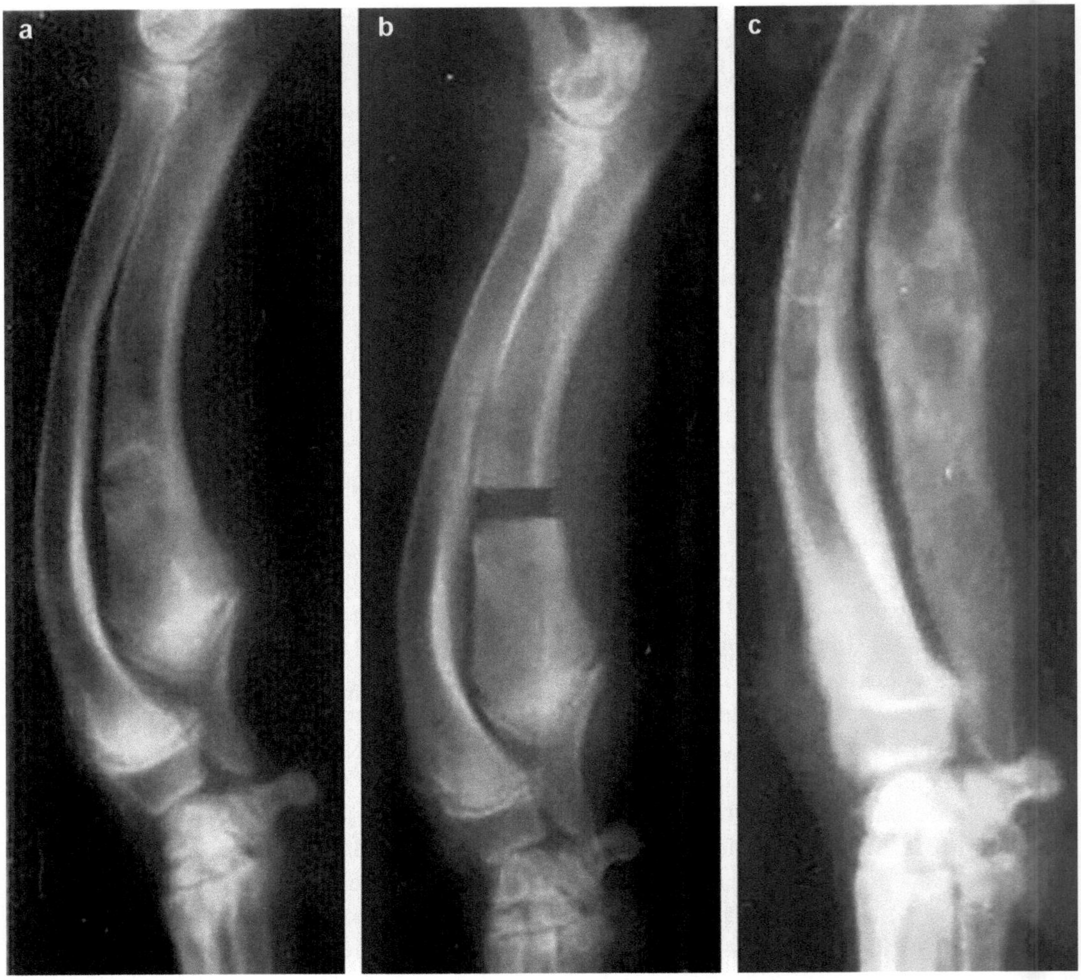


**Fig. 10.1** Distal ulnar physeal premature closure in a growing dog showing bowing of radius (**a**), surgically corrected by performing ulnar ostectomy (**b**), and relieving of the pressure on the radius resulted in straightening of the bones (**c**)

to premature closure of distal radial physis [33–36]. The limb affected with closure of distal radial growth plate may appear significantly shorter than the normal contralateral limb with varied degrees of lameness. The severity of lameness would depend on the degree of abnormality in the joint. If the closure of lower growth plate of the radius is symmetrical, the limb may remain straight mediolaterally, but there may be caudal bow of radius and ulna with a widened space in radial carpal joint (Fig. 10.4). When medial lower growth plate of the radius has asymmetrical closure, the foreleg may be rotated or bent inward toward the center of the body (varus deformity) and occasionally twisted inward. When lateral lower growth plate of the radius is closed, which is more common, the foreleg would be twisted or bent outward away from the center of the body (valgus deformity) with external rotation.

Surgically an osteotomy of the radius is done so that pressure on the distal ulna can be relieved, which may allow the radial head to realign with the humerus. Removal of a piece of the radius will help move the proximal radius automatically (Fig. 10.1); otherwise a distraction device may be used to realign the proximal radius. If the distal radius is involved in a significant deformity, a corrective osteotomy should be performed followed by application of distraction (using an ESF) along the radius. If a young dog is presented

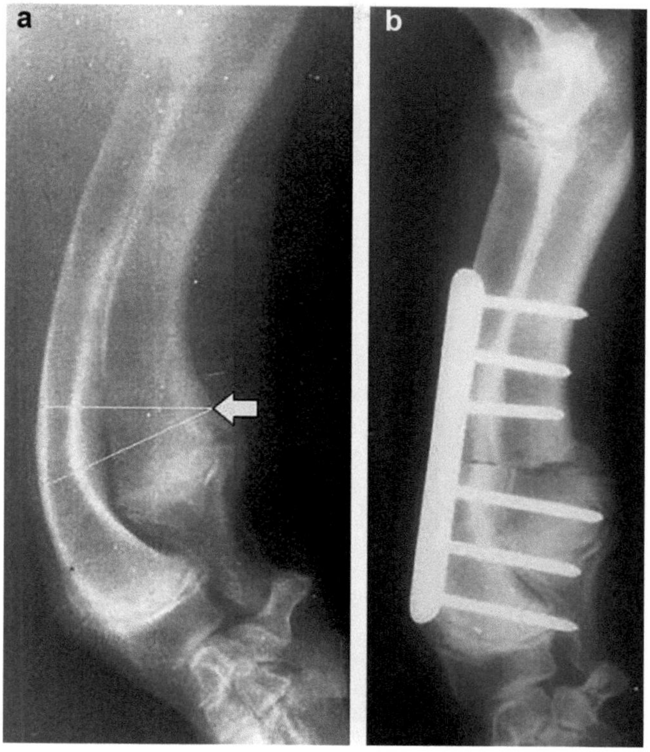


**Fig. 10.2** Distal ulnar physeal premature closure in a grown-up dog showing bowing of radius (**a**), surgically corrected by performing wedge osteotomy and surgical fixation using a bone plate and screws (**b**). Arrow shows the site of wedge osteotomy

with a significantly shortening of the limb, both the radius and ulna can be transected, and distraction should be applied (1–2 mm a day) to correct the shortening and to allow for continued growth. In adult dogs, single radial osteotomy may be performed for straightening of the distal radius, and slow distraction may be provided using an ESF, which will help align the radial head with the humerus.

## 10.3 Closure of Proximal Radial Physis

Closure of proximal radial physis is rarely seen and is usually due to a trauma [9]. Clinically, the dog may show progressive lameness, which may be exacerbated on direct manipulation of the elbow joint. Generally, there will not be any deformity of the forelimb. The space between the radial head and the distal lateral humeral condyle will be increased that can be appreciated radiographically. Occasionally, lateral curvature of the proximal radius, lateral displacement of the radial head, and oblique angulation of the radial joint surface may also be observed.

When diagnosed, the corrective surgery should be undertaken as early as possible, since continued instability in the elbow may result in degenerative joint disease. Proximal radial osteotomy may correct mild subluxation of radial head automatically. In cases of severe ventral subluxation of radius, transverse osteotomy along with cortical bone grafting and rigid internal fixation is indicated. If there is lateral displacement or angulation of the radial head is present, care is to be taken to properly angle the proximal fragment of the radius for articulation before fixing the bone.

## 10.4 Closure of Both Growth Plates: Distal Radius and Ulna

At times, closure of both distal radial and ulnar growth plates may occur secondary to trauma [9, 10]. If it happens at an early age, it can result in marked shortening of the limb. The clinical

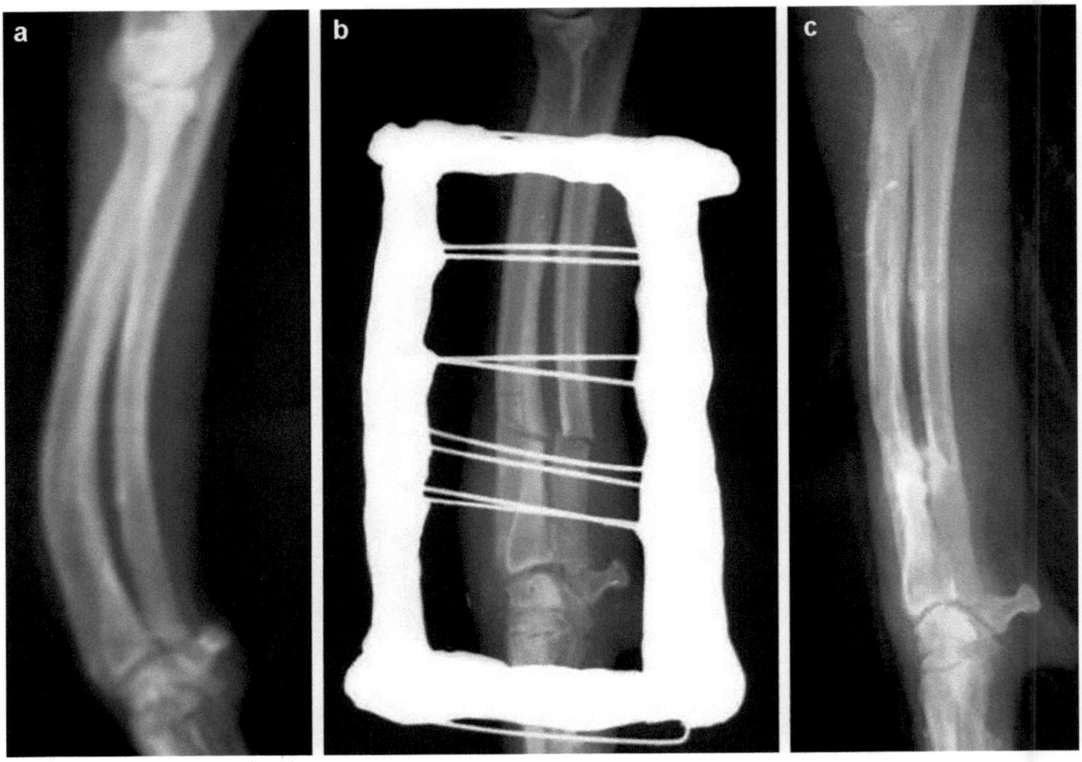


**Fig. 10.3** Angular deformity of radius and ulna secondary to an old fracture (**a**), treated by wedge osteotomy, and fixation using epoxy-pin ESF shows good bone reduction and alignment (**b**), and radiograph made one year post-fixation shows almost complete healing and correction of the deformity (**c**)

outcome may be similar to a distal ulnar closure, as the proximal radial physis contributes relatively more toward overall longitudinal growth of the bone than the proximal ulnar physis. The condition can be best treated by osteotomy of both the radius and the ulna, and providing distraction using an ESF (circular), especially in young growing dogs, would help further. In case of premature healing of the osteotomy gap before the end of normal growth, a second osteotomy followed by continued distraction may be required.

## 10.5 Postoperative Care, Management, and Prognosis

Postoperative care and management include restriction of the animal's movement by allowing only leashed walking for short distances, strict care of external skeletal fixator, and physiotherapy and exercises to allow elbow and carpus range of motion. Periodic examinations should be done to evaluate arthritic status, and anti-inflammatory therapy may be administered as per the need. Nutraceuticals such as glucosamine may help control cartilage damage and subsequent development of arthritis. In case of a metabolic cause, the treatment should also be directed toward correcting the metabolic disturbances, such as mineral imbalance.

Early initiation of surgical treatment would generally lead to a better prognosis. By correcting angular and rotational deformities of the carpus/distal radius-ulna, improving elbow congruence, and lengthening the radius/ulna when needed, a functional recovery of the limb can be achieved. By avoiding breeding of susceptible breeds and by preventing dietary over-supplementation in

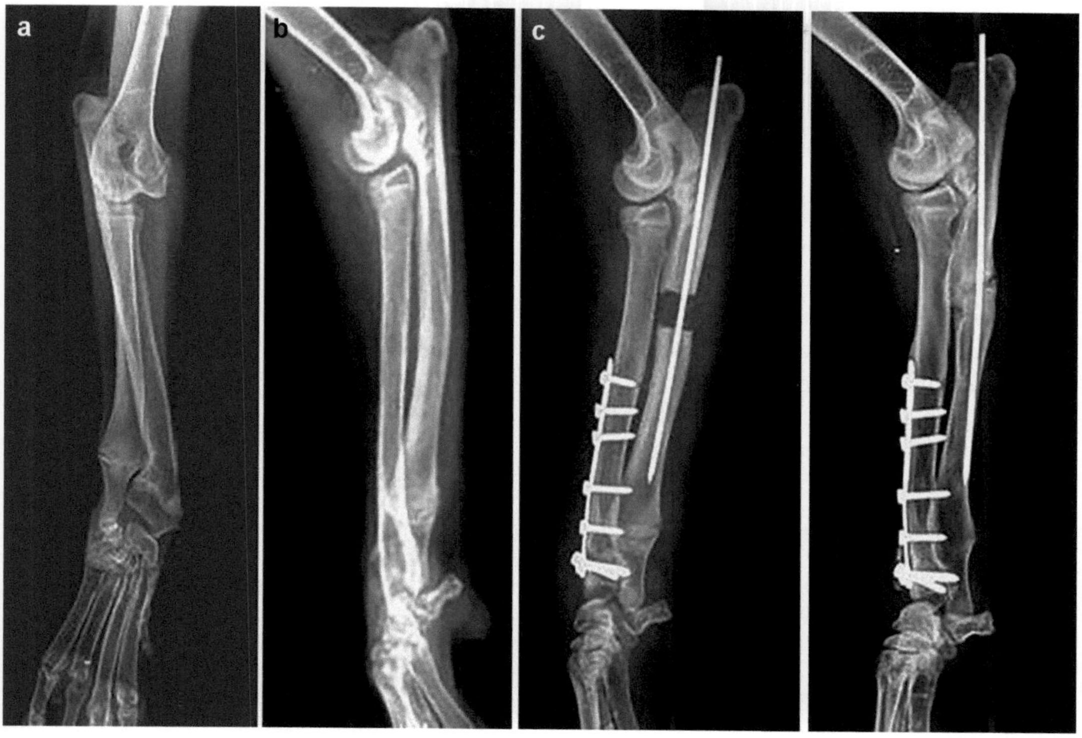


**Fig. 10.4** Carpal valgus with elbow subluxation secondary to trauma in a dog shows asymmetrical physeal closure of right distal radius and subluxation of carpal and elbow joints (**a** and **b**) and its surgical correction by ulnar ostectomy and T-plate fixation of distal radial wedge osteotomy, and (**c**) 60 day postoperative radiograph shows straightened radius, normal humero-radial and humero-ulnar joints, and healed ulnectomy site (Source: Shahid Hussain Dar et al., Carpal valgus with elbow sub-luxation secondary to trauma and its surgical treatment by ulnar ostectomy and T-plate fixation of distal radial wedge osteotomy in a Labrador dog. Indian J. Vet. Surg. 42 (2), 2021)

rapidly growing giant-breed dogs, the incidences of the condition may be prevented/reduced.

## Chapter 10: Sample Questions

### Question No. 1: Mark the correct answer

1. In growth plate deformities, the principles of treatment are to
   (a) Prevent, reduce, and/or correct the angular deformity,
   (b) Preserve the joint congruity
   (c) Maintain the bone length
   (d) All the above
2. In closure of both distal radius and ulnar physes, the recommended surgical treatment is
   (a) ostectomy of the ulna
   (b) Ostectomy of the radius
   (c) Osteotomy of both the radius and ulna
   (d) None of these
3. Distal physis of ulna contributes to its longitudinal growth up to
   (a) 5%
   (b) 15%
   (c) 50%
   (d) 85%
4. Surgical treatment of premature closer of distal ulna in young growing dogs include ostectomy of
   (a) Radius
   (b) Ulna
   (c) Both radius/ulna
   (d) None of the above

### Question No. 2: State true or false

1. Distal ulnar growth plate deformity is more common than that of distal radius often leading to antebrachial deformities.
2. The conical shape of the distal ulnar physis makes it more susceptible for the stress concentration leading to injuries.
3. Wedge osteotomy at the point of greatest deformity in the radius including ulna is the method of choice to correct the antebrachial deformity in young growing dogs.
4. Incongruity of the elbow joint can occur in either a distal ulnar or distal/proximal radial closure.

### Question No. 3: Fill up the blanks

1. The most common location of angular limb deformity in dogs is in the ________________________.
2. About ______________ of longitudinal growth of ulna occurs from the distal physis, whereas distal radial physis contributes for about __________________ of the growth; this disparity in growth between the two bones predisposes this area to ________________________.

### Question No. 4: Write short note on the following

1. Causes for premature closure of distal ulnar growth plate
2. Wedge osteotomy for correction of antebrachial deformities

## References


1. Carrig, C.B. 1983. Growth abnormalities of the canine radius and ulna. *The Veterinary Clinics of North America. Small Animal Practice* 13 (1): 91–115.
2. Fox, S.M. 1984. Premature closure of distal radial and ulnar physes in dog. Part I. pathogenesis and diagnosis. *Compendium on Continuing Education for the Practicing Veterinarian* 6 (2): 128–139.
3. Johnson, J.A., C. Austin, and G.J. Breur. 1994. Incidence of canine appendicular musculoskeletal disorders in 16 veterinary teaching hospitals from 1980 to 1989. *Veterinary and Comparative Orthopaedics and Traumatology* 7: 56–69.
4. Kushwaha, R.B., H.P. Aithal, P. Kinjavdekar, Amarpal, A.M. Pawde, G.R. Singh, and H.C. Setia. 2006. Premature closure of physis in growing dogs: clinical, haemato-biochemical and radiographic changes. *Indian Journal of Veterinary Surgery* 27: 30–32.
5. Ramadan, R.O., and L.C. Vaughan. 1978. Premature closure of the distal ulnar growth plate in dogs: A review of 58 cases. *The Journal of Small Animal Practice* 19: 647.
6. Singh, K., P. Kinjavdekar, H.P. Aithal, A. Gopinathan, Amarpal, and A.M. Pawde. 2008. Occurrence of antebracheal deformities in growing dogs. *The Indian Journal of Animal Sciences* 78: 1373–1375.
7. Weigel, J.P. 1987. Growth deformities. *The Veterinary Clinics of North America. Small Animal Practice* 17: 905–922.
8. Egger, E.L. 1993. Fractures of the radius and ulna. In *Textbook of small animal surgery*, ed. D.H. Slatter, vol. 2, 2nd ed., 1736–1757. Philadelphia: WB Saunders.
9. Newton, C.D. 1985. Radial and ulnar osteotomy. In *Textbook of small animal orthopaedics*, ed. C.D. Newton and D.M. Nunamaker, 533–544. Philadelphia: J.B. Lippincott.
10. Johnson, A.L. 1990. Correction of radial and ulnar growth deformities resulting from premature physeal closure. In *Current techniques in small animal surgery*, ed. M.J. Bojrab, 3rd ed., 793–801. Philadelphia: Lea & Febiger.
11. Marcellin-Little, D. 2020. Limb deformities in dogs: the role of the primary care veterinarian. ISVMA – November 2020. 17 pages. https://www.isvma.org
12. Carlson, R.L., C.L. Lohse, L.A. Eld, and F.G. Hughbanks. 1972. Correction of angular limb deformities by physeal stapling. *Modern Veterinary Practice* 53: 41–42.
13. Fox, D.B., J.L. Tomlinson, J.L. Cook, and L.M. Breshears. 2006. Principles of uniapical and biapical radial deformity correction using dome osteotomies and the center of rotation of angulation methodology in dogs. *Veterinary Surgery* 35 (1): 67–77.
14. Franklin, S.P., R.K. Dover, N. Andrade, and D. Rosselli. 2017. Correction of antebrachial angulation-rotation deformities in dogs with oblique plane inclined osteotomies. *Veterinary Surgery*. https://doi.org/10.1111/vsu.12706.
15. Knapp, J.L., J.L. Tomlinson, and D.B. Fox. 2016. Classification of angular limb deformities affecting the canine radius and ulna using the center of rotation of angulation method. *Veterinary Surgery* 45 (3): 295–302.
16. Bordelo, J.P.A., M.I.R. Dias, L.M.M.L. Cardoso, J.M.F. Requicha, C.A.A. Viegas, and J.F. Bardet. 2018. A 3D printed model for radius curvus surgical treatment planning in a dog. *Pesquisa Veterinaria Brasileira* 38 (6). https://doi.org/10.1590/1678-5150-pvb-5209.

17. Dismukes, D.I., D.B. Fox, J.L. Tomlinson, and S.C. Essman. 2008. Use of radiographic measures and three- dimensional computed tomographic imaging in surgical correction of an antebrachial deformity in a dog. *Journal of the American Veterinary Medical Association* 232 (1): 68–73.
18. Leong, N.L., G.A. Buijze, E.C. Fu, F. Stockmans, and J.B. Jupiter. 2010. Distal radius Malunion (DiRaM) collaborative group. Computer-assisted versus non-computer-assisted preoperative planning of corrective osteotomy for extra-articular distal radius malunions: a randomized controlled trial. *BMC Musculoskeletal Disorders* 11: 282.
19. Balfour, R.J., R.J. Boudrieau, and B.R. Gores. 2000. T-plate fixation of distal radial closing wedge osteotomies for treatment of angular limb deformities in 18 dogs. *Veterinary Surgery* 29 (3): 207–217.
20. Cappellari, F., L. Piras, E. Panichi, A. Ferretti, and B. Peirone. 2014. Treatment of antebrachial and crural septic nonunion fractures in dogs using circular external skeletal fixation: a retrospective study. *Veterinary and Comparative Orthopaedics and Traumatology* 27: 297–305.
21. Dar, S.H., et al. 2021. Carpal valgus with elbow sub-luxation secondary to trauma and its surgical treatment by ulnar ostectomy and T-plate fixation of distal radial wedge osteotomy in a Labrador dog. *Indian Journal of Veterinary Surgery* 42 (2): 148–149.
22. Fox, S.M., J.C. Bray, S.R. Guerin, and H.M. Burbridge. 1995. Antebrachial deformities in the dog: treatment with external fixation. *The Journal of Small Animal Practice* 36 (7): 315–320.
23. Lewis, D.D., R.M. Radasch, B.S. Beale, J.T. Stallings, O.I. Lanz, R.D. Welch, and M.L. Samchukov. 1999. Initial clinical experience with the IMEXTM circular external skeleton fixation system. Part II: use in bone lengthening and correction of angular and rotational deformities. *Veterinary and Comparative Orthopaedics and Traumatology* 12 (2): 118–127.
24. MacDonald, J.M., and D. Matthiesen. 1991. Treatment of forelimb growth plate deformity in 11 dogs by radial dome osteotomy and external coaptation. *Veterinary Surgery* 20 (6): 402–408.
25. Marcellin-Little, D.J. 2003. External Skeletal Fixation. In *Textbook of small animal surgery*, ed. D.H. Slatter, 3rd ed., 1818–1834. Philadelphia: W.B. Saunders.
26. Rovesti, G.L., G. Schwarz, and P. Bogoni. 2009. Treatment of 30 angular limb deformities of the antebrachium and the crus in the dog using circular external fixators. *The Open Veterinary Science Journal* 3: 41–54.
27. Sereda, C.W., D.D. Lewis, R.M. Radasch, C.W. Bruce, and K.A. Kirkby. 2009. Descriptive report of antebrachial growth deformity correction in 17 dogs from 1999 to 2007, using hybrid linear-circular external fixator constructs. *The Canadian Veterinary Journal* 50: 723–732.
28. Singh, K., P. Kinjavdekar, H.P. Aithal, A. Gopinathan, Amarpal, and A.M. Pawde. 2008. Comparison of dynamic compression plate with circular external skeletal fixator for correcting angular deformity after wedge osteotomy of canine antebrachium. *Indian Journal of Veterinary Surgery* 29: 87–92.
29. Singh, K., P. Kinjavdekar, H.P. Aithal, A. Gopinathan, Amarpal, A.M. Pawde, and G.R. Singh. 2012. Comparative evaluation of different internal fixation techniques to correct ante-brachial deformities in growing dogs. *Indian Journal of Veterinary Surgery* 33: 27–30.
30. Theyse, L.F., G. Voorhout, and H.A. Hazewinkel. 2005. Prognostic factors in treating antebrachial growth deformities with a lengthening procedure using a circular external skeletal fixation system in dogs. *Veterinary Surgery* 34: 424–435.
31. Skaggs, S., M.P. DeAngelis, and H. Rosen. 1973. Deformities due to premature closure of the distal ulna in fourteen dogs: a radiographic evaluation. *Journal of the American Animal Hospital Association* 9: 496–500.
32. Craig, E. 1981. Autogenous fat grafts to prevent recurrence following surgical correction of growth deformities of the radius and ulna in the dog. *Veterinary Surgery* 10: 69–76.
33. Bigham, A.S., and Z. Shafiei. 2008. Unilateral premature closure of distal radial growth plate due to hematogenous osteomyelitis in a German shepherd dog. *Comparative Clinical Pathology* 17: 275–277.
34. Jaeger, G. 2017. Case study: approach to premature closure of the distal radial physis. https://www.vrcmalvern.com
35. Olson, N.C., W.O. Brinker, and C.B. Carrig. 1980. Premature closure of the distal radial physis in two dogs. *Journal of the American Veterinary Medical Association* 176 (9): 906–910.
36. Vandewater, M.S.A., and M.L. Olmstead. 2008. Premature closure of the distal radial physis in the dog a review of eleven cases. *Veterinary Surgery* 12 (1): 7–12.

# 11 Joint Luxations

**Learning Objectives**

You will be able to understand the following after reading this chapter:

- Clinical signs, diagnosis, and conservative and surgical treatment of various joint luxations, such as shoulder luxation, elbow luxation, carpal luxation, coxofemoral luxation, stifle luxation, patellar luxation, and tarsal luxation in small animals
- Clinical signs, diagnosis, and management of shoulder luxation, coxofemoral luxation, patellar luxation, carpal and tarsal luxations, and metacarpophalangeal and metatarsophalangeal luxations in large animals


**Summary**

- A joint luxation (dislocation) is a complete separation of bone ends articulating within a joint, whereas subluxation is a partial separation. In dogs, hip and elbow joints are most commonly luxated.
- General principles of open reduction of a joint include replacement of the dislocated bone back to its normal position, suturing the joint capsule and repairing the torn ligaments (using screws, pins, or washers) to hold the joint in place, and providing an external coaptation to maintain the joint stability.
- Shoulder joint in dogs is most frequently luxated medially; the common causes are trauma and congenital malformation. Transposition of the biceps brachii tendon can be used for its successful repair.
- In luxation of the elbow joint in dogs, the radius and ulna are generally displaced laterally to the humerus (relatively larger medial condyle of the humerus prevents the medial displacement of radius-ulna). The luxated elbow can be surgically reduced and fixed by drilling holes in the proximal radius and distal humerus and stabilizing the joint using two screws, washers, and wire.
- Coxofemoral joint luxation is common in dogs as well as cattle; the femoral head is most frequently displaced craniodorsally relative to the acetabulum, whereas it is relatively rare in


(continued)


H. P. Aithal et al., *Textbook of Veterinary Orthopaedic Surgery*,
https://doi.org/10.1007/978-981-99-2575-9_11

horses due to the strong ligamentous support to the joint.

- Hip joint luxation in dogs can be surgically treated by replacement of the round ligament (toggle pin), by reconstruction or substitution of the torn joint capsule (capsulorrhaphy, extracapsular suture stabilization) or by creation of muscular support around the hip joint to maintain reduction (translocation of the greater trochanter).
- Excision of femoral head and neck excision is commonly indicated in severe degeneration of hip and avascular necrosis and non-reconstructable fractures of the femoral head. Implantation of hip prosthesis may be considered in suitable cases.
- The medial luxation of patella is more common in dogs, whereas lateral luxation is often recorded in horses. In large ruminants (more in buffaloes), intermittent upward luxation of patella is common; however, in horses, upward fixation of the patella is not a true luxation (horses can keep standing for a long period of time due to their ability to lock their patella in upward position to conserve energy), but often the patella may fail to get unlocked causing lameness.
- Patellar luxation in immature patients (mostly in dogs and in horses) can be treated by giving release incisions on the side of luxation and imbrication of the lax tissues on the opposite side. Trochleoplasty is used to create adequate depth and width in the trochlear groove to safely secure the patella within the trochlear ridges while gliding. Tibial tuberosity transposition technique is used to treat patellar luxation by correcting the abnormal line of the quadriceps-patella-patellar tendon mechanism in a straight line.
- In cattle, upward luxation of patella can be easily treated by performing medial patellar desmotomy, which can dislodge the patella from medial trochlear ridge to allow free movement of the stifle joint.
- Metacarpophalangeal or metatarsophalangeal (fetlock) joint luxation may be accompanied by fracture in cattle/buffaloes and horses and can be managed using external fixation techniques in most cases.

## 11.1 Small Animals

A joint is a structure where two or more bones unite together and are stabilized with the help of a thick layer of fibrous joint capsule. Most joints are also provided with additional ligaments, which are connected between the bones and allow the joint movements within normal ranges. During a trauma to the joint, these structures may be damaged to a varied extent.

A joint luxation or dislocation is characterized by complete separation of bony ends that would normally articulate to form a joint. On the other hand, subluxation refers to the partial dislocation of the joint. The hip and elbow are the most commonly subluxated joints in dogs; however, any joint may get affected. Trauma, due to automobile accidents, is the most common etiology of sudden or acute joint luxations in animal patients. Certain breeds of dogs, like Labrador retrievers and German shepherds, are more predisposed to the conditions like hip dysplasia leading to chronic joint subluxations due to conformational or anatomical anomalies. The smaller breeds of dogs like miniature poodles are more predisposed to shoulder joint luxation.

The clinical signs of joint luxation may vary depending on the joint involved. Usually the dogs will exhibit the signs of lameness or limping in the affected limb that may progress gradually, if not treated. The dog may show reluctance to walk due to pain. The pain may be pronounced on touching or moving the joint. Swelling may be seen around the joint. Other signs such as loose hanging of the affected limb with movement of joint in unusual directions, flexion of the affected joint and shortening of limb may also be observed as per the involved joint.

Complete physical examination and radiography of the affected joint will help determine the extent of joint luxation and may reveal the presence of associated fractures if any. Management of joint luxations in dogs and cats includes complete assessment and treatment of the existing life-threatening injuries, apart from early reduction, stabilization, and return to joint function. The luxated joint can be managed by either closed or open reduction and stabilization. In closed reduction, the joint is returned to its normal location without requiring surgical opening of the joint. The procedure, however, requires general anesthesia to induce muscle relaxation. A radiograph may be made following the reduction to confirm the correct position of the joint. If the ligaments in and around the joint are damaged, surgical correction would be required to repair the joint. Once the dislocated bones are repositioned back to their original position, the joint capsule is sutured to support the joint. The use of screws, pins, or washers may be required to repair the torn ligaments and hold in position, depending upon the extent of the damage. Joint stability is maintained by external coaptation or internal stabilization methods, depending on the degree of laxity present after reduction. The physical activity of the animal is restricted for several weeks to prevent further relaxation of the joint. Once joint stability is achieved, physiotherapy is done to establish normal joint function. Reluxation, persistence of lameness, and degenerative joint disease are possible complications of traumatic joint luxations. The prognosis is usually good in acute or traumatic joint subluxations, provided the injury is treated immediately.

### 11.1.1 Shoulder Luxation

The shoulder (scapulohumeral) joint is composed of a spherical humeral head that articulates with a shallow glenoid fossa of the scapula, and it is the most mobile of all the limb joints. The shoulder joint, unlike other major appendicular joints in canine and feline, does not possess collateral ligaments and is supported mainly by the medial and lateral glenohumeral ligaments. These ligaments are merely capsular thickenings. The joint stability of the shoulder is maintained by the 'rotator cuff' muscles that originate at the scapula and insert on the proximal humerus. The four cuff muscles are the supraspinatus, infraspinatus, teres minor, and subscapularis. The rotator cuff tendons together with the joint capsule as well as glenohumeral ligaments and regional muscles support the shoulder during movement [1].

Luxation of the shoulder joint is not common in dogs and rarely reported in cats; however, if it occurs, medial luxation is the most frequently observed, followed by lateral and cranial, but caudal luxations are rarely seen [2] (Fig. 11.1). The most common causes are trauma and congenital malformation. In small dog breeds, medial luxation of the shoulder is frequently congenital, but clinical signs are usually apparent in about 4 months (between 3 and 8 months) of age and it may be bilateral. While in large breed dogs, most often lateral luxation occurs after a trauma.

The important clinical signs of traumatic shoulder luxation include non-weight-bearing lameness and flexion of the limb with external rotation [3]. On the other hand, clinical signs of congenital luxation include an intermittent to continuous lameness, which may be progressive in nature. Dissymmetry of the greater tubercle and the acromial process may be evident on palpation. Manipulation of the joint can be used to assess flexion, extension, abduction, craniocaudal translation and rotational stability of the shoulder joint. The ability to abduct the limb for $>30°$ angle generally indicates joint instability. Radiographic examination is done to confirm the diagnosis. The craniocaudal radiographic view of the shoulder in cases of medial or lateral luxation will be more diagnostic than the lateral view. On a mediolateral view, the glenoid is seen overlapping the humeral head in cases of medial luxation. Careful radiographic examination will also help to detect any fracture of the medial glenoid rim. Mild cases

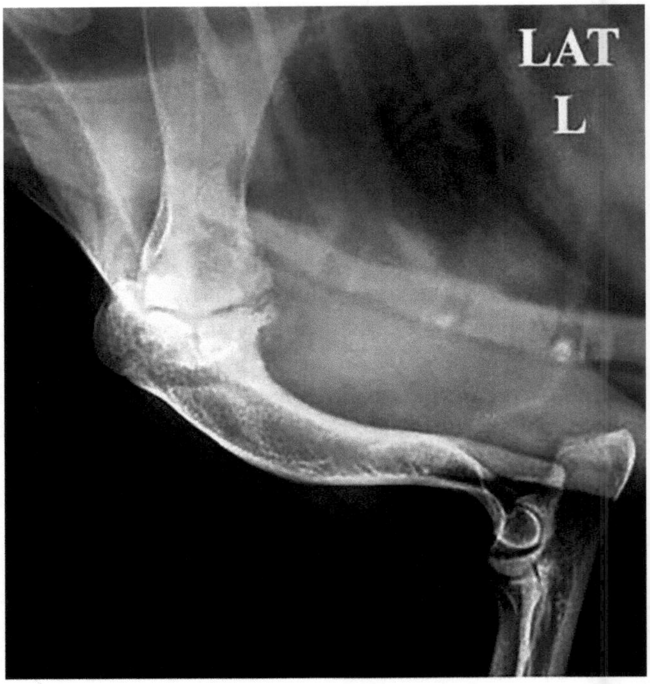


**Fig. 11.1** Lateral radiograph of the left shoulder region shows flattened articular surfaces of scapula and proximal humerus with osteophyte formation at the caudal aspect of shoulder joint indicating shoulder luxation (congenital) (Source: Praveen Kumar et al., Radiographic diagnosis of congenital and developmental orthopedic diseases in 50 dogs, Indian J. Vet. Surg. 35 (2): 116–120, 1014)

of shoulder instability are difficult to diagnose by radiography, and they would require CT/MRI scan or arthroscopy for definitive diagnosis.

The dogs with congenital shoulder luxation are usually managed by restricting their activity and using analgesic, anti-inflammatory drugs. The surgical correction is not generally undertaken as the bony components of the shoulder are not structurally normal; and surgery would require reshaping of the glenoid before attempting reduction and stabilization, which would result in ankylosis or degenerative arthritis. However, arthrodesis or glenoid excision may be considered to correct congenital shoulder luxation, if pain is a major complaint.

Closed reduction and external fixation have been recommended for acute traumatic luxations of the shoulder [3]. Under general anesthesia, the shoulder is extended manually using one hand while the humeral head is seated into the position with the free hand. Generally reduction can be accomplished easily in fresh cases without much complication. If a capsular flap falls between the humeral head and glenoid, or any organized haematoma or fibrous mass is filled in the glenoid cavity (as in old cases), closed reduction may not be achieved easily, necessitating open reduction. If the reduction is found to be stable on gentle extension and flexion, the correct positioning of the limb may be confirmed by radiography and the limb should be bandaged. A Velpeau sling should be used for medial luxation, but a non-weight-bearing bandage maintaining the limb in physiologic position can be applied for lateral luxation taking care to hold the shoulder in a stable position [4, 5]. Excessive internal rotation of the humeral head should be avoided as it may cause redislocation. If gentle manipulation of the joint after reduction and splintage results in reluxation, open reduction and stabilization are necessary. The sling/bandage should be retained for about 2–3 weeks. The success of closed reduction and fixation will depend on the time of stabilization (earlier the better), the extent of soft tissue trauma, the retention of the sling/bandage, and the owner's compliance.

Open reduction followed by surgical fixation should be practised in the dogs with shoulder luxation that cannot be reduced and stabilized by closed method. Different techniques of open reduction and fixation have been described [6–9]. A technique of transposition of the biceps brachii tendon is generally practised and found to be successful for treatment of medial, lateral, or cranial luxation of the shoulder. The approached to the shoulder may be made by acromial osteotomy and deltoid reflection, deltoid splitting laterally, deltoid retraction craniolaterally or separation of deltoid head caudolaterally. In the medial approach, the insertion of both heads of the pectoral muscles has to be severed.

#### 11.1.1.1 Transposition of Biceps Brachii Tendon

The biceps brachii tendon originates on the supraglenoid tubercle of scapula and crosses the shoulder joint craniomedially and then runs through the intertubercular groove of the humerus, where it is secured by the transverse ligament.

In medial luxation of the shoulder, a caudomedial transposition of the biceps brachii tendon can be performed [2, 3, 10, 11]. To approach the site, a craniomedial incision is made starting at about 3–4 cm dorsal to the shoulder joint and extending up to mid-diaphysis of the humerus. After incising the skin and the subcutaneous tissues, the medial border of the brachiocephalicus muscle is separated from the superficial pectoral muscle and retracted laterally to expose superficial and deep pectoral muscles, supraspinatus muscle, and distal branch of the cephalic vein. To expose the deep pectoral muscle, superficial pectoral muscle is transected at its insertion down up to the border of the distal branch of the cephalic vein and is pulled medially. The deep pectoral muscle is then incised along the length of its insertion on the humerus and is pulled medially. Further, the fascial attachments present between the supraspinatus and deep pectoral muscles are incised to expose the medial aspect of the shoulder joint. It will visualize the insertion of the subscapularis muscle tendon crossed by the coracobrachialis muscle tendon and the medial aspect of the joint capsule. Subscapularis muscle is then elevated and detached from its insertion on the lesser tubercle to reflect it medially and so also the coracobrachialis muscle tendon lying craniomedially. The soft tissue over the bicipital groove and the intertubercular ligament is resected, and the joint capsule surrounding the bicipital tendon is incised dorsally to allow mobilization of the bicipital tendon from the intertubercular groove and visualization of the joint. The tendon of biceps brachii is then fixed in its new position using a screw and a washer or a staple taking care not to compress and damage the tendon. The joint capsule on the medial aspect is freshened and closed routinely. The free end of the subscapularis muscle is advanced cranially toward the crest of the greater tubercle, tightened, and sutured close to the insertion of the deep pectoral muscle. Thereafter, the deep pectoral muscle is sutured to the fascia over the greater tubercle on the lateral surface of the crest and the deltoid insertion. Similarly, the superficial pectoral muscle should be closed over the deep pectoral muscle, and the brachiocephalicus muscle is sutured to the superficial pectoral muscle. The closure of subcutaneous tissues and skin is accomplished in standard manner.

In cases of lateral luxation of the shoulder, the technique of biceps tendon transplantation is almost similar to the method that is used for correction of medial luxation; however, in lateral luxation, the tendon is repositioned on the lateral aspect of the shoulder joint to provide lateral collateral support [2, 11]. After retraction of the superficial tissues through skin incision, the brachiocephalicus muscle is retracted medially to expose the cranial aspect of the proximal humerus and the insertions of the supraspinatus, deltoideus, and superficial and deep pectoral muscles. The superficial pectoral muscle is detached from its insertion site down up to the border of the distal communicating branch of the cephalic vein and is retracted medially so that the insertion of the deep pectoral muscle is exposed. Similarly, the deltoideus muscle is also transected. The deep pectoral muscle is elevated from its insertion at the humerus and retracted medially to expose the biceps brachii muscle and tendon in the intertubercular groove. The intertubercular ligament is then incised to disengage the biceps tendon from the surrounding fascia and joint capsule. The greater tubercle is carefully osteotomized, and the intact tendon of the supraspinatus muscle is reflected dorsomedially. The joint capsule is incised at the dorsal aspect to free the biceps brachii tendon, which is then transpositioned laterally on the opposite side of the greater tubercle. The osteotomized portion of the greater tubercle is then replaced and fixed in its position with two K-wires. The incised dorsal joint capsule is closed routinely and the capsular attachments near the intertubercular groove are sutured. The bicipital tendon and the tendinous insertions of infraspinatus supraspinatus and teres minor muscles are sutured to immobilize the tendon firmly. The muscles are reattached as described above for medial luxation.

In cases of cranial luxation of the shoulder, the biceps tendon is transposed cranially at the osteotomy site of the greater tubercle, and then secured by returning the osteotomized tubercle to its initial position and fixing it with K-wires and tension band wire [12]. The caudal luxation of the shoulder can be corrected by imbrication of the lateral and caudolateral joint capsule generally.

In cases of severe shoulder instability, the joint can be reduced to a normal anatomical position and fixed using a Steinmann pin/K-wire driven through the humeral head from cranially below the greater tubercle, across the joint space, and anchored firmly in the glenoid. The rationale behind this technique is to hold the joint in reduction until the joint capsule and surrounding muscles heal by scar formation, which will ultimately help support the joint, and the pin can then be removed. Common complications of this technique include decreased range of motion, arthritis leading to pain and loss of joint function. Hence, the technique should be used only as the last resort for salvage.

Following reduction and stabilization, a Velpeau sling is to be applied in cases of medial luxation, whereas a non-weight-bearing bandage is to be applied in cases of lateral luxation, for about 2–3 weeks. Open reduction and fixation of luxated shoulder joint using biceps tendon transposition for the simple cases without concurrent fractures or joint abnormality will generally lead to satisfactory outcome with return to near normal function of the shoulder. However, in cases with osteoarthritic changes, dysplasia of the glenoid cavity or excessive instability or in cases of recurrent luxations after corrective surgical fixation, excision arthroplasty or arthrodesis of the joint is recommended as salvage procedures.

#### 11.1.1.2 Shoulder Arthrodesis and Excision Arthroplasty

Shoulder arthrodesis is indicated in cases of severe shoulder instability as in cases of congenital luxation with marked remodeling of the glenoid or painful joint with secondary degenerative joint disease after failure of the other treatment [13]. Often shoulder arthrodesis is done as the first-choice treatment rather than the tendinous or muscular transposition. The joint can be reduced to the normal anatomical position and fixed using a Steinmann pin/K-wire driven through the humeral head from cranial aspect below the greater tubercle, across the joint space, and is anchored firmly in the glenoid. The rationale behind this technique is to hold the joint in reduction until the joint capsule and surrounding muscles heal by scar formation, which will ultimately help support the joint, and the pin can then be removed. Common complications of this technique include decreased range of motion and arthritis leading to pain and loss of joint function. Hence, the technique should be used only as the last resort for salvage.

Excision of the glenoid and a portion of humeral head can also be done as a salvage procedure [14, 15]. A lateral approach can be used for osteotomy of both the humeral head and the glenoid. The teres minor muscle is inserted between the cut ends of bones and sutured to the biceps brachii tendon. There is no need of bandaging postoperatively.

### 11.1.2 Elbow Luxation

Complete luxation of the elbow joint is usually associated with trauma (automobile accidents, infighting, falling from a height), wherein the radius and ulna are displaced laterally in relation to the humerus [16–19] (Fig. 11.2). Relatively larger medial condyle of the distal humerus prevents the radius and ulna from displacing medially. Caudal luxation of the elbow is very

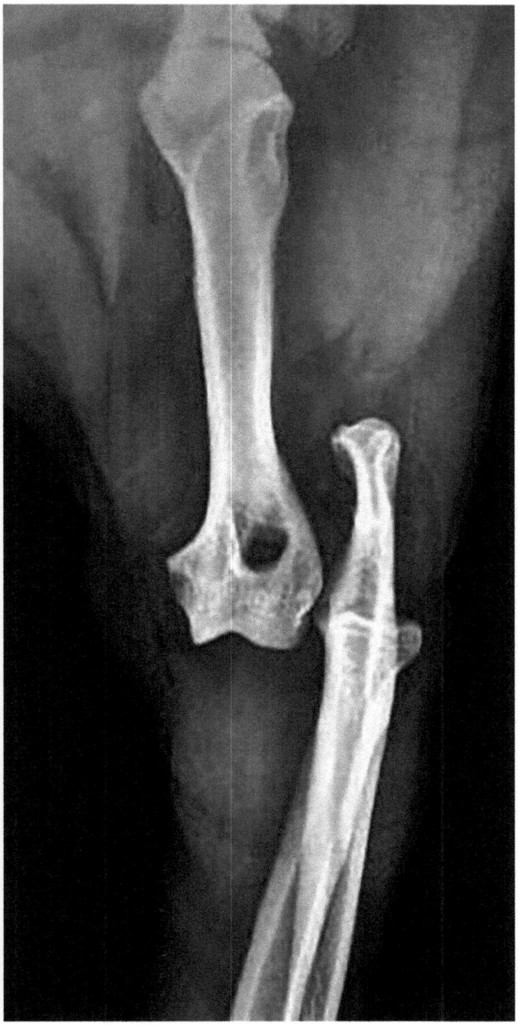

**Fig. 11.2** Craniocaudal radiograph of the left elbow joint shows complete luxation of radius and ulna (lateral) from the humeral condyles (congenital elbow luxation) (Source: Praveen Kumar et al., Radiographic diagnosis of congenital and developmental orthopedic diseases in 50 dogs, Indian J. Vet. Surg. 35 (2): 116–120, 1014)

rare [20]. There is no specific age, breed, or sex predisposition for elbow luxation in dogs; however, the younger dogs would get fractured at the growth plates of their long bones rather than developing a luxation.

Most dogs with elbow luxation are presented with a history of trauma and an abrupt onset of profound lameness in the forelimb. Clinical examination may reveal complete instability of the involved joint with deformity and pain. Palpation of the joint may show prominent medial condyle with absence of normal features of the joint on the lateral surface. The affected dogs show non-weight-bearing lameness and carrying of the limb. The animal may hold its leg in abduction with outward rotation. Craniocaudal view of the radiograph will help confirm the diagnosis, wherein there will be lateral movement/displacement of the radius and ulna. Radiographs should also be carefully examined for any fractures and avulsion injuries.

Treatment of elbow luxation can be done either by closed or open method [18, 21]. The closed reduction of a dislocated elbow could be difficult or even impossible if the injury is more than a few days old or there could be severe damage to the collateral ligaments that stabilize the joint. It should not be attempted if there is severe swelling, and prolonged manipulation should be avoided if reduction is unsuccessful during the initial attempts. Closed reduction (of the lateral luxation of the elbow joint) is accomplished by flexing the joint to 90° and rotating the anconeal process medially to fix into the supratrochlear foramen. The limb is then gradually extended while applying force to the radial head (lateral to medial) and medial condyle of the humerus (medial to lateral); simultaneously, the radius and ulna bones are rotated internally after hooking the anconeal process beak into the trochlear groove. Once the elbow has been reduced, extension and flexion of the joint will show a full range of motion. Radiographs are made to confirm that the elbow is in place. If found completely stable (flexion and extension do not result in reluxation), a Roberts Jones bandage should be applied to include the elbow joint so that the joint movement is restricted and the limb remains in extension. If unstable (reluxation results during flexion), the joint may be immobilized using a modified Thomas splint for about two weeks. Usually the elbow joint will become stable due to healing (fibrosis) of soft tissues around the joint. If there is recurrence after closed reduction and external fixation, open reduction and fixation should be attempted. Surgical stabilization of traumatic elbow luxation generally produces better outcomes compared to closed reduction [21].

Different techniques reported for surgical repair include reconstruction of the collateral structures with sutures and/or anchoring of distal humerus with proximal radius/ulna using different techniques and immobilizing the joint to allow for healing [18, 22–25]. Open reduction of the luxated elbow can be done through the anconeus muscle by a lateral incision to the joint. Once opened, the joint is debrided and cleaned, and reduction can be carried out as described above for closed reduction. If needed, a periosteal elevator should be used within the joint surface to facilitate reduction. The proximal ulnar diaphyseal osteotomy will allow easy reduction of the luxated elbow. Once reduced, the bones are secured in place by meticulously suturing the soft tissues around. In case of an unstable joint, screws, washers, or pins can be used to hold the joint under reduction or to reconstruct/replace the ligaments holding the elbow in appropriate position (Fig. 11.3). Holes are drilled in the proximal radius and distal humerus; and the joint is then stabilized using two screws, washers, and wire, with further augmentation with monofilament nonabsorbable suture material if required (Fig. 11.4). Suturing of the lateral collateral ligament is then performed when possible. Post-fixation, the limb is immobilized in extension using external bandage application for about two weeks.

Congenital luxation of the elbow may occur in the small breeds of dogs [26, 27]. It may exhibit complete luxation of both radius and ulna or luxation of the radial head with an intact ulnar articulation/ulnar subluxation or an intact radio-humeral articulation with subluxation/complete dislocation of the ulna. In dogs, the congenital luxation of the elbow is generally associated with hypoplasia or aplasia of the medial collateral ligament and a functionally annular ligament. The treatment in these cases is aimed to achieve reasonable functional recovery of the limb. If the absence of associated soft tissues makes reconstruction impossible, arthrodesis might be undertaken to achieve functional recovery. If radial-humeral joint is intact, the proximal ulnar diaphyseal osteotomy is done to reposition the ulna. The ulnar segment is then stabilized with the proximal radius by fixing the pins or small screws. If the radial head is luxated, proximal ulnar osteotomy is performed (at the level of maximum curvature), and the radial head is repositioned [28]. If the radial head has spherical joint surface, it has to be contoured appropriately before reduction.

In developmental dislocation, subluxations occur at first, often leading to complete dislocation, and trauma is the primary cause [29, 30]. Premature closure of the ulnar distal physis may lead to elbow luxation and/or fracture of the anconeal process. Treatment in such cases includes osteotomy of the proximal ulnar diaphysis reducing the luxation and thus stabilization of the ulna to the radius. If this condition is treated after 4 months of age, the outcome is generally successful. However, if the dislocation occurs before 4 months of age, repeated corrections may be needed, and the results are not generally good. In cases of trauma to the proximal or distal growth plates of the radius, subluxation and dislocation of the elbow would occur distally. In growing animals, the condition is treated by radial osteotomy and distraction osteosynthesis using an external skeletal fixator.

Following the correction of an elbow luxation, the range of motion is usually fair to good. If joint stiffness and arthritis develop, the prognosis is generally poor. The overall functional recovery is poor in the unstable elbow, especially in large breeds of dog.

### 11.1.3 Carpal Luxation

The carpus is a complex joint formed by seven carpal bones including the radial carpal and ulnar carpal bones in proximal row and first (I), second (II), third (III), and fourth (IV) carpal bones in distal row [31]. The accessory carpal bone is located at the caudolateral surface of the joint. The joint has three major articulations as follows:

(i) The antebrachiocarpal joint formed by the distal radius-ulna and the radial and ulnar carpal bones. It is primarily stabilized by a medial collateral ligament (radial) and a lateral collateral ligament (ulnar). This joint is involved in most

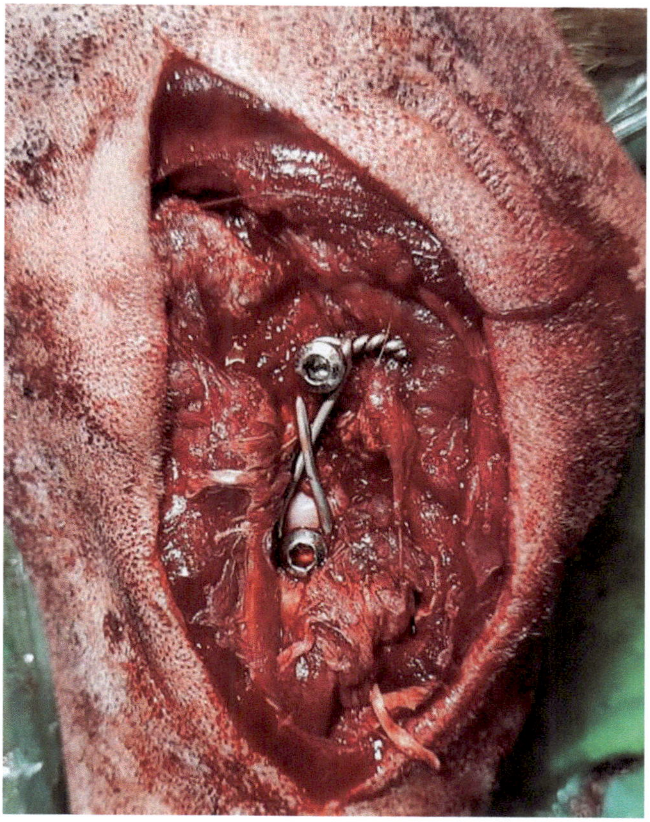

**Fig. 11.3** Surgical fixation of the luxated elbow: screws are fixed in the proximal radius and distal humeral condyle and the joint stabilized using orthopedic wire fixation in figure 8 fashion

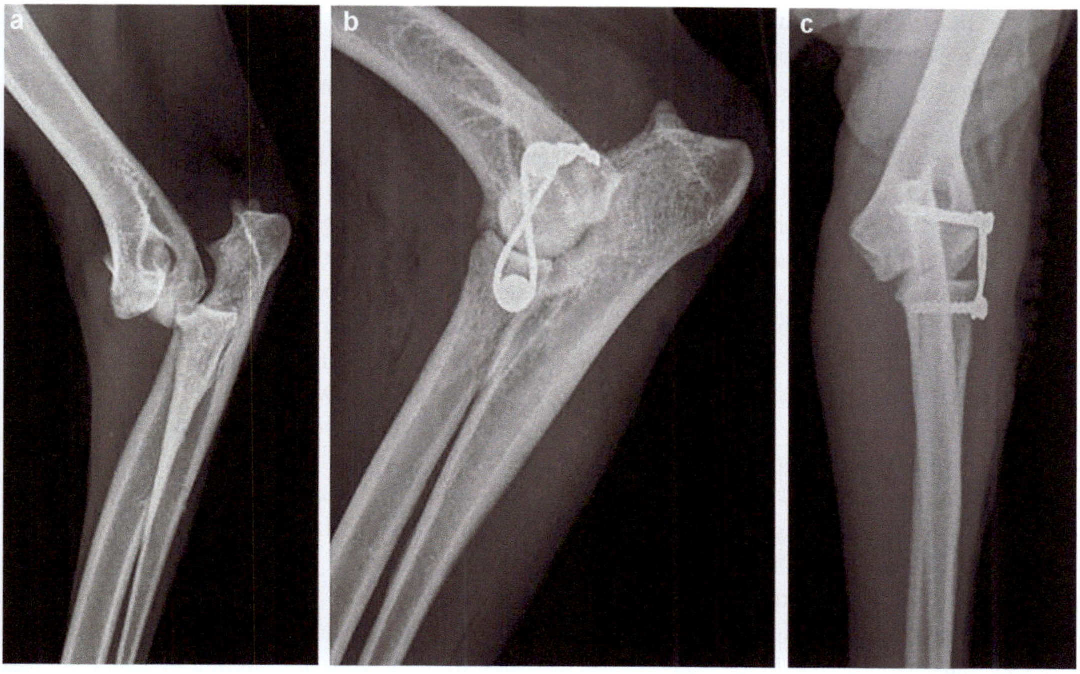


**Fig. 11.4** Radiographs show complete luxation of the elbow in a dog (a), adequately reduced elbow joint after fixation using screws and wire—lateral view—(b) craniocaudal view (c)

(80–90%) of the carpal movements. (ii) The middle carpal joint is formed by the radial-ulnar carpal bones and distal row (I, II, III, IV) of carpal bones.

(iii) The carpometacarpal joint is formed between I, II, III, and IV (distal row) carpal bones and the base of I, II, III, IV, and V metacarpal bones.

The middle carpal joint and the carpometacarpal joint are supported by numerous short ligaments. The accessory carpal bone is located on the caudolateral surface of the joint and articulates with ulnar carpal bone and styloid process of the ulna. It is held by short ligaments connecting to the ulnar carpal bone and long ligaments connecting to the base of IV and V metacarpal bones.

Luxation or subluxation of individual carpal bone is relatively rare, but there are a few reports, mostly of radiocarpal bone luxation [32–37]. Luxation can occur at different levels of carpal joint, that is, antebrachiocarpal, middle carpal, carpometacarpal or multiple luxations. Palmar dislocation occurs most common; however, dorsal, medial, lateral, valgus or varus displacement may also be seen. Carpal subluxation or luxation occurs most commonly due to automobile trauma, fall or jumping from a height. Clinically the animals are presented with carrying the affected limb (acute cases) or plantigrade walking on the affected limb (chronic cases). Radiography should be done with the joint in stressed position to help demonstrate the lesion in subluxations, and in complete dislocation, a dorsopalmar view will help detect abnormal bony alignment.

Closed reduction of luxated carpus can usually be achieved easily. Maintenance of reduction using external fixation may support soft tissue healing, leading to maintenance of normal position. External fixation, however, rarely results in success [35].

Carpal joint is surgically approached through dorsal exposure using a skin incision over the dorsum of carpus extending from the distal end of radius to the metacarpal bones. The incision is deepened to expose and retract the tendons of the extensor carpi radialis and the common digital extensor muscles. The antebrachiocarpal joint is approached through transverse arthrotomy incision to expose the radial carpal as well as ulnar carpal bones. Similarly, I, II, III, and IV carpal bones can be visualized through a transverse arthrotomy at the middle carpal joint. However, the accessory carpal bone is surgically exposed through a lateral incision made directly over the bone.

Surgical repair of the medial and/or lateral collateral ligaments followed by stabilization of the joint by external fixation would result in successful outcome in a large number of cases. However, most animals require arthrodesis. Arthrodesis of antebrachiocarpal joint, middle carpal joint or carpometacarpal joint may be enough in most cases of respective joint subluxations or luxations. In multiple level luxation, panarthrodesis of the entire carpal joint is performed [38, 39]. In successful cases, the affected animal would have near normal functional recovery (80–90% normal movement) following surgery.

Subluxation or luxation of individual carpal bones (radial carpal bone or I and II carpal bones are commonly involved) may also occur wherein the bones are usually displaced dorsally. Closed reduction and external immobilization are unlikely to provide good results, with recurrent subluxations leading to instability and degenerative joint disease. Open reduction and fixation using screws, multiple pins or wires generally result in failure, and only carpal arthrodesis will provide satisfactory results.

Luxation along with proximal displacement of the accessory carpal bone may occur if the two ligaments attaching the bone to the base of IV and V metacarpals are damaged. This is commonly seen along with luxation of the antebrachiocarpal joint. Animals show a plantigrade posture, with muscular laxity in the flexor carpi ulnaris muscle. Radiography shows proximal displacement of accessory carpal bone. Mostly the bone is seen to hinge on its dorsal-proximal end and rarely gets distracted proximally away from the carpus. External immobilization of the limb may not help reduce the bone. Open surgical repair involving suturing of the palmar carpal fibrocartilage or wiring caudal tip of accessory carpal bone to the base of V metacarpal or both may result in good outcome. If it fails, panarthrodesis is necessary to stabilize the joint.

### 11.1.4 Hip (Coxofemoral) Luxation

Hip (coxofemoral) luxation is characterized by dislocation of the coxofemoral joint leading to displacement of the femoral head from the acetabular socket. Most frequently (>90%), femoral head is displaced craniodorsally relative to the acetabulum (Fig. 11.5). Dislocation results in rupture of the joint capsule and disruption of other supportive structures of the joint, including ligaments and often bone. Luxation of the hip is generally caused by trauma, but joint degeneration may also increase the risk for developing hip luxation [40].

Clinical signs of coxofemoral luxation may include lameness, pain on manipulation of the hip joint and a shortened length of the limb as a result of dorsal displacement of the femur. Partial dislocation of the hip joint (subluxation) can also occur many times and may be associated with joint degeneration as in case of hip dysplasia. Usually subluxation associated with degeneration of joint is bilateral (but the extent of subluxation may vary); however bilateral hip luxation due to trauma is rare. Radiography is useful to confirm the luxation, assessing the direction and extent of dislocation, and detecting the presence of bony fractures in the femoral neck, head or acetabulum.

Numerous techniques, both closed or open reduction and fixation, can be used for management of hip luxation in dogs. Closed reduction could be the procedure of choice in the initial stage but considered in only those cases that do not have hip dysplasia, arthritis, or fracture of the hip [41, 42]. It should be attempted at the earliest point of time after the injury and prognosis will be poorer if it is done after 3–4 days of trauma. In a closed reduction, the femoral head is replaced back in the acetabular cavity by internal rotation and abduction of luxated femur bone under general anesthesia and maintained with non-weight-bearing Ehmer sling application and subsequent confinement for about 4 weeks. Closed reduction may be successful in approximately 50% cases, if undertaken early.

If the hip cannot be reduced or the hip does not feel stable (femur head comes out of the joint with minimal force), and concurrent pelvic fractures are present, surgical fixation is recommended. The surgical treatment includes replacement of the hip by open reduction and restoration of the supporting structures. Supporting implants may be placed to provide additional mechanical support to the hip during the healing period. A large variety of techniques, such as reconstruction of round ligament, transarticular pinning, toggle rod fixation, capsulorrhaphy, surgical anchors and trochanteric transposition have been described [43–57]. The femoral head and neck ostectomy, wherein the femoral head and neck are removed to produce a false joint, can be used as last option; it usually provides satisfactory results except in heavy animals. Functional recovery is generally very good, and the risk of implant-related complications and recurrent luxation is eliminated with the use of this technique. Total hip replacement, wherein the femoral head and the acetabulum (ball and socket) are replaced with synthetic implants, can be undertaken whenever feasible.

#### 11.1.4.1 Open Reduction and Fixation of the Femoral Head

Several surgical techniques have been documented for treatment of hip luxation in the dog. The primary aim of surgery is to replace the femoral head into the acetabulum and secure the joint with artificial ligaments and suturing the torn joint capsule. This can be achieved by several methods such as replacement of the round ligament (toggle pin), reconstruction or substitution of the torn joint capsule (capsulorrhaphy, extracapsular suture stabilization), the creation of muscular support around the hip joint so that the reduction is maintained (translocation of the greater trochanter), etc.

In the 'toggle' technique, a hole is drilled in the acetabular wall at the site of attachment of the round ligament, and a bone tunnel is drilled through the femoral neck from the subtrochanteric region of the lateral femur to the point of the fovea capitis of the femoral head [46, 47, 51, 56]. A strong suture material or an orthopedic wire attached to a toggle pin is first threaded through the acetabular hole and

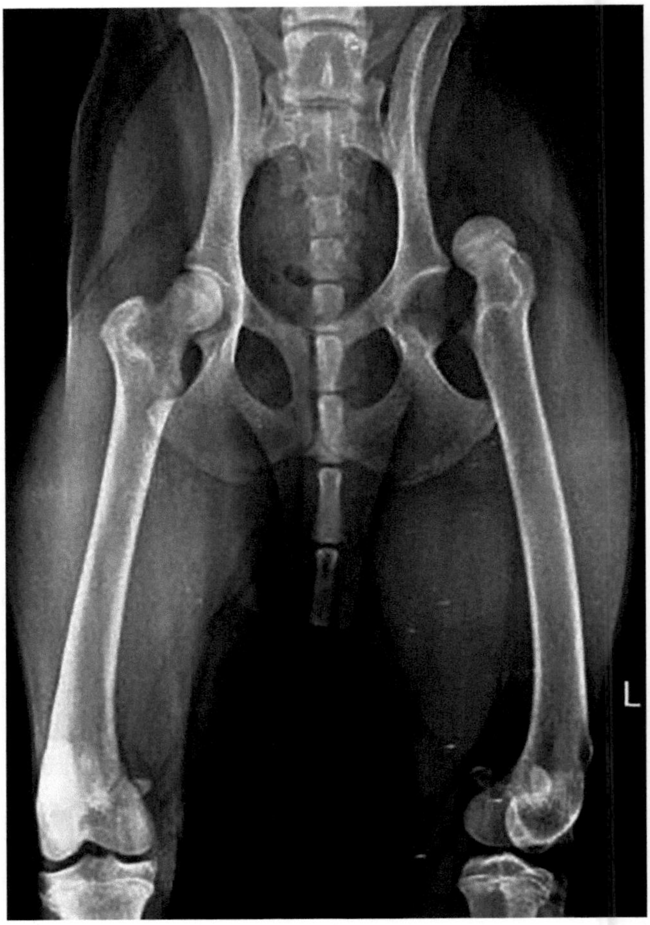


**Fig. 11.5** VD view of pelvic region shows complete dorsolateral luxation of left coxofemoral joint

tensioned to pull the toggle pin against the medial wall of the acetabulum tightly (Fig. 11.6). The suture is then pulled or pushed through the femur bone tunnel to exit the lateral femur and tensioned while the femur head is replaced into the acetabulum. After verifying that the femur head is firmly seated in the acetabular socket, the suture ends are tied to a toggle pin on the femoral surface (Fig. 11.7). Subsequently, the torn joint capsule is sutured as much as possible.

The technique of capsulorrhaphy with trochanteric transposition can be done in cases with sufficient intact joint capsule to allow primary closure and intact gluteal musculature to permit internal rotation and abduction. In this technique, the joint capsule is reconstructed and the greater trochanter is repositioned caudodistally while maintaining the hip in reduction, flexion, abduction, and internal rotation.

In cases with extensive damage to the joint capsule, where capsulorrhaphy cannot be performed, additional support to the joint capsule is provided by extracapsular suture stabilization. The range of motion of the femoral head can be reduced by applying two mattress sutures of heavy suture material between the tendons of insertion of the muscles psoas minor and the gluteus medius. This stabilization technique has shown encouraging results in preventing reluxation.

In modified synthetic capsule technique [58], two small cortical screws are inserted into the dorsal rim of the acetabulum about 5 mm away from the edge of the acetabulum at 10 and 12 o'clock positions in the left hip and 12 and 2 o'clock positions in the right hip, and a monofilament nonabsorbable suture material should be tied to the screw heads (Fig. 11.8). A transverse

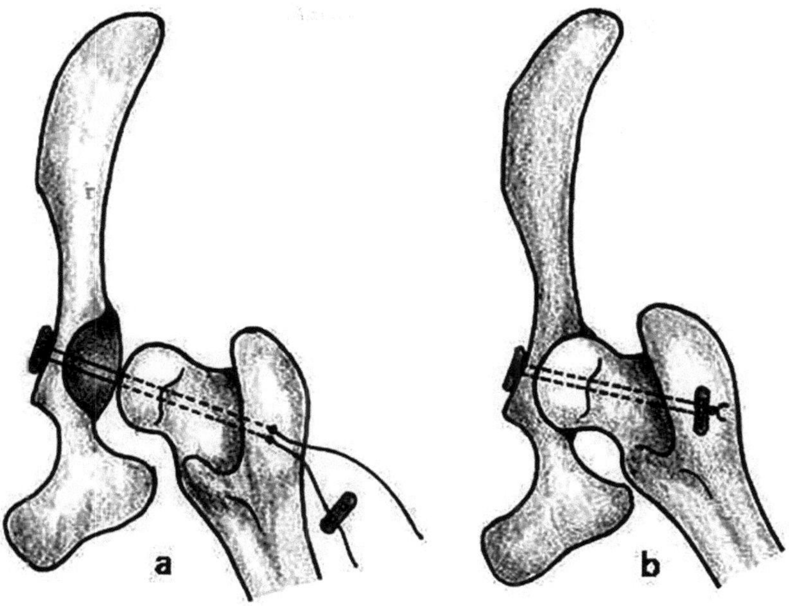


**Fig. 11.6** The 'toggle-pin' technique to reduce the dislocated hip joint: a hole is drilled in the acetabular wall at the site of the round ligament, and another hole is drilled through the femoral neck from the subtrochanteric region to the point of fovea capitis. A strong thread/suture material attached to a toggle pin is inserted through the acetabular hole and tensioned to pull the toggle pin against the medial acetabular wall; the thread is then pulled through the femur bone tunnel to exit the lateral femur (**a**); the suture ends are then tensioned while the femur head is replaced into the acetabulum and tied to a toggle pin (**b**)

hole is then drilled in the greater trochanter, and the suture ends secured to the screw heads are passed through this transverse tunnel in the trochanter major crosswise and tied on the greater trochanter by ensuring that the femoral head is placed within the acetabular cavity.

Post-fixation of the hip joint using any of the surgical techniques, an Ehmer sling is advised for about two weeks to prevent direct weight bearing on the limb. Although animals can use the limb immediately following surgical repair, restricted activity is mandatory for 8–10 weeks after the surgery to allow the healing of the joint capsule and the surrounding musculature.

Rehabilitation therapy can be started at four weeks postoperatively to achieve early return of the limb to function. Reluxation rate following surgical repair is very low. In most cases, prognosis is good with early weight bearing and functional recovery of the limb when reductions are successful either with closed or open methods and are maintained postoperatively.

#### 11.1.4.2 Femoral Head and Neck Excision (Ostectomy)

Excision of femoral the head and neck is most often an indicated procedure in severe osteoarthritis of the hip joint, Legg-Calve-Perthes disease (avascular necrosis of the femoral head) and non-reconstructable fractures of the femoral head. Occasionally, femoral head and neck osteotomy is performed in cases of traumatic luxation of the hip to relieve pain and regain functional recovery of the limb [40]. The procedure can be done in both large and small breed dogs; however, the results are more satisfactory in smaller dogs and cats (procedure detailed in Chap. 9). Total hip replacement surgery is also recommended in chronic cases of coxofemoral joint luxations [59].

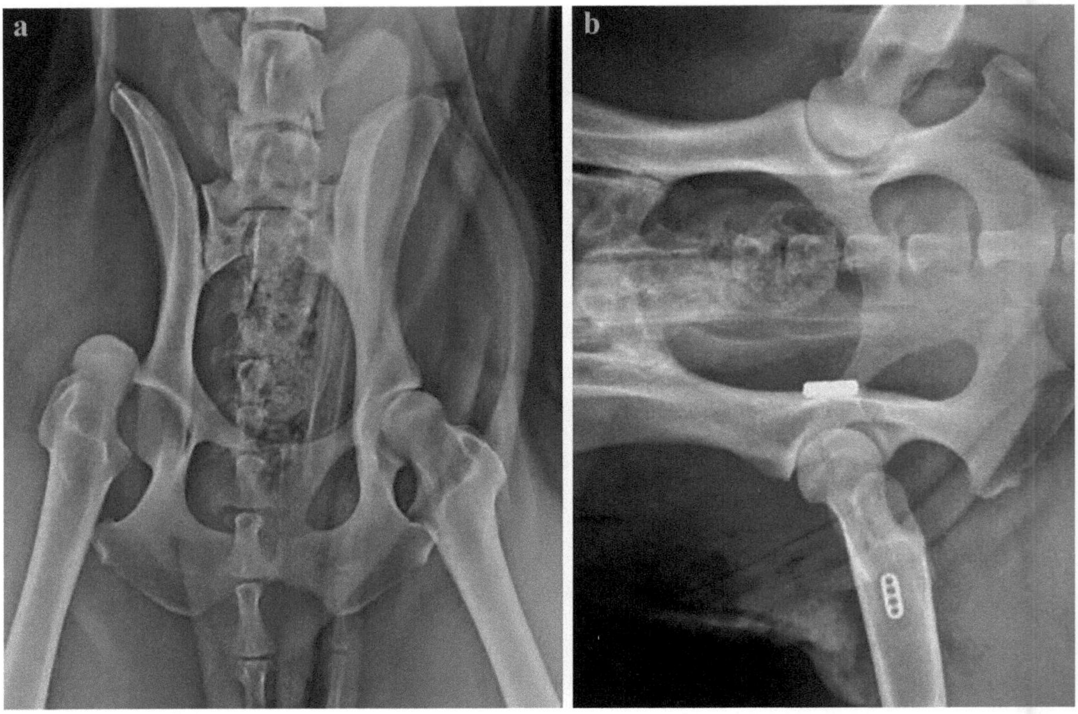


**Fig. 11.7** VD radiograph of pelvic region of a dog shows complete luxation of the hip joint (**a**), adequate reduction and fixation with 'toggle' technique (**b**) (Courtesy: Dr Drona Patil, Mumbai, India)

### 11.1.5 Stifle Luxation

Luxation of the stifle joint is a less common condition but may result from severe trauma but can be potentially devastating, if more than one of the primary or secondary stabilizing structures are damaged. The stifle joint is generally well protected by soft tissue structures within and around the joint, which include the cranial and caudal cruciate ligaments, the medial and lateral collateral ligaments, the patella tendon and the quadriceps muscle cranially and the oblique popliteal, hamstring and gastrocnemius muscles caudally. At many instances, dislocations may be open and accompanied by fractures and injury to the menisci and joint capsule and often with injury to the popliteal artery and peroneal nerve [60].

The goal of treatment of stifle luxation is to stabilize the joint so as to restore anatomical alignments, limit further damage to the articular surface and maintain normal joint movements. This includes two types of repair: primary reconstruction of the damaged ligaments and the use of internal or external supports to provide functional stability [61–67]. In cats and small dogs, extraarticular stabilization along with external coaptation using modified Robert Jones bandage may provide good to excellent results in many cases. However, it is often difficult to get and maintain adequate reduction by closed reduction with external coaptation, especially in heavy animals.

Open reduction with reconstruction of extraarticular or intraarticular ligament along with transarticular pin fixation or external skeletal fixation has been used successfully for treatment of stifle joint luxations [60, 64, 65, 67, 68] (Fig. 11.9). Through a standard lateral parapatellar incision, the stifle joint is approached and lateral arthrotomy done to visualize the intraarticular and periarticular tissue damage. All the ligaments are carefully inspected, and remnants of the damaged ligaments, if any, are removed. If cruciate ligaments are damaged, they are repaired/replaced using extraarticular sutures

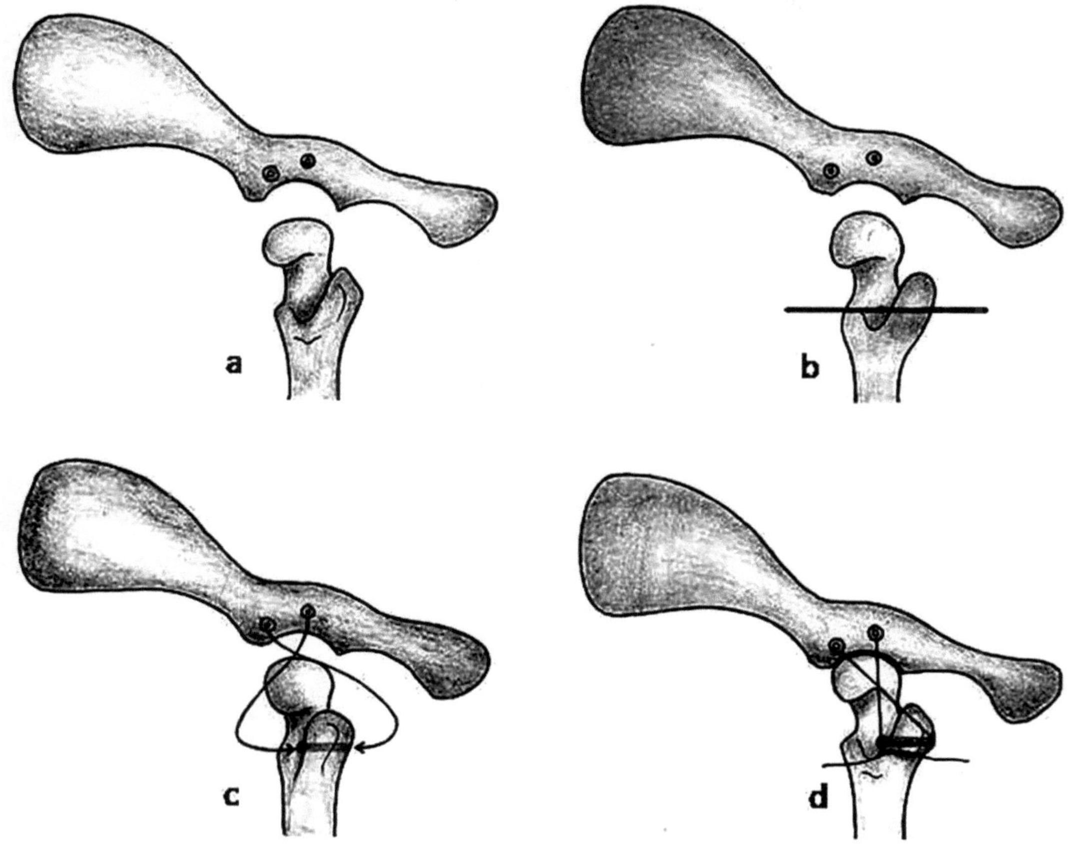


**Fig. 11.8** Modified synthetic capsule technique for reduction of hip joint: two small cortical screws are inserted into the dorsal rim of the acetabulum at 10 and 12 o'clock positions (**a**), a transverse hole is drilled in the greater trochanter (**b**), a monofilament nonabsorbable suture material secured to the screw heads is passed through the transverse tunnel in the trochanter major crosswise (**c**) and tied on the greater trochanter after ensuring that the femoral head is replaced back within the acetabular cavity (**d**)

or intraarticular reconstruction (procedures detailed in Chap. 12). In cases with meniscal tears or avulsions, partial meniscectomy is performed. The damaged collateral ligaments are repaired and reconstructed. Then the joint can be stabilized using multiple extraarticular sutures along with transarticular external skeletal fixation, which would provide rigid stabilization. Generally good to excellent functional outcome can be seen in all sizes of dogs and cats with this technique. Transarticular pin fixation has also been used to achieve stability of the stifle joint, wherein the stifle is fixed in a functional angle of about 135–140°. Although this technique is quick, easy to perform and inexpensive as compared to other techniques, it may be difficult to achieve stable fixation in large dogs, and complications such as pin migration and reduction in range of motion of the stifle joint after surgery are its limitations. The outcome of surgical reduction and stabilization is generally very good, and primary arthrodesis may be done only after attempts at reconstruction have failed. Arthrodesis may be performed using pinning, plating, or external skeletal fixation even in cases with severely damaged joint with arthritic changes. Some prosthetic devices have also been developed for extracapsular applications. The Simitri™ (New Generation Devices, Glen Rock, New Jersey, USA) implant was one such device

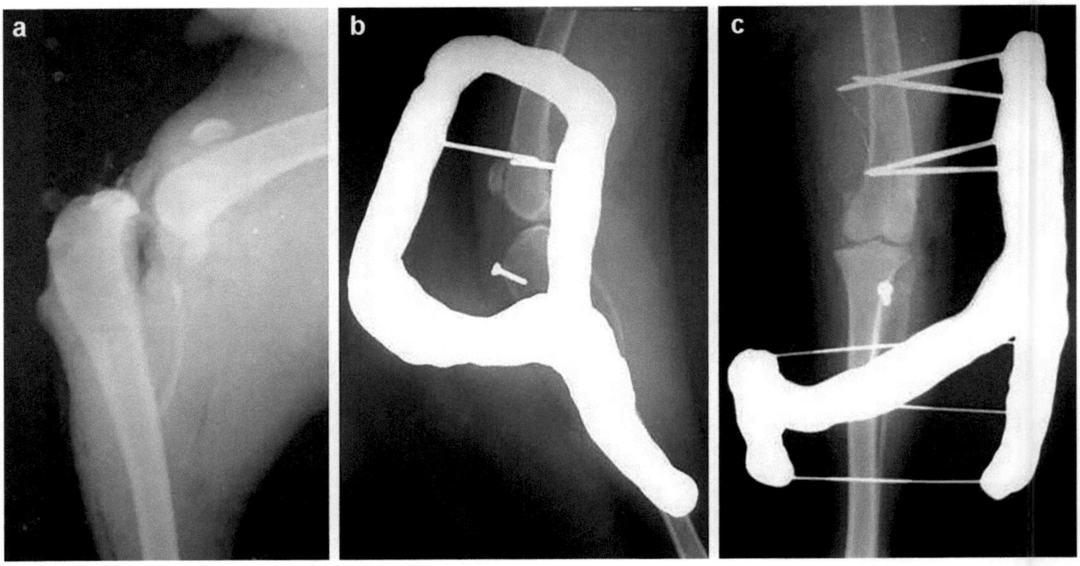


**Fig. 11.9** Open luxation of stifle (femoro-tibial) joint with avulsion of patellar ligament in a dog (**a**), fixation of ligament using a lag screw and stabilization of joint by epoxy-pin ESF (**b** and **c**)

designed to provide a completely extracapsular means of stifle stabilization, which can also be used as an adjunct with primary repair of damaged collateral ligaments to allow normal stifle movements and to help facilitate early mobilization of the affected limb [68].

### 11.1.6 Patellar Luxation

The patella is a sesamoid bone buried in the tendon of the quadriceps muscles of the thigh and it glides in a groove within the femoral condyles. The patellar tendon attaches on the tibial crest. The quadriceps muscle, the patella and its tendon that are normally well aligned to each other form the extensor mechanism [69]. During patellar luxation (dislocation), the patella glides outside the femoral condylar groove during the knee flexion. The cause for patellar luxation can be congenital, hereditary, developmental, or traumatic [70, 71]. Although patellar luxation is mostly regarded as a developmental disease, its exact pathogenesis is obscure. Developmental patellar luxation can be attributable to complex skeletal abnormalities that affect the overall alignment of the limb. These abnormalities may include abnormal conformation of the hip joint (decreased tilting of the femoral head and neck), abnormal shape of the femur or tibia, tibial crest deviation, tightness/atrophy of the quadriceps muscles or a too long patellar ligament; thus it may be the result of structural abnormalities involving any part of the hindlimb [72].

Congenital or hereditary luxation of the patella is a common orthopedic condition in dogs, reported in about 7% of puppies. The condition is more common in small breeds of dogs, including Chihuahuas, Boston, and Yorkshire terriers, Pomeranians and miniature poodles. Medial luxation occurs in about 75–80% of cases, and small breed dogs are mostly affected [69, 70, 73–75]. Even in cats, medial patellar luxation is more common than lateral luxation [76–78]. Lateral luxation is less common but can be seen in giant breeds (St. Bernard) [69, 79]. In certain cases, the patella may luxate both medially and laterally. The incidence of bilateral patellar luxation is about 20–50%, and female animals have been reported to be about 1.5 times more susceptible than males. There is also an association between medial patellar luxation and rupture of cranial cruciate ligament, and it is found that at least 15–20% of dogs with patellar luxation would finally have rupture of their cranial cruciate ligament [70].

Based on physical examination, patellar luxation can be classified in grades 0–4: In grade 0, patella will not luxate during the physical examination. In grade 1, the patella tends to luxate on application of digital pressure (with the stifle in extension) but returns to its normal position as the pressure is released. In grade 2 luxation, the patella readily luxates on application of digital pressure and tends to remain luxated even on release of the pressure; however, it can be returned to its normal position and would remain in trochlear groove most of the time. In grade 3, the patella remains in the luxated position most of the time, but it can be brought to its normal position with digital pressure, temporarily. And in grade 4, the patella remains in the luxated position permanently and cannot be returned to the normal position. Many small dogs with grade 1 luxation never show the signs of lameness; however, large breed dogs having grade 1–4 luxation and will be clinically affected, and nearly all dogs affected with grade 3 and 4 luxation exhibit the signs of lameness and disability.

Patellar luxation can be diagnosed by careful physical examination while the animal is in standing position or in lateral recumbent position. During the examination, the stifle joint is observed for the instability and range of motion, presence or absence of crepitus, location of the patella, grade of patella luxation, extent of deviation of tibial tuberosity and angulation of the limb, and presence or absence of drawer movement (to determine the associated cruciate ligament rupture). The patella is located by following the patellar ligament starting at its attachment on the tibial tuberosity. It is then caught by the thumb and index finger of one hand, and using the other hand, the tibia is grasped and lifted above the floor. The stifle joint is manipulated by flexion, extension, and rotation (internal and external), and it is tried to manually displace the patella in lateral and medial directions to identify the direction and degree of luxation. After luxating the patella, the depth of the trochlear groove is assessed by palpation. To assess the status of cranial cruciate ligament, cranial drawer and tibial thrust examinations are carried out (detailed in Chap. 12). Radiographic examination includes standard lateral and craniocaudal views and skyline/tangential projection (Fig. 11.10). In lateral view, the patella is seen missing from its normal position (superimposed over the femoral condyles), whereas in craniocaudal view, the patella can be seen displaced either medially or laterally (Figs. 11.11 and 11.12). The skyline radiographic projection is used to better visualize the patella and trochlear groove; the radiograph can be made either by horizontal (by positioning the animal in dorsal recumbency using a V-trough and by flexing the pelvic limbs) or vertical (by positioning the animal in ventral recumbency with the affected limb flexed and pushed craniolaterally and the tibia positioned under the femur) x-ray projection.

Conservative treatment is recommended in grade 1 luxations with no clinical signs, which may include rehabilitation to enhance quadriceps mechanism [70, 80]. Similarly, if lameness is mild and infrequent, with mild non-progressive osteoarthritis, conservative treatment is indicated. In cases of grade 3 or grade 4 luxation, however, surgical management is needed at early stage of the disease. In very young animals with significant potential for growth, a two-stage repair may be contemplated; in the first stage, only soft tissue reconstruction and trochlear chondroplasty techniques may be performed, and other techniques may be undertaken once the patient reaches skeletal maturity.

The principle of surgical management of luxation of patella is the quadriceps mechanism realignment and patellar stabilization within the femoral trochlear groove. Even though different soft tissue maneuvers and osseous procedures can be used to achieve this goal, soft tissue techniques alone are more likely to fail, but along with osseous techniques, they will provide more satisfactory results [70, 72, 78, 80, 81].

**Soft tissue techniques** can be used as the first choice of treatment for traumatic patellar

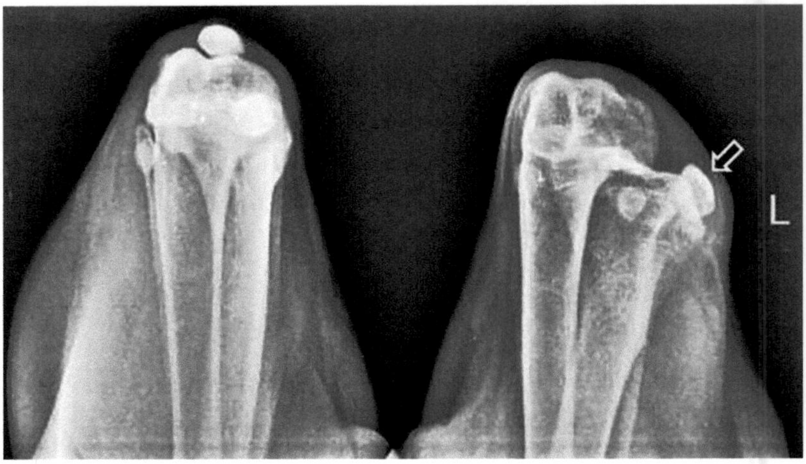


**Fig. 11.10** Skyline/tangential radiographic projection of stifle joint showing lateral displacement of left patella from the trochlear groove, suggesting lateral patellar luxation

luxations. These procedures include release of musculature, desmotomy, imbrications, and antirotational sutures. Basically the technique involves giving incisions to release the contracted tissues on the side of the luxated patella and imbrication (overlapping sutures) of the lax tissues on the opposite side. These procedures may be applied in the immature patients to modify the abnormal forces on growing bones, but in mature patients, they are used to supplement bony procedures.

In medial patellar luxation, medial retinacular release (fascia and other fibrous tissues attached to the patella) is done by giving an incision on the

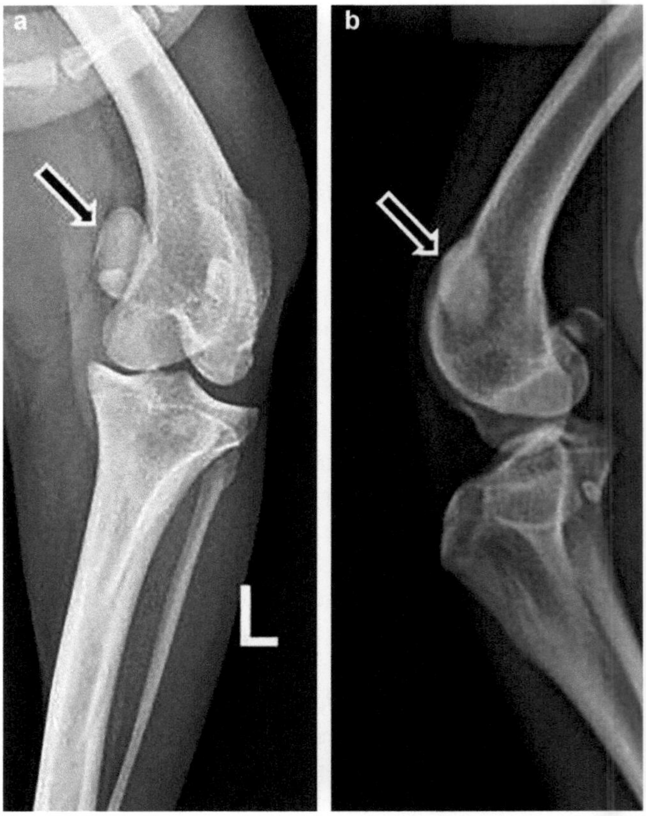


**Fig. 11.11** Oblique (**a**) and lateral (**b**) views of stifle showing medial displacement of patella (arrow)

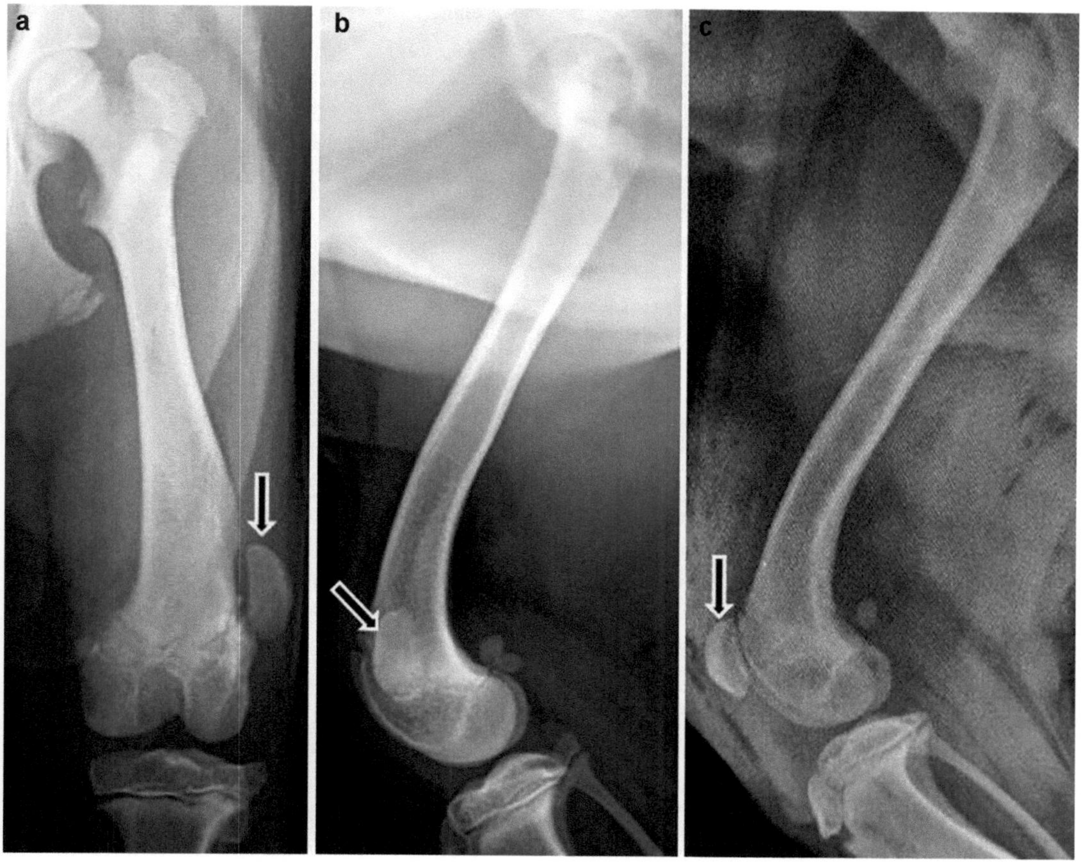


**Fig. 11.12** Craniocaudal (**a**) and lateral (**b**) radiographic views of stifle joint showing laterally displaced patella (arrow); radiograph made after fixation of patella by soft tissue imbrication method shows patella in its normal position (**c**)

medial aspect, starting from the point where the patellar ligament is attached to the tibial crest, continuing proximally until the patella is relieved of the tension. The incision is left open without suturing. The patella along with the patellar ligament is pulled to replace the patella back in the trochlear groove and stabilized on the lateral side by imbrication of the soft tissues. Lateral imbrication should be done hand in hand with desmotomy, which includes 'gathering sutures' to tighten up the soft tissues on the opposite side of the luxation using synthetic monofilament absorbable sutures. If the joint capsule is abundant and laxed, a strip of joint capsule can be removed (partial capsulectomy) and the edges are apposed in a 'vest-over-pants' fashion, or mattress sutures can be applied in the lateral periarticular soft tissues without arthrotomy. Soft tissue imbrication technique alone may not be adequate in grade 3 and 4 luxations, but it can be applied as the first stage of repair in immature animals. Placing a non-absorbable suture from the lateral fabella to the distal part of the straight patellar ligament (antirotational sutures) may help in early correction of rotation of the tibia in immature animals and reduce the severity of deformity. Alternatively, the suture can be passed in figure of '8' fashion around the patella after anchoring behind the lateral fabella. Muscle release procedures can be performed in a variety of ways. The rectus femoris muscle may be freed, at least up to the level of the mid diaphysis of the femur, to relieve medially directed tension on the patella. As an alternative, the origins of the rectus femoris muscle (at the caudal portion of the ilium), or the cranial part of the sartorius muscle (at the cranial wing of the ilium), can be transplanted more laterally to help reduce medial pull on the patella. Medial pull on patella can be reduced by elevation of the origin of the rectus femoris muscle (without transplantation) especially in puppies. However, in mature adult animals, these techniques are unlikely to correct medial patellar luxation by themselves and are useful only if used along with other osseous techniques.

The techniques that modify the bony structures of the stifle joint and around it provide more reliable surgical correction for patellar luxation; they include augmentation of the trochlear groove and transplantation of the tibial tuberosity.

**Trochleoplasty** is a commonly practised osseous technique for the correction of medial patellar luxation [70, 72, 81]. This technique modifies the shape of the trochlear groove to create enough depth and width to safely secure the patella within the trochlear ridges while gliding (which should allow approximately 50% of the patella to protrude above the trochlear ridges). **Trochlear sulcoplasty** is a simple technique, wherein the articular cartilage along with several millimeters of subchondral bone is removed with bone rongeurs. This technique may be successful in small dogs, but the complications such as quadriceps femoris muscle atrophy, crepitus on palpation and severe erosion of the patellar cartilage are common. The functional recovery is slower in this technique as compared to other techniques. **Trochlear chondroplasty** is a technique in which a rectangular flap of cartilage is elevated from the groove and then the subchondral bone is removed from underneath it, and subsequently the flap is pressed back into the deepened groove. This technique may be useful only in growing puppies aged up to about six months; however, in mature animals, flap dissection is difficult as the cartilage is thinner and more adhered to the subchondral bone. **Trochlear wedge recession** is another technique [82], wherein a V-shaped wedge is removed from the trochlear groove with a saw. Then the defect in the trochlea is further widened by cutting at one edge to remove another piece of bone [75]. Then the bone wedge cut earlier is replaced back into the defect; thus a deeper trochlear groove covered with hyaline cartilage may be created (Fig. 11.13). The osteochondral wedge will remain in place due to the friction between the cancellous surfaces of the two cut bony edges and the compressive force of the patella (Fig. 11.4b). In **trochlear block recession** technique [83], two parallel incisions are made in the cartilage and subchondral bone using a saw (far enough to accommodate the patella), taking care to maintain the trochlear ridges. Fresh cuts are made connecting the previously made lateral cuts at just proximal to the site of the origin of the caudal cruciate ligament and the proximal aspect of the trochlea. This segment of the bone and cartilage is cut and removed and wrapped in a sterile moist gauze sponge. The trabecular bone is then removed from the femur to recess the block. Alternatively, the proximal aspect of the segment may be kept attached, and the cartilaginous segment is flipped proximally so that recession of the trochlea can be done. The lateral cuts may be deepened (2–3 mm) by removing another layer of cancellous bone using an osteotome. The cartilage segment with the subchondral bone is then pressed back into the recessed femur. If necessary, cancellous graft may be packed into the gaps along the sides of the segment to prevent wobbling. This technique is better than trochlear wedge recession in preventing patellar luxation in an extended position.

**Tibial tuberosity transposition (TTT):** TTT is used to reposition the quadriceps-patella-patellar tendon mechanism in a normal straight line [70, 72, 74, 81]. Lateral transplantation of the osteotomized fragment is done in cases of medial patellar luxation. The fragment of the bone should be large enough to accept two K-wires of appropriate size or a lag screw. The periosteum along the proposed line of osteotomy on the medial aspect of the tibia is incised. The osteotomy is done starting at a point midway between the insertion site of the patella tendon and the cranial aspect of the tibial plateau and extended up to the distal aspect of the tibial crest, preferably leaving the distal periosteal attachment intact. Then the

a

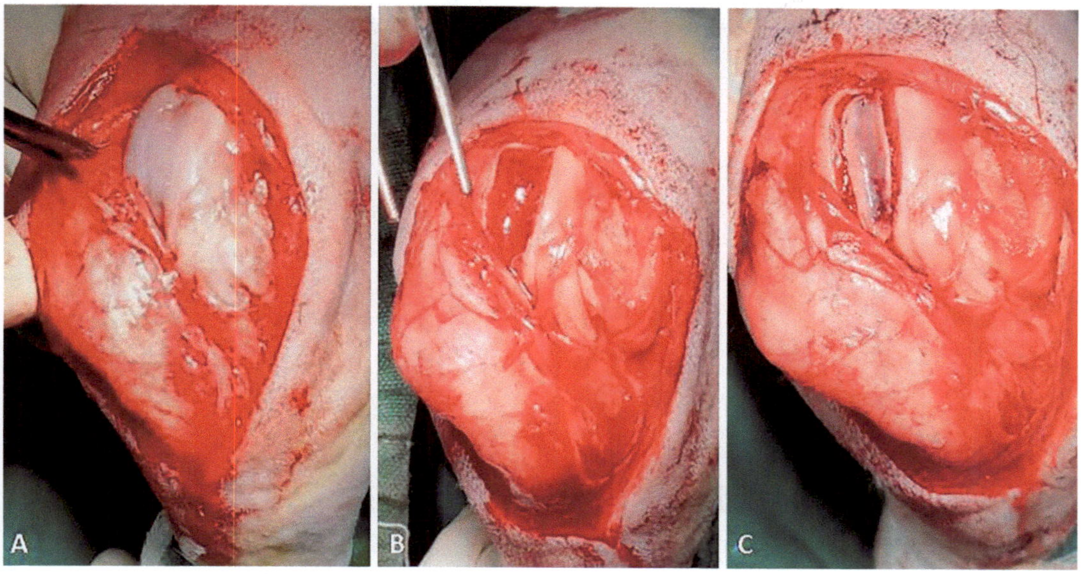


**Fig. 11.13** (**A**) Lateral patellar luxation in dog: shallow trochlear groove (**a**) and deepening of trochlear groove by removing V-shaped wedge (**b**), and the cartilage flap cut earlier is replaced back into the defect (**c**) (Courtesy: Dr. M Raghunath, College of Veterinary Science, Tirupati, Andhra Pradesh, India). (**B**) Radiographs showing lateral patellar luxation in dog with shallow trochlear groove (**a** and **b**), postoperative radiograph made on day 0 shows proper placement of patella in the patellar groove (**c**) and day 65 radiograph shows retention of patella in the normal place (**d**). Note: the animal showed normal functional recovery (Courtesy: Dr. M Raghunath, College of Veterinary Science, Tirupati, Andhra Pradesh, India)

tuberosity is transposed laterally to make realignment between the quadriceps muscle, patella, patellar ligament, and tibial tuberosity by keeping the stifle in extended position having the dog positioned in dorsal recumbency for easy evaluation. The tibial tuberosity is then fixed in the new position using two K-wires of adequate size fixed in a slightly distal and caudomedial direction. It is important that the wires are placed proximal to the point of insertion of the patellar ligament. However, in small dogs, where the distal periosteum has not been removed, placement of a tension band wire is not needed. If the transaction of the tibial tuberosity has been made distally, a tension band wire is needed to counteract the distractive forces of the patellar ligament, especially in larger, active dogs. TTT is the most useful surgical procedure performed in the majority of the cases of medial patellar luxation [75].

Postoperatively adequate analgesia is provided, and activity of the animal is restricted for first few days. Periodical radiographic examination of the stifle joint is done to evaluate correction of the patellar luxation and proper positioning of the implant. If the patient is progressing well and the osteotomy is healing, then the animal would gradually return to normal activity in 6–8 weeks. Complications of medial patellar luxation may include patellar reluxation, infection, delayed union, fixation failure, and osteoarthritis [81, 84]. Larger dogs of over 20 kg weight and high-grade luxations are more prone to such complications. Surgical correction involving tibial tuberosity transposition, femoral trochleoplasty, and soft tissue techniques will reduce postoperative risks. In severe deformities, early correction is indicated to ensure good functional outcome. Generally prognosis is good, and treatment can be successful in more than 90% cases up to grade 3 patellar luxation and poor in grade 4 luxation [71, 80, 84, 85].

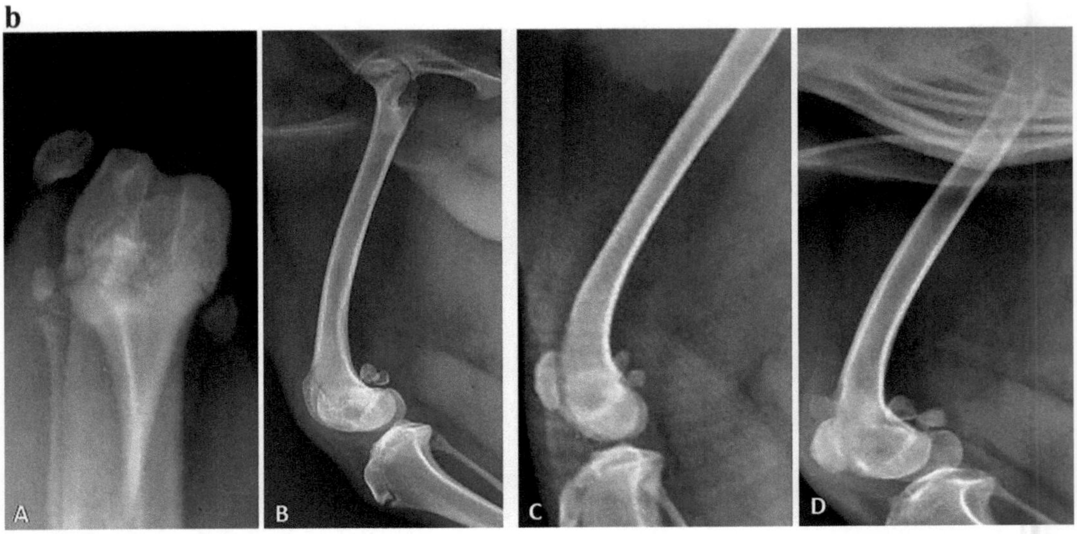


**Fig. 11.13** (continued)

### 11.1.7 Tarsal Luxation

The tarsal joint has seven major bones in dog. The tibial tarsal bone articulates with the distal surface of the tibia and attached to the tibia by the medial collateral ligament. The fibular tarsal bone attaches to the fibular malleolus by the lateral collateral ligament. It has a large prominence called the calcaneal tuber or tuber calcaneus. The central tarsal bone located distal to the tibial tarsal bone articulates with II, III, and IV tarsal bones. A small tarsal bone I articulates with the central tarsal, II tarsal and I metatarsal bones. Tarsal bone II articulates proximally with the central tarsal bone, laterally with III tarsal bone, medially with I tarsal bone and distally with II metatarsal bone. Tarsal bone III is larger than the I or II, and it articulates with the central tarsal bone proximally, with III metatarsal bone distally, with the II tarsal and metatarsal bones medially and with IV tarsal bone laterally. The IV tarsal bone is the largest among the numbered tarsal bone, which articulates with the fibular tarsal bone proximally, with IV and V metatarsal bones distally and with the central tarsal and III tarsal bones medially. The tarsal bones are supported by many short ligaments running between the bones within the joint and the medial and lateral collateral ligaments spanning along the length of the joint. Caudally, the joint is supported by the plantar ligament. The tarsal joint has many articulations, of which the talocrural joint allows the highest degree of movement [86].

The luxation of tibiotarsal joint is common in small animals (Fig. 11.14). The tarsal joint can be exposed through many approaches. With intact collateral ligaments, it is difficult to approach the joint through medial or lateral incisions, and thus the joint is approached through small incisions. The tibial tarsal and the fibular tarsal bones are better exposed through an osteotomy of either the medial or the lateral malleolus. The collateral ligament can be reconstructed by tension band wiring of the malleolus. The fibular tarsal can be approached by a medial or lateral incision made over the bone. Similarly, the central tarsal bone can be exposed through a dorsomedial incision made over the bone.

Complete or partial luxation of the talocrural, intertarsal, or tarsometatarsal joints is common in dogs and cats. It is commonly seen following a trauma, such as severe twisting of the tarsus or hyperextension of the talocrural joint. The injury may cause tearing of the ligaments (collateral, intertarsal, or plantar) and often with fracture of the malleoli or tarsal bones. Clinically, animals

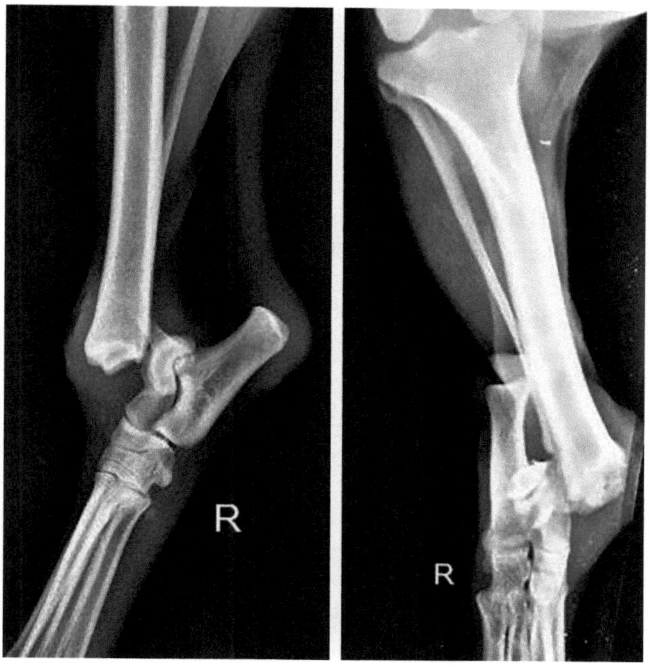


**Fig. 11.14** Orthogonal x-ray views showing fracture-luxation of tibio-tarsal joint

with luxation of the tarsal joint may carry the affected limb with non-weight-bearing lameness and show swinging of the lower part of the limb. On palpation complete or partial instability may be noticed. If bony crepitus is evident, fracture of malleoli or tarsal bones is suspected. Most animals with intertarsal or tarsometatarsal luxation show abnormal prominence on plantar aspect of the tarsus. Manipulation of the site will reveal instability mainly in a dorsoplantar direction. Radiography will help in detecting the extent of the injury and the presence of fracture, if any.

Several techniques of closed and open reduction and fixation of tarsal luxation have been described [87–94]. Closed reduction can be done easily in many cases; however, maintaining the reduction may be difficult. Once reduced, a cranial half cast or long leg cast may be tried, but usually it will fail as it is not rigid enough to allow ligament healing. However, application of external skeletal fixation may provide stable fixation. If fracture is present, open reduction should be attempted, along with internal fixation or external skeletal fixation. Fixation without removing articular cartilage often fails to provide desired effect. Fixation can be done using a bone plate applied across the luxation site either on the lateral or on the plantar surface [93–95]. Only complete arthrodesis of the joint with cancellous bone grafting will lead to permanent fixation.

In case of ligament tears, torn ligaments must be repaired as much as possible and fixed using a suture, screw, K-wire, or staple. Following this, external splint and bandage is applied for 4–6 weeks, to allow fibrosis of the torn ligaments, which may lead to functional recovery of the joint. In case of fractures (like in malleolar fracture), the bone fragments should be reduced and fixed rigidly using a fixation technique such as tension band wiring. In severe cases of fracture luxation, joint arthrodesis is recommended.

Complications are generally not common. Arthrodesis may fail if there is inadequate debridement or inadequate amount of bone graft. Prognosis is good if anatomical reduction is possible. Arthrodesis of talocrural joint generally leads to gait abnormalities; however, intertarsal or tarsometatarsal joint arthrodesis will have excellent prognosis and return to normal function.

## 11.2 Large Animals

Luxation of joints is relatively uncommon in large animals, maybe due to heavy muscle mass and inherently strong tendon and ligament structures [96]; however, luxation can occur in any joint. Luxations of proximal limb joints like scapula-humeral, humero-radial, coxofemoral, and femoro-tibial joint luxations are difficult to treat and are mostly managed conservatively with little success, especially in heavy animals. Luxations of lower limb joints can be better managed using closed reduction and external fixation or by external skeletal fixation.

### 11.2.1 Shoulder Luxation

Luxation of the scapulohumeral joint is a rare injury that can cause severe lameness in large animals [55, 97]. As the scapulohumeral joint does not possess ligaments for support, stability of the joint depends on the surrounding musculature and tendons. Luxation usually results from trauma such as an automobile injury or a fall with the shoulder joint in flexed position. Clinical signs include acute lameness, shortening of the affected limb, swelling in the shoulder region and, in long-standing cases, muscle atrophy from disuse of the limb. Extension and flexion of the affected limb may allow palpation of the tuberosity and the head of the humerus cranial to the glenoid cavity. The lateral lip of the glenoid cavity may be palpable in the case of medial luxation; and in lateral luxations, the proximolateral prominences of the humerus can be easily palpated. Radiography will help confirm the diagnosis.

Closed reduction of humeral head luxations can be attempted under deep sedation or general anesthesia [98, 99]. The affected limb may be held suspended from a sling to achieve relaxation of shoulder muscles and facilitate reduction. Muscle relaxants may also be used, if required. Reduction is done by manipulation at the site of luxation concurrent with limb traction. Some reports show improved outcome with a combination of closed reduction and arthroscopy [100]. Prognosis is generally favorable if the case is fresh and soft tissue damage is minimal. In cases of shoulder joint luxation and concurrent fractures, prognosis is generally poorer than those with shoulder joint luxation alone [101].

### 11.2.2 Elbow Luxation

The luxation of the elbow joint is rarely reported in cattle as well as in horses [102–104]. The condition is more commonly observed in young animals, but it can also occur in adults. In many cases, the condition is associated with concomitant fracture of radius and/or ulna, due to trauma causing severe limb abduction. In most cases, the proximal end of radius-ulna is displaced laterally, but often it can displace medially (Fig. 11.15). Elbow luxation is frequently accompanied with tearing of collateral ligaments, more often the lateral collateral ligament.

Fresh cases of elbow luxation in young animals are generally treated by close reduction and fixation. Under general anesthesia, the luxated joint is reduced manually by flexing the elbow and carpal joints, simultaneously by rotating the forearm medially by strongly pressing the radial head and olecranon. Post-reduction, the animals are given stall rest and external support for a few days. Usually the animals recover with good functional outcome [103]. Surgical techniques described include fixation of screws in the radial head and humeral condyle and stabilization with monofilament non-absorbable sutures like nylon or orthopedic wire in a figure of 8 pattern or placement of prosthetic collateral ligaments. In heavy animals, it is difficult to achieve satisfactory results either by external or internal stabilization technique, postoperative complications are common or prognosis is generally guarded.

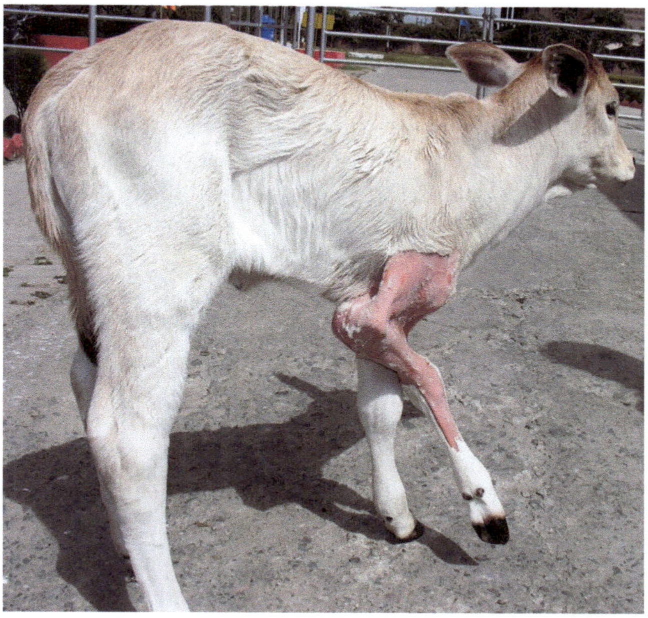

**Fig. 11.15** A calf showing complete luxation of the right elbow joint with medial displacement of radius-ulna

### 11.2.3 Coxofemoral Luxation

The femoral head displacement outside the acetabulum is called a coxofemoral luxation (commonly known as hip luxation). It is the most common joint luxation in cattle, whereas it is relatively uncommon in horses due to the strong ligamentous support to the joint provided by the round ligament and the accessory femoral ligament and also by the fibro-cartilaginous lip surrounding the acetabulum. Luxation of coxofemoral joint occurs usually in craniodorsal (upward) direction and mostly unilateral but often can be bilateral [105–107]. Hip luxation is more commonly seen in cattle aged 2–5 years, often seen around parturient period; the cause is attributed to slipping or any other forms of trauma and hypocalcemia. In horses, luxations are more frequently reported in small ponies, usually due to upward fixation of the patella, often accompanied with fracture of the dorsal acetabular rim.

Clinical signs may vary depending on the direction, extent, and duration of hip luxation. Heavy cattle may be unable to get up and lie holding the affected leg in abduction. If the animal is able to stand, the affected limb may appear shorter than the contralateral normal limb. The animal will show acute onset of non-weight-bearing lameness with the affected leg resting on the toe with outward rotation. During walk, the animal may appear dragging one foot behind the other [105]. Muscle atrophy and pelvic asymmetry may also be noticed. The condition has to be differentiated from fracture of the femoral neck or slipped capital femoral epiphysis, greater trochanter fracture or pelvic fracture. Radiography and ultrasonography will help confirm the diagnosis [96, 108].

Closed reduction of the hip joint in craniodorsal luxations is possible in early cases (if attempted within first 1–2 days, prognosis more favorable if the duration is less than 12 h), provided that there is no fracture of femoral head or the acetabular rim [106, 109]. Reduction should be attempted only under deep sedation and high epidural analgesia or general anesthesia. With the affected leg positioned on the upper side, a strong rope is looped around the groin region and secured by tying around a fixed object such as a tree. Another rope is tied at the pastern/hoof region and traction applied by pulling the rope to extend the limb. Simultaneously by applying downward pressure to the hock, it is rotated outward and upward forcefully until the femoral head slips back into the acetabulum [105, 110]. Many times it is necessary to apply traction at different angles to reduce the femur head. Caudodorsal luxations can be easily reduced by applying straight ventral traction. In other types of luxation (such as cranioventral or medial luxation), repositioning of the hip is extremely difficult by manipulation especially when the femur head gets jammed in the obturator foramen [110]. To achieve close reduction, the femur head should be first moved dorsally by flexing the stifle (with rotating outwards) and hock joints (with rotating inwards) and slowly lifting the leg pushing upwards. Then it is reduced as described for dorsal luxation. In any case, once the hip joint is reduced, it should be checked for the correct fit in the acetabular cavity by feeling for crepitus while flexing and extending the leg, and checking for any outward rotation of the stifle, and symmetry of greater trochanter on both sides. Once confirmed of right placement of the hip, the gluteal muscles may be beaten (using a batten) to bruise the muscles and produce spasm that help holding the joint tight and reduce the chances of reluxation. Subsequently the animal should be encouraged/assisted to get up and walk around.

The surgical reduction through a cranio-lateral or dorso-caudal approach has been somewhat successful especially in smaller animals [107, 108]. If left alone without treatment (in unilateral cases), a pseudoarthrosis may develop. But it is difficult to achieve functional recovery, as lameness may persist and the animal may gradually lose weight. In horses, stall rest can be the best choice of treatment; and if the luxation is mild, extended rest may help heal the condition. In most cases, however, only stall rest will not help stabilize the luxated coxofemoral joint, as arthritis may set in. Medications can help control the pain of an arthritic horse, but eventually the quality of life will deteriorate and euthanasia is recommended. Joint replacement surgery is neither advised nor gives satisfactory results in heavy animals. Treatment can be more successful in craniodorsal luxations than caudodorsal luxations; similarly prognosis is more successful in young animals than in heavy adults [107, 109].

### 11.2.4 Patellar Luxation

Fixation of the patella intermittently on the upper part of the femoral trochlea is a common condition in large ruminants. It can be unilateral or bilateral (symptoms in one limb may be more severe than the other) and can be permanent or recurrent in nature. The condition is more common in buffaloes but also seen frequently in young working bullocks. It also occurs in horses but most frequently seen in young ponies working on hills and having a faulty conformation of the hindlimbs. Patellar luxation can be acquired, developmental, or congenital [111–119].

In cases of recurrent dorsal fixation, the clinical signs are not apparent when animal is at rest, where the patella may occupy its normal position in the femoral trochlea. During progression, it can be manifested by intermittent fixation of the patella due to the hooking of the medial patellar ligament over the upper extremity of the trochlear ridge. During forced walk, the condition becomes evident by characteristic jerky action of one or both hindlimbs. As the condition worsens, the symptoms would become more frequent and apparent with obvious gait abnormality and lameness (Fig. 11.16). The limb remains in caudal extension (with fixed/locked stifle and hock joints) for a longer period than normal and may be seen dragging for a few steps before clicking forward to a normal posture. In animals with permanent dorsal fixation of patella (usually chronic cases), forced walking may lead to carrying of their legs rigidly with flexed fetlock and dragging of the toe on the ground with the weight bearing on the flexed digits. Gradually the animal may adapt its gait by swinging the limb forward

Fig. 11.16 Bilateral medial patellar luxation in a calf with locked stifle and hock joints

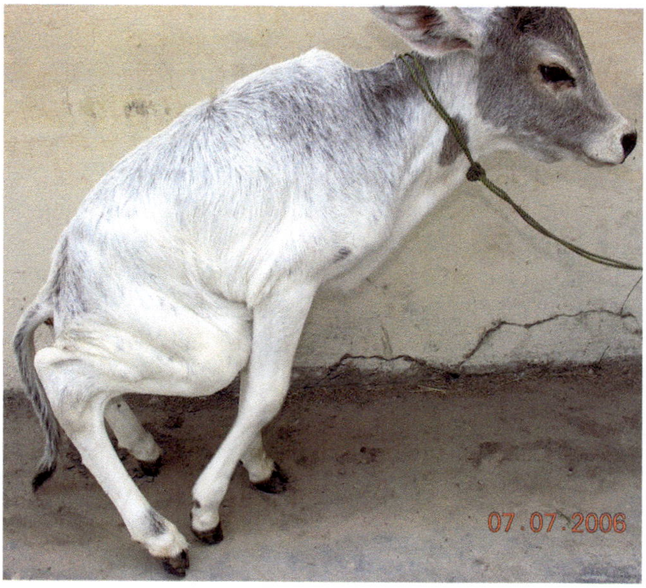


in abduction, without flexing the hock and stifle joints. The animal may refuse to move backwards when forced attempts are made. The symptoms may be exaggerated by circling the animal with the affected limb on the inner side, while circling in the opposite direction may lessen the symptoms.

In young animals, the condition may get resolved spontaneously. For luxations that do not resolve, surgical correction (medial patellar desmotomy) should be performed; its main aim is to disengage the patella from medial trochlear ridge to allow free movement of the stifle joint. Desmotomy can be performed in standing animal or in lateral recumbent position, with closed or open method.

In standing animals, using the index finger, the site of surgical incision can be determined by feeling a small depression between the middle and medial patellar ligaments proximal to their insertion at the tibial tuberosity. The surgical site is prepared aseptically, and 2% lignocaine (2–5 ml) is injected over and around the medial patellar ligament subcutaneously. Just proximal to the tibial tuberosity, a small incision is made in the skin between the middle and medial patellar ligaments. Care should be taken to avoid penetration of the joint capsule. A tenotome/No. 11 BP blade (small curved edge) is then inserted through the skin incision under the medial patellar ligament, near the ligament insertion at the tibial tuberosity. The cutting edge of the tenotome is kept in vertical direction. Once the correct position is ascertained, the cutting edge of the blade is directed toward the ligament and pressed strongly against the ligament to transect it. Care is taken to avoid the severance of the middle patellar ligament or collateral ligaments. Severance of the medial ligament can be confirmed by observing a deep depression developed at its normal position between the cut ends. If the depression is not felt, the procedure should be repeated to completely transect the ligament. Penetration of joint should be avoided during the entire surgical procedure. Subsequently, an antiseptic solution such as betadine may be injected into the incision site, which can be left unsutured.

If the animal is agile or excited, it is better to perform desmotomy in the animal restrained under lateral recumbency keeping the affected limb positioned downside [120]. The upper hindlimb is tied together with both the forelimbs and affected limb is extended backwards by pulling at the rope tied to the fetlock region. The hock joint is pushed downwards to rotate the stifle for better exposure of the incision site. By taking the cranial tibial tuberosity and the medial tibial prominence as points of reference, the groove between the middle and medial patellar ligaments is palpated using the index finger. The medial patellar ligament is then severed in the similar manner as described above. A less experienced surgeon may identify and resect the patellar ligament by open method. In this method, the site is prepped for aseptic surgery, and under local infiltration analgesia, about 3-cm-long incision is made about 0.5 cm lateral to the medial patellar ligament close to its insertion at the tibial tuberosity. Using artery forceps, the medial patellar ligament is exteriorized by separating the underlying fascia by blunt dissection. The ligament is then cut transversely using a BP blade, and the skin incision is closed with a few interrupted sutures after injecting an antiseptic solution at the site of incision.

Immediately after successful surgical resection of the medial patellar ligament, the animal will start walking without a limp. Once the animal gets up, it is made to walk backwards to help break any string of ligament that may be intact. Postoperatively, antiseptic dressing and a course of antibiotic may be given for a few days. The results are excellent in fresh cases with early surgical resection of the ligament; and in long-standing cases, complete recovery (walk without lameness) may take longer time due to adhesions and incomplete separation and resection of the ligament.

Upward fixation of patella is not a true luxation in horses. Horses can keep standing for a long period of time due to their ability to lock their knee (patella) in upward position, which conserves energy. If the patella is unable to be unlocked and the leg stays stiff and unable to bend back to normal position, it can cause problems. Lateral luxation of patella has been described in horses and ponies (Fig. 11.17), and medial luxation is very rarely reported [121]. Lateral luxation of patella in foals is most commonly caused due to expression of a recessive gene, and in adult horses, it may be traumatic in origin. Hypoplasia of the lateral trochlear ridge of the femur predisposes horses and foals to lateral

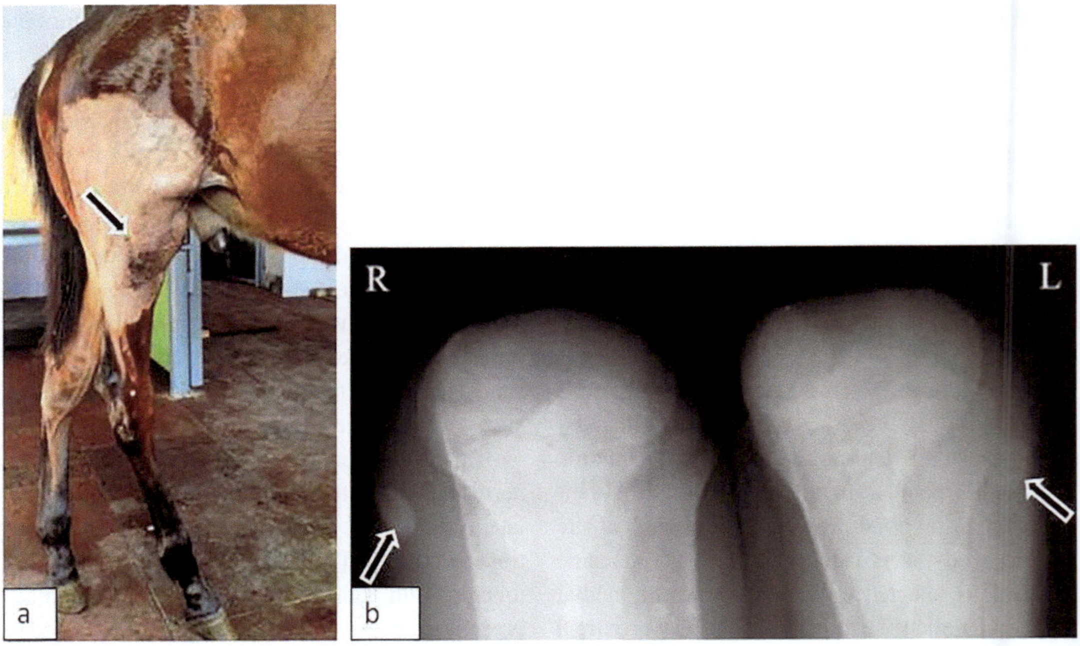


**Fig. 11.17** A horse showing swelling on the right of stifle joint (arrow) suggesting laterally luxated patella (**a**); oblique radiographic view of both stifle joints show bilateral patellar luxation (arrows), with signs of trochlear ridge hypoplasia and shallow trochlear groove (**b**) (Source: Samaneh Ghasemi et al., Iranian J. Vet. Surg. 2015; 10 (1); Serial No: 22)

luxation of patella. The condition may vary from intermittent luxation that can be reduced rapidly to persistent luxation that cannot be reduced and it may be unilateral or bilateral. Miniature horses are known to be more predisposed to patellar luxation.

In horses with no or minor anatomical abnormalities, release of fascia and imbrications techniques can be used [121], while cases with major anatomical abnormalities require reconstructive procedures along with release and imbrication techniques. In lateral patellar luxation, the release techniques are applied to the lateral retinacular structures, and imbrication is performed on the medial side of the joint capsule and vice versa in medial luxation. The use of release and imbrication technique alone was more successful in miniature breed horses (75% cases) than in larger breeds. The wedge recession trochleoplasty (described for dogs) in combination with medial imbrications has been used successfully in the management of lateral patellar luxation in foals. The modified recession trochleoplasty with the attachment maintained proximally has been found advantageous over the technique of complete wedge recession or chondroplasty, as it provided a smooth articular surface proximally and excellent stability of the construct [122, 123]; but the technique is more demanding and time consuming. If surgery is performed in young animals, the distal femur and patella adapt to normal movement, and the functional outcome will be better. The operated animals should be discouraged for breeding to prevent the disease. In traumatic cases with severe damage to the collateral ligaments of patella, reconstruction of femoropatellar ligaments may be done using any strong implant. Ideal attachment point in femur for lateral ligament is lateral epicondyle (just proximal to lateral collateral ligament) and for medial ligament is just proximal to the medial epicondyle (just proximal to medial collateral ligament). In patella, the attachment point is lateral border of patella (for lateral ligament) and medial parapatellar fibrocartilage (for medial ligament).

### 11.2.5 Carpal and Tarsal Luxations

Luxation of tarsal joint is relatively more common than carpal luxations in cattle and buffaloes [96], whereas luxation or subluxation of the carpal or tarsal joint is reported to be infrequent in horses [124, 125]. Severe trauma due to automobile accidents, sudden fall or slip can lead to closed or open luxation of carpal/tarsal joints at different levels. Often it is accompanied with fractures of carpal/tarsal bones and injury to the surrounding ligament structures. Under general anesthesia, reduction of luxated joint can be achieved easily due to less soft tissue covering around the joints. Once reduced, closed luxations can be immobilized by applying a full limb cast for 6–8 weeks. In open cases, transarticular external skeletal fixation will be useful to provide stable fixation. Restricted range of motion of the joint and progressive osteoarthritis may be the complications.

### 11.2.6 Metacarpophalangeal and Metatarsophalangeal Luxations

Metacarpophalangeal or metatarsophalangeal (fetlock) joint luxation either alone or along with fracture is often seen both in cattle/buffaloes and horses. Fetlock fracture/dislocation is common during the animal crossing the fence, fall or a vehicular trauma leading to a crush injury. Luxation of fetlock may be medial or lateral and it can be closed or open. Tranquilization or light anesthesia facilitates replacement of dislocated structures. Reduced joint can be immobilized using a cast application for 3–6 weeks. Apposition of a ruptured collateral ligament may be attempted, and in open cases, after debridement of soft tissues and joint lavage, an external skeletal fixation may be used to provide stable fixation of the joint (Fig. 11.18). Whether closed or open, fetlock luxations have a good prognostic normal functional recovery.

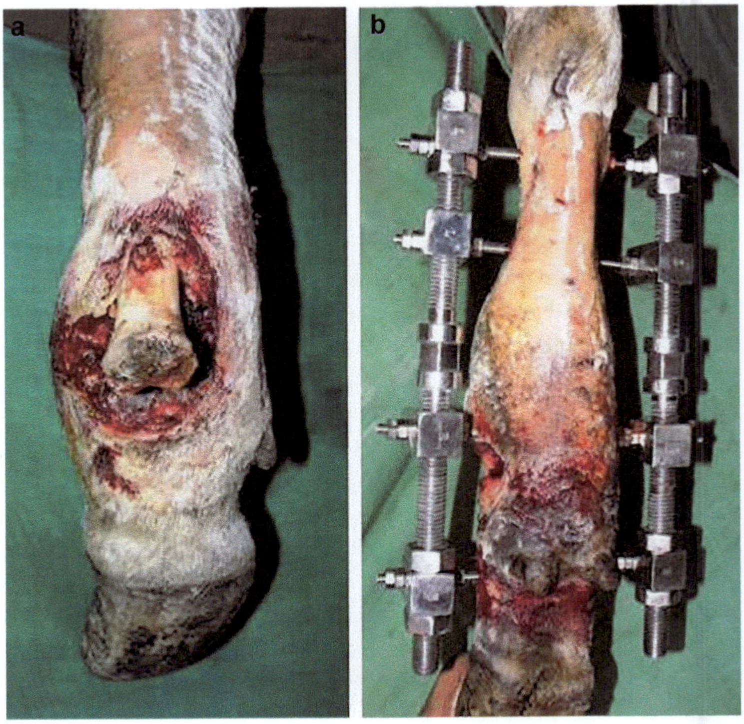


**Fig. 11.18** Open fracture-luxation of fetlock joint in cattle (**a**), stabilized with fixation of a novel bilateral linear fixation device (**b**)

## Chapter 11: Sample Questions

### Question No. 1: Mark the correct answer

1. The most common type of shoulder luxation noticed in dogs is
   (a) cranial (b) lateral (c) medial (d) caudal
2. During the surgical fixation of luxated hip joint, the greater trochanter is repositioned in the following direction to maintain the hip in reduction, flexion, abduction, and internal rotation.
   (a) craniodorsally (b) craniodistally (c) caudodorsally (d) caudodistally
3. During femoral head and neck excision, the partial tenotomy of the following muscle tendon is performed to access the femoral neck
   (a) biceps femoris (b) vastus lateralis (c) superficial gluteus (d) deep gluteus
4. Upward patellar luxation in cattle can be surgically treated by desmotomy of
   (a) medial patellar ligament (b) middle patellar ligament (c) lateral patellar ligament (d) caudal patellar ligament
5. Which of the muscle is not a component of rotator calf muscle in dog
   (a) supraspinatus (b) infraspinatus (c) teres minor (d) teres major

### Question No. 2: State true or false

1. Caudal luxation of shoulder is most frequently observed in dogs and cats.
2. Smaller breeds of dogs such as miniature poodles are more predisposed to shoulder joint luxation.
3. In management of lateral luxation of shoulder, a caudomedial transposition of the biceps brachii tendon is performed.
4. Closed reduction and fixation of the luxated hip can only be successful if attempted soon after the injury and prognosis will be poorer if it is done after 3–4 days of trauma.
5. In dogs, medial patellar luxation is common and is more often seen in small breeds of dog.
6. Hip joint luxation is more common in cattle than horses.
7. Medial patellar luxation is common in cattle.
8. Upward fixation of the patella is not a true luxation in horses.

9. Luxation of shoulder joint is common in cats.
10. Tibial plateau leveling osteotomy is used for the correction of medial patellar luxation in dog.

**Question No. 3: Fill up the blanks**

1. Complete separation of bone ends that normally articulate to form a joint is called ______________________________, whereas partial separation of joint is termed as ______________________________.
2. The surgical technique generally practised and found successful for treatment of luxated shoulder is ______________________________ ______________________________ ______.
3. ______________________ condyle of the distal humerus is relatively larger, preventing the radius and ulna from moving __________ __________ and more often leading to their ______________________ displacement.
4. *The* ______________________________-______ joint is responsible for most (about 80–90%) of the carpal motion in dogs.
5. In hip luxation, most frequently femoral head is displaced in ______________________ ____ direction relative to the acetabulum.
6. Complete hip luxation is commonly unilateral and caused by ______________________ _, while subluxation of the hip is typically associated with ______________________ ______ and is bilateral.
7. The commonly practised osseous technique that modifies the shape of the trochlear groove to secure the patella within the trochlear ridges for the correction of patellar luxation is called as ______________________________.

**Question No. 4: Write short note on the following:**

1. Surgical correction of the luxated elbow in dogs
2. Difference between hip dislocation and hip dysplasia
3. Tibial tuberosity transposition technique for correction of patellar luxation
4. Toggle pin technique for surgical fixation of luxated hip
5. Transposition of biceps brachii tendon for shoulder luxation

## References


1. Evans, H.E., and G.C. Christensen. 1979. Shoulder joint. In *Miller's anatomy of the dog*, 240–243. Philadelphia: W.B. Saunders.
2. Genevois, J.P. 2004. The lax shoulder in the dog: Surgical Management. World Small Animal Veterinary Association World Congress Proceedings, 2004. https://www.vin.com
3. Newton, C.D. 1985. Dislocation of the shoulder. In *Textbook of small animal orthopaedics*, ed. C.D. Newton and D.M. Nunamaker, 343–355. Philadelphia: J.B. Lippincott.
4. Denny, H.R. 1980. Dislocation of the shoulder. In *A guide to canine surgery*. Oxford: Blackwell Scientific Publications.
5. Olin, F.H. 1965. Luxation of the shoulder joint in a toy poodle. *Veterinary Medicine* 60: 17.
6. Craig, E., R. Hohn, and W. Anderson. 1980. Surgical stabilisation of traumatic medial shoulder dislocation. *Journal of the American Animal Hospital Association* 1: 93–102.
7. Pucheu, B., and B. Duhautois. 2008. Surgical treatment of shoulder instability. A retrospective study on 76 cases (1993-2007). *Veterinary and Comparative Orthopaedics and Traumatology* 21: 368–374.
8. Purohit, N.R., R.J. Choudhary, D.S. Chouhan, and C.K. Sharma. 1985. Surgical repair of scapulohumeral luxation in goats. *Modern Veterinary Practice* 66: 758–759.
9. Slocum, B., and T.D. Slocum. 1998. Suture stabilisation for luxations of the shoulder. In *Current techniques in small animal surgery*, ed. M.J. Bojrab, 1079–1081. Philadelphia: Lea and Febiger.
10. Hohn, R.B., H. Rosen, and A.J. Bianco Jr. 1973. Luxation of the shoulder. *Journal of the American Animal Hospital Association* 1973: 467.
11. Wolff, E.F. 1974. Transposition of the biceps brachii tendon to repair luxation of the canine shoulder joint. *Veterinary Medicine, Small Animal Clinician* 1: 51–53.
12. Barber, L.N., D.D. Lewis, E.G. Porter, and L.H. Elam. 2020. Long-term outcome following cranial biceps brachii tendon transposition in a dog with a traumatic cranial scapulohumeral luxation. *Open Veterinary Journal* 10 (4): 400–406.
13. Fowler, J.D., K.R. Presnell, and D.L. Holmberg. 1988. Scapulohumeral arthrodesis: results in 7 dogs. *Journal of the American Animal Hospital Association* 24: 667–672.

14. Bruecker, K.A., and D.L. Piermattei. 1988. Excision arthroplasty of the canine scapulohumeral joint: report of three cases. *Veterinary and Comparative Orthopaedics and Traumatology* 01 (03/04): 134–140.
15. Montasell, X., J. Dupuis, L. Huneault, and G.R. Ragetly. 2018. Short- and long-term outcomes after shoulder excision arthroplasty in 7 small breed dogs. *The Canadian Veterinary Journal* 59 (3): 277–283.
16. Dassler, C., and P.B. Vasseur. 2002. Elbow luxation. In *Textbook of small animal surgery*, ed. D. Slatter, vol. 2, 1919–1927. Philadelphia, PA: W.B. Saunders.
17. Mitchell, K.E. 2011. Traumatic elbow luxation in 14 dogs and 11 cats. *Australian Veterinary Journal* 89 (6): 213–216.
18. O'Brien, M.G., R.J. Boudrieau, and G.N. Clark. 1992. Traumatic luxation of the cubital joint (elbow) in dogs: 44 cases (1978-1988). *Journal of the American Veterinary Medical Association* 201 (11): 1760–1765.
19. Schaeffer, I.G.F., P. Wolvekamp, B.P. Meij, L.F.H. Theijse, and H.A.W. Hazewinkel. 1999. Traumatic luxation of the elbow in 31 dogs. *Veterinary and Comparative Orthopaedics and Traumatology* 12 (2): 33–39.
20. Hamilton, K. 2014. Caudal elbow luxation in a dog managed by temporary transarticular external skeletal fixation. Case reports. *Veterinary Medicine* 2014. Article ID 498329. https://doi.org/10.1155/2014/498329.
21. Mccartney, W.T., K. Kiss, and F. McGovern. 2010. Surgical stabilisation as the primary treatment for traumatic luxation of the elbow joint in 10 dogs. *The International Journal of Applied Research in Veterinary Medicine* 8: 97–100.
22. Billings, L.A., P.B. Vasseur, R.J. Todoroff, and W. Johnson. 1992. Clinical results after reduction of traumatic elbow luxation in nine dogs and one cat. *Journal of the American Animal Hospital Association* 28: 137–142.
23. Farrell, M., D. Draffan, T. Gemmill, D. Mellor, and S. Carmichael. 2007. In vitro validation of a technique for assessment of canine and feline elbow joint collateral ligament integrity and description of a new method for collateral ligament prosthetic replacement. *Veterinary Surgery* 36 (6): 548–556.
24. Rahal, S.C., F. de Biasi, L.C. Vulcano, and F.J.T. Neto. 2000. Reduction of humeroulnar congenital elbow luxation in 8 dogs by using the transarticular pin. *The Canadian Veterinary Journal* 41 (11): 849–853.
25. Schwartz, Z., and D.J. Griffon. 2008. Nonrigid external fixation of the elbow, coxofemoral, and tarsal joints in dogs. *Compendium on Continuing Education for the Practising Veterinarian* 30 (12): 648–653.
26. Fafard, A.R. 2006. Unilateral congenital elbow luxation in a dachshund. *The Canadian Veterinary Journal* 47 (9): 909–912.
27. Harasen, G. 2012. Congenital radial head luxation in a bulldog puppy. *The Canadian Veterinary Journal* 53 (4): 439–441.
28. Nunamaker, D.M. 1985. Fractures and dislocation of the elbow. In *Textbook of small animal orthopaedics*, ed. C.D. Newton and D.M. Nunamaker, 365–372. Philadelphia: J.B. Lippincott.
29. Mason, T.A., and M.J. Baker. 1978. The surgical management of elbow joint deformity associated with premature growth plate closure in dogs. *The Journal of Small Animal Practice* 19: 639.
30. Newton, C.D., D.M. Nunamaker, and C.R. Dickinson. 1975. Surgical management of radial physeal growth disturbance in dogs. *Journal of the American Veterinary Medical Association* 167: 1011.
31. Miller, M.E., G.C. Christensen, and H.E. Evans. 1964. Ligaments and joints of the thoracic limb. In *Miller's anatomy of the dog*, 73–74. Philadelphia: W.B. Saunders.
32. Guilliard, M.J., and A.K. Mayo. 2001. Subluxation/luxation of the second carpal bone in two racing greyhounds and a Staffordshire bull terrier. *The Journal of Small Animal Practice* 42: 356–359.
33. Kaya, D.A. 2018. Bilateral radial carpal bone luxation and its treatment in a dog. *Turkish Journal of Veterinary and Animal Sciences* 42 (4): 366–369.
34. Miller, A., S. Carmichael, T.J. Anderson, and I. Brown. 1990. Luxation of the radial carpal bone in four dogs. *The Journal of Small Animal Practice* 31: 148–154.
35. Palierne, S., C. Delbeke, E. Asimus, P. Meynaud-Collard, D. Mathon, A. Zahra, and A. Autefage. 2008. A case of dorso-medial luxation of the radial carpal bone in dog. *Veterinary and Comparative Orthopaedics and Traumatology* 21: 171–176.
36. Pitcher, G.D. 1996. Luxation of the radial carpal bone in a cat. *The Journal of Small Animal Practice* 37: 292–295.
37. Punzet, G. 1974. Luxation of the os carpi radiale in the dog – pathogenesis, symptoms, and treatment. *The Journal of Small Animal Practice* 15: 751–756.
38. Guerrero, T.G., and P.M. Montavon. 2005. Medial plating for carpal panarthrodesis. *Veterinary Surgery* 34: 153–158.
39. Newton, C.D. 1985. Fracture and dislocation of the carpus. In *Textbook of small animal orthopaedics*, ed. C.D. Newton and D.M. Nunamaker, 381–386. Philadelphia: J.B. Lippincott.
40. Nunamaker, D.M. 1985. Fractures and dislocations of the hip joint. In *Textbook of small animal orthopaedics*, ed. C.D. Newton and D.M. Nunamaker, 403–414. Philadelphia: J.B. Lippincott.
41. Duff, S.R., and D. Bennett. 1982. Hip luxation in small animals: an evaluation of some methods of treatment. *The Veterinary Record* 111 (7): 140–143.

42. LeFloch, M.D., and G.S. Coronado. 2022. Outcome of coxofemoral luxation treated with closed reduction in 51 cats. *Journal of Feline Medicine and Surgery* 24 (8): 709–714.
43. Adamiak, Z. 2012. Treatment of bilateral hip luxation in dogs with the Shani-Johnston-Shahar technique: case report. *Revue de Medecine Veterinaire* 163 (2): 76–78.
44. Ash, K., D. Rosseli, A. Danielsli, M. Farrell, M. Hamilton, and N. Fitzpatrick. 2012. Correction of craniodorsal coxofemoral luxation in cats and small breed dogs using a modified Knowles technique with the braided polyblend TightRope™ systems. *Veterinary and Comparative Orthopaedics and Traumatology* 25: 54–60.
45. Bennett, D., and S.R. Duff. 1980. Transarticular pinning as a treatment for hip luxation in the dog and cat. *The Journal of Small Animal Practice* 21 (7): 373–379.
46. Cetinkaya, M.A., and B. Olcay. 2010. Modified Knowles toggle pin technique with nylon monofilament suture material for treatment of two caudoventral hip luxation cases. *Veterinary and Comparative Orthopaedics and Traumatology* 23: 114–118.
47. Demko, J.L., B.K. Sidaway, K.M. Thieman, D.B. Fox, C.R. Boyle, and R.M. McLaughlin. 2006. Toggle rod stabilization for treatment of hip joint luxation in dogs: 62 cases (2000–2005). *Journal of the American Veterinary Medical Association* 229 (6): 984–989.
48. Galga, L.H., J.A.T. Pigatto, C.L. Constanti, et al. 2016. Ilium-femoral suture technique using wire of polydioxanone for hip joint stabilization in a dog with traumatic hip dislocation. *Acta Scientiae Veterinariae* 44: 1–6.
49. Haburjak, J.J., T.M. Lenehan, J. Harari, R. Gurevitch, B. Rivers, G.B. Tarvin, and P.D. Constable. 2001. Treatment of traumatic coxofemoral luxation with triple pelvic osteotomy in 19 dogs (1987-1999). *Veterinary and Comparative Orthopaedics and Traumatology* 14: 69–77.
50. Harasen, G. 2005. Coxofemoral luxations - part 2: surgical options. *The Canadian Veterinary Journal* 46: 546–547.
51. Kieves, N.R., P.J. Lotsikas, K.S. Schulz, et al. 2014. Hip toggle stabilization using the TightRope® system in 17 dogs: technique and long-term outcome. *Veterinary Surgery* 43: 515–522.
52. Martini, M.F., B. Simonazzi, and M. Del Bue. 2001. Extra-articular absorbable suture stabilization of coxofemoral luxation in dogs. *Veterinary Surgery* 30: 468–475.
53. Meij, B.P., H.A. Hazewinkel, and R.C. Nap. 1992. Results of an extra-articular stabilization following open reduction of coxofemoral luxation in dogs and cats. *The Journal of Small Animal Practice* 33: 320–326.
54. Rocha, A.G., R.C. Costa, G.O. Morato, D.G. Chung, J.G. Padilha-Filho, B.W. Minto, and L.G.G.G. Dias. 2020. Iliofemoral technique modification using an anchor screw as treatment of canine traumatic hip luxation - case report. *Arquivo Brasileiro de Medicina Veterinária e Zootecnia* 72 (06). https://doi.org/10.1590/1678-4162-12037.
55. Shani, J., D.E. Johnston, and R. Shahar. 2004. Stabilization of traumatic luxation with extra-capsular suture from the greater trochanter to the origin of the rectus femoris. *Veterinary and Comparative Orthopaedics and Traumatology* 17: 12–16.
56. Trostel, C.T., and D.B. Fox. 2020. Coxofemoral joint luxation in dogs treated with toggle rod stabilization: a multi-institutional retrospective review with client survey. *Journal of the American Animal Hospital Association* 56 (2): 83–91.
57. Venturini, A., S. Pinna, and R. Tamburro. 2010. Combined intra extra-articular technique for stabilization of coxofemoral luxation. Preliminary results in two dogs. *Veterinary and Comparative Orthopaedics and Traumatology* 23: 182–185.
58. Belge, A., Z. Bozkan, M. Sarierler, and R. Yaygingul. 2014. The treatment of coxofemoral luxation by modified synthetic capsule technique in dogs: 6 cases. *Kafkas Universitesi Veteriner Fakultesi Dergisi* 20 (3): 337–343.
59. Yoon, J.W., S.Y. Heo, S.M. Jeong, and H.B. Leel. 2019. Total hip replacement for treatment of chronic coxofemoral joint dislocation in 7 dogs. *Journal of Veterinary Clinics* 36 (4): 229–232.
60. Nunamaker, D.M. 1985. Fractures and dislocations of the stifle. In *Textbook of small animal orthopaedics*, ed. C.D. Newton and D.M. Nunamaker, 433–437. Philadelphia: J.B. Lippincott.
61. Aron, D.N. 1988. Traumatic dislocation of the stifle joint: treatment of 12 dogs and one cat. *Journal of the American Animal Hospital Association* 24: 333–340.
62. Bruce, W.J. 1998. Multiple ligamentous injuries of the canine stifle joint: a study of 12 cases. *The Journal of Small Animal Practice* 39: 333–340.
63. Hulse, D.A., and P.K. Shires. 1986. Multiple ligament injury of the stifle joint in the dog. *Journal of the American Animal Hospital Association* 22: 105–110.
64. Jaeger, G.H., M.A. Wosar, D.J. Marcellin-Little, and B.D.X. Lascelles. 2005. Use of hinged transarticular external fixation for adjunctive joint stabilization in dogs and cats: 14 cases (1999-2003). *Journal of the American Veterinary Medical Association* 227: 586–591.
65. Keely, B., M. Glyde, S. Guerin, and R. Doyle. 2007. Stifle joint luxation in the dog and cat: the use of temporary intraoperative transarticular pinning to facilitate joint reconstruction. *Journal of Veterinary and Comparative Orthopaedics and Traumatology* 3: 198–203.

66. Laing, E.J. 1993. Collateral ligament injury and stifle luxation. *The Veterinary Clinics of North America. Small Animal Practice* 23: 845–853.
67. Welches, C., and T. Scavelli. 1990. Transarticular pinning to repair luxation of the stifle joint in dogs and cats: a retrospective study of 10 cases. *Journal of the American Animal Hospital Association* 26: 207–214.
68. Embleton, N.A., and V.J. Barkowski. 2015. Surgical treatment of canine stifle disruption using a novel extracapsular articulated stifle stabilizing implant. *The Canadian Veterinary Journal* 56 (2): 144–148.
69. Pérez, P., W.T. Chelsea, and P. Lafuente. 2014. Management of medial patellar luxation in dogs: what you need to know. *Irish Veterinary Journal* 4: 636–640.
70. Gibbons, S.E., C. Macias, M.A. Tonzing, G.L. Pinchbeck, and W.M. Mackee. 2006. Patellar luxations in 70 large breed dogs. *The Journal of Small Animal Practice* 47: 3–9.
71. Remedios, A.M., A.W.P. Basher, C.L. Runyon, and C.L. Fries. 1992. Medial patellar luxation in 16 large dogs: a retrospective study. *Veterinary Surgery* 21: 5–9.
72. L'Eplattenier, H., and P. Montavon. 2002. Patellar luxation in dogs and cats: pathogenesis and diagnosis. *Small Animals Exotics* 24: 234–240.
73. Hayes, A.G., R.J. Boudrieau, and L.L. Hungerford. 1994. Frequency and distribution of medial and lateral patellar luxation in dogs: 124 cases (1982-1992). *Journal of the American Veterinary Medical Association* 57: 105–109.
74. Nagaoka, K., H. Orima, M. Fujita, and H. Ichiki. 1995. A new surgical method for canine congenital patellar luxation. *The Journal of Veterinary Medical Science* 57: 105–109.
75. Roush, J.K. 1993. Canine patellar luxation. *The Veterinary Clinics of North America. Small Animal Practice* 23: 855–868.
76. Engvall, P.D., and N. Bushnell. 1990. Patellar luxation in Abyssinian cats. *Feline Practice* 18: 20–22.
77. Houlton, J.E.F., and S.E. Meynink. 1989. Medial patellar luxation in the cat. *The Journal of Small Animal Practice* 30: 349–352.
78. Johnson, M.E. 1986. Feline patellar luxation: a retrospective case study. *Journal of the American Animal Hospital Association* 22: 835–838.
79. Olmstead, M.L. 1993. Lateral luxation of the patella. In *Disease mechanism in small animal surgery*, ed. M.J. Bojrab, 2nd ed., 818–820. Philadelphia: Lea & Febiger.
80. Loughlin, C.A., S.C. Kerwin, G. Hosgood, P.B. Ringwood, J. Williams, J.D. Stefanacci, and R.J. McCarthy. 2006. Clinical signs and results of treatment in cats with patellar luxation: 42 cases. *Journal of the American Veterinary Medical Association* 228: 1370–1375.
81. Wandgee, C. 2013. Evaluation of surgical treatment of medial patellar luxation in Pomeranian dogs. *Veterinary and Comparative Orthopaedics and Traumatology* 26: 435–439.
82. Slocum, B., and T. Devine. 1985. Trochlear recession for correction of luxating patella in the dog. *Journal of the American Veterinary Medical Association* 186 (4): 365–369.
83. Talcott, K.W., R.L. Goring, and J.J. de Haan. 2000. Rectangular recession trochleoplasty for treatment of patellar luxation in dogs and cats. *Veterinary and Comparative Orthopaedics and Traumatology* 13: 39–43.
84. Arthurs, G.I., and S.J. Langley-Hobbs. 2006. Complications associated with corrective surgery for patellar luxation in 109 dogs. *Veterinary Surgery* 35: 559–566.
85. DeAngelis, M., and R.B. Hohn. 1970. Evaluation and surgical correction of canine patellar luxation in 142 cases. *Journal of the American Veterinary Medical Association* 156: 587–594.
86. Miller, M.E., G.C. Christensen, and H.E. Evans. 1964. *Anatomy of the dog*. Philadelphia: W.B. Saunders.
87. Barnes, D.C., C.S. Knudsen, M. Gosling, M. McKee, R.G. Whitelock, G.I. Arthurs, M.G. Ness, H. Radke, and S.J. Langley-Hobbs. 2013. Complications of lateral plate fixation compared with tension band wiring and pin or lag screw fixation for calcaneoquartal arthrodesis. *Veterinary and Comparative Orthopaedics and Traumatology* 26: 445–452.
88. Dyce, J., R.G. Whitelock, K.V. Robinson, F. Forsythe, and J.E.F. Houlton. 1998. Arthrodesis of the tarsometatarsal joint using a laterally applied plate in 10 dogs. *The Journal of Small Animal Practice* 39: 19–22.
89. Harasen, G. 2002. Arthrodesis - part II: the tarsus. *The Canadian Veterinary Journal* 43: 806–808.
90. Hudson, C.C., and A. Pozzi. 2012. Minimally invasive repair of central tarsal bone luxation in a dog. *Veterinary and Comparative Orthopaedics and Traumatology* 25 (1): 79–82.
91. Lorinson, D., and K. Grosslinger. 2001. Central tarsal bone luxation in three non-racing dogs. *Veterinary and Comparative Orthopaedics and Traumatology* 14 (4): 229–231.
92. Newton, C.D. 1985. Fracture and luxation of the tarsus and metatarsus. In *Textbook of small animal orthopaedics*, ed. C.D. Newton and D.M. Nunamaker, 445–452. Philadelphia: J.B. Lippincott.
93. Theoret, M.C., and N.M.M. Moens. 2007. The use of veterinary cuttable plates for carpal and tarsal arthrodesis in small dogs and cats. *The Canadian Veterinary Journal* 48: 165–168.
94. Wilke, V.L., T.M. Robinson, and R.T. Dueland. 2000. Intertarsal and tarsometatarsal arthrodesis using a plantar approach: a carpal arthrodesis plate or dynamic compression plates: four arthrodeses in three dogs. *Veterinary and Comparative Orthopaedics and Traumatology* 13: 28–33.

95. Campbell, J.R., D. Bennett, and R. Lee. 1976. Intertarsal and tarsometatarsal subluxation in the dog. *The Journal of Small Animal Practice* 17: 427.
96. Singh, A.P., and R. Tayal. 2020. Section C: joints; the musculoskeletal system. In *Ruminant surgery, a textbook of the surgical diseases of cattle, buffaloes, camels, sheep and goats*, ed. G. Singh, S. Singh, and R.P.S. Tyagi. 2nd ed., 444–465. New Delhi: CBS Publishers and Distributors.
97. Hubert, J., and T.S. Stashak. 2011. Luxation of the scapulohumeral (shoulder) joint. In *Adams and Stashak's lameness in horses*, ed. G.M. Baxter, 6th ed., 717–718. Ames: Willey-Blackwell.
98. Hahn, J.A., F. Geburek, P. Stadler, and A.K. Rötting. 2011. Closed reduction of scapulohumeral joint luxation in an Icelandic horse after general anaesthesia. *Equine Veterinary Education* 23: 163–168.
99. Mizuguchi, Y., D. Miyakoshi, and M. Maeda. 2017. Scapulohumeral joint luxation in a thoroughbred racehorse during recovery from general anesthesia. *The Japanese Journal of Veterinary Research* 65 (2): 89–93.
100. Madison, J.B., D. Young, and D. Richardson. 1991. Repair of shoulder luxation in a horse. *Journal of the American Veterinary Medical Association* 198 (3): 455–456.
101. Semevolos, S.A., A.J. Nixon, L.R. Goodrich, and N.G. Ducharme. 1998. Shoulder joint luxation in large animals: 14 cases (1976-1997). *Journal of the American Veterinary Medical Association* 213 (11): 1608–1611.
102. Bottegaro, N.B., J. Gotic, H. Capak, and D. Huber. 2017. Elbow joint luxation in a ten month old Arabian colt- a case report. *Acta Veterinaria* 67 (3): 441. https://doi.org/10.1515/acve-2017-0036.
103. Devaux, D., J. Müller, M.A. Butty, A. Steiner, and K. Nuss. 2019. Lateral radioulnar subluxation in three cattle: clinical findings, treatment, and outcome. *Veterinary Surgery* 48 (7): 1271–1277.
104. Rubio-Martínez, L.M., F.J. Vázquez, A. Romero, and J.R. Ormazábal. 2008. Elbow joint luxation in a 1-month-old foal. *Australian Veterinary Journal* 86: 56–59.
105. Greenough, P.R. 2015. *Coxofemoral luxation in cattle*. Rahway, NJ: MSD Veterinary Manual. Merck & Co., Inc.
106. Larcombe, M.T., and J. Malmo. 1989. Dislocation of the coxo-femoral joint in dairy cows. *Australian Veterinary Journal* 66: 351–354.
107. Tulleners, E.P., D.M. Nunamaker, and D.W. Richardson. 1987. Coxofemoral luxations in cattle: 22 cases (1980-1985). *Journal of the American Veterinary Medical Association* 191: 569–574.
108. Starke, A., K. Herzog, J. Sohrt, V. Haist, A. Höhling, W. Baumgärtner, and J. Rehage. 2007. Diagnostic procedures and surgical treatment of craniodorsal coxofemoral luxation in calves. *Veterinary Surgery* 36 (2): 99–106.
109. Jubb, T., J. Malmo, G. Anderson, and G. Davis. 1989. Prognostic factors for recovery from coxofemoral dislocation in cattle. *Australian Veterinary Journal* 66: 354–358.
110. Reynolds, I.B. 1996. Reduction of dislocated hips. *The Bovine Practitioner* 30: 46–48.
111. Baird, A.N., K.L. Angel, H.D. Moll, et al. 1993. Upward fixation of the patella in cattle: 38 cases (1984-1990). *Journal of the American Veterinary Medical Association* 202: 343.
112. Dass, L.L., P.N. Sahay, and M. Ehsan. 1983. A report on the incidence of upward fixation of patella (stringhalt) in bovines of Chota Nagpur hilly terrain. *The Indian Veterinary Journal* 60: 628.
113. Greenough, P.R., F.J. Maccallum, and A.D. Weaver. 1972. Patellar luxation. In *Lameness in cattle*, ed. P.R. Greenough, F.J. Maccallum, and A.D. Weaver, 260. Philadelphia: Lippincott.
114. Johnson, R., and N.K. Ames. 1983. Upward fixation of the patella in a Holstein cow. *Agricultural Practice* 4: 13.
115. Leitch, M., and M. Kotlikoff. 1980. Surgical repair of congenital luxation of the patella in the foal and calf. *Veterinary Surgery* 9: 1.
116. Pallai, M.R. 1944. A note on chronic luxation of patella among bovines with special references to its etiology. *The Indian Veterinary Journal* 21: 48.
117. Philip, R.G. 1970. Lateral luxation of the patella in a calf. *The Veterinary Record* 86: 190.
118. Rahimuddin, M. 1944. Chronic luxation of the patella in cattle - an investigation. *The Indian Veterinary Journal* 21: 55.
119. Weaver, A.D. 1972. Surgical correction of lateral and medial patellar luxation in calves. *The Veterinary Record* 90: 567.
120. Singh, K., A. Gangwar, S. Devi, and N. Singh. 2015. Studies on incidence and evaluation of the closed medial patellar desmotomy in lateral recumbency in bovines. *Veterinary World* 8 (2): 221–224.
121. Ghasemi, S., K. Sardari, A. Mohamadnia, F. Alipour, A. Mirshahi, and M. Rajabioun. 2015. Surgical repair of lateral patellar luxation in two foals. *Iranian Journal of Veterinary Surgery* 10 (1): 59–63.
122. Abu-Seida, A.M. 2021. Luxation of the patella in foals: a treatment challenge. *Equine Veterinary Education*. https://doi.org/10.1111/eve.13475.
123. Hart, J.C.A., H.W. Jann, and V.J. Moorman. 2009. Surgical correction of a medial patellar luxation in a foal using a modified recession trochleoplasty technique. *Equine Veterinary Education* 21: 307–311.
124. Bailey, J.V., S.M. Barber, P.B. Fretz, and K.A. Jacobs. 1984. Subluxation of the carpus in thirteen horses. *The Canadian Veterinary Journal* 25 (8): 311–314.
125. Moll, H.D., D.E. Slone, J.M. Humburg, and J.E. Jagar. 1987. Traumatic tarsal luxation repaired without internal fixation in three horses and three ponies. *Journal of the American Veterinary Medical Association* 190 (3): 297–300.

# 12 Arthritis

**Learning Objectives**

You will be able to understand the following after reading this chapter:

- Traumatic arthritis—clinical signs, diagnosis, and treatment
- Septic (infectious) arthritis—causes, clinical signs, diagnosis and treatment, follow-up care, management, complications, and prognosis
- Osteoarthritis—pathophysiology, predisposing factors, clinical signs, diagnosis, and management
- Rheumatoid arthritis—clinical signs, diagnosis, and treatment


**Summary**

- Arthritis is an inflammation of a joint with secondary changes leading to pain, lameness, cartilage degeneration and reduced joint mobility. The most common form of arthritis in animals is osteoarthritis; other types include traumatic arthritis, septic arthritis and rheumatoid arthritis. Many times, a traumatic, septic, or immune mediated arthritis can progress to osteoarthritis.
- Traumatic arthritis is an inflammation of the joint following an injury to any structure of a joint, whereas septic arthritis is caused by an infective agent, most commonly bacteria.
- Septic arthritis is more common in dogs than cats and medium to large breed dogs aged 4–7 years are more prone. In small animals, common cause is direct exposure of joint after a traumatic injury or a surgical intervention, whereas the common route of joint infection in large animals is haematogenous spread.
- The aim of treatment in septic arthritis is early control of infection (administration of antibiotics- systemic or intra-articular) and inflammation (opioids and NSAIDs [non-steroidal anti-inflammatory drugs]), removal of infected joint fluid and debris (joint lavage) and restoration of joint function.
- Osteoarthritis or degenerative joint disease is caused by progressive degeneration of the joint cartilage leading to inflammation, pain and development of bone spurs and reduced joint range of motion. Predisposing factors include large or giant breeds, middle to old age, poor body conformation, abnormal joint


(continued)


H. P. Aithal et al., *Textbook of Veterinary Orthopaedic Surgery*,
https://doi.org/10.1007/978-981-99-2575-9_12

development, trauma or repetitive stress, improper nutrition, and genetic factors.
- Osteoarthritis cannot be cured; treatment should be aimed to slow down the progression of the disease and to control the pain and inflammation, thereby improving the quality of life. Surgical repair is recommended in severe cases of arthritis; it includes smoothening or realigning the joint surfaces through standard arthrotomy or arthroscopy and replacement of joint by a prosthetic implant.
- Rheumatoid arthritis, an autoimmune disease, is a chronic, progressive, destructive inflammatory arthropathy usually affecting several joints. Typical rheumatoid arthritis commonly seen in humans is rarely detected in animals, and it does not seem to cause severe problem in pet and domestic animals.

Arthritis is a common joint illness occurring in humans and animals alike [1–5]. Arthritis can be defined as inflammation of a joint with secondary changes leading to pain and reduced joint mobility. Typically, hyaline cartilage lines the ends of the bone at the joint, and the space in between is filled with joint fluid, which acts as a cushion for the bone ends and allows free movement of the joint without friction. Inflammation of joint can lead to swelling, pain, loss of joint mobility and lameness.

Among different pet and domestic animals, dogs and cats more often suffer from arthritis, but it is also common in all domestic animals. Like in human beings, the most common form of arthritis in animals is osteoarthritis (degenerative joint disease). The other types are categorized as traumatic arthritis, septic (infectious) arthritis and rheumatoid (immune-mediated) arthritis. Many times, a traumatic, septic, or immune-mediated arthritis can progress to osteoarthritis.

## 12.1 Traumatic Arthritis

Traumatic arthritis refers to inflammation of the joint (synovial membrane, synovitis, joint capsule, capsulitis) following an injury to the bone, cartilage (chip fractures) or ligament (tears) near or within a joint. Traumatic arthritis may be seen in any animal but more common in athletic animals. The condition may occur after a sudden trauma or due to prolonged stress, leading to inflammation and degradation of the articular cartilage. Mild inflammation of joint normally subsides on its own due to normal repair response of the body. Prolonged inflammation, either from acute or chronic injury, results in cascade of events. The inflammatory enzymes break down the synovial fluid (which becomes thin), and loss of integrity of proteoglycans and collagen fibers diminishes the cartilage's ability to retain the lubricating water. This further promotes inflammation, causing accumulation of fluid within the joint capsule, leading to pain and stiffness in the joint. The sharp increase in inflammatory enzymes further breaks down the synovial fluid, leading to degradation of the cartilage. Progressive loss of articular cartilage may lead to osteoarthritis, which can be the consequence of any traumatic injury to the joint [6].

### 12.1.1 Clinical Signs

Arthritis in general results in pain and alteration in the joint function. In early stages, excess accumulation of joint fluid leads to swelling and warmth in and around the joint, and palpation of the joint may elicit pain. In chronic cases, there can be thickening and fibrosis of connective tissue, leading to reduced range of the joint motion, varied degrees of lameness and gait abnormalities.

### 12.1.2 Diagnosis

Radiography can help to differentiate traumatic arthritis from other conditions such as osteochondral fractures or disease. In chronic cases of severe osteoarthritis, radiography may demonstrate loss of joint space, subchondral sclerosis and formation of osteophytes (Figs. 12.1 and 12.2). Arthroscopy may help visualize osteoarthritis in very early stage, and it is often used to diagnose tearing of ligaments or cartilage.

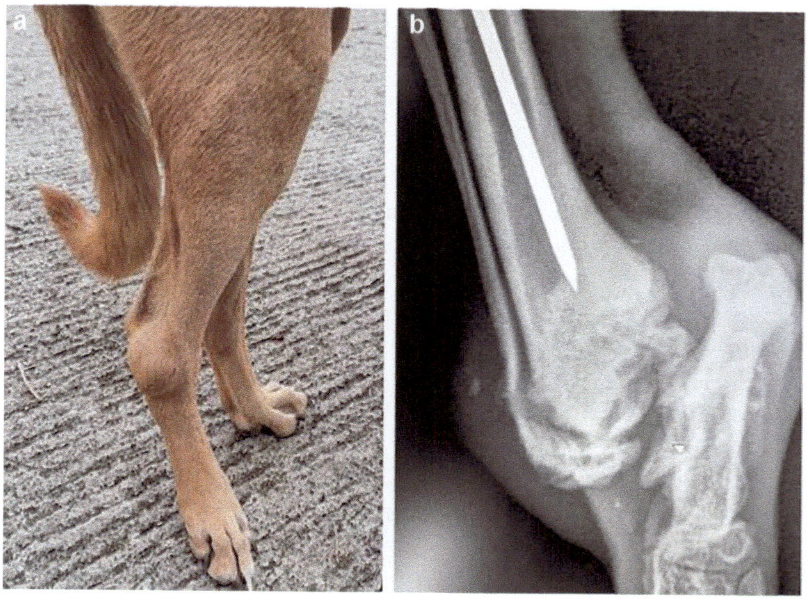


**Fig. 12.1** Traumatic injury to the joint leading to osteoarthritis of the hock joint of a dog: hard swelling around the joint (**a**), lateral radiograph showing subchondral bone lysis and degenerative changes (**b**). Note that the animal also had diaphyseal fracture of tibia stabilized with IM pin

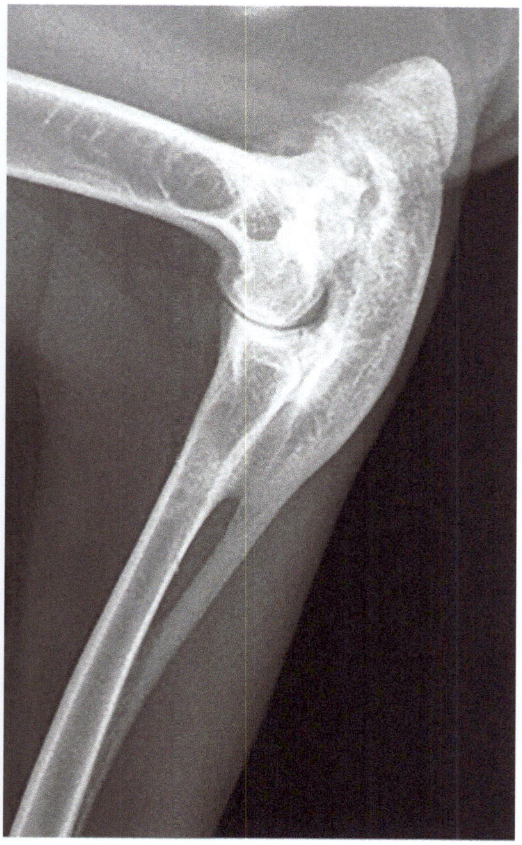

**Fig. 12.2** Lateral radiographic view of the elbow joint of a dog shows severe degenerative changes, attributed to old traumatic injury/fracture

### 12.1.3 Treatment

Providing rest and physical therapy protocols like cold water or ice treatment, passive joint motion and swimming are recommended in acute traumatic arthritis cases. Administration of non-steroidal anti-inflammatory drugs such as phenylbutazone or corticosteroids will help to relieve pain and inflammation. Lameness generally improves within 24–48 h.

The joint lavage is recommended to remove the inflammatory products and debris present in the synovial fluid. Intra-articular administration of corticosteroids has been found effective in treatment of acute traumatic arthritis cases (betamethasone and triamcinolone acetonide can be effective without any deleterious effect, whereas methylprednisolone acetate is longer acting and more potent but can cause significant adverse effects on the articular cartilage). Intra-articular injection of sodium hyaluronate has a chondroprotective effect in mild to moderate synovitis cases but it may be less effective in severe cases especially when intra-articular fractures are present. Polysulphated glycosaminoglycans can be effective in controlling synovitis and preventing ongoing degeneration of articular cartilage and are used frequently in traumatic arthritis cases.

Arthroscopic surgery is recommended to remove fragments of the bone and cartilage (most common in the carpus and fetlock joints in horses) and to minimize the chances for development of osteoarthritis. After the surgery, the animal should be rested for 4–6 months, and physiotherapy regimens followed during the recovery period. If the surgical correction is performed in the early stages with minimal osteoarthritic changes, the success is high with good prognosis.

## 12.2 Septic (Infectious) Arthritis

Septic or infectious arthritis is an inflammation of joint caused by an infective agent, most commonly bacteria [3, 7], but other microorganisms such as virus, fungi, and protozoa can also cause joint infection. Septic arthritis can be differentiated from other forms of arthritis by the presence of a pathogenic microorganism within the joint fluid.

Among the pets, septic arthritis is more common in dogs and is rare in cats. German shepherd, Doberman Pinschers and Labrador retrievers and other medium to large breeds of dog are more often affected. Although septic arthritis has been reported in all age groups, the dogs aged between four and seven years are more frequently affected. Male dogs are more frequently affected by the disease than the female dogs. Commonly, infection of a single joint is seen, but more than one joint may get affected in some cases. Septic arthritis is also common in both cattle and horses [8–10].

### 12.2.1 Causes of Infection

The most common source and route of joint infection are debated and are variable depending on the case. In small animals, septic arthritis is usually seen after an injury directly exposing the joint to external contamination and after a surgical intervention or intra-articular injection [11, 12]. However, contrary to the general belief, they are not always secondary to a trauma, but often the microorganisms can enter the joints from the blood stream [7, 13]. Infection of gastrointestinal tract, urinary tract, skin, and ear or other body systems can be a source of the microorganisms' gaining entry into the joint. Pre-existing joint diseases such as osteoarthritis, rheumatoid arthritis or even blunt trauma can predispose to haematogenous spread of infection. Dogs with immune suppression, diabetes mellitus or hypoadrenocorticism are at higher risk of developing septic arthritis. Intra-articular injections, especially of steroids, may further enhance the risk of developing septic arthritis.

However, the common route of joint infection is haematogenous spread both in adult and young large animals. The source of infection in adult animals (bovines) could be the postpartum diseases such as retained placenta, endometritis, mastitis, and endocarditis or concurrent orthopedic diseases. In young animals, umbilical infection (navel ill) is the most common source of joint infection, along with diarrhea and pneumonia [14]. Septic arthritis in foals is often accompanied with osteomyelitis. Other causes of joint infection are direct traumatic injury and iatrogenic infection through injections, arthrocentesis, or surgery. Usually only one joint is affected in adult animals; polyarthritis is more common in young calves and foals.

The most common bacteria isolated from joint infections in canines include aerobic bacteria such as *Staphylococcus* species (*S. aureus*, *S. intermedius*), *Streptococcus* species (*S. pyogenes*) and *Pasteurella*, apart from anaerobic bacteria like *Propionibacterium*, *Peptostreptococcus*, *Fusobacterium*, and *Bacteroides* [7, 11, 12]. In cattle, the most common bacteria isolated included *A. pyogenes*, *Streptococci*, *Staphylococci*, *E. coli* and *Bacteroides* sp. [8]. Often infectious agents such as *Brucella* and *Mycoplasma* have been found to cause polyarthritis.

Once the infectious agent enters the synovial space, it elicits severe inflammatory and immunological responses. Bacteria can directly damage the articular cartilage and the synovial membrane altering the composition of the joint fluid. Further, inadequate nutrition and enzymatic degradation leads to degeneration of the articular cartilage; the break-down products further cause synovitis. This vicious cycle continues until proper treatment is initiated to control the infection.

### 12.2.2 Clinical Signs

The history in most cases reveals acute onset of lameness involving a single joint (monoarticular arthritis), and rarely multiple joints are involved (if four or fewer joints are involved, it is called as pauciarticular arthritis, and if five or more joints are involved, it is known as polyarticular arthritis). Lameness is typically associated with warm swollen joints (increased joint effusion and soft tissue swelling), pain on manipulation and decreased range of joint motion [7]. Systemic illness is uncommon with an infected joint, but often the animal may show increased body temperature, anorexia, and lethargy. In some cases, the lameness can be less severe and chronic. But generally there is prolonged lameness that often worsens with time.

### 12.2.3 Diagnosis

Animals presented with symptoms of lameness and joint swelling give an indication of arthritis. History of any previous injury or illness and a detailed physical examination of the animal can help to establish the involvement of one or more joints, but they do not provide a definitive diagnosis of septic arthritis. Radiography/ultrasonography, synovial fluid analysis and other laboratory findings will help arrive at definitive diagnosis of septic arthritis [13, 15].

Synovial fluid analysis of joint is a simple but important diagnostic test for infectious arthritis. Under sedation and fully aseptic conditions, synovial fluid is collected by performing a joint tap (arthrocentesis). Cytological analysis can be made directly on smeared slides while sampling or from analysis of synovial fluid collected in vials containing EDTA (ethylenediamine tetraacetic acid). Synovial fluid sample is also subjected to bacterial culture examination. Grossly there will be increased volume of synovia along with change in its color (yellowish to reddish brown) and odor, reduced viscosity, increased turbidity and fibrin content. Cytological examination may reveal an increased level of WBCs (white blood cells) (>25,000/ µl), especially neutrophils (polymorphonuclear cells) (>80%) and total protein (>4.5 g/dl) [11, 16]. Bacterial culture and antibacterial sensitivity testing would confirm the diagnosis, but unfortunately culture is not always successful, and only in 50–80% cases bacteria can be isolated [16, 17]. Synovial membrane biopsy, which is more invasive, however, produces much more reliable culture results.

Complete blood count, blood biochemistry profile and urinalysis may be indicated to rule out any concurrent disease. The results of these tests in cases of septic arthritis are usually normal, except for the complete blood count (neutrophilia), which may indicate the presence of infection and inflammation in the body. The acute phase protein, serum or synovial fluid serum amyloid A (SAA), has been found to have potential to be used as an adjunct in diagnosis of septic arthritis in the horse, and it can be useful for monitoring the progression of the disease and response to treatment [18, 19]. In patients where septic arthritis is suspected to be associated with infection of other body systems, blood and urine samples may be subjected to culture examination, which may help in establishing the diagnosis and planning treatment.

Radiographic changes in septic arthritis may vary with the type and duration of infection. In the early stages of acute infection, there may be evidence of joint effusions, soft tissue swelling around the joint, accumulation of gas in the joint and widening of the joint space (due to fluid accumulation) (Fig. 12.3). In later stages (after about two weeks), there can be periosteal bone reaction around the joint and subchondral bone lysis [7] (Fig. 12.4). In chronic cases, more severe changes related to bone destruction, irregular or narrowing of joint space due to loss of cartilage,

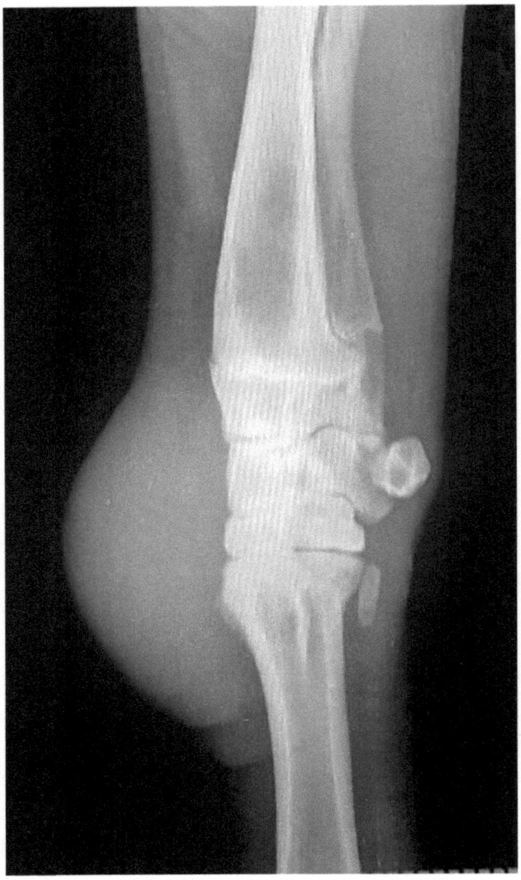

**Fig. 12.3** Lateral radiograph of carpal joint of a calf with early stage of infectious arthritis showing a large soft tissue swelling on the cranial aspect (Courtesy: Dr. RV Suryawanshi, KNPCVAS, Shirwal, Satara, Maharashtra, India)

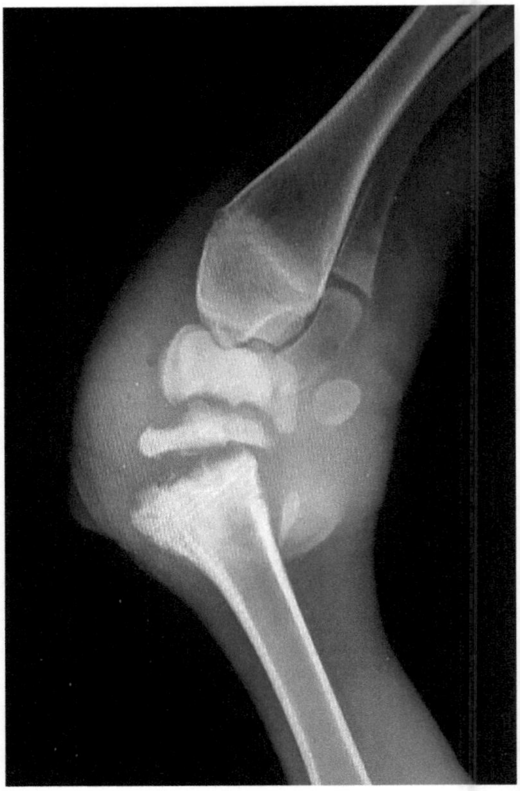

**Fig. 12.4** Lateral radiograph of carpal joint of a calf with septic arthritis shows soft tissue swelling around the joint and lytic changes in the joint. (Courtesy: Dr. RV Suryawanshi, KNPCVAS, Shirwal, Satara, Maharashtra, India)

and abnormal bone formation within the joint and the surrounding soft tissues can be visible. In more advanced cases, subluxation of the joint may be appreciable due to severe soft tissue damage. Ultrasonography will be more useful to evaluate changes in soft tissues including synovial membrane, joint fluid and periarticular tissues.

### 12.2.4 Treatment

Prompt recognition (diagnosis and cause) of the joint infection and initiation of treatment will facilitate early recovery and return to function. The aim of treatment in septic arthritis is early control of infection and inflammation, removal of infected joint fluid and debris and restoration of joint function. In majority of cases, surgery may not be required and can be managed medically with a good prognosis and functional recovery [11].

In principle, administration of antibiotic should be initiated as early as the joint infection is diagnosed or suspected [7, 10]. Ideally, antibiotic should be selected based on culture and sensitivity testing. Broad-spectrum antibiotics (cefuroxime or amoxicillin/clavulanate, cephalosporins, gentamicin or ampicillin) should be administered systemically (by IM or IV route) at the earliest, until microbial culture results are obtained. Subsequently antibiotic should be changed as per the culture results. However, due to higher intra-articular pressure and viscosity, reduced pH and presence of peri-articular oedema, MIC (minimum inhibitory concentration) of an antibiotic is difficult to reach within the joint cavity when administered systemically. Hence systemic antibiotic administration should be accompanied with intra-articular injections. Intra-articular administration has the advantage of attaining good concentration of drug at the site of infection even with reduced dose, thus causing minimal systemic side effects; however, its disadvantage is the need for repeated joint pricks. Gentamicin is the drug most often used for intra-articular injections. Intra-articular injection should be preceded by joint lavage, when possible though the same punctured needle. Simultaneously the primary source of infection should also be detected and treated aggressively. Antibiotic treatment should be continued for 4–8 weeks or until 2 weeks after resolution of clinical signs. Generally a positive response will be noticed within 5–10 days of initiation of treatment.

Joint lavage is indicated to remove the infected synovial fluid and other debris [11]. This can be achieved either by repeated aspiration and irrigation through the same needle or by through and through lavage using two or more needles (16–20G needles and 20–50 mL syringes). In any case, the joint is thoroughly irrigated/flushed using sterile Ringers/lactated Ringers solution (1–2 L) until there is complete flushing of infected joint fluid and clear fluid comes out. Initially joint lavage should be carried out once daily for 3–4 days; by then the signs of improvement are generally seen. If needed later, it can be repeated once every alternate day until the condition improves and the WBC count recedes. Arthroscopic lavage and repeated intra-articular administration of antibiotic in adult horses and foals with septic arthritis has been shown to decrease the synovial nucleated cell counts and total protein concentrations [20]. The studies have shown that sodium hyaluronate with antibiotic therapy and joint lavage appears to be more beneficial than lavage alone for treatment of septic arthritis [21].

Endoscopy/arthroscopy can be used to examine the joint structures, to remove the debris and fibrin clots and also to curette the lytic bone [10, 15, 22]. It is always done under general anesthesia. When arthroscopy is not feasible (either due to non-availability or cost considerations), an arthrotomy can be considered [23], wherein slightly elongated incision is given to allow visual examination and drainage. Arthrotomy incision can be either primarily closed or left as such to allow drainage and heal by second intention.

The decision whether to go for conservative lavage or surgical drainage of joint by arthrotomy or arthroscopy should be taken based on the stage of arthritis/tenosynovitis. In mild infection with serous to serofibrinous synovial fluid, lavage therapy may be chosen, whereas in severe arthritis with fibrinous, purulent or putrid joint fluid, surgical treatment may be preferred to get better results. In chronic cases, which do not respond to lavage and antibiotic treatment and restoration of joint function is difficult, ankylosis of the joint may be performed.

Even though administration of antibiotic and drainage of joint fluid are the important approaches to treat joint infection, non-steroidal anti-inflammatory drugs (and opioids) may be given in the acute cases to reduce inflammation and control pain. However, prolonged administration of NSAIDs should be avoided to prevent cartilage damage and development of ulcers, especially in young animals. Ice packs may be applied for 10–15 min 4–6 times a day to reduce acute swelling and pain (warm packs are contraindicated in infected tissues and in acute stage). The animal's activity and movement should be restricted to prevent further damage to the articular cartilage and the surrounding soft tissues. Joint immobilization (application of cast or splints) may provide comfort to the animal (minimize the movement and pain) and facilitate healing of joint but should be used only for limited period.

The animals should be monitored regularly by clinical signs and regular fluid analyses to assess the effectiveness of treatment. Prognosis of joint infection depends on the chronicity of the condition; good outcome can be achieved in early cases by prompt diagnosis and proper treatment.

### 12.2.5 Follow-Up Care, Management, Complications, and Prognosis

Close monitoring and follow-up are vital in cases of joint infection. Treatment protocol should be properly followed, while keeping a close watch on the signs and symptoms of infection. Joint fluid should be subjected to microscopic evaluation every 1–2 weeks to assess response to therapy and ensure that the infection does not rebound. Antibiotic therapy should be extended for at least two weeks even after resolution of the signs of infection to prevent possible recurrence.

Physiotherapy with passive range of motion may be adopted, which will help prevent muscle contracture and cartilage degeneration and maintain joint mobility. It is also recommended to apply alternating cold and heat packs on the affected joint to enhance blood circulation, decrease swelling and thus promote healing and recovery.

Persistence of joint inflammation may be observed in some patients even after bacterial infection is subsided, which may be attributed antigen-antibody deposition or residual antigenic bacterial fragments. In such cases it has been recommended to use low dose of steroids (prednisolone 0.1–0.2 mg/kg PO once daily), but steroid treatment should be given only after ensuring that the culture results are negative.

Complications of infectious arthritis may include development of degenerative joint disease, persistence or recurrence of joint infection, restricted range of motion of affected joints, generalized infection spreading to other parts of the body from the septic joint, and bone infection or osteomyelitis.

Prognosis of the infectious arthritis depends on the type of infection and also its chronicity. Acute cases diagnosed early may respond well within 24–48 h to antibiotic therapy, and in chronic cases with delayed diagnosis and treatment, response is guarded. Medical and/or surgical treatment may help resolve infection in most cases, but often it is unsuccessful in restoring full joint function [11].

## 12.3 Osteoarthritis

Osteoarthritis is a degenerative joint disease (DJD) caused by progressive deterioration in the joint cartilage leading to inflammation, pain, development of bone spurs and reduced joint range of motion [1, 5, 24]. It is considered to be the most common cause of chronic pain both in pets and domestic animals. It has been documented that at least 20% of dogs above 1 year and about 90% of cats over 12 years of age are known to develop osteoarthritis. Even though osteoarthritis can be seen in animals of any age group, middle-aged and older animals are often affected. The condition most commonly affects the limb joints and the lower spine. Commonly affected joints in dogs include the hip, elbow, and shoulder, followed by the stifle, carpus, tarsus, and spine (Figs. 12.5 and 12.6), whereas the commonly affected joints in cats are the shoulder, hip, elbow, carpus, and tarsus. In working/athletic equines, osteoarthritic changes are more commonly reported in the fetlock and pastern joints (Fig. 12.7). In cattle and buffaloes, hind limb joints are commonly affected [14, 25].

### 12.3.1 Pathophysiology

Typical synovial joints consist of synovial membrane (joint capsule, made up of dense connective tissue), synovial fluid (a clear viscous fluid) and articular cartilage (hyaline cartilage). The synovial fluid secreted by the synovial membrane (synoviocytes) predominantly consists of hyaluronic acid and glycosaminoglycans (proteins that impart viscosity to the fluid), acts as a lubricant and also provides nutrition to the articular cartilage. The articular cartilage is avascular, and it consists of chondroblasts and chondrocytes embedded in extracellular matrix essentially consisting of collagens and proteoglycans. The presence of abundant collagen type II in the cartilage matrix acts as a shock absorber by distributing load over the subchondral bone. In normal conditions, any small injuries to the cartilage are healed naturally

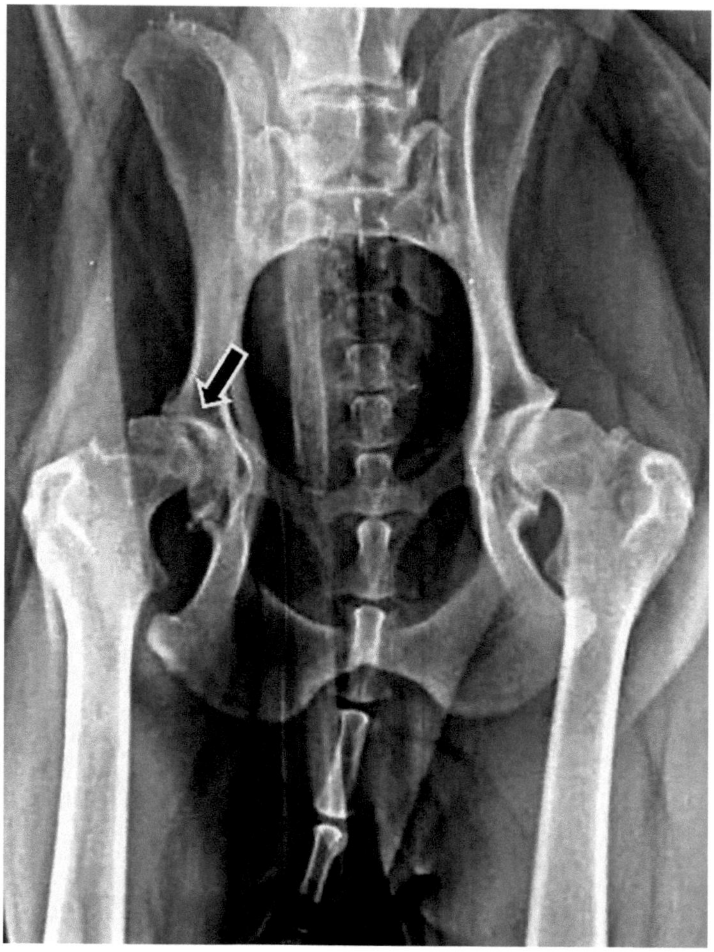

**Fig. 12.5** VD radiographic view of hip joints of a dog with chronic hip dysplasia shows severe degenerative changes such as subchondral bone lysis, osteophyte formation, irregular flattened surfaces of femoral head and acetabulum and luxation of coxo-femoral joint, more pronounced on one side (arrow)

with a fine balance between chondroblast and chondroclast activity. In arthritis, this balance is disturbed and there is overproduction of osteoblasts causing pain and inflammation.

Four different progressive stages have been described for osteoarthritis. In the first stage (initial), due to changes in the chondrocytes' metabolism, there is increased production of lytic enzymes metalloproteinases (MMPs), initiating breakdown of cartilage matrix. This leads to increased friction, instability, and development of bone spurs resulting in inflammation and pain in joint. In the second stage (mild), continued damage and erosion of cartilage lead to the release of proteoglycans and collagen fragments into the synovial fluid. Erosion of subchondral bone occurs causing osteophyte (bone spur) formation, which will further increase pain and affect the joint motion. In the third stage (moderate), due to loss of cartilage cushion, the distance between the adjacent bones gets narrowed (reduced joint space) causing fraction between the subchondral bones and fragments of the cartilage and bone may be seen floating in the joint space (joint mice). Synovial macrophages start releasing MMPs, cytokines, and tumor necrosis factor-alpha, causing further destruction of tissues. In the fourth stage (severe), due to complete destruction of joint cartilage and more new bone formation, joint space is drastically reduced, and the joint movement is severely affected.

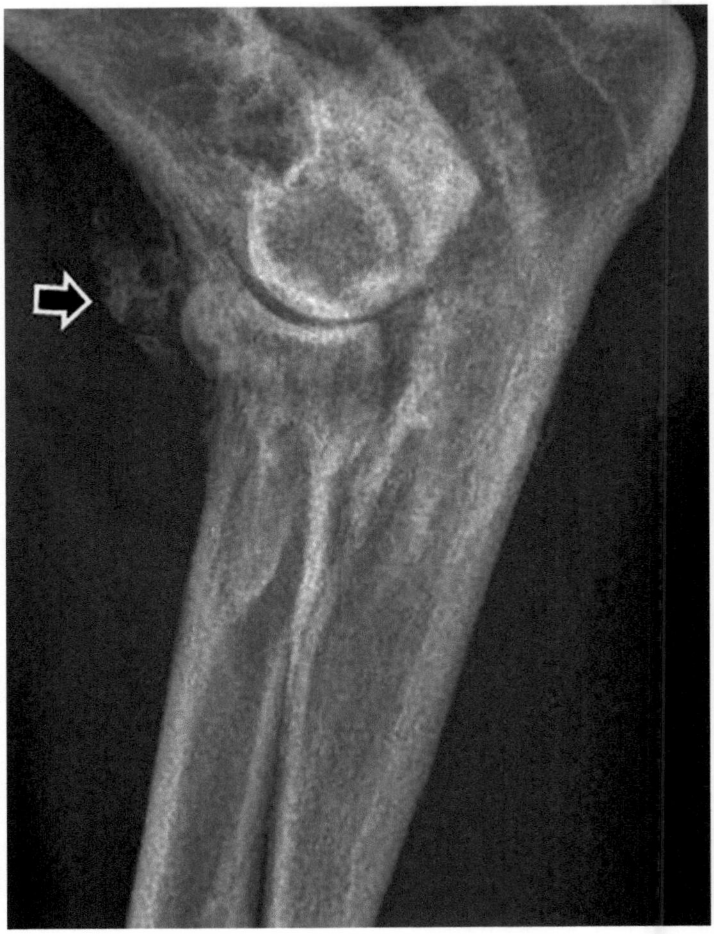

**Fig. 12.6** Lateral radiographic view of the elbow joint of a dog showing degenerative changes with osteophyte formation on the cranial surface (arrow)

### 12.3.2 Predisposing Factors

While any dog can develop osteoarthritis, there are some factors which predispose the dog to develop this condition [6, 26]. Large or giant breeds (such as German shepherds, Golden retrievers and Labrador retrievers) and middle-age to old-age dogs are more susceptible. Poor body conformation (overweight or obese), abnormal joint development (hip or elbow dysplasia, luxating patella, etc.), history of trauma (old fracture, ligament or muscle injury, joint infection, etc.) or repetitive stress (such as agility, jumping, or diving), improper nutrition and genetic factors (some cat and dog breeds are more prone) can predispose to arthritis [27]. In large animals, it is usually the end stage of most of other diseases such as traumatic and infectious arthritis.

### 12.3.3 Clinical Signs

Symptoms of osteoarthritis are often difficult to recognize in the early stages. Mild symptoms in the initial stages may not be noticed, but as the condition worsens with the time, the symptoms become obvious even when the animal is resting. Animals with arthritis can exhibit many different signs, but they may not necessarily demonstrate all the signs at the same time. There may be varying extent of synovial effusion and enlargement of joint, joint stiffness and diminished mobility. The animals may feel difficulty in getting up and down and show varying degrees of lameness/limping in one or more legs [28]. The lameness is usually progressive over a period of time, and often it improves after exercise. Sometimes the animals may not exhibit lameness and

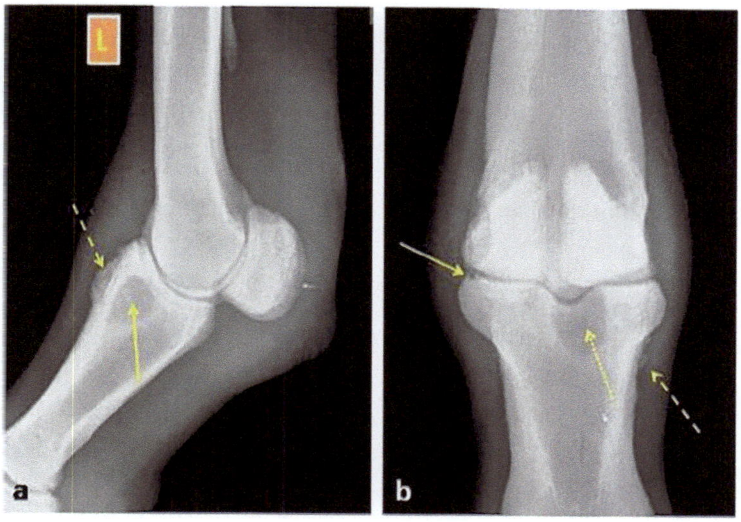


**Fig. 12.7** Latero-medial radiograph of a 15-year-old horse shows irregular periosteal reaction on the dorso-proximal aspect of the first phalanx extending up to the articular cartilage (dashed arrow) (**a**). On dorso-palmar view (**b**), spur-like bony projection is visible on the medial articular part of first phalanx (dashed arrow); enthesiophytes can be seen on the lateral border of first phalanx where lateral sesamoidean ligaments insert (dotted arrow). Periosteal reaction is observed in the depression of the medial collateral ligament attachment region (dashed dot arrow). An oval lytic lesion measuring 1 cm can also be seen in the proximal aspect of the first phalanx in both the views suggesting a bone cyst (line arrow). These findings are suggestive of osteoarthritis involving the metacarpophalangeal joint (Source: K. Balamurugan et al., Radiographic and Ultrasonographic Evaluation of Osteoarthritic Metacarpophalangeal joints in Working Equines, Indian J Vet Surg 41(1): 53–55, 2020)

move normally even when the arthritic changes are visible in radiographs. Local nerve blocks can be used to confirm the lameness and localize the site of pain. Other signs may include abnormal posture, stiff walking, hesitation to climb up or down stairs, reluctance to jump up or down, stiff and swollen joint(s), muscle atrophy (due to inactivity), pain on palpation and movement of the joint, loss of appetite, lethargy, depression, weight gain, loss of stamina (get tired easily), and change in behavior with unexpected aggression (bite, snap, or vocalize).

### 12.3.4 Diagnosis

Osteoarthritis is diagnosed through a combination of physical examination, clinical and laboratory tests and diagnostic imaging techniques. Physical examination such as palpation will help to localize the site of pain and determine its intensity. Laboratory analysis of body fluids (blood, urine, and joint effusions) will help determine the type of arthritis. A multitude of blood tests such as erythrocyte sedimentation test, complete blood counts (non-specific), c-reactive protein quantity, presence of antinuclear antibody (ANA) and estimation of rheumatoid factor (specific) can be used to diagnose arthritis. Radiography can help visualize the bone damage and bone spur formation [29]. As X-rays cannot directly visualize the cartilage, radiography may not show early arthritic changes, but they are usually used to monitor the progression of the disease, whereas computerized tomography (CT) can help visualize changes in both the bone and the surrounding soft tissues. Magnetic resonance imaging (MRI) produces detailed cross-sectional images of the soft tissues such as cartilage, tendons, and ligaments. CT scans are usually recommended for the elbow, tarsus, and carpus joints, and MRIs are used more often for the shoulder, stifle, and spine. Ultrasonography can be useful to image soft tissues and fluid-containing structures near the joints (bursae) and cartilage, and it can be used to guide placement of the needle for fluid aspirations and joint injections. Arthroscopy or arthrotomy can help to directly visualize the arthritic changes in the joint.

### 12.3.5 Management

Osteoarthritis is a progressive disease that cannot be cured by treatment, but it has to be 'managed' by slowing the progression of the disease by controlling pain and inflammation and improving quality of life. Management of osteoarthritis is usually multimodal [28, 30], which includes confinement and rest (which can be the first line of treatment in an arthritic animal, as it helps preventing more damage to the inflamed tissues), medication to control pain and inflammation, proper diet, exercise, and the use of protective joint supplements to improve the joint strength and function.

*Medications:* Analgesics such as acetaminophen can be used to control pain. In cases of severe pain, opioids such as tramadol, oxycodone, or hydrocodone may be given, but their prolonged use should be avoided. The use of non-steroidal anti-inflammatory drugs (NSAIDs – phenylbutazone, meclofenamic acid and ketoprofen), which reduce both pain and inflammation (oral, parenteral administration or local application of creams or gels), is more beneficial [2]. Some counter-irritant creams and ointments containing menthol or capsaicin may be applied over the affected joint to reduce the transmission of pain signals and thus help relieve pain. Corticosteroids (prednisone and dexamethasone), which reduce inflammation and suppress the immune system, are also recommended to treat osteoarthritis (administered orally or injected directly into the affected joint). Intra-articular injections of hyaluronic acid and glycosaminoglycans have been found beneficial to control inflammation within the joint and help re-build the lubricating fluid. Gabapentin, which is known to reduce pain (which acts differently from NSAIDs or corticosteroids), has also been used to treat chronic osteoarthritic pain, especially in older patients who are unable to take a NSAID.

Anti-rheumatic, immune suppressant drugs such as methotrexate and hydroxychloroquine used to treat rheumatoid arthritis have also been found beneficial in osteoarthritis cases. Genetically engineered drugs (targeting protein molecules involved in the immune reaction) such as tumor necrosis factor inhibitors (etanercept and infliximab) are commonly prescribed. Other medications targeting other substances involved in inflammation, including interleukin-1 (IL-1) and interleukin-6 (IL-6), have been found beneficial. Disease-modifying osteoarthritis drug (DMAOD) such as sodium pentosan polysulphate (semi-synthetic, polysulphated polysaccharide) having anti-inflammatory and anti-arthritis properties has been recommended for injection into the joint (at 5–7-day intervals); it is known to inhibit MMPs and maintain the cartilage structure and integrity.

Miscellaneous treatments such as acupuncture, massage, and stem cell therapy are also becoming popular to treat osteoarthritis in dogs. Mesenchymal stem cells are known to release anti-inflammatory chemicals that are thought to repair the damaged cartilage, though their mode of their action is little known. Stem cell therapy seems to be beneficial in treatment and prevention of osteoarthritis in human and animal patients. Even though many classes of drugs have been found beneficial and can be used in osteoarthritic cases, a suitable combination of drugs is generally used based on the case situation.

*Diet and supplements:* Several diets or dietary supplements (nutraceuticals) containing essential fatty acids (omega 3 fatty acids, which reduce inflammation), glycosaminoglycans (which are known to be building blocks of cartilage) and antioxidants have been recommended in arthritic animals. Glucosamine and chondroitin are two common ingredients used in joint supplements for both human and animal patients. These supplements are often used to reduce inflammation, promote healing, increase water retention in the cartilage and thus slow the progression of joint damage.

*Exercise:* Exercise is recommended for treatment of arthritis as it has several beneficial effects. Exercise can stimulate the production of joint fluid, which lubricates and nourishes joint cartilage. Exercise can also improve range of motion of the joint and strengthen the muscles, tendons and ligaments surrounding joints and thus prevents worsening of arthritis. It also helps to maintain the body weight of arthritic animals and prevents them from becoming obese and reduces the extra load on joints.

*Other modalities:* Several physiotherapy modalities such as therapeutic LASER (light amplification by stimulated emission of radiation), therapeutic exercise, joint mobilization, hydrotherapy, and acupuncture [31, 32] have also been used in the treatment of arthritis in animals.

*Surgical treatment*: In some cases such as traumatic injuries with fractures involving the joint or ligament tears, surgery might be required at initial diagnosis to slow down the progression of arthritis. However, surgical repair is commonly recommended in severe cases of arthritis when conservative measures do not improve the condition. Through standard arthrotomy incision or arthroscopy, the joint surfaces can be smoothened or realigned to minimize pain and increase joint function. Surgical replacement of the damaged joint by a prosthetic implant has also been recommended wherever possible (hip and knee joints most common). Arthrodesis (fusion of joints) can be performed as a last resort in certain lower limb joints. Fetlock arthrodesis can be successful in valuable animals (breeding cattle and horses) making them comfortable and breeding fit. However, arthrodesis of distal tarsal joint and pastern joint may affect athletic soundness of animals.

Management of arthritic dog needs a holistic approach; apart from hospital treatment, day-to-day management by the animal owner is also equally important. The arthritic patient should be housed in non-skid floor with soft padded bedding. Food and water may be provided in raised (elbow height) platforms. A ramp may be provided to walk up or down the stairs or vehicles. Regular medication, diet, and exercise schedule should be followed to improve joint functioning and to provide comfort to the patient. With proper management, an animal with osteoarthritis can live a normal life, but it is important to remember that its activities have to be modified and adjusted as per the changing body conditions. The prognosis is generally not favorable in chronic severe cases but in low-grade arthritic cases treated appropriately may respond favorably without any recurring signs of pain and lameness.

## 12.4 Rheumatoid Arthritis

It is an autoimmune disease, wherein the body starts attacking its own proteins mistakenly considering them as foreign subjects eventually leading to erosion of the cartilage and subchondral bone. It is a chronic, progressive, destructive inflammatory joint disease, usually affecting several joints simultaneously. Rheumatoid arthritis is very common in humans, but it is rarely detected in animals and it does seem to cause severe problem in pet and domestic animals [33–39].

The cause of rheumatoid arthritis is unknown, just like in human beings. In dogs, it sometimes appears as a complication of other diseases such as canine distemper. Rheumatoid arthritis can be either 'idiopathic' or 'erosive' type. Idiopathic disease can occur in all dogs, but most commonly, it affects small breeds such as Miniature Poodle and Shetland sheepdog; and it is mostly observed in dogs aged 2–4 years. Whereas erosive disease affects Greyhounds, mostly young animals aged below 2–2½ years of age. Both types of rheumatoid arthritis affect male and female dogs equally. In cats, feline progressive polyarthritis, which resembles human rheumatoid arthritis, occurs due to an autoimmune dysfunction that causes destruction of the joint cartilage and subchondral bone, resulting in swelling, pain, and joint deformation. Even in horses, a true immune-mediated rheumatoid arthritis is not often diagnosed; a very similar inflammatory process causing inflammation of synovial membrane and joint swelling has been commonly observed. Rheumatoid-like arthritis has also been reported in calves.

### 12.4.1 Clinical Signs

Symptoms of rheumatoid arthritis in animals can vary greatly and may include lameness, stiffness, fever, joint pain and swelling [33]. Often lameness is the only clinical sign noticed, but it can shift from one leg to another and sometimes may disappear completely. Usually multiple joints may show the symptoms of pain and swelling. Other non-specific symptoms may include muscle wasting, inappetence, enlarged lymph nodes, tonsillitis, etc.

### 12.4.2 Diagnosis

Diagnosis of rheumatoid arthritis is difficult as the occurrence is rare in animals and symptoms are non-specific. Radiography may help to detect joint swelling and bony changes in chronic cases. Radiographs may also show generalized reduction in bony mass. Blood tests may help to detect inflammatory changes and the rheumatoid factor; however, the rheumatoid factor (RF) may not be detected in all the animals having rheumatoid arthritis [33]. Measurement of IgA-RF may be useful to diagnose rheumatoid arthritis in dogs [40]. Analysis of synovial fluid may reveal arthritic changes.

### 12.4.3 Treatment

The aim of treatment in rheumatoid arthritis is only to reduce pain and provide comfort to the patient, as the condition cannot be cured. Treatment often includes administration of anti-inflammatory drugs, steroids, and other immunosuppressive drugs [35, 36]. Drugs such as methotrexate, cyclosporine, cyclophosphamide, and azathioprine used for the treatment of rheumatoid/immune-mediated arthritis in human beings can also be used in dogs [37, 41]. In recent years, various novel therapeutics such as B-cell depletion agents, tumor necrosis factor-α inhibitors, interleukin-6 receptor blockers and T-cell co-stimulatory blockers are used as disease-modifying antirheumatic drugs (DMARDs) for the treatment of rheumatoid arthritis [36]. Prognosis is generally guarded. Routine physical exercise, especially low-impact exercise such as swimming, is indicated. Providing warmth at the place of stay will provide comfort to the animal. Relapse of arthritic symptoms is relatively common.

## Chapter 12: Sample Questions

**Question No. 1: Mark the correct answer**

1. The most common form of arthritis in animals is osteoarthritis
   (a) degenerative arthritis (b) infectious arthritis (c) traumatic arthritis (d) rheumatoid arthritis
2. Inflammation of the synovial membrane and articular surfaces, resulting from localisation of microbes, is called as
   (a) degenerative arthritis (b) infectious arthritis (c) traumatic arthritis (d) rheumatoid arthritis
3. Radiographic signs of chronic severe osteoarthritis does not include
   (a) Increase in joint space (b) decrease in joint space (c) subchondral sclerosis (d) osteophyte formation
4. Methotrexate can be used for the treatment of
   (a) traumatic arthritis (b) septic arthritis (c) osteoarthritis (d) rheumatoid arthritis

**Question No. 2: State true or false**

1. A traumatic, septic, or immune-mediated arthritis can often progress to osteoarthritis.
2. Septic arthritis is more common in cats and is rare in dogs.
3. Usually only one joint is affected in young calves and foals, whereas polyarthritis is more common in adult animals.

4. Bacterial culture and isolation may confirm the diagnosis of infectious arthritis, and failure to isolate bacteria can rule out septic arthritis.
5. Narrowing of the joint space is a common sign in the early stages of infectious arthritis, and in later stages, widening of joint space is characteristic.
6. Intra-articular administration of antibiotic can result in good concentration of drug at the site of infection even with reduced dose.
7. Rheumatoid arthritis is very common in humans, but it is rarely detected in animals.

**Question No. 3: Fill up the blanks**

1. The common route of joint infection in large animals is ________________________________.
2. In young calves, the most common source of joint infection is ________________________________.
3. Infectious arthritis can be diagnosed using a simple test of ________________________________.
4. Mild infection with serous to serofibrinous synovial fluid can be treated by ________________________, whereas in severe arthritis with fibrinous, purulent or putrid joint fluid, ________________________ is generally preferred.
5. Persistence of joint inflammation even after bacterial infection is subsided may be attributed to ________________________ or ________________________.
6. The synovial fluid predominantly consisting of ________________________ and ________________________ acts as a lubricant and also provides nutrition to the articular cartilage.
7. Anti-rheumatic and immune suppressant drugs used to treat rheumatoid arthritis and osteoarthritis are ________________________ and ________________________.
8. Rheumatoid arthritis in dogs can be either ________________________ or ________________________ type.

**Question No. 4: Write short note on the following:**

1. Differentiate between infectious and degenerative arthritis
2. Pathophysiology of osteoarthritis
3. Management of infectious arthritis
4. Rheumatoid arthritis in animals

## References


1. Bland, S.D. 2015. Canine osteoarthritis and treatments: a review. *Veterinary Science Development* 5. https://doi.org/10.4081/vsd.2015.5931.
2. Goodrich, L.R., and A.J. Nixon. 2006. Medical treatment of osteoarthritis in the horse - a review. *Veterinary Journal* 171 (Suppl.1): 51–69.
3. May, C. 2005. Diagnosis and management of bacterial infective arthritis in dogs and cats. *In Practice* 27 (6): 316–321.
4. Meeson, R.L., R.J. Todhunter, G. Blunn, G. Nuki, and A.A. Pitsillides. 2019. Spontaneous dog osteoarthritis – a one medicine vision. *Nature Reviews Rheumatology* 15: 273–287.
5. Nichols, S., and H. Lardé. 2014. Noninfectious joint disease in cattle. *The Veterinary Clinics of North America. Food Animal Practice* 30 (Suppl.1): 205–223.
6. Martinez, S.A., and G.S. Coronodo. 1997. Acquired conditions that lead to osteoarthritis in the dog. *The Veterinary Clinics of North America. Small Animal Practice* 27 (4): 759–775.
7. Bennett, D., and D.J. Taylor. 1988. Bacterial infective arthritis in the dog. *The Journal of Small Animal Practice* 29 (4): 207–230.
8. Constant, C., S. Nichols, A. Desrochers, M. Babkine, G. Fecteau, H. Lardé, J.H. Fairbrother, and D.J. Francoz. 2018. Clinical findings and diagnostic test results for calves with septic arthritis: 64 cases (2009-2014). *American Veterinary Medical Association* 252 (8): 995–1005.
9. Morton, A.J. 2005. Diagnosis and treatment of septic arthritis. *The Veterinary Clinics of North America. Equine Practice* 21: 627–649.
10. Mulon, P.Y., A. Desrochers, and D. Francoz. 2016. Surgical management of septic arthritis. *The Veterinary Clinics of North America. Food Animal Practice* 32 (3): 777–795.
11. Marchevsky, A.M., and R.A. Read. 1999. Bacterial septic arthritis in 19 dogs. *Australian Veterinary Journal* 77 (4): 233–237.

12. Schneider, R., L. Bramlage, R. Moore, L.M. Mecklenburg, C.W. Kohn, and A.A. Gabel. 1992. A retrospective study of 192 horses affected with septic arthritis/tenosynovitis. *Equine Veterinary Journal* 24: 436–442.
13. Constant, C., I. Masseau, M. Babkine, S. Nichols, D. Francoz, G. Fecteau, E. Marchionatti, H. Larde, and A. Desrochers. 2018. Radiographic study of haematogenous septic arthritis in dairy cows. *Veterinary and Comparative Orthopaedics and Traumatology* 31: 252–260.
14. Singh, A.P., and R. Tayal. 2020. Section C - joints, the musculoskeletal system. In *Ruminant surgery: a textbook of the surgical diseases of cattle, buffaloes, camels, sheep and goats*, ed. J. Singh, S. Singh, and R.P.S. Tyagi, 2nd ed., 444–465. New Delhi: CBS Publishers and Distributors Pvt. Ltd.
15. Desrochers, A., and D. Francoz. 2014. Clinical management of septic arthritis in cattle. *The Veterinary Clinics of North America. Food Animal Practice* 30 (1): 177–203.
16. Mielke, B., E. Comerford, K. English, and R. Meeson. 2018. Spontaneous septic arthritis of canine elbows: twenty-one cases. *Veterinary and Comparative Orthopaedics and Traumatology* 31 (6): 488–493.
17. Scharf, V.F., S.T. Lewis, J.F. Wellehan, H.L. Wamsley, R. Richardson, D.A. Sundstrom, and D.D. Lewis. 2015. Retrospective evaluation of the efficacy of isolating bacteria from synovial fluid in dogs with suspected septic arthritis. *Australian Veterinary Journal* 93 (6): 200–203.
18. Jacobsen, S., and P. Andersen. 2007. The acute phase protein serum amyloid A (SAA) as a marker of inflammation in horses. *Equine Veterinary Education* 19: 38–46.
19. Ludwig, E.L., R.B. Wiese, M.R. Graham, A.J. Tyler, J.M. Settlage, S.R. Werre, C.S. Petersson-Wolfe, I. Kanevsky-Mullarky, and L.A. Dahlgren. 2016. Serum and synovial fluid serum amyloid: a response in equine models of synovitis and septic arthritis. *Veterinary Surgery* 45: 859–867.
20. Matthieu, C., John, D.S., Cyril, T. And Florent, D. 2017. Effect of arthroscopic lavage and repeated intra-articular administrations of antibiotic in adult horses and foals with septic arthritis. Veterinary Surgery 46(7): 1008–1016
21. Bruise, R., K. Sullins, N.A. White 2nd, P.C. Coffin, G.A. Parker, M.R. Anver, and J.L. Rosenberger. 1992. Evaluation of sodium hyaluronate therapy in induced septic arthritis in the horse. *Equine Veterinary Journal* 24: 18–23.
22. Wright, I., M. Smith, D. Humphrey, T.C.J. Eaton-Evans, and M.H. Hillyer. 2003. Endoscopic surgery in the treatment of contaminated and infected synovial cavities. *Equine Veterinary Journal* 35: 613–619.
23. Heppelmann, M., C. Staszyk, J. Rehage, and A. Starke. 2012. Arthrotomy for the treatment of chronic purulent septic gonitis with subchondral osteolysis in two calves. *New Zealand Veterinary Journal* 60: 310–314.
24. Johnston, S.A. 1997. Osteoarthritis. Joint anatomy, physiology, and pathobiology. *The Veterinary Clinics of North America. Small Animal Practice* 27: 699–723. https://doi.org/10.1016/S0195-5616(97)50076-3.
25. Barbosa, J.D., D.H.S. Lima, A.S. Belo-Reis, C.P. Pinheiro, M.G.S. Sousa, J.B. Silva, F.M. Salvarani, and C.M.C. Oliveira. 2014. Degenerative joint disease in cattle and buffaloes in the Amazon region: a retrospective study. *Pesquisa Veterinaria Brasileira* 34 (9). https://doi.org/10.1590/S0100-736X2014000900007.
26. Anderson, K.L., H. Zulch, D.G. O'Neill, R.L. Meeson, and L.M. Collins. 2020. Risk factors for canine osteoarthritis and its predisposing arthropathies: a systematic review. *Frontiers in Veterinary Science* 7: 220. https://doi.org/10.3389/fvets.2020.00220.
27. Clements, D.N., S.D. Carter, J.F. Innes, and W.E. Ollier. 2006. Genetic basis of secondary osteoarthritis in dogs with joint dysplasia. *American Journal of Veterinary Research* 67: 909–918.
28. Pettitt, R.A., and A.J. German. 2015. Investigation and management of canine osteoarthritis. *In Practice* 37 (S1): 1–8.
29. Balamurugan, K., Shammi Mala, George Ravi Sundar, T.A. Kannan, and R. Sivashankar. 2020. Radiographic and ultrasonographic evaluation of osteoarthritic metacarpophalangeal joints in working equines. *Indian Journal of Veterinary Surgery* 41 (1): 53–55.
30. Sanderson, R.O., C. Beata, R.M. Flipo, J.-P. Genevois, C. Macias, S. Tacke, A. Vezzoni, and J.F. Innes. 2009. Systematic review of the management of canine osteoarthritis. *The Veterinary Record* 164: 418–424.
31. Pawde, A.M., O.P. Gupta, G.R. Singh, H.P. Aithal, and H.C. Setia. 2004. Radiographic estimation of soft tissue swelling in electroacupuncture treated arthritic buffalo calves (*Bubalus bubalis*). *Indian Journal of Veterinary Surgery* 25: 112–113.
32. Pawde, A.M., O.P. Gupta, G.R. Singh, P. Kinjavdekar, H.P. Aithal, and Amarpal. 2008. Haematological and serum electrolyte changes in arthritic buffalo calves treated with electroacupuncture. *The Indian Journal of Animal Sciences* 78: 168–169.
33. Bennett, D. 1987. Immune-based erosive inflammatory joint disease of the dog: canine rheumatoid arthritis. *The Journal of Small Animal Practice* 28 (9): 779–797.
34. Halliwell, R.E., R.B. Lavelle, and K.M. Butt. 1972. Canine rheumatoid arthritis- a review and a case report. *The Journal of Small Animal Practice* 13 (5): 239–248.
35. Heuser, W. 1980. Canine rheumatoid arthritis. *The Canadian Veterinary Journal* 21 (11): 314–316.
36. Kalil, M.A. 2014. Modern treatment of rheumatoid arthritis in cows. *Journal of Veterinary Science and Technology* 5: 202. https://doi.org/10.4172/2157-7579.1000202.

37. Pedersen, N.C., J.J. Castles, and K. Weisner. 1976. Noninfectious canine arthritis: rheumatoid arthritis. *Journal of the American Veterinary Medical Association* 169 (3): 295–303.
38. Stull, J.W., M. Evason, A.P. Carr, and C. Waldner. 2008. Canine immune-mediated polyarthritis: clinical and laboratory findings in 83 cases in western Canada (1991-2001). *The Canadian Veterinary Journal* 49: 1195–1203.
39. Ward, R. 1880. Rheumatoid arthritis in the horse. *Veterinary Jouranl of Annals Comparative Pathology* 10 (4): 245–248.
40. Bell, S.C., S.D. Carter, C. May, and D. Bennett. 1993. IgA and IgM rheumatoid factors in canine rheumatoid arthritis. *The Journal of Small Animal Practice* 34 (6): 259–264.
41. Rhoades, A.C., W. Vernau, P.H. Kass, M.A. Herrera, and J.E. Sykes. 2016. Comparison of the efficacy of prednisolone and cyclosporine for treatment of dogs with primary immune-mediated polyarthritis. *Journal of the American Veterinary Medical Association* 248: 395–404.

# Common Tendon and Ligament Injuries 13

**Learning Objectives**

You will be able to understand the following after reading this chapter:

- Principles and techniques of management of common tendon injuries like Achilles tendon, superficial and deep digital flexor tendons, contracted flexor tendons, and principles and techniques of tendon suturing
- Principles and techniques of the management of common ligament injuries like cranial cruciate ligament, patellar ligament and collateral ligaments
- Postoperative care and management in cases of tendon and ligament injuries

**Summary**

- Tendons present at the ends of skeletal muscles attach them onto the bones at specific locations and help in locomotion, whereas ligaments connect bones at joints and help to stabilize joints and control range of motion.
- Achilles tendon is the most commonly torn tendon in dogs, cats, and horses. The superficial digital flexor tendon injuries are the most common type of tendon injuries in horses (mostly attributed to racing) and cattle (caused by accidents involving farm machinery).
- The aim of tendon repair is to create a favorable environment for satisfactory healing with minimal adhesions with sufficient strength at the apposed cut ends of tendon permitting frictionless glide.
- Non-absorbable monofilament materials such as prolene have been preferred for tendon suturing (over non-absorbable braided synthetic suture materials) as they cause minimal friction and tendon deformation than braided sutures.
- Double- or triple-interlocking-loop or three-loop pulley suture using nylon, polydioxanon, or polyglyconate can provide stable repair of tendons.
- Different bioscaffolds have been used to support and enhance tendon repair, which include autogenous flaps such as free fascia lata grafts, fascial flaps of the surrounding musculature, tendon transposition and muscle transfer and allogenic grafts of porcine small intestinal submucosa and acellular human dermal tissue matrix.

(continued)


H. P. Aithal et al., *Textbook of Veterinary Orthopaedic Surgery*,
https://doi.org/10.1007/978-981-99-2575-9_13

- Contracted flexor tendon is a common congenital defect observed in large animals, especially in cattle. Apart from inheritance, other causes may include intra-uterine mal-positioning, oversized fetus and manipulation during dystocia. Mild and moderate flexural deformities may respond well to conservative treatment, but in cases of severe flexural deformities of the fetlock, surgical treatment (tenotomy) is recommended.
- Cranial cruciate ligament (CCL) injuries are the common orthopedic problems causing lameness in dogs. Sudden, severe limping on one of the hindlimbs is the most common sign of cruciate ligament rupture; other signs may include joint swelling, effusion, crepitation, cranial drawer sign and increased internal rotation of tibia.
- Traditionally, extracapsular technique has been used for surgical repair of ruptured CCL. In this technique, after removing the damaged ligament, a large, strong suture is passed through a hole drilled in the cranial tibia and tightened around the fabella behind the knee to replace the cruciate ligament.
- The tibial plateau leveling osteotomy (TPLO) is the most popular surgical technique to repair CCL rupture, by altering the mechanism of the knee joint and allowing it to function normally without a cruciate ligament. In this technique, a cut is made in the tibial plateau, which is rotated to change the angle and then stabilized with a plate and screws so that it gradually heals in its new position.
- Avulsion/tearing of the patellar ligament from the tibial tuberosity can occur during a sudden and extreme flexion of the knee; with contraction of the quadriceps, it can be treated by applying a tension band wire between the patella and the tibial tuberosity.

Tendon and ligaments are dense connective tissues [1]. Tendons occur at the ends of skeletal muscles and insert them onto the bones at specific locations. A tendon helps in transmission of the force of a muscle contraction to be bone across a joint and prevents muscle trauma by absorbing the forces transmitted through it. The digital flexor tendons in horses also help to absorb shock and support weight-bearing joints and store energy. Whereas ligaments connect bones at joints and help them to hold together in position, their main functions are to stabilize joints and control range of motion. Tendons and ligaments can get ruptured, torn or lacerated due to injury or trauma and often accompanied by bone fractures, which can affect the functional ability of the limb. Early and proper treatment to achieve strong repair and immobilization is important to restore the most function.

## 13.1 Tendon Injuries

### 13.1.1 Achilles Tendon

The Achilles tendon is the most frequently ruptured tendon in dogs and cats (Fig. 13.1). It is a bunch of three tendons made of insertion of tendinous part of five muscles: gastrocnemius tendon is the main tendon component and attaches to the heel (calcaneus bone); the superficial digital flexor tendon attaches collaterally to the proximal part of calcaneal bone and then passes over it and runs distally to attach to the digits [2–4].

The Achilles tendon can rupture either partially or completely. Partial rupture generally involves only gastrocnemius tendon, and the clinical signs include dropped hock, curled toes and varied degrees of lameness. Complete rupture involves all three tendons and is usually caused by a laceration injury. The animal with complete rupture of Achilles tendon shows completely dropped hock with severe lameness. The condition can be easily diagnosed by physical examination. Radiography will help to rule out a fracture, while ultrasonography will help confirm the diagnosis [4, 5].

The treatment option for injured Achilles tendon depends on the severity of the injury

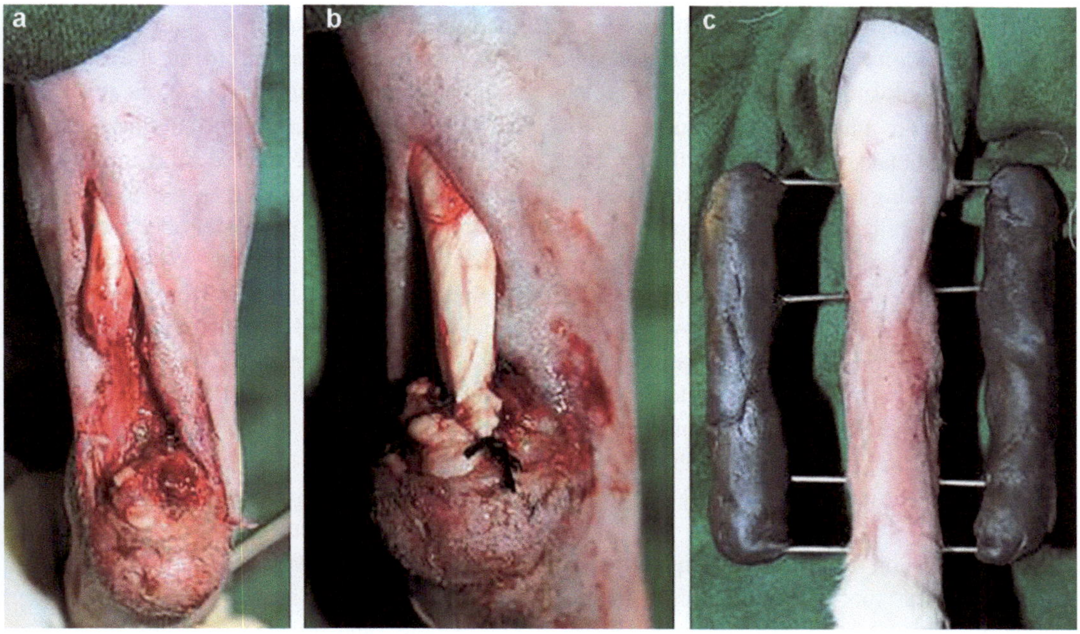


**Fig. 13.1** Achilles tendon rupture in a cat (**a**), repaired with end-to-end anastomosis (**b**) and the tarsal joint immobilized with epoxy-pin ESF (**c**). The cat showed good functional recovery

[6]. Often, the injury to the tendons can be managed by just providing plenty of rest to the dog and administration of anti-inflammatory drugs until complete healing. If a minor tear is present, splinting may be enough. In a complete tear, surgical repair is recommended. Surgical repair of Achilles tendon can be accomplished by primary apposition of the cut ends using a locking-loop suture. A monofilament suture can be used in a locking-loop or a three-loop pulley pattern [7, 8]. If the gastrocnemius tendon is torn off of the calcaneus bone, the sutures are secured through a hole drilled into the bone for stability. If a gap exists at the site of trauma, the defect site may be bridged using an autograft such as fascia lata graft, transposition of tendons such as deep digital flexor tendon or tissue-engineered bioactive scaffolds [9, 10].

Post-fixation, the dog must be supported for about two months, using either a cast, a combination of trans-calcaneotibial screw and cast or an external skeletal fixator (epoxy-pin ESF) [11]. The involved joints should be immobilized (with the hock joint in extension) to protect the primary injury. The cast or the external fixator may be removed after two months and a soft padded bandage may be applied for another two weeks. The surgical outcome is generally good if the dog is treated within 1–2 days of the injury. Potential complications may include pressure sores from the cast, infection, and breakdown of the support device.

Rupture of the gastrocnemius muscle or tendon is relatively rare in cattle [12, 13]. Lacerating injury is the primary cause; however, deficiencies of calcium, phosphorus, and vitamin D may predispose to this condition. Prolonged recumbency, myositis, and struggling to rise often precipitate rupture of Achilles tendon. Occasionally, pyelonephritis may lead to myositis and weakening of the muscle enough to cause rupture, or injections of irritant medicines may also cause necrosis and rupture of the gastrocnemius muscle.

The affected cattle are normally presented with flexed hock. In case of complete rupture, the animal rests the hock (rabbit leg) and distal portion of the limb on the ground while standing or during a walk, which is diagnostic. Cases of incomplete rupture may be treated conservatively by applying a full limb cast that maintains the hock in extension. In cattle the treatment of gastrocnemius tendon rupture is recommended only for young, lightweight animals, and complete rupture cases are unlikely to be successful in heavy adult animals. After suturing the cut ends of the tendon using a very strong suture, the joint should be immobilized using a full limb cast or an external fixator. Supplementation of adequate vitamins and minerals along with proper nursing may be useful for a successful recovery, which may require a prolonged period. In cases of complete rupture of gastrocnemius muscle or disruption of the calcaneal tendon, the prognosis is poor for the animals weighing less than about 500 kg and grave for the animals weighing more than 500 kg.

Achilles tendon is the most frequently torn tendon in horses too [14]. The equine Achilles tendon is formed by the gastrocnemius tendon, the tarsal tendon of the biceps femoris, semitendinosus and gracilis muscles, tendon of superficial digital flexor and the soleus muscle tendon [15]. The main component is the gastrocnemius; when this tendon is damaged/ruptured, the limb will collapse with severe lameness because it connects the heel to the upper hock. Partial rupture Achilles tendon is limited to the damage to the gastrocnemius tendon alone, whereas complete rupture would include rupture of all the tendons. Injury/rupture is commonly caused by road traffic accidents or sporting trauma. Tendon injury may be caused by direct injury by the kick or blow, and indirect injury due to loading or unloading accidents may also cause tendon injury.

Injury to the gastrocnemius tendon can be diagnosed by comprehensive physical examination, including checking for lameness, movement, conformation, flexion test and hoof testing. The confirmatory diagnosis, however, can be made by ultrasonography, contrast radiography, CT scanning, bone scanning and MRI [16].

Treatment for gastrocnemius tendon injury depends on the age of the horse and general health and the nature of the animal and severity of the condition [16, 17]. A young and healthy horse with a partial/incomplete rupture would recover completely with the support of only a splint or bandage along with complete stall rest for more than two months, depending on the injury. In cases of complete rupture, the surgical repair is the only option. Under general anesthesia, the cut ends of the tendon are sutured using locking-loop technique. External support is provided using a cast or a screw and cast or an external skeletal fixator (circular) to protect and support the repaired tendon by immobilizing the involved joints for about 2–3 months. In adult horses, stall rest or application of full limb cast or modified Thomas splint-cast combination can be used [17].

### 13.1.2 Superficial and Deep Digital Flexor Tendons

The tendons (and ligaments) present on the palmar or plantar aspect of the distal limb are most often injured in horses [18]. Superficial digital flexor tendon (SDFT) in the forelimb of the horse originates from the superficial flexor muscle that originates at the caudal aspect of the humerus above the elbow, and in the hindlimb in horse, it originates from the back of the femur bone above the stifle. The tendon runs downwards and inserts on the first phalanx and second phalanx in each limb. The deep digital flexor tendon (DDFT) in the forelimb arises from three different locations, that is, humerus, radius and ulna, and it then runs down the carpus and passes over the navicular bone and then inserts at the back of the third phalanx (coffin bone which lies beneath the SDFT and just over the suspensory ligament). DDFT in the hindlimb originates from two locations at the tibia and inserts on the third phalanx.

The SDFT injuries are the most common types of tendon injuries in horse. Apart from genetic predisposition, its cause is mostly attributed to racing, especially repetitive high speed races with jumps and obstacles. DDFT injuries are most frequently recorded within the hoof capsule and the tendon sheath, and the likely cause is repetitive excessive loading, whereas in cattle, injury to the flexor tendons is most commonly caused by accidents involving farm machinery,

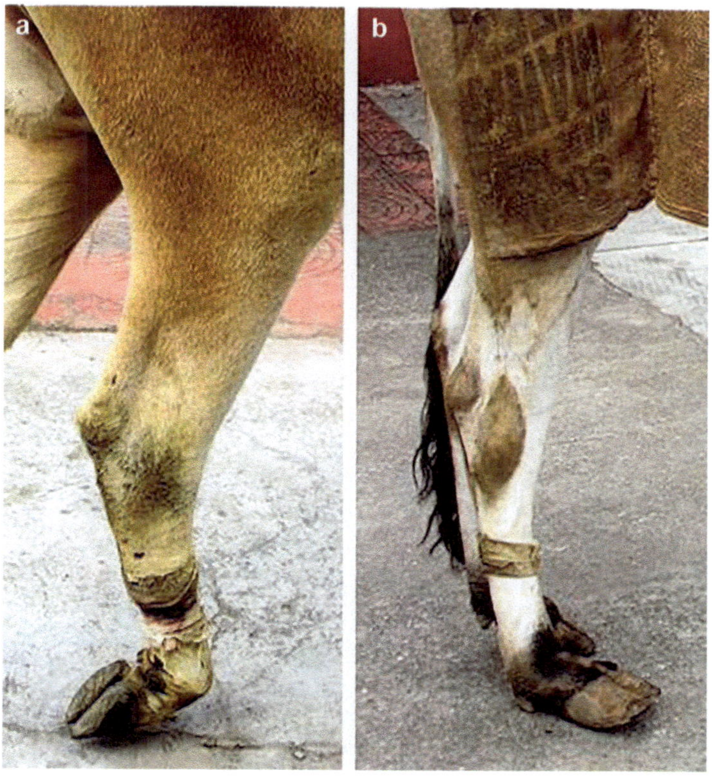


**Fig. 13.2** Rupture of digital extensor (**a**) and flexor (**b**) tendons in cattle leading to hyperflexion and hyperextension of fetlock joints, respectively

leading to laceration or complete rupture (Fig. 13.2). Tendon laceration is uncommon and occurs mostly when the cow kicks a sharp object or falls onto it. Such injury most commonly affects one of the hindlimbs at the level of the mid-metatarsus. Flexor tendon rupture also commonly occurs secondary to sepsis of peritendinous tissues, septic tendinitis and necrosis of the tendon [19]. Spontaneous tendon rupture may also occur at the muscle fibers and tendon junction during breeding accidents, bull fights or post-parturient neuropathy. Avulsion of the DDF tendon from its insertion point at the solar surface of the third phalanx is also common in cattle, which occurs secondary to P3 sepsis and necrosis of the DDF tendon insertion (solar abscess, ulcers septic pedal osteitis or septic arthritis of the distal interphalangeal joint).

The tendon injuries can be diagnosed by collecting history, clinical signs (lameness, increased sensitivity to the touch, increased temperature at the site, tendon swelling or thickening and a bowed or convex appearance), radiography (fasciagraphy) and ultrasonographic evaluation (preferably done after 7–10 days, by then the inflammatory signs subside) [18, 19]. MRI and tenoscopy will help in effective diagnosis, especially of DDFT injuries.

Tendon laceration can be treated by administration of anti-inflammatory drugs, stall rest, application of a cast, surgical repair and corrective farriery, depending on the location, tendon involved and the extent of injury [20, 21]. Apart from anti-inflammatory drugs such as phenylbutazone and corticosteroids, dimethyl sulfoxide (DMSO) and polysulphated glycosaminoglycans (PSGAGs) have been widely used [18]. In incomplete lacerations, stall confinement and rest or external coaptation with a cast may be adequate, which allows tendon healing by scarring (second intention). During cast application, the fetlock may be flexed to bring the cut ends of the tendon closer and release tension. Splints may be reinforced on the compression as well as the tension sides of the limb to provide additional strength to the fixation. Ruptured tendons may be sutured (tenorrhaphy) in addition to providing external coaptation, to achieve rapid healing.

Three-loop pulley suture or double- or triple-interlocking-loop sutures using nylon, polydioxanon, or polyglyconate are known to provide stable repair of tendons [22]. Various implant materials used to repair lacerated tendons include carbon fiber, polyester, autologous tendon grafts, absorbable tendon splints and poly-L-lactic acid [23]. Several growth factors such as insulin-like growth factor-I, equine recombinant growth factor, transforming growth factor-ß, platelet-rich plasma and mesenchymal stem cells have been shown to enhance tendon healing [18]. In cases of avulsion injuries, treatment should also be directed toward treating the inciting disease, including surgical debridement, lavage, and administration of broad-spectrum antibiotics and anti-inflammatory drugs. As the avulsion of DDF tendon occurs at its origin at the distal phalanx, ankylosis of distal interphalangeal joint provides stability to the limb [19].

The prognosis is generally good in large animals for tendon rupture involving the SDF tendon alone. However, the chances of long-term survival and functional recovery of the cattle and horses with traumatic rupture of the superficial or deep digital flexor tendon are fair to good. In cases of ruptures involving both SDF and DDF tendons, lameness may persist for longer time often with delayed recovery. Ultrasonographic examination will help evaluate tendon healing and assess prognosis.

### 13.1.3 Contracted Flexor Tendons

Contracted flexor tendon is one of the common congenital defects observed in large animals, especially in cattle [19, 24–26] (Fig. 13.3). Apart from inheritance, other causes may include intra-uterine mal-positioning, oversized fetus and manipulation during dystocia. The condition can be seen normally within the first few days after the birth. Often the contracted tendons are associated with other congenital abnormalities like cleft palate, dwarfism, and arthrogryposis. Generally carpal or fetlock joints are affected with variable extent of the deformity.

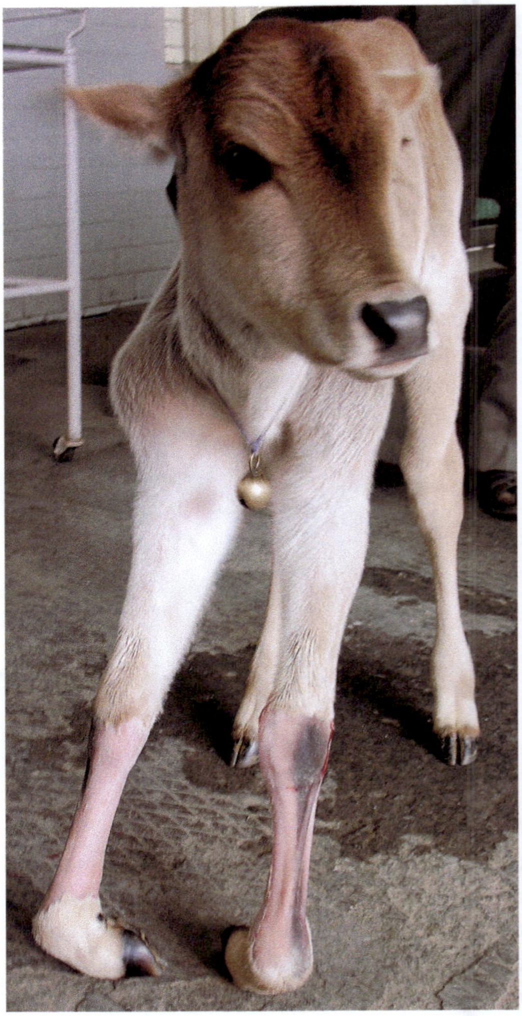

**Fig. 13.3** Contracted flexor tendon (congenital) involving the fetlock joints in a bovine calf

Treatment of contracted tendon would depend on the severity and site of the condition. Congenital deformities should be treated as soon as possible, as it becomes less responsive in older animals. Mild flexural deformities generally respond well to physical therapy and manual stretching of the joints and tendons. Moderate deformity cases can be treated by using a splint-bandage or a cast along with administration of a NSAID (non-steroidal anti-inflammatory drugs). The splint (made of bamboo or PVC (polyvinyl chloride) pipe) should be applied on the palmar or plantar aspect, extending from the hoof up to the elbow in forelimbs and in the hindlimb from the hoof up to the point of the hock. The use of a fiberglass cast may provide better support than the POP (plaster of Paris) cast, especially in calves with carpal deformity. Splint-bandage or cast should be removed every 2–4 days initially, and subsequently the interval of change may be prolonged so that the limb can be examined regularly. Intravenous administration of a single high dose of oxytetracycline (about 40–50 mg/kg body weight) has been recommended for treatment of flexed tendons in early stages [27]. It has been thought to relax the muscles by calcium chelating effect. However, care should be taken to inject the drug slowly to avoid any acute effect on the heart and kidneys.

In cases of severe flexural deformities of the fetlock (which do not show improvement to application of splint-bandage or a cast), surgical intervention is recommended. Tenotomy is done in the midmetacarpal or midmetatarsal region if the fetlock is primarily affected and tenotomy is done proximal to the carpus, if the carpus is affected. Sometimes tenotomy may be required at both the locations. Through a small incision, all the tensed tendinous tissues are severed until the tension on the tendons in relieved and the limb can be extended fully. If desired effect is not achieved, the periarticular tissues may also be severed to ensure proper extension of the affected limbs. Postoperatively splint/cast is applied to hold the limb in extended position. It may be required to change the splint/cast as per the need (at least once in a week) and maintained for about 2–4 weeks until the cut ends of the tendons are healed by fibrous tissue formation.

Arthrogryposis is a congenital condition, wherein there is persistent contracture of joint present at birth [28–30]. The condition is normally hereditary in nature affecting any one leg or all four legs (Fig. 13.4). Unlike in cases of contracted tendons wherein there is no rotation of the limb and the joints are aligned properly, in calves with arthrogryposis, the articular and osseous changes may be permanent in most cases. The condition can be surgically treated by incising contracted periarticular soft tissues including performing desmotomy and tenotomy of the involved ligaments and tendons. It may be necessary to transact all the structures present at the palmar surface of the carpus (except blood vessels and nerves). Postoperatively, external support is given by application of a cast for a prolonged period of about 6–8 weeks. In severe cases, which do not respond to this treatment, arthrodesis of the carpus is advised.

### 13.1.4 Principles and Techniques of Tendon Suturing

Surgical repair of tendon is quite challenging. The aim of tendon repair should be to achieve sufficient strength at the apposed cut ends of tendon permitting glide and allowing satisfactory healing with minimal adhesions [31]. Various standard and modified techniques, including those described by Bunnel, Kessler, Becker, Tajima, Lee, Tsuge, and others, have been used to repair a ruptured tendon [32–39] (Fig. 13.5). Traditional tendon sutures employ two core strands to bridge the gap between the tendon ends. They are simple and least traumatic techniques; the repair site is initially weaker, but they result in more rapid healing. By increasing the number of core sutures and anchor points, the strength can be increased, but it will also increase the bulk at the repair site and gliding resistance due to the complexity of multiple tendon passes. Further, increased tendon passes (as in Bunnell technique) may lead to decreased microcirculation and a high occurrence of gap formation at the site of repair. Tendon repairs with a gap of 3 mm or more may have a greater risk of rupture as compared to those with less than 1 mm gap. Hence the surgeon should select the technique as per the requirement of the case and must be prepared to modify the technique when needed. Several techniques have been described for lengthening or shortening the tendon (Figs. 13.6 and 13.7).

Traditionally, non-absorbable braided synthetic suture materials, which have the advantages of greater strength and increased frictional force, have been used for tendon repair. However, more recently non-absorbable monofilament materials such as prolene have been preferred as they have been shown to cause less friction and tendon

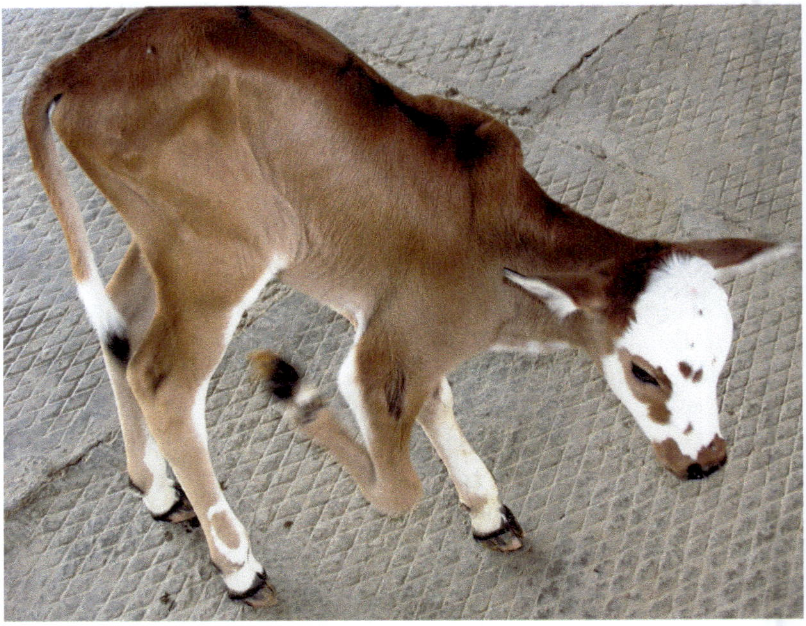

**Fig. 13.4** A calf showing signs of arthrogryposis of right carpal joint, a congenital condition with articular and osseous changes

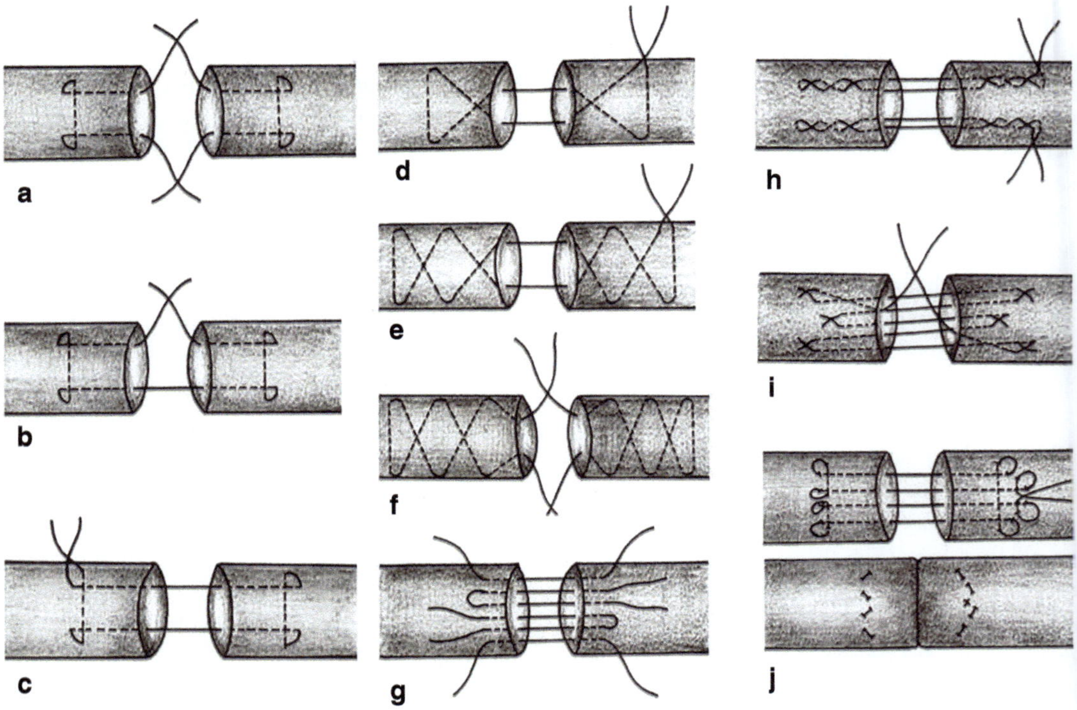


**Fig. 13.5** Different techniques of tendon suturing: (**a**) Kessler-Tajima, (**b**) modified Kessler-1, (**c**) modified Kessler-2, (**d**) Bunnell, (**e**) Bunnell technique with two loops in each segment, (**f**) Bunnell-Mayer, (**g**) interrupted mattress, (**h**) augmented Becker, (**i**) Savage and (**j**) double-locking loop technique

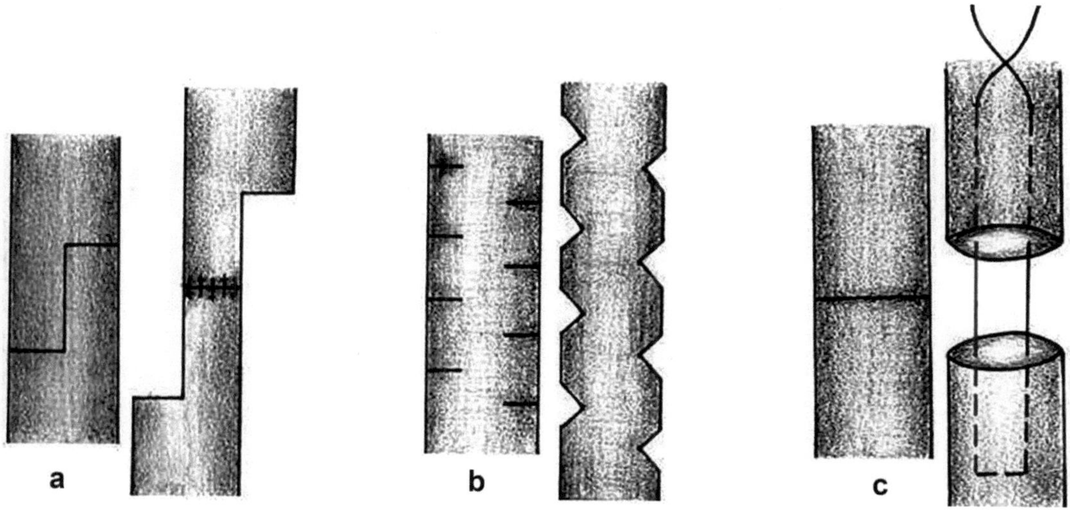


**Fig. 13.6** Different suturing techniques of tendon lengthening (Z-plasty, accordion technique and Lange techniques)

deformation than braided sutures. Placement of sutures may also influence the repair strength. Internal suture repairs have lower gliding resistance, but they have concerns on acellularity and ischaemia. Application of peripheral circumferential sutures in addition to core sutures will ensure that the tendon ends meet laterally (reduce gap) and also provide additional strength to repair. Sutures placed at volar or plantar surface have been shown to minimize interruption of blood flow, but the pull-out strength is about 50% lesser than dorsally placed sutures. Hence suture placement must also be considered as per the individual patient needs.

## 13.2 Ligament Injuries

### 13.2.1 Cranial Cruciate Ligament

The knee (stifle) is a complex joint composed of distal femur (proximally) and proximal tibia (distally), patella (cranially) and small bean-shaped bone fabella (caudally). The medial and lateral

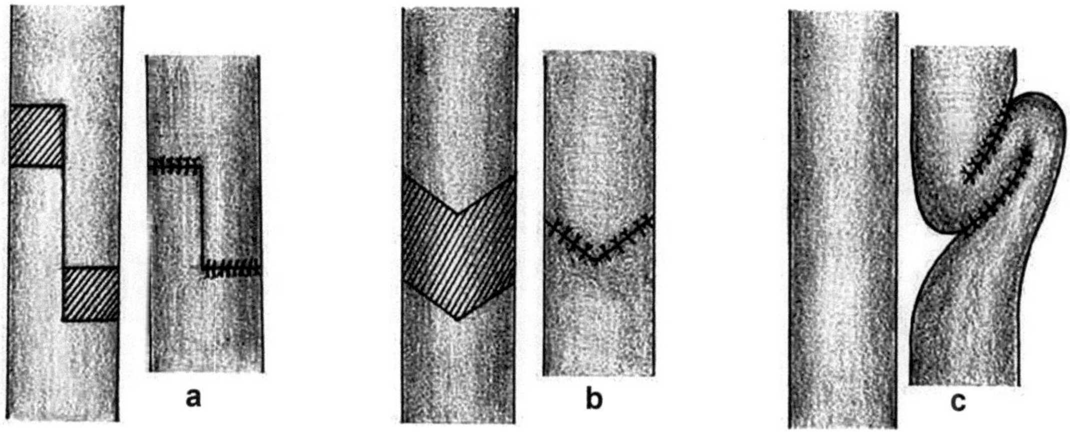


**Fig. 13.7** Different suturing techniques of tendon shortening (Z tenotomy, segment excision and doubling over methods)

menisci (cartilage) cushion the bones, and ligaments hold the structures in position and enable the joint to function properly. The cranial and caudal cruciate ligaments are two important stabilizing ligaments that cross over one another inside the knee joint. Cranial cruciate ligament (CCL) injuries are one of the most commonly seen orthopedic problems, causing discomfort and lameness in dogs [40–42] (Fig. 13.8).

Injury to cruciate ligaments can result in a partial or complete rupture of any of the two cruciate ligaments. However, injury to the cranial cruciate ligament is more frequently reported than to the caudal cruciate ligament, leading to free movement of the tibia resulting in pain and abnormal gait. In healthy young dogs, it can be caused by a simple athletic injury due to wrong landing while running, jumping, or turning sharply. Overweight animals with weakened joints are more prone to the injury. Often CCL rupture is accompanied with patellar luxation [43]. Additionally, some large dog breeds such as Neapolitan Mastiffs, Newfoundlands, Akitas, Saint Bernards, Rottweilers, terriers, retrievers (Chesapeake Bay, Labrador and golden retrievers) and German shepherds are at a higher risk of cruciate ligament injuries than the other breeds [44–46]. The incidence of CCL injuries may be higher in dogs, which are neutered early (before 12 months) [47]. Further it has been seen that nearly 50% of the dogs having rupture of the CCL in one leg would eventually develop the condition in the contralateral limb. In old-age dogs, cruciate ligaments may be weakened due to degenerative changes, and the joint may become unstable, predisposing the ligament to rupture even during day-to-day normal activities. Other joint abnormalities and diseases like arthritis of the knee joint may also put unusual stress on the cruciate ligaments, leading to weakness and tearing. Genetic factors may also contribute to the occurrence of CCL rupture in dogs, irrespective of dog breeds [48, 49].

Sudden onset of severe limping in one of the hindlimbs may be the most common symptom of cruciate ligament rupture. In most cases, the dogs may experience severe pain and may not bear weight on the affected limb after an injury. If the injury remains untreated, arthritic changes may start quickly, resulting in long-term lameness and discomfort. Other signs may include joint swelling (on medial side), effusion, crepitation, cranial drawer sign (increased cranial laxity of the proximal tibia in relation to the distal femur) and apparent internal rotation of the tibia. The absence of the drawer sign, however, does not rule out damage to the CCL. The tibial compression test (on flexion of the hock, the proximal tibia moves forward) can also indicate CCL laxity. Dogs with partial tear in the CCL may experience milder or intermittent limping and an increased cranial laxity, which may be more pronounced in flexion. In medial meniscal injury, a clicking sound is characteristic during locomotion or extension and flexion of the joint. Radiography may reveal joint effusion and fracture (avulsion of the ligament, common in immature dogs) or indicate degenerative joint disease (in chronic cases). Arthrocentesis may show mild increase in the cells and haemarthrosis. Arthroscopy may be used (done under anesthesia) to confirm a cruciate ligament rupture and assess the integrity of menisci, which may be damaged in cases of cruciate ligament rupture.

Partial cruciate ligament tear in an early stage may be managed conservatively with restriction of activities in combination with anti-inflammatory therapy (steroids or NSAIDs). Activity restriction may be needed for a prolonged period of up to six weeks. A few dogs, especially small dogs, may recover with cage rest [50]. Prolotherapy, a method of tightening up a loose, unstable, and hyper-mobile joint by injecting a natural sclerosing agent in and around the joint, has also been used. This results in thickening of the ligaments and the joint capsule, eventually leading to their contraction and relief from joint pain. Other modalities that are recommended include pulse magnetic therapy and soft laser therapy, which will help in decreasing the pain and the joint would recuperate. Stem cell and platelet-rich plasma therapy has also shown promising effects in the treatment of early partial CCL ruptures in dogs [51]. Recently, the use of custom-made canine stifle orthotics is emerging as a non-surgical means of managing

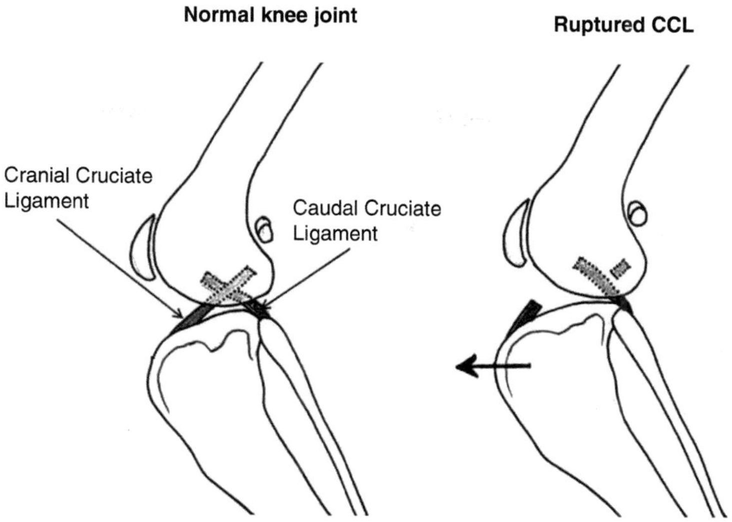


**Fig. 13.8** Schematic presentation of normal stifle joint with intact or ruptured cranial cruciate ligament. Ruptured CCL results in cranial drawer sign with increased cranial laxity of proximal tibia

patients with cranial cruciate ligament insufficiency [52]. If conservative treatment fails, surgical fixation is recommended. The prolonged instability of the stifle joint following rupture of the CCL can lead to injury to medial meniscus, joint effusion, osteophyte formation and fibrosis of the joint capsule. Hence, the best method for treatment of cruciate ligament injury is the surgical repair.

Surgical correction is recommended in most cases of complete cruciate ligament tears as well as many partial injuries, especially in active dogs. Different surgical procedures have been developed to correct cruciate ligament injuries [42, 53, 54]. Extracapsular techniques for surgical repair of CCL rupture include fascial suturing, fabella to tibial tuberosity imbrication sutures, cranial transposition of the fibular head, tibial plateau leveling osteotomy, tibial tuberosity advancement osteotomy and implantation of synthetic grafts. The intracapsular techniques include suturing of the fascia lata or patellar tendon grafts over the top of the lateral condyle of the femur.

Traditionally, extracapsular imbrication suture technique has been used for surgical repair of ruptured CCL [55] (Fig. 13.9). In this technique, the damaged ligament as well as the damaged portion of the meniscus is removed. Then a large, strong suture passed through a hole drilled in the cranial tibia and tightened around the fabella behind the knee to replace the cruciate ligament. In due course of time, the suture may break, but the healed tissue would stabilize the knee. The technique is uncomplicated and relatively quick and has been found to be successful especially in smaller dogs. The long-term success, however, is not generally good and many dogs may show the signs of recurrence. In the intracapsular repair method, the cruciate ligament is replaced with a connective tissue strip that can be sutured in place or anchored to an implant.

The tibial plateau leveling osteotomy (TPLO) is a complex surgical procedure, but it is the most popular surgical technique for the management of CCL rupture [56, 57] (Fig. 13.10). TPLO is done to alter the mechanism of the knee joint that allows it to function properly without a cruciate ligament. In this technique, a cut is made in the tibial plateau including the adequate part of proximal tibia, which is rotated anticlockwise to reduce the tibial plateau angle and then stabilized with a plate and screws (Fig. 13.11). Gradually, the bone heals in its new position. It may take several months for full recovery under cage rest. The long-term recovery is generally very good with rare chances of re-injury. The tibial tuberosity advancement (TTA) is another technique, which may facilitate the knee to function without a cruciate ligament [56, 58]. It repositions the tibial tuberosity more cranially by cutting and then anchoring it with implants (Figs. 13.12 and 13.13).

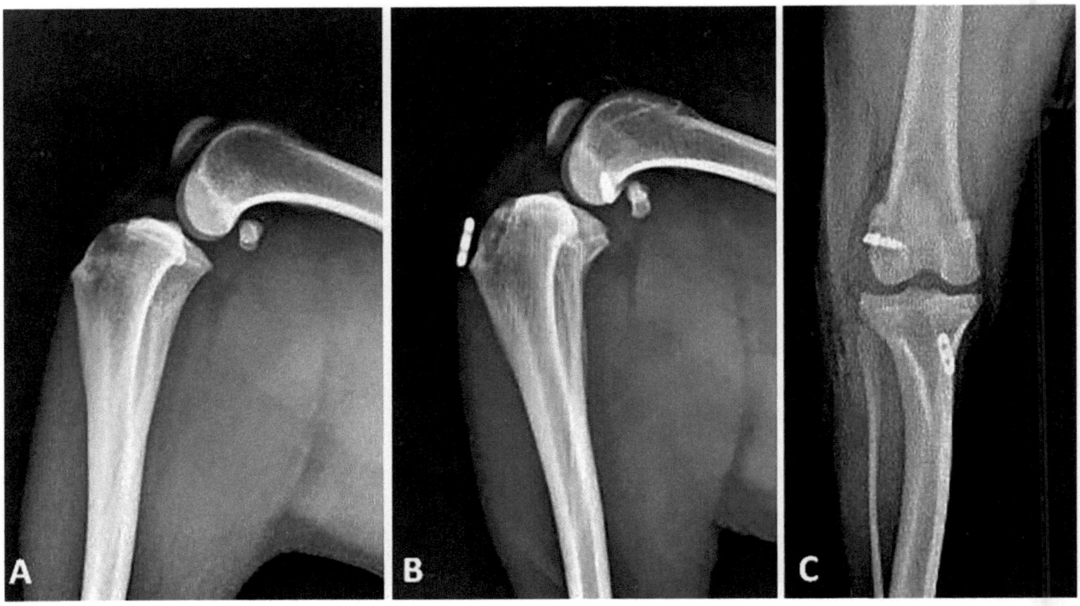


**Fig. 13.9** Repair of CCL rupture using extra-capsular technique in a dog (23.6 pounds): preoperative radiograph shows increased radio-opacity in the stifle joint space, with evidence of joint effusion and very mild osteoarthritic changes (**a**); surgical treatment included debridement and lavage of stifle joint through miniarthrotomy and lateral imbrications was done using an Arthrex FASTak placed at isometric points on the femur and tibia with the tensioning device set at 5 lbs. (**b** and **c**). Postoperatively excellent range of motion and stability was noticed (Courtesy: Dr. Suresha Basavaraj, DVM, Ontario, L4S 4B8, Canada)

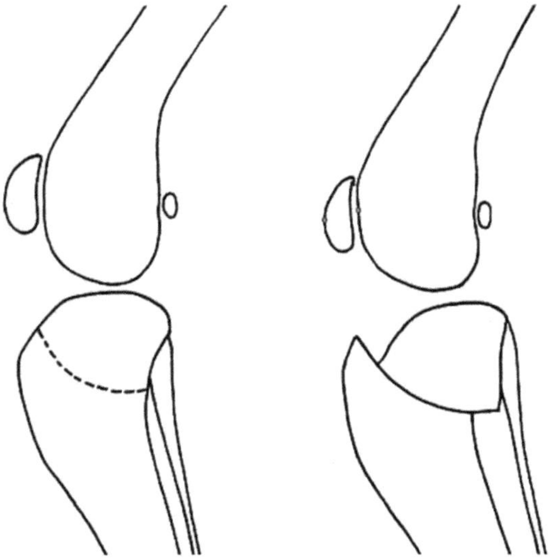

**Fig. 13.10** Schematic presentation of TPLO technique for treatment of CCL rupture: a semicircular cut is made through the proximal end of tibia and the proximal segment is displaced and rotated caudally and fixed in position using a plate

Postoperatively 6–8 weeks of rest (restriction of excessive mobility and activity) is crucial to achieve clinical healing. Physiotherapy is usually recommended postoperatively and can be extremely beneficial for recovery from cruciate repair surgery [59–61]. Swimming/hydrotherapy is an effective method of exercise for the injured dogs [62]. It is also important to check the weight, gained by the dog which is likely to happen when the routine activity of the dog is interrupted. Overweight dogs are difficult to recover from a cruciate ligament injury, and there could be injury to the contralateral knee in such dogs. Supplementation of the diet with glucosamine-chondroitin combinations may benefit the dogs with cruciate ligament injuries; some may require prolonged therapy with anti-inflammatory drugs. Most dogs recover well from CCL injury if the condition is treated appropriately and adequate postoperative care is done. Preoperative low-level laser therapy has shown to improve the postoperative recovery following TPLO

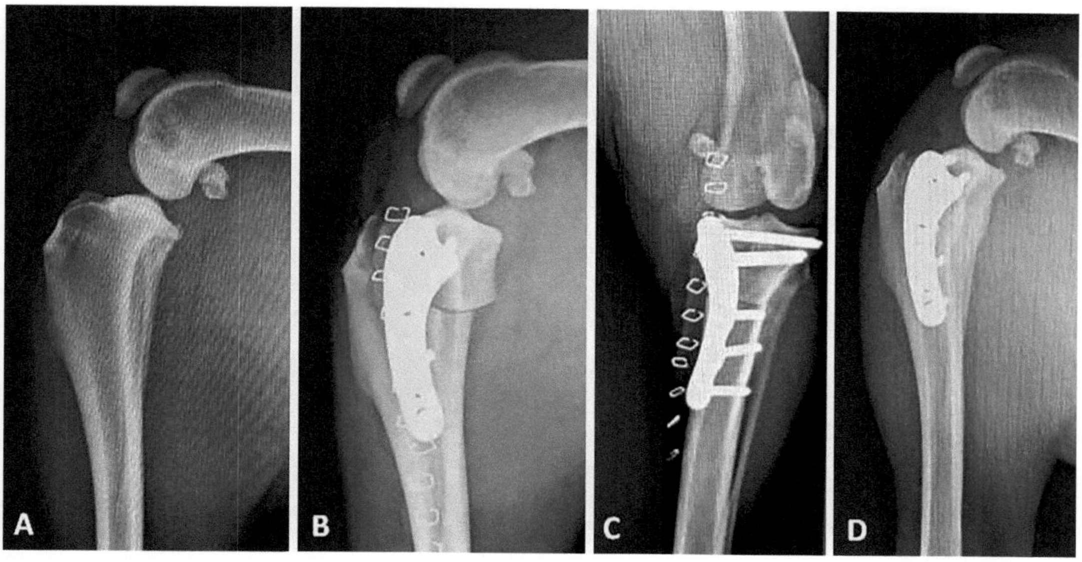


**Fig. 13.11** TPLO surgery in a 106-pound dog [surgical plan included preoperative radiograph to determine the tibial rotation]. Through a medial approach, a curvilinear incision was made from 1 cm cranial to the patella up to 3 cm distal to the distal portion of the tibial tubercle. All fascia undermined and reflected. The pes anserinus incised and reflected both cranially and caudally exposing the medial proximal surface of the tibia. Meniscus was inspected via arthroscopy, found to be normal. The joint capsule was apposed with a 2–0 PDS suture. A 3.5 standard biomedtrix TPLO plate was placed 3.5 mm screws placed in order. After perfect alignment was determined, all screws were tightened. Area thoroughly flushed, pes anserinus apposed to the cranial fascia with No-0 PDS. Fascia and subcutaneous tissues apposed, skin apposed with staples: preoperative lateral radiographic view of stifle joint (**a**), radiographic views made soon after surgery (**b**), and at eight weeks postoperatively (**c**) with excellent functional recovery (Courtesy: Dr. Suresha Basavaraj, DVM, Ontario, L4S 4B8, Canada)

**Fig. 13.12** Schematic presentation of TTA technique for treatment of CCL rupture: a cut is made through cranial part of the tibia and the cranial segment is advanced to make room for the spacer. By keeping the spacer in place, the displaced segment is secured in place by fixing a special bone plate

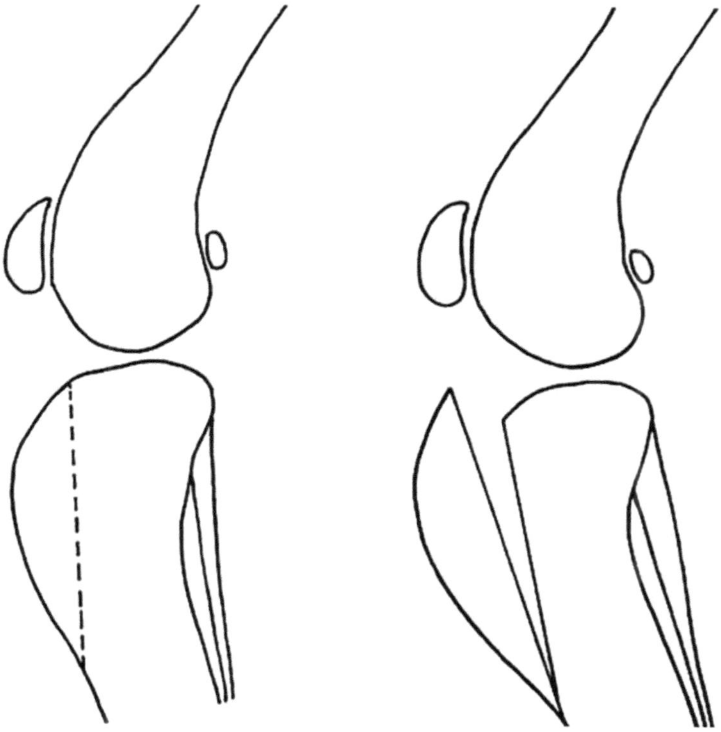

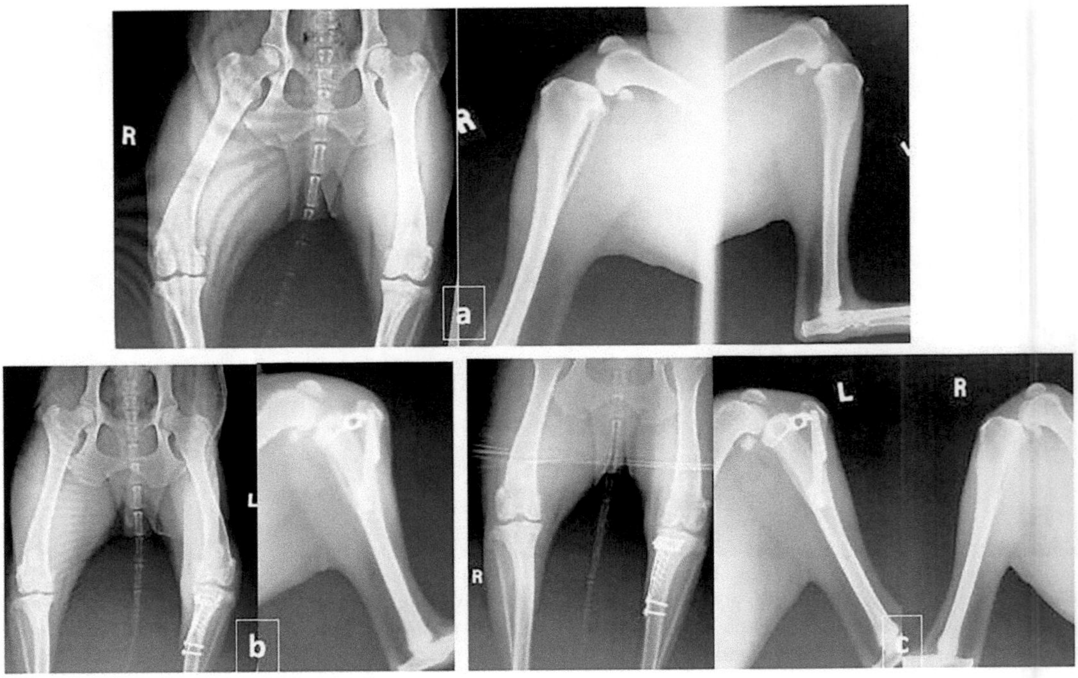


**Fig. 13.13** TTA surgery in a dog [Surgical technique included preoperative radiograph showing fat pad displacement consistent with rupture of CCL. Through the medial approach, medial osteotomy is done along the tibial tuberosity. Placed six-hole tension band plate and fork. Placed 12 mm advancement cage with a 6 mm medial spacer at the cranial ear of the cage. Joint lavaged, sutured with 2–0 PDS and skin sutured with staples]: preoperative craniocaudal and lateral radiographic views of stifle joint (**a**), radiographic views made soon after surgery (**b** and **c**), 8 weeks postoperative radiographs (**d**), excellent functional recovery achieved (Courtesy: Dr. Suresha Basavaraj, DVM, Ontario, L4S 4B8, Canada)

surgery [63]. Some dogs, however, may develop complications such as arthritis in due course of time; however, with proper care and compliance to the advice of the veterinarian, the dog can live a healthy and comfortable life.

In large ruminants (cattle, buffaloes) and horses, complete rupture of cranial and/or caudal cruciate ligament are often seen following a catastrophic injury resulting in joint instability and lameness, leading to secondary osteoarthritic changes in the articular cartilage [64–67]. Incomplete rupture or strains of cruciate ligaments may result in a variable degree of lameness, depending on the severity of the injury. Intraarticular injection of local anesthetic may improve the lameness. Clinical examination may reveal marked effusion in the femoropatellar joint. Craniocaudal instability could be elicited in animals under general anesthesia; however, the anterior drawer test is technically difficult to perform in large animals. Radiographically considerable amount of joint effusion may be evident, and osteophyte formation (at the sites of attachment of ligaments) or focal areas of radiolucency may be seen [64, 68, 69]. Avulsion fracture of the medial intercondylar eminence is one of the common findings in most of the horses with cruciate rupture [70]. Ultrasonographic imaging of ligaments in the stifle is very difficult in large animals, and arthroscopy is the best technique available to confirm the diagnosis.

The ligament rupture can be treated conservatively by offering rest and administration of systemic NSAIDs and intra-articular corticosteroids. If the condition does not improve, the surgical stabilization techniques to manage the injured cranial cruciate ligament can be tried. In horses, surgical stabilization by placing a row of Lembert sutures in both the lateral and medial retinacular tissues and additional imbrication suture placed from the lateral femorotibial ligament to the lateral or middle patellar ligament (imbrication method) has improved the condition in some cases [67]. Externally a modified Robert Jones/Thomas-Schroeder splint can be applied to provide additional support. Arthroscopic surgery may be done to debride the loose and torn fibers of the ligament. Replacement of ruptured cranial cruciate ligament has been tried using facial graft or patellar ligament graft [65, 66, 71, 72]. In this technique, the torn cruciate ligament is replaced by a graft attached to the tibial crest, passed between the condyles and secured to the lateral condyle (over the top). Reconstruction of the ligament using braided nylon or a nitinol prosthesis has also shown promising results [73, 74]. In general, the outcome of the case would depend on the severity of the condition; in cases of complete ligament rupture, the prognosis is poor especially in heavy adult animals, whereas in mild injuries, the prognosis is generally fair.

### 13.2.2 Patellar Ligament

Rupture of patellar ligament is not very common in dogs and cats [75–77]. Sudden and extreme flexion of the knee, along with contraction of the quadriceps, often results in avulsion of the patellar ligament from the tibial tuberosity or tearing of the patellar ligament [78]. Patellar ligament tear may also occur due to laceration injury during an automobile trauma and glass cuts or can be iatrogenic (following surgical repair of patellar luxation) [76]. Affected animals generally exhibit lameness and pain on palpation at the stifle. When the stifle joint is flexed and palpated, laxity of the patellar ligament can be easily detected cranio-dorsally to the tibial crest. The patella is usually positioned more proximally, which can be clearly visualized radiographically. Treatment of patellar ligament rupture includes primary apposition of the ligament and application of a tension band wire between the patella and the tibial tuberosity. It can be achieved by passing a wire proximally via a transverse hole drilled through the patella or the wire looped over the top of the patella to secure patellar attachment and distally by passing the wire through a transverse hole made in the tibial tuberosity [76, 79, 80]. The wire loops are then tensioned (tension band wiring) until the cut ends of the patellar ligament appose each other. Instead of orthopedic wire, nylon, polypropylene, or polydioxanone sutures can be used, as they do not require surgical removal [75, 76, 81]. The ligament is then repaired by applying a large tension suture and simple interrupted sutures at the cut ends. If the cut ends of the ligament do not meet each other and if the gap persists, a strip of fascia lata may be used to bridge the gap by suturing into the defect.

Postoperatively a soft supportive bandage is applied for 8–10 days along with exercise restriction. Stifle may be immobilized by transarticular application of an ESF [75, 80]. Exercise should be limited to leash walking for an additional 2–3 weeks following removal of the bandage/fixator. It is better to remove the orthopedic wire if used to approximate the cut ends of the tendon at a later date to prevent its breakage and subsequent complications.

Patellar ligament injuries are rare in large animals but may be seen especially in jumping horses, the middle patellar ligament being the most commonly affected. Lateral patellar ligament injuries are also often seen at the mid to insertional portion [82]. Clinically the affected animals may exhibit variable degrees of lameness, which may be severe in acute cases. Other signs may include joint effusion, edema, and periligamentous thickening. Ultrasonography will help in confirmatory diagnosis [83]. The condition is generally managed conservatively by providing prolonged rest.

### 13.2.3 Collateral Ligaments

Collateral ligaments are short, relatively inelastic structures connecting the bones, found both on the medial and lateral sides of major limb joints in both small and large animals [78]. Extreme bending of the joints in varus/valgus directions, rotation or traumatic injury may lead to ligament tear (sprain). Injuries to the collateral ligaments of the carpal, tarsal, metacarpophalangeal, and metatarsophalangeal joints are common.

The significance of collateral ligament injuries is often underestimated. Repair of injured collateral ligaments is difficult as they are very short structures and the prognosis is guarded especially for athletic soundness [84]. Stress radiography and ultrasonography can help to diagnose ligament injuries in animals with acute lameness and joint swelling [85]. Surgical reconstruction by primary suturing of the torn ligaments is rarely possible. Rigid external fixation of the joint in its normal position for 6–8 weeks may allow healing through fibrous union. However, this technique will not be successful in most cases. Spiked washers may be used to fix the ligament into its near normal anatomical location. Alternatively, collateral ligament tears are reconstructed using wire or nylon sutures to mimic the collateral function to support the joint [78, 86–89]. This can be achieved by placing a cortical screw at each attachment point of the collateral ligament and connecting them through an orthopedic wire or nylon suture. The wire/suture is then sufficiently tightened (but prevent crushing the opposing cartilage surface) to give stability to the joint. In due course of time, the collateral ligament heals by scar formation to achieve stable repair, and then the wire or nylon suture may be removed to prevent any complications from breakage.

Postoperatively a soft bandage is applied to provide external support, which is kept for about 8–10 days. Prolonged immobilization should be avoided as it will lead to joint stiffness. Once the external support is removed, the animal should be allowed only leash walking for additional 2–3 weeks.

### 13.2.4 Postoperative Care and Management of Tendon/Ligament Injuries

In an acute tendon or ligament injury, anti-inflammatory and analgesic drug administration should be started immediately after an injury/surgery along with cage/stall rest to minimize further injury and inflammation. Steroids and/or NSAIDs exert strong anti-inflammatory action; polysulphated glycosaminoglycan (PSGAG) may also be administered to offer soft tissue anti-inflammatory effects. The use of therapeutic ultrasound, acupuncture, and other physiotherapeutic modalities like low-level laser therapy can improve blood supply and stimulate fibroblast proliferation [90, 91].

Different regenerative therapies have been described for tendon and ligament injuries, especially in horses [92–96]. Platelet-rich plasma (PRP) is known to contain bioactive factors such as PDGF, VEGF, and transforming growth factor-β (TGF- β). PRP injected at the site of tendon/ligament injury can provide high levels of growth factors for early healing. It has been reported to enhance proliferation of cells around the injured tendon, increase collagen (types I and III) production and increase the strength of the repaired tendon. Stem cell (undifferentiated cells) treatment is currently the most popular method to treat a tendon/ligament injury. Stem cell therapy appears to improve healing of the tendon by increasing fibroblast proliferation and collagen deposition and facilitating organization of the collagen fibers. The best effects are achieved if treatment is done once the inflammatory phase of healing passed but significant fibrosis has not developed.

Different bioscaffolds (autogenous, allogenous, and synthetic materials) have been used to support and enhance tendon repair. Among the autogenous flaps, free fascia lata, fascial flaps of the surrounding musculature and muscle and tendon transposition transfer have been advocated to strengthen repaired tendons. Among the allogenic grafts, porcine small intestinal submucosa and acellular dermal tissue matrix are commonly used. Porous tantalum interposed with tendon has been used to reattach tendons in place with a screw experimentally.

Prolonged immobilization after a tendon/ligament injury may damage the articular cartilage; therefore an early sub-maximal loading of the repaired tendon or ligament is recommended. Physical therapy with a controlled exercise regimen may be started as early as possible in specific cases.

## Chapter 13: Sample Questions

**Question No. 1: Mark the correct answer**

1. The main component of equine Achilles tendon is
   (a) gastrocnemius muscle tendon (b) biceps femoris muscle tendon (c) semitendinosus muscle tendon (d) superficial digital flexor tendon
2. Preferred suture material for tendon suturing is
   (a) non-absorbable braided synthetic suture (b) non-absorbable monofilament synthetic suture (c) absorbable braided suture (d) absorbable monofilament suture
3. What is not true with respect to cruciate ligament (CL) rupture
   (a) The cranial CL is more commonly affected than the caudal CL, (b) overweight and large breed dogs are more prone (c) the incidence is higher in non-neutered dogs (d) the dogs that rupture the cranial CL in one leg are more likely to develop the condition in the opposite leg
4. Repair and surgical reconstruction of collateral ligaments is difficult as
   (a) they are very short (b) difficult to approach surgically (c) structurally weak (d) present intra-articularly
5. In cranial cruciate ligament rupture, joint swelling is most often seen on the
   (a) cranial side (b) caudal side (c) medial side (d) lateral side

**Question No. 2: State true or false**

1. The most commonly ruptured tendon in dogs and cats is the Achilles tendon.
2. Ultrasonography is generally not useful to evaluate tendon healing and assess prognosis.
3. In contracted flexor tendon affecting the fetlock joints, tenotomy is performed in the midmetacarpal or midmetatarsal region.
4. Sutures placed at volar or plantar surface of tendon affect the blood flow but can increase the pull-out strength as compared to dorsally placed sutures.
5. Injury to the cranial cruciate ligament is more frequently reported than to the caudal cruciate ligament.
6. The tibial plateau leveling osteotomy alters the mechanism of the knee joint and allows it to function properly without a cruciate ligament.

**Question No. 3: Fill in the blanks**

1. ________________ occur at the ends of skeletal muscles and function to insert muscles onto the bones in specific locations, whereas ________________ connect bones at joints and help them to hold together in position.
2. Completely dropped hock with severe lameness is a characteristic clinical sign with complete rupture of ________________ tendon.
3. The flexor tendon injuries in horse are mostly attributed to ________________-_, whereas in cattle, it is commonly caused due to ________________ ________.
4. Contracted flexor tendon is one of the common congenital defects observed in large animals, especially in cattle, generally affecting ________________ or ________________ ________ joints.
5. A congenital, hereditary condition, usually showing permanent changes in the articular and osseous structures in any one leg or all four legs, is ________________ _____.
6. Pathognomonic clinical signs of cranial cruciate ligament rupture are ________________- ________ and ________________ ________________.

**Question No. 4: Write short note on the following:**

1. Surgical treatment of Achilles tendon rupture in cattle
2. Principles of tendon suturing
3. Diagnosis of cranial cruciate ligament rupture in dog
4. The tibial plateau leveling osteotomy

## References


1. Johnston, D.E. 1985. Tendons, skeletal muscles, and ligaments in health and disease. In *Textbook of small animal orthopaedics*, ed. C.D. Newton and D.M. Nunamaker, 65–76. Philadelphia: J.B. Lippincott.
2. Evans, H.E., and G.C. Christensen. 1979. *Miller's anatomy of the dog*, 392–402. Philadelphia: W.B. Saunders.
3. Harasen, G. 2006. Ruptures of the common calcaneal tendon. The Canadian Veterinary Journal 47(12): 1219–1220
4. King, M., and R. Jerram. 2003. Achilles tendon rupture in dogs. *Compendium on Continuing Education for the Practising Veterinarian* 25: 613–620.
5. Swiderski, J., R.B. Fitch, A. Staatz, and J. Lowery. 2005. Sonographic assisted diagnosis and treatment of bilateral gastrocnemius tendon rupture in a Labrador retriever repaired with fascia lata and polypropylene mesh. *Veterinary and Comparative Orthopaedics and Traumatology* 4: 258–263.
6. Fahie, M.A. 2005. Healing, diagnosis, repair, and rehabilitation of tendon conditions. *The Veterinary Clinics of North America. Small Animal Practice* 35: 1195–1211.
7. Berg, R.J., and E.L. Egger. 1986. In vitro comparison of the three loop pulley and locking loop suture patterns for the repair of canine weight bearing tendons and collateral ligaments. *Veterinary Surgery* 15: 107–114.
8. Moores, A.P., M.R. Owen, and J.F. Tarlton. 2004. The three-loop pulley suture versus two locking-loop sutures for the repair of canine Achilles tendons. *Veterinary Surgery* 33: 131–137.
9. Shani, J., and R. Shahar. 2000. Repair of chronic complete traumatic rupture of the common calcaneal tendon in a dog, using a fascia lata graft. *Veterinary and Comparative Orthopaedics and Traumatology* 13: 104–108.
10. Spinella, G., R. Tamburro, G. Loprete, J.M. Vilar, and S. Valentine. 2010. Surgical repair of Achilles tendon rupture in dogs: a review of the literature, a case report and new perspectives. *Veterinární Medicína* 55 (7): 303–310.
11. Guerin, S., H. Burbridge, E. Firth, and S. Fox. 1998. Achilles tenorrhaphy in five dogs: a modified surgical technique and evaluation of a cranial half cast. *Veterinary and Comparative Orthopaedics and Traumatology* 11: 205–210.
12. Altug, N., C. Ozkan, N. Yuksek, A. Karasu, I. Keles, Z.T. Agaoglu, and F. Ilhan. 2007. Rupture of the gastrocnemius muscle in a cow two months after twin birth. *Bulletin of the Veterinary Institute in Pulaway* 51: 615–619.
13. Mori, A.P., C.I. Schwertz, L.C. Henker, F.A. Stedille, R. Christ, M.P. Lorenzett, F. Broll, and R.E. Mendes. 2017. Bilateral gastrocnemius muscle rupture in a bovine. Acta. *Veterinary Sciences* 45 (Suppl. 1): 189. (5 pages).
14. Jesty, S.A., J.E. Palmer, E.J. Parente, T.P. Schaer, and P.A. Wilkins. 2005. Rupture of the gastrocnemius muscle in six foals. *Journal of the American Veterinary Medical Association* 227: 1965–1968.
15. Budras, K.D., W.O. Sack, S. Rock, A. Horowitz, and R. Berg. 2004. *Anatomy of the horse*. Hannover: Schlutersche Verlagsgesellschaft mbH & Co. KG.
16. Sato, F., R. Shibata, M. Shikichi, K. Ito, H. Murase, T. Ueno, H. Furuoka, and K. Yamada. 2014. Rupture of the gastrocnemius muscle in neonatal thoroughbred foals: A report of three cases. *Journal of Equine Science* 25 (3): 61–64.
17. Lescun, T.B., J.F. Hawkins, and J.J. Siems. 1998. Management of rupture of the gastrocnemius and superficial digital flexor muscles with a modified Thomas splint-cast combination in a horse. *Journal of the American Veterinary Medical Association* 213: 1457–1459.
18. Smith, R.K.W. 2008. Tendon and ligament injury. *AAEP Proceedings* 54: 475–501.
19. Anderson, D.E., A. Desrochers, and St. Jean, G. 2008. Management of tendon disorders in cattle. *Veterinary Clinics of North America: Food Animal Practice* 24: 551–566.
20. Jann, H.W., and R.R. Stecke. 1989. Treatment of lacerated flexor tendons in a dairy cow, using specialized farriery. *Journal of the American Veterinary Medical Association* 195 (6): 772–774.
21. Stashak, T.A. 1987. Lameness. In *Adam's lameness in horses*, ed. T.S. Stashak, 4th ed., 764–767. Philadelphia: Lea and Febiger.
22. Jann, H.W., L.E. Stein, and J.K. Good. 1990. Strength characteristics and failure modes of locking-loop and three loop pulley suture patterns in equine tendons. *Veterinary Surgery* 19: 28–33.
23. Eliashar, E., M.C. Schramme, J. Schumacher, et al. 2001. Use of a bioabsorbable implant for the repair of severed digital flexor tendons in four horses. *The Veterinary Record* 148: 506–509.
24. Anderson, D.E., and St. Jean, G. 1996. Diagnosis and management of tendon disorders in cattle. *The Veterinary Clinics of North America. Food Animal Practice* 12 (1): 86–116.
25. Leipold, H.W., T. Hirarga, and S.M. Dennis. 1993. Congenital defects of the bovine musculoskeletal system and joints. *The Veterinary Clinics of North America. Food Animal Practice* 9: 93–104.

26. Schoiswohl, J., J. Eiter, H. Schwarzenbacher, and J. Kofler. 2019. Congenital flexural deformity in 93 calves- appearance, treatment techniques and results of pedigree analysis. *Schweizer Archiv für Tierheilkunde* 2019: 677–688. https://doi.org/10.17236/sat00230.
27. Madison, J.B., J.L. Garber, B. Rice, A.J. Stumf, A.E. Zimmer, and E.A. Ott. 1994. Effect of oxytetracycline on metacarpophalangeal and distal interphalangeal joint angles in new born foals. *Journal of the American Veterinary Medical Association* 204: 246–249.
28. Kumar, S., A.C. Mathur, and S.K. Jana. 2017. Surgical correction of congenital arthrogryposis of carpal joint in calves. *Exploratory Animal and Medical Research* 7 (1): 110–112.
29. Van Huffel, X., and A. DeMoor. 1987. Congenital multiple arthrogryposis of the forelimb in calves. *Compendium on Continuing Education for the Practising Veterinarian* 9 (10): F333–F339.
30. Verschooten, F., A. DeMoor, P. Desmet, et al. 1969. Surgical treatment of arthrogryposis of the carpal joint associated with contraction of the flexor tendons in calves. *The Veterinary Record* 85: 140–171.
31. Butler, H.C. 1985. Surgery of tendinous injuries and muscle injuries. In *Textbook of small animal Orthopaedics*, ed. C.D. Newton and D.M. Nunamaker, 835–842. Philadelphia: J.B. Lippincott.
32. Bunnell, S. 1940. Primary repair of severed tendons. *American Journal of Surgery* 47: 502–510.
33. Cao, Y., and J.B. Tang. 2010. A new variant of four-strand tendon repairs. *The Journal of Hand Surgery (European Volume)* 35 (6): 513–515.
34. Chen, J., K. Wang, F. Katirai, and Z. Chen. 2014. A new modified Tsuge suture for flexor tendon repairs: the biomechanical analysis and clinical application. *Journal of Orthopaedic Surgery and Research* 9: 136.
35. Lee, H. 1990. Double loop locking suture: a technique of tendon repair for early active mobilization. Part I: evolution of technique and experimental study. *The Journal of Hand Surgery* 15 (6): 945–952.
36. Pennington, D.G. 1979. The locking loop tendon suture. *Plastic and Reconstructive Surgery* 63 (5): 648–652.
37. Rawson, S., S. Cartmell, and J. Wong. 2013. Suture techniques for tendon repair; a comparative review. *Muscles, Ligaments and Tendons Journal* 3 (3): 220–228.
38. Soejima, O., E. Diao, J.C. Lotz, and J.S. Hariharan. 1995. Comparative mechanical analysis of dorsal versus palmar placement of core suture for flexor tendon repairs. *The Journal of Hand Surgery* 20: 801–807.
39. Wu, Y.F., Y. Cao, Y.L. Zhou, and J.B. Tang. 2011. Biomechanical comparisons of four-strand tendon repairs with double-stranded sutures: effects of different locks and suture geometry. *The Journal of Hand Surgery* 36 (1): 34–39.
40. Baker, L.A., and P. Muir. 2018. Epidemiology of cruciate ligament rupture. In *Advances in the canine cranial cruciate ligament*, ed. P. Muir, 2nd ed., 109–114. Hoboken, NJ: Wiley-Blackwell.
41. Harasen, G. 2003. Canine cranial cruciate ligament rupture in profile. *The Canadian Veterinary Journal* 44: 845–846.
42. Spinella, G., G. Arcamone, and S. Valentine. 2021. Cranial cruciate ligament rupture in dogs: review of biomechanics, etiopathogenic factors and rehabilitation. *Veterinary Science* 8 (9): 186. https://doi.org/10.3390/vetsci809018.
43. Candela Andrade, M., P. Slunsky, K.G. Klass, and L. Brunnberg. 2022. Patellar luxation and concomitant cranial cruciate ligament rupture in dogs- A review. *Veterinární Medicína Czech* 67: 163–178.
44. Nečas, A., J. Zatloukal, H. Kecová, and M. Dvořák. 2000. Predisposition of dog breeds to rupture of the cranial cruciate ligament. *Acta Veterinaria* 69: 305–310.
45. Taylor-Brown, F.E., R.L. Meeson, D.C. Brodbelt, D.B. Church, P.D. McGreevy, P.C. Thomson, and D.G. O'Neill. 2015. Epidemiology of cranial cruciate ligament disease, diagnosis in dogs attending primary-care veterinary practices in England. *Veterinary Surgery* 44: 777–783.
46. Whitehair, J.G., P.B. Vasseur, and N.H. Willits. 1993. Epidemiology of cranial cruciate ligament rupture in dogs. *Journal of the American Veterinary Medical Association* 203: 1016–1019.
47. Slauterbeck, J.R., K. Pankratz, K.T. Xu, S.C. Bozeman, and D.M. Hardy. 2004. Canine ovariohysterectomy and orchiectomy increase the prevalence of ACL injury. *Clinical Orthopaedics and Related Research* 429: 301–305.
48. Baird, A.E.G., S.D. Carter, J.F. Innes, W. Ollier, and A. Short. 2014. Genetic basis of cranial cruciate ligament rupture (CCLR) in dogs. *Connective Tissue Research* 55: 275–281.
49. Baker, L.A., B. Kirkpatrick, G.J.M. Rosa, D. Gianola, B. Valente, J.P. Sumner, W. Baltzer, Z. Hao, E.E. Binversie, N. Volstad, et al. 2017. Genome-wide association analysis in dogs implicates 99 loci as risk variants for anterior cruciate ligament rupture. *PLoS One* 2017 (12): e0173810.
50. Vasseur, P.B. 1985. Clinical results following nonoperative management for rupture of the cranial cruciate ligament in dogs. *Veterinary Surgery* 13: 243–246.
51. Canapp, S.O., C.S. Leasure, C. Cox, V. Ibrahim, and Carr B. Jean. 2016. Partial cranial cruciate ligament tears treated with stem cell and platelet-rich plasma combination therapy in 36 dogs: A retrospective study. *Frontiers in Veterinary Science* 14: 112. https://doi.org/10.3389/fvets.2016.00112.
52. Jean Carr, B., S.O. Canapp, S. Meilleur, S.A. Christopher, J. Collins, and C. Cox. 2016. The use of canine stifle orthotics for cranial cruciate ligament insufficiency. *Veterinary Evidence* 2016: 1. https://doi.org/10.18849/ve.v1i1.10.
53. Jerram, R.M., and A.M. Walker. 2003. Cranial cruciate ligament injury in the dog: pathophysiology,

diagnosis, and treatment. *New Zealand Veterinary Journal* 51: 149–158.
54. Kirkness, H. 2020. Management of cranial cruciate ligament ruptures in dogs. *Veterinary Nursing Journal* 35: 235–237.
55. Jerre, S. 2009. Rehabilitation after extra-articular stabilisation of cranial cruciate ligament rupture in dogs. *Veterinary and Comparative Orthopaedics and Traumatology* 22: 148–152.
56. Boudrieau, R.J. 2009. Tibial plateau leveling osteotomy or tibial tuberosity advancement? *Veterinary Surgery* 38: 1–22.
57. Slocum, B., and T.D. Slocum. 1993. Tibial plateau leveling osteotomy for repair of cranial cruciate ligament rupture in the canine. *Veterinary Clinics of North America: Small Animal Practice* 23: 777–795.
58. Lafaver, S., N.A. Miller, W.P. Stubbs, R.A. Taylor, and R.J. Boudrieau. 2007. Tibial tuberosity advancement for stabilization of the canine cranial cruciate ligament deficient stifle joint: surgical technique, early results and complications in 101 dogs. *Veterinary Surgery* 36: 573–586.
59. Berté, L., A. Mazzanti, F.Z. Salbego, D.V. Beckmann, R.P. Santos, D. Polidoro, and R. Baumhardt. 2012. Immediate physical therapy in dogs with rupture of the cranial cruciate ligament submitted to extracapsular surgical stabilization. *Arquivo Brasileiro de Medicina Veterinária e Zootecnia* 64: 1–8.
60. Marcellin-Little, D.J., and C.J. Arnoldy. 2018. Rehabilitation for dogs with cruciate ligament rupture. In *Advances in the canine cranial cruciate ligament*, ed. P. Muir, 2nd ed., 343–351. Hoboken, NJ: Wiley-Blackwell.
61. Monk, M.L., C.A. Preston, and C.M. McGowan. 2006. Effects of early intensive postoperative physiotherapy on limb function after tibial plateau leveling osteotomy in dogs with deficiency of the cranial cruciate ligament. *American Journal of Veterinary Research* 67: 529–536.
62. Wild, S. 2017. Canine cranial cruciate ligament damage and the use of hydrotherapy as a rehabilitation tool. *Veterinary Nursing Journal* 32: 228–234.
63. Rogatko, C.P., W.I. Baltzer, and R. Tennant. 2017. Preoperative low level laser therapy in dogs undergoing tibial plateau levelling osteotomy: a blinded, prospective, randomized clinical trial. *Veterinary and Comparative Orthopaedics and Traumatology* 30: 46–53.
64. Ducharme, N.G. 1996. Stifle injuries in cattle. *The Veterinary Clinics of North America. Food Animal Practice* 12 (1): 59–85.
65. Hamilton, G.F., and O.R. Adams. 1971. Anterior cruciate repair in cattle. *Journal of the American Veterinary Medical Association* 158: 178.
66. Hofmeyr, C.F.B. 1968. Reconstruction of the anterior cruciate ligament in the stifle of a bull. *The Veterinarian* 5: 89.
67. Nelson, D.R., and D.B. Koch. 1982. Surgical stabilization of the stifle in cranial cruciate injury in cattle. *The Veterinary Record* 111: 259.
68. Huhn, J.C., S.K. Kneller, and D.R. Nelson. 1986. Radiographic assessment of cranial cruciate ligament rupture in dairy cow: a retrospective study. *Veterinary Radiology* 27: 184.
69. Lee, H., S.H. Yun, J.O. Park, S.J. Kim, Y.S. Kwon, and K.H. Jang. 2014. Anterior cruciate ligament rupture in a Korean native cattle. *J Vet Clin* 31 (1): 54–56.
70. Prades, M., B.D. Grant, T.A. Turner, A.J. Nixon, and M.P. Brown. 1989. Injuries to the cranial cruciate ligament and associated structures: summary of clinical, radiographic, arthroscopic and pathological findings from 10 horses. *Equine Veterinary Journal* 21 (5): 354–357.
71. Crawford, W.H. 1990. Intra-articular replacement of bovine cranial cruciate ligaments with an autogenous fascial graft. *Veterinary Surgery* 19: 380–388.
72. Moss, E.W., D.M. McCurnin, and T.H. Ferguson. 1988. Experimental cranial cruciate replacement in cattle using a patellar ligament graft. *The Canadian Veterinary Journal* 29: 157.
73. Constant, C., V.B. MIng, E.W. BIng, Y.P. BIng, A. Desrochers, and S. Nichols. 2021. Biomechanical evaluation of bovine stifles stabilized with an innovative braided superelastic nitinol prosthesis after transection of the cranial cruciate ligament. *Veterinary Surgery* 50 (7): 1398–1408.
74. Niehaus, A.J., D.E. Anderson, J.K. Johnson, and J.J. Lannutti. 2013. Comparison of the mechanical characteristics of polymerized caprolactam and monofilament nylon loops constructed in parallel strands or as braided ropes versus cranial cruciate ligaments of cattle. *American Journal of Veterinary Research* 74 (3): 381–385.
75. Das, S., R. Thorne, S. Langley-Hobbs, K.L. Perry, N.J. Burton, and J.R. Mosley. 2015. Patellar ligament rupture in the cat: repair methods and patient outcomes in seven cases. *Journal of Feline Medicine and Surgery* 17 (4): 348–352.
76. Das, S., R. Thorne, N. Lorenz, S. Clarke, M. Madden, S. Langley-Hobbs, K.L. Perry, N.J. Burton, A.L. Moores, and J.R. Mosley. 2014. Patellar ligament rupture in the dog: repair methods and patient outcomes in 43 cases. *The Veterinary Record* 175 (15): 370.
77. Johnson, M.D., D.R. Sobrino, D.D. Lewis, and J. Shmalberg. 2018. Surgical repair of a proximal patellar tendon avulsion in a dog utilizing triple patellar bone tunnels and modified tendon repair technique. *Open Veterinary Journal* 8 (3): 256–264.
78. Farrow, C.S., and C.D. Newton. 1985. Ligamentous injury (sprain). In *Textbook of small animal Orthopaedics*, ed. C.D. Newton and D.M. Nunamaker, 843–851. Philadelphia: J.B. Lippincott.
79. Sarierler, M., I. Akin, A. Belge, and N. Kiliç. 2013. Patellar fracture and patellar tendon rupture in a dog.

*Turkish Journal of Veterinary and Animal Sciences* 37: 121–124.
80. Shipov, A., R. Shahar, R. Joseph, and J. Milgram. 2008. Successful management of bilateral patellar tendon rupture in a dog. *Veterinary and Comparative Orthopaedics and Traumatology* 21 (2): 181–184.
81. Smith, M., J. de Haan, J. Peck, and S. Madden. 2000. Augmented primary repair of patellar ligament rupture in three dogs. *Veterinary and Comparative Orthopaedics and Traumatology* 13 (3): 154–157.
82. Gottlieb, R. M.B. Whitcomb, B. Vaughan, L.D. Galuppo and M. Spriet. 2015. Ultrasonographic appearance of normal and injured lateral patellar ligaments in the equine stifle. *Equine Veterinary Journal* 48: 299–306.
83. Dyson, S.J. 2002. Normal ultrasonographic anatomy and injury of the patellar ligaments in the horse. *Equine Veterinary Journal* 34: 258–264.
84. Lamb, L., C. Zubrod, B. Hague, J. Brakenhoff, and M. Major. 2012. Clinical outcome of collateral ligament injuries of the tarsus. *The Canadian Veterinary Journal* 53 (5): 518–524.
85. Tenney, W.A., and M.B. Whitcomb. 2008. Rupture of collateral ligaments in metacarpophalangeal and metatarsophalangeal joints in horses: 17 cases (1999-2005). *Journal of the American Veterinary Medical Association* 233 (3): 456–462.
86. Bell, C., K. Torske, and B. Lobb. 2016. Collateral ligament reconstruction in two horses following traumatic avulsion fracture using a knotless suture anchor construct. *Equine Veterinary Education* 30 (7): 360–366.
87. Rodgerson, D.H., and M.A. Spirito. 2001. Repair of collateral ligament instability in 2 foals by using suture anchors. *The Canadian Veterinary Journal* 42 (7): 557–560.
88. Rothlisberger, J., P. Schawalder, P. Kircher, and A. Steiner. 2001. Collateral ligament prosthesis for the repair of subluxation of the metatarsophalangeal joint in a Jersey cow. *The Veterinary Record* 146 (22): 640–643.
89. Sanders-Shamis, M., and A.A. Gabel. 1988. Surgical reconstruction of a ruptured medial collateral ligament in a foal. *Journal of the American Veterinary Medical Association* 193 (1): 80–82.
90. Demir, H., P. Menku, M. Kirnap, M. Calis, and I. Ikizceli. 2004. Comparison of the effects of laser, ultrasound, and combined laser + ultrasound treatments in experimental tendon healing. *Lasers in Surgery and Medicine* 35 (1): 84–89.
91. Enwemeka, C., O. Rodriguez, and S. Mendosa. 1990. The biomechanical effects of low-intensity ultrasound on healing tendons. *Ultrasound in Medicine & Biology* 16 (8): 801–807.
92. Fortier, L.A., and R.K.W. Smith. 2008. Regenerative medicine for tendinous and ligamentous injuries of sport horses. *Veterinary Clinics: Equine Practice* 24: 191–201.
93. Geburek, F., and P. Stadler. 2011. Regenerative therapy for tendon and ligament disorders in horses. Terminology, production, biologic potential and in vitro effects. *Tierärztliche Praxis. Ausgabe G, Grosstiere/Nutztiere* 39 (6): 373–383.
94. Romero, A., L. Barrachina, B. Ranera, A.R. Remacha, B. Moreno, I. de Blas, A. Sanz, F.J. Vázquez, A. Vitoria, C. Junquera, P. Zaragoza, and C. Rodellar. 2017. Comparison of autologous bone marrow and adipose tissue derived mesenchymal stem cells, and platelet rich plasma, for treating surgically induced lesions of the equine superficial digital flexor tendon. *Veterinary Journal* 224: 76–84.
95. Siddiqui, N.A., J.M.L. Wong, W.S. Khan, and A. Hazlerigg. 2010. Stem cells for tendon and ligament tissue engineering and regeneration. *Journal of Stem Cells* 5 (4): 187–194.
96. Spaas, J.H., D.J. Guest, and G.R. Van de Valle. 2012. Tendon regeneration in human and equine athletes. *Sports Medicine* 42 (10): 871–890.

# Bone Tumors

# 14

**Learning Objectives**

You will be able to understand the following after reading this chapter:

- Common bone tumors, their clinical signs, diagnosis, treatment (use of analgesics, radiation therapy, bisphosphonates, chemotherapy, excision of tumor and amputation of limb) and prognosis

**Summary**

- Bone tumors are more commonly reported in dogs, osteosarcoma is the most common primary bone tumor and large giant breed dogs are more susceptible.
- Most common clinical signs in dogs and cats with tumors of the appendicular skeleton are lameness and swelling around the affected bone. Pathognomonic radiographic signs include the lytic lesion in the bone giving sunburst appearance mostly at the metaphyseal region of long bones (the lesion does not cross the joint space to affect other bones in the joint, unlike in osteomyelitis or osteoarthritis).
- Analgesics and radiation therapy are primarily used as palliative treatment option for osteosarcoma.
- Different chemotherapeutic drugs or combinations used for osteosarcoma are *cisplatin* (IV, every 3–4 weeks for three times), *carboplatin* (IV, every 3–4 weeks for four times), *doxorubicin* (IV, every two weeks for five times) and a combination of *doxorubicin* and *cisplatin* (IV, together every three weeks for four times).
- Limb amputation is considered as the gold standard for the surgical treatment of primary bone tumors; it can be combined with chemotherapy (starting at two weeks after surgery) to control metastasis and recurrence and improve the survival time significantly.

Skeletal (bone) tumors can occur in any domestic animal, but it is more commonly reported in dogs. It can be benign or malignant and primary or secondary (metastases from other soft tissues). Osteosarcoma is reported to be the most common primary tumor of the bone [1–7].



H. P. Aithal et al., *Textbook of Veterinary Orthopaedic Surgery*,
https://doi.org/10.1007/978-981-99-2575-9_14

## 14.1 Dogs and Cats

The most commonly reported primary bone tumor is osteosarcoma, accounting for more than 95% of all bone tumors in dogs. It usually involves the limb bones (75–85%) of large breed dogs [3, 8]. Other tumors reported are chondrosarcoma, squamous cell carcinoma and synovial cell sarcoma. The majority of primary bone tumors arise spontaneously without any apparent cause. But tumors can occur at sites of old fracture or at the implant site; however, the incidence of bone tumor after a fracture or fracture repair is rare. Large giant breeds of dog such as German shepherd, Great Dane, Saint Bernard, Boxer, Labrador, retriever, Irish setter and Doberman pinscher are more susceptible for developing osteosarcoma, but small dogs can also be affected. Some breeds like Scottish Deerhounds are found to be genetically predisposed for occurrence of osteosarcoma, but other large breeds of dog like Rottweiler can also be affected frequently. Most of the reports show more prevalence of osteosarcoma in male dogs [8]. Osteosarcoma or other tumors of bony tissue can occur at any age but older dogs are more commonly affected. The most common sites are distal radius-ulna, proximal humerus and distal end of tibia and femur; however, the tumors are often recorded at the proximal end of the tibia and femur as well.

Primary bone tumors are less common in cats than in dogs, but osteosarcoma is still the most common tumor in cats [6, 9]. In cats, osteosarcoma occurs with almost equal frequency in the axial and appendicular skeleton, with no gender predilection [10]. In the appendicular skeleton, the prevalence is more in hind limbs, mostly at the distal femur, the proximal tibia, the humerus and the digits; and among the flat and irregular bones, skull is the most common site. In another study, a large number of osteosarcomas (38%) arose from extraskeletal sites in cats [11]. Osteosarcoma associated with osteosynthesis has also been reported in cats [10, 12]. About one-third of bone tumors in cats are benign in contrast to the dog, where majority of bone tumors are malignant. Even though osteosarcomas in felines and canines have similar histologic characteristics, they have different prognostic characteristics [13]. Osteosarcoma is generally less aggressive in cats than in dogs.

### 14.1.1 Clinical Signs

The most common signs in dogs and cats affected with tumor of appendicular skeleton are lameness and swelling of the affected bone [3–5, 10]. The progression and extent of lameness can be variable. Generally a slow onset of lameness is reported, which may progress rapidly over a short period of time (within 1–2 months); however, an acute lameness with no weight bearing on the affected limb can be present if a fracture occurs at the site of tumor. There will be soft tissue swelling at the site of bone tumor, and the dogs with metastatic lung lesions may also show diffuse swelling of all four limbs especially at the distal extremity (suggestive of hypertrophic osteopathy) along with generalized weakness and breathing difficulties. In cases of primary tumors of the bones of axial skeleton (like in the skull or jaw), the clinical signs may depend on the bone involved, and in most of the cases, an observable swelling or mass may be the first sign of tumor. Other signs may include difficulty in eating (jaw tumors), neurologic signs (skull or vertebral tumors), respiratory difficulties (rib tumors), etc.

### 14.1.2 Diagnosis

History and clinical signs most often give an indication of bone tumor, and radiography will confirm diagnosis in most cases [14]. The lytic lesion in the bone gives sunburst appearance, wherein the tumor grows outwards and outer bone is pushed away (Fig. 14.1). A pathological fracture may also be seen at the site of lesion. Osteosarcoma grows rapidly but does not affect the other bones across the joint (unlike in osteomyelitis or osteoarthritis). Physical appearance, location, and radiographic signs of osteosarcoma are classical, and radiography is confirmatory in

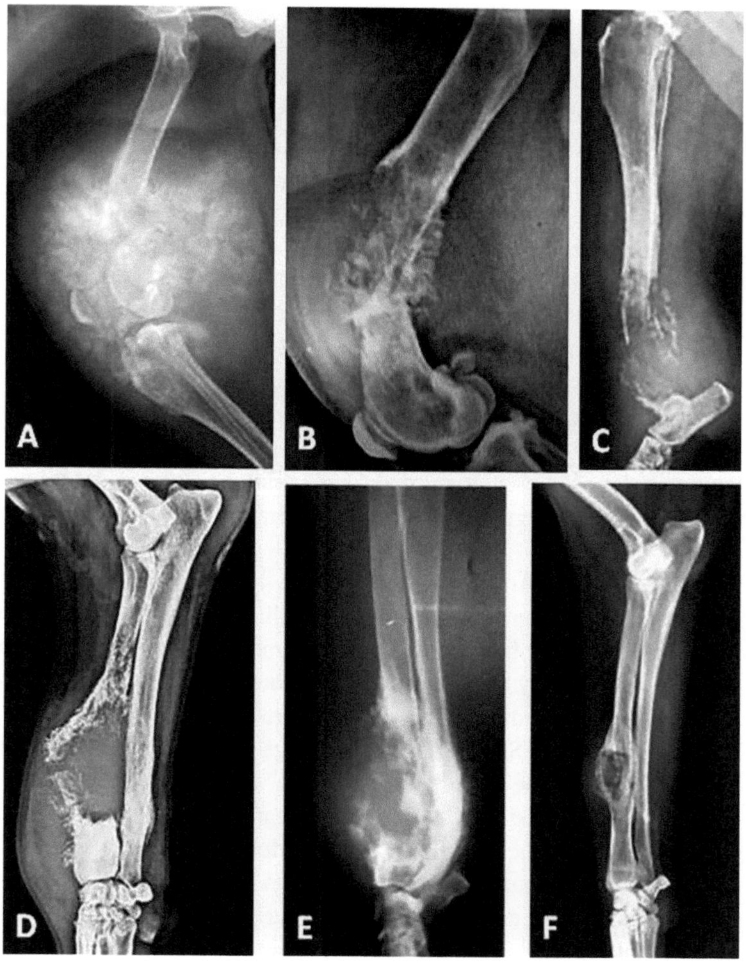


**Fig. 14.1** Radiographs showing osteosarcoma at different locations in dogs: femur (**a** and **b**), tibia (**c**) and distal radius-ulna (**d–f**). Cardinal radiographic signs of lytic changes in the bone with sunburst appearance can be seen

most cases. The condition is generally easily diagnosed, but there are a few other conditions that may show similar signs in the limb. Differential diagnosis of osteosarcoma may be done from chondrosarcoma, squamous cell carcinoma and fungal infection mainly through radiographic examination. *Chondrosarcoma* is a tumor of cartilage tissue, which generally affects the flat bones such as that of ribs or skull, and it is not as malignant as osteosarcoma. The *squamous cell carcinoma* is a tumor of the periosteum. It is also a destructive tumor locally but it spreads at a relatively slow speed. *Synovial cell sarcoma* is a tumor of the joint capsule, which affects both bones of the joint, but generally with better prognosis. The fungal infection grows rapidly but does not show typical lytic lesions of osteosarcoma. Because osteosarcoma spreads quickly to the lungs, chest radiography or CT scan may be necessary for detection of possible lung metastasis. If there is already visible tumor spread, it is recommended to go for a whole-body nuclear imaging, if possible, to identify the spread of the tumor to other bones.

It is also necessary to confirm diagnosis by histopathological examination of the tissue obtained by either biopsy or by needle aspiration cytology [14]. Biopsy sample may be more useful if the clinical signs are not typical (like small breed, middle-aged dog, multiple lesions, lesion located in mid diaphysis of long bones, etc.) or if any other diseases like osteomyelitis or a fungal bone infection is suspected. Minimally invasive ultrasound-guided needle aspiration biopsy can be an effective technique for diagnosis of bone tumors [15].

### 14.1.3 Treatment

Treatment options available for management of bone tumors of appendicular skeleton can be grouped into two main categories, the palliative and the curative treatments [16]. The purpose of the palliative treatment is to control the pain and improve the quality of life but it may not necessarily prolong life. The curative treatment, however, is administered to control the spread of tumor metastasis in an effort to cure the tumor and provide a prolonged good quality of life. The use of analgesics and radiation therapy are primarily used as palliative treatment option; and limb amputation is used as palliative and curative treatment option often along with chemotherapy.

#### 14.1.3.1 Use of Analgesics

A large variety of analgesic drugs are available for use in dogs with bone tumor. A single medication, however, may not be very effective; hence a combination of medications may be required to have desired effect. Several groups of drugs are available that can be used in combination with added effects. Non-steroidal anti-inflammatory drugs (NSAIDs) such as carprofen, etodolac, deracoxib, meloxicam, firocoxib, etc. can be given once or twice daily in patients having good liver and kidney functions. They can be effective initially; however, stronger analgesic drugs or drug combinations may be needed in later stages of tumor. Narcotic analgesics even though do not possess anti-inflammatory activity, they are good analgesics and are particularly useful in chronic pain. Other drugs such as gabapentin and amantadine can be used as adjunct pain killers in cases of animals having chronic pain.

#### 14.1.3.2 Radiation Therapy

Limb amputation controls pain completely in all cases; however, when amputation is not an option, radiation therapy is used often as a palliative treatment [17]. Various protocols of radiation therapy have been recommended for the management of bone tumors [18–21]. The most common protocol comprised of 3–4 exposures of radiation at weekly interval or at monthly interval depending upon the condition of the animal. The beneficial effects of radiation therapy usually become evident in a few weeks and usually last for 2–4 months. Several studies have shown improvement in the quality of life and increased survival time after radiation therapy [22]. If pain returns back, radiation therapy can be repeated again, if considered appropriate based on the evaluation of the patient at that time. Radiation therapy can also be combined with analgesic drugs and cancer chemotherapy for added advantages.

#### 14.1.3.3 Bisphosphonates

Use of biphosphonates is the standard treatment protocol in human patients of bone tumors, and it has also been found useful in pain management in dogs with osteosarcoma. They inhibit bone destruction (osteoclastic activity); thus they are useful to control bone damage and in turn control pain in bone tumor cases [23–25]. The common bisphosphonates used in dogs are pamidronate, zoledronate, and alendronate. It is given as an intravenous drip slowly over a period of 2 h every 3–4 weeks. Bisphosphonates are particularly important in controlling pain in patients who have not undergone amputation.

#### 14.1.3.4 Chemotherapy

Osteosarcoma is a fast-spreading tumor, and by the time it is diagnosed, the tumor would have spread to other organs, especially to the lungs. If lung metastasis is detected on chest radiographs, the only option to change the course of tumor is chemotherapy. The purpose of chemotherapy is to destroy the tumor cells and to improve the quality of life. Different drugs or combination of drugs have been tried [8, 26, 27]. *Cisplatin* given intravenously every 3–4 weeks for three times has been shown median survival time of 400 days and 30–60% survival at one year and 7–21% survival at two years. *Cisplatin* should not be used in kidney patients as it is nephrotoxic. *Carboplatin* given intravenously every 3–4 weeks for four times has also shown to give similar results. *Carboplatin* is more expensive but not toxic to kidneys. Doxorubicin given intravenously at

15 days' interval for 5 times has shown median survival time of 365 days and 10% survival at 2 years, but it is toxic to heart. Combination of *doxorubicin* and *cisplatin* administered intravenously at three weeks' interval for four times has been shown to provide about 50% survival at one year time and 30% survival at two-year duration.

The majority of dogs (>85%) can tolerate chemotherapy protocol with no or minimal problems. Some of the common side effects of chemotherapy include generalized weakness and nausea that may last for 1–2 days; some dogs may show signs of bone marrow suppression and infection. Chemotherapy does not usually result in hair loss in animals, but dog breeds known for continuously growing coats, such as poodles, Scottish terriers, etc., may suffer from hair loss. The complications and severity of side effects associated with chemotherapy are more often drug and dose dependent. Some studies have also suggested that dual-agent protocols do not improve the survival times; hence it is advised to use a single-agent protocol, which is equally effective with less toxicity [28, 29].

In recent years, the use of nanotechnology has been proposed as a new approach to avoid multidrug resistance and reduce the adverse toxic reactions of chemotherapeutic agents for the treatment of osteosarcoma in both human and veterinary medicines [30]. In one such study involving doxorubicin-loaded lipid nanoparticles coated with calcium phosphate, there was an increase in drug uptake and cytotoxicity for calcium phosphate-coated nanoparticles, suggesting potential applications of nano-drug delivery in human and canine osteosarcoma therapy [31].

#### 14.1.3.5 Excision of Tumor (Limb-Sparing Surgery)

Even though amputation of the limb is recommended in most of the limb tumors, often due to animal owners' reluctance, limb-sparing techniques are used by surgically excising the tumor mass (including the surrounding normal tissues) and either replacing the gap by a bone graft or re-growing the bone-by-bone transport osteogenesis. In this technique, the joint nearest the tumor is allowed to fuse (ankylose). Limb-sparing technique should not be adopted in animals where the tumor has affected more than 50% of the bone and/or if neighboring soft tissue is involved. This technique is better suited for tumors of the distal radius, if diagnosed early. In tumors involving proximal bones such as humerus or hind limbs, the prognosis is generally not good. Further, except for preservation of limb function, the limb-sparing surgery does not provide any advantage over the benefits of limb amputation. Complication rate is relatively high (as compared to limb amputation), which may include bone infection, implant failure, tumor recurrence, etc. For better results, limb-sparing surgery is performed along with chemotherapy.

#### 14.1.3.6 Amputation of the Limb

The gold standard for the surgical treatment of primary bone tumors is limb amputation as complications associated with the surgery are very few. Patients having one tumor in a leg with no visible tumor spread/metastasis are considered as good candidates for limb amputation. The patients suffering from arthritis in the other limb or having tumor spread in the lungs should not be considered for amputation, and such patients may be given palliative treatment by using pain killers along with radiotherapy. It should also be kept in mind that limb amputation alone is only palliative and may not prolong survival time. Limb amputation with chemotherapy has been shown to improve the survival time significantly as compared to the survival time recorded after surgery alone, and it is recommended to start chemotherapy in about two weeks after surgery, at the time of suture removal [26, 32–35]. Limb amputation and chemotherapy, when followed by immunotherapy, have been shown to further increase the survival time [36]. Immunotherapy could be a prudent treatment strategy to transform the management of metastatic bone tumors in man and animals [37].

In cats with primary bone tumor of the limb, amputation and limb-sparing surgery are the treatment options [9]. The most of the primary bone tumors of cats have limited potential to metastasize, and therefore postoperative chemotherapy is not required after successful surgery.

In the axial skeleton, the tumor does not spread as rapidly as do in the appendicular skeleton (except osteosarcoma of the rib, which grows aggressively); thus the tumor may be present there for as long as two years without being detected. Metastatic potential of axial bone tumors is also lower than the appendicular skeleton tumors. The primary bone tumors of the axial skeleton are treated depending on the size and location of the tumor [38]. Tumors of the jaw are surgically treated by mandibulectomy or maxillectomy, skull tumors may require craniectomy, vertebral tumors may need partial vertebrectomy and rib tumors may require chest wall resection and reconstruction. Similarly, pelvic tumors may be treated by removing involved part the pelvis, and scapular tumors may be treated by subtotal or total scapulectomy. If surgery is not wanted or possible, tumors of axial skeleton may be managed using analgesic drugs, radiation therapy and chemotherapy. The outcome of surgical treatment of axial bone tumors depends on the location and type of tumor and the extent to which the tumor mass is removed by surgery.

### 14.1.4 Prognosis

Prognosis in cases of any bone tumor is generally guarded. While untreated animals do not generally survive for more than a few months, a two-fold increase in survival time has been seen after amputation and chemotherapy. The dogs with limb osteosarcoma usually survive for 90–175 days following palliative treatment, but 45–50% of dogs may survive up to 6 months and 15–20% dogs may live even up to 12 months after diagnosis. Palliative radiation therapy and chemotherapy can prolong median survival time up to approximately 300 days. The usual median survival time after curative surgery can be 235–366 days, but 33–65% of dogs alive can live up to 12 months and 16–28% dogs up to 2 years.

## 14.2 Large Animals

In horses, bone tumor (osteosarcoma) is rare, with the majority of reported cases occurring in the maxilla and mandible of young horses, without metastatic lesions [2, 39–41]. However, few cases have also been reported in the vertebral column as well as in appendicular skeleton (Fig. 14.2). In one report, seven of eight cases of osteosarcoma in horses were recorded in male horses aged more than seven years, mostly in the mandible or maxilla, and were predominant fibroblastic osteosarcoma [2]. In bovines also osteosarcoma has been reported more often in mandible, maxilla, and nasal or skull region (Fig. 14.3) [42–45], and rarely it has been recorded in other places like coccygeal vertebrae [7]. Despite being locally very aggressive, the tumors in cattle do not normally metastasize to other body parts. Radiation therapy and chemotherapy following aggressive surgical excision are not considered practical and economical in large animals, and such animals are generally euthanized.

## Chapter 14: Sample Questions

**Question No. 1: Mark the correct answer**

1. Common bone tumor in animals is
   (a) osteoma, (b) osteochondroma, (c) osteosarcoma, (d) enchondroma
2. Most aggressive bone tumor is
   (a) chondrosarcoma, (b) osteosarcoma, (c) squamous cell carcinoma, (d) synovial cell sarcoma
3. Biphosphonates are used in dogs with bone tumors as they can
   (a) inhibit bone destruction and control pain, (b) kill tumor cells, (c) prevent cell multiplication, (d) none of these
4. Chondrosarcoma is primarily a tumor of
   (a) bone, (b) cartilage, (c) fibrous tissue, (d) haemopoietic tissue

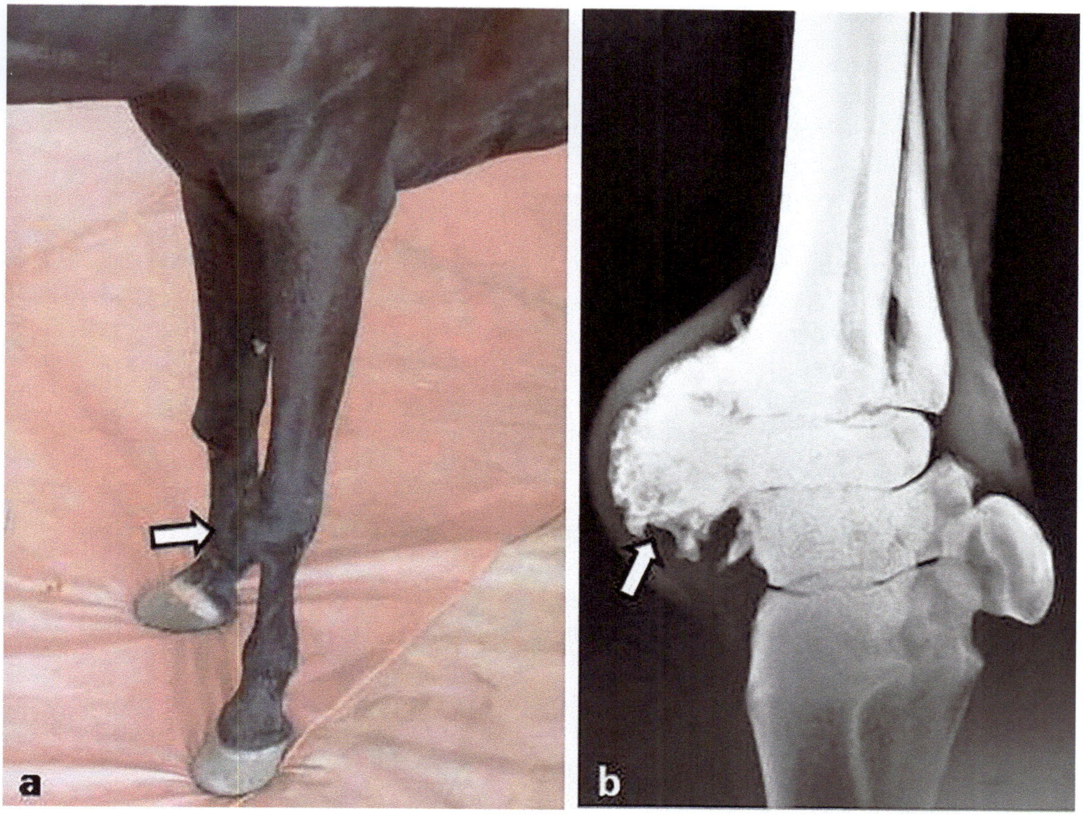


**Fig. 14.2** A hard tumor mass at cranial aspect of knee joint (arrow) in a five-year-old stallion (**a**); radiograph shows sunburst appearance of bony growth (arrow) at the distal radius and radiocarpal bone (**b**). Histological examination revealed fibroblastic osteosarcoma. (Source: J. Khurma et al., Surgical management of osteosarcoma in a horse. Indian J. Vet. Surg. 38 (1): 70–71, 2017)

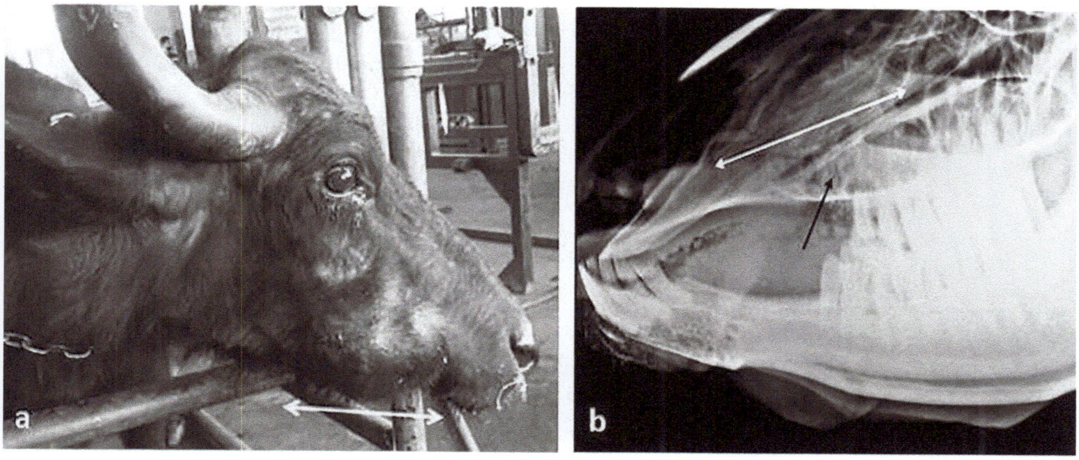


**Fig. 14.3** A 13-year-old, 3-month pregnant buffalo shows a hard swelling in the right maxillary region (**a**); lateral radiograph shows rarefaction of the bone at the maxillary region (arrow) (**b**). Histological examination confirmed chondrosarcoma. (Source: Deepti Sharma et al., Maxillary chondrosarcoma in a buffalo, Indian J. Vet. Surg. 40 (2): 141, 2019)

**Question No. 2: State true or false**

1. Bone tumor is more common in large giant breed dogs.
2. More often bone tumors are recorded at the diaphyseal region of long bones.
3. Osteosarcoma is more aggressive in cats than dogs.
4. Unlike in osteomyelitis or osteoarthritis, osteosarcoma may cross the joint space and affect adjoining bones in the joint.
5. Chondrosarcoma generally occurs on flat bones such as ribs or skull bones.
6. Limb amputation without chemotherapy is palliative and may not prolong survival time in cases of osteosarcoma.
7. Axial bone tumors are more aggressive and metastatic than the appendicular bone tumors.
8. In large animals, osteosarcoma is rare but often can be seen in the maxilla and mandible without metastatic lesions.

**Question No. 3: Fill in the blanks**

1. Among the different domestic animals, bone tumors are most common in ______________ __________, and the most common primary bone tumor is ________________________ ________.
2. ____________________________________-__ breed of dogs is genetically predisposed for developing osteosarcoma.
3. The condition with diffuse swelling at the distal extremity of all four limbs with metastatic lung lesions in dogs is called as _________ ______________________________________ __.
4. Characteristic radiographic sign of osteosarcoma is ______________________________ _______________.
5. __________________________ and ___________________________________ are primarily used as palliative treatment options, and ______________________________ along with ____________________________ ___ is used as curative treatment for osteosarcoma.
6. __________________________ analgesics, which do not have anti-inflammatory properties, are potent analgesics useful particularly in chronic pain cases of bone tumor.

**Question No. 4: Write short note on the following:**

1. Clinical and radiographic signs of osteosarcoma
2. Chemotherapy of bone tumors
3. Radiation therapy for bone tumors

## References


1. Alexander, J.W., and C.S. Patton. 1983. Primary tumors of the skeletal system. *The Veterinary Clinics of North America. Small Animal Practice* 13: 181–195.
2. Bush, J.M., R.L. Fredrickson, and E.J. Ehrhart. 2007. Equine osteosarcoma: a series of 8 cases. *Veterinary Pathology* 44 (2): 247–249.
3. Goldschmidt, M.H., and D.E. Thrall. 1985. Malignant bone tumours in the dog. In *Textbook of small animal orthopaedics*, ed. C.D. Newton and D.M. Nunamaker, 887–898. Philadelphia: J.B. Lippincott.
4. Goldschmidt, M.H., and D.E. Thrall. 1985. Primary and secondary bone tumours in the cat. In *Textbook of small animal orthopaedics*, ed. C.D. Newton and D.M. Nunamaker, 911–913. Philadelphia: J.B. Lippincott.
5. Maiti, S.K., A.M. Pawde, N. Kumar, G.R. Singh, H.P. Aithal, and H.C. Setia. 2003. Clinical management of osteosarcoma in dogs. *The Journal of Canine Development & Research* 3: 77–79.
6. Quigley, P.J., and A.H. Leedale. 1983. Tumors involving bone in the domestic cat: a review of fifty eight cases. *Veterinary Pathology* 20: 670–686.
7. Sangwan, V., K. Gill, N. Tandia, A. Kumar, and K. Gupta. 2021. Bovine coccygeal osteosarcoma – a report of three cows. *Large Animals Review* 28: 41–45.
8. Chun, R., and L.P. de Lorimier. 2003. Update on the biology and management of canine osteosarcoma. *The Veterinary Clinics of North America. Small Animal Practice* 33: 491–516.
9. Bitetto, W.V., A.K. Patnaik, S.C. Schrader, and S.C. Mooney. 1987. Osteosarcoma in cats: 22 cases (1974–1984). *Journal of the American Veterinary Medical Association* 190 (1): 91–93.
10. Kessler, M., M. Tassani-Prell, D. von Bomhard, and U. Matis. 1997. Osteosarcoma in cats: epidemiological, clinical and radiological findings in 78 animals (1990-1995). *Tierärztliche Praxis* 25 (3): 275–283.
11. Heldmann, E., M.A. Anderson, and C. Wagner-Mann. 2000. Feline osteosarcoma: 145 cases (1990-1995).

*Journal of the American Animal Hospital Association* 36 (6): 518–521.
12. Baum, J.I., O.T. Skinner, and S.E. Boston. 2018. Fracture-associated osteosarcoma of the femur in a cat. *The Canadian Veterinary Journal* 59 (10): 1096–1098.
13. Dimopoulou, M., J. Kirpensteijn, H. Moens, and M. Kik. 2008. Histologic prognosticators in feline steosarcoma: a comparison with phenotypically similar canine osteosarcoma. *Veterinary Surgery* 37 (5): 466–471.
14. Thrall, D.E., and M.H. Goldschmidt. 1985. Radiography and biopsy of bony neoplasia. In *Textbook of small animal orthopaedics*, ed. C.D. Newton and D.M. Nunamaker, 875–885. Philadelphia: J.B. Lippincott.
15. Britt, T., C. Clifford, A. Barger, S. Moroff, K. Drobatz, C. Thacher, and G. Davis. 2007. Diagnosing appendicular osteosarcoma with ultrasound-guided fine-needle aspiration: 36 cases. *The Journal of Small Animal Practice* 48: 145–150.
16. Jeglum, K.A. 1985. Treatment of bone tumors. In *Textbook of small animal orthopaedics*, ed. C.D. Newton and D.M. Nunamaker, 915–920. Philadelphia: J.B. Lippincott.
17. Mayer, M., and C.K. Grier. 2006. Palliative radiation therapy for canine osteosarcoma. *The Canadian Veterinary Journal* 47 (7): 707–709.
18. Bateman, K.E., P.A. Catton, P.W. Pennock, and S.A. Kruth. 1994. 0–7–21 radiation therapy for the palliation of advanced cancer in dogs. *Journal of Veterinary Internal Medicine* 8 (6): 394–399.
19. Green, E.M., W.M. Adams, and L.J. Forrest. 2002. Four fraction palliative radiotherapy for osteosarcoma in 24 dogs. *Journal of the American Animal Hospital Association* 38: 445–451.
20. McEntee, M.C., R.L. Page, C.A. Novotney, and D.E. Thrall. 1993. Palliative radiotherapy for canine appendicular osteosarcoma. *Veterinary Radiology & Ultrasound* 34: 367–370.
21. Ramirez, O. III, R.K. Dodge, R.L. Page, G.S. Price, M.L. Hauck, T.A. LaDue, F. Nutter, and D.E. Thrall. 1999. Palliative radiotherapy of appendicular osteosarcoma in 95 dogs. *Veterinary Radiology & Ultrasound* 40: 517–522.
22. Tollett, M.A., L. Duda, D.C. Brown, and E.L. Krick. 2016. Palliative radiation therapy for solid tumors in dogs: 103 cases (2007-2011). *Journal of the American Veterinary Medical Association* 248 (1): 72–82.
23. Farese, J.P., J. Ashton, R. Milner, L.L. Ambrose, and J. Van Gilder. 2004. The effect of the biphosphonate alendronate on viability of canine osteosarcoma cells in vitro. *In Vitro Cellular & Developmental Biology. Animal* 40 (3/4): 113–117.
24. Milner, R.J., J. Farese, C.J. Henry, K. Selting, T.M. Fan, and L.P. de Lorimier. 2004. Bisphosphonates and cancer. *Journal of Veterinary Internal Medicine* 18: 597–604.
25. Tomlin, J.L., C. Sturgeon, M.J. Pead, and P. Muir. 2000. Use of the bisphosphonate drug alendronate for palliative management of osteosarcoma in two dogs. *The Veterinary Record* 147 (5): 129–132.
26. Berg, J. 1996. Canine osteosarcoma: amputation and chemotherapy. *The Veterinary Clinics of North America. Small Animal Practice* 26: 111–121.
27. Straw, R.C., S.J. Withrow, and B.E. Powers. 1990. Management of canine appendicular osteosarcoma. *The Veterinary Clinics of North America. Small Animal Practice* 20: 1141–1161.
28. Chun, R., L.D. Garrett, C. Henry, M. Wall, A. Smith, and N.M. Azene. 2005. Toxicity and efficacy of cisplatin and doxorubicin combination chemotherapy for the treatment of canine osteosarcoma. *Journal of the American Animal Hospital Association* 41: 382–387.
29. Lane, A., M. Black, and K. Wyatt. 2012. Toxicity and efficacy of a novel doxorubicin and carboplatin chemotherapy protocol for the treatment of canine appendicular osteosarcoma following limb amputation. *Australian Veterinary Journal* 90: 69–74.
30. Liu, Y., Q. Li, Q. Bai, and W. Jiang. 2021. Advances of smart nano-drug delivery systems in osteosarcoma treatment. *Journal of Materials Chemistry B* 9: 5439–5450.
31. Chirio, D., S. Sapino, G. Chindamo, E. Peira, C. Vercelli, C. Riganti, M. Manzoli, G. Gambino, G. Re, and M. Gallarate. 2022. Doxorubicin-loaded lipid nanoparticles coated with calcium phosphate as a potential tool in human and canine osteosarcoma therapy. *Pharmaceutics* 14 (7): 1362. https://doi.org/10.3390/pharmaceutics14071362.
32. Mauldin, G.N., R.E. Matus, S.J. Withrow, and A.K. Patnaik. 1988. Canine osteosarcoma. Treatment by amputation versus amputation and adjuvant chemotherapy using doxorubicin and cisplatin. *Journal of Veterinary Internal Medicine* 2: 177–180.
33. Phillips, B., B.E. Powers, W.S. Dernell, R.C. Straw, C. Khanna, G.S. Hogge, et al. 2009. Use of single-agent carboplatin as adjuvant or neoadjuvant therapy in conjunction with amputation for appendicular osteosarcoma in dogs. *Journal of the American Animal Hospital Association* 45: 33–38.
34. Shapiro, W., T.W. Fossum, B.E. Kitchell, C.G. Couto, and G.H. Theilen. 1988. Use of cisplatin for treatment of appendicular osteosarcoma in dogs. *Journal of the American Veterinary Medical Association* 192: 507–511.
35. Thompson, J.P., and M.J. Fugent. 1992. Evaluation of survival times after limb amputation, with and without subsequent administration of cisplatin, for treatment of appendicular osteosarcoma in dogs: 30 cases (1979-1990). *Journal of the American Veterinary Medical Association* 200: 531–533.
36. MacEwen, E.G., and I.D. Kurzman. 1996. Canine osteosarcoma. Amputation and chemoimmunotherapy. *The Veterinary Clinics of North America. Small Animal Practice* 26: 123–133.

37. Wycislo, K.L., and T.M. Fan. 2015. The immunotherapy of canine osteosarcoma: a historical and systematic review. *Journal of Veterinary Internal Medicine* 29 (3): 759–769.
38. Straw, R., B. Powers, J. Klausner, R. Henderson, W. Morrison, D. McCaw, et al. 1996. Canine mandibular osteosarcoma: 51 cases (1980-1992). *Journal of the American Animal Hospital Association* 32: 257–262.
39. Daffner, R., K.R. Fox, and K.R. Galey. 2002. Fibroblastic osteosarcoma of the mandible. *Skeletal Radiology* 31: 107–111.
40. Leite, R.O., V.E. Fabris, E.S. Monteiro da Silva, G.M. Nogueira, and D.J. Zanzarini Delfiol. 2019. Sinonasal osteosarcoma in a horse. *Acta Scientiae Veterinariae* 47. https://doi.org/10.22456/1679-9216.90022.
41. Leonardi, L., F. Roperto, M. Sforna, G. Angeli, and R. Gialletti. 2012. Parosteal fibrous maxillary osteosarcoma in a horse: a case report. *Veterinary Science Research* 3 (1): 44–47.
42. Micheloud, J.F., M.G. Guidi, and E.J. Gimeno. 2014. Ostosarcoma in the skull of a Holstein heifer. *Brazilian Journal of Veterinary Pathology* 8 (1): 10–13.
43. Peixoto, T.C., D.N. Silva, B.R. Araújo, S.S. de Farias, M.P.R. Pinto, L.G.T. Requião, C. Muramoto, and K.M. Madureira. 2016. Mandibular chondroblastic osteosarcoma in a bovine - Case report. *Revista Brasileira de Medicina Veterinária* 38 (Supl.1): 60–64.
44. Prins, D.G.J., T. Wittek, and D.C. Barrsett. 2012. Maxillary osteosarcoma in a beef suckler cow. *Irish Veterinary Journal* 65 (1): 15.
45. Yoshimoto, K., M. Komagata, S. Chiba, M. Hiro, Y. Kobayashi, K. Matsumoto, and H. Inokuma. 2011. A case of nasal osteosarcoma in a Holstein cow. *Journal of the Japan Veterinary Medical Association* 64: 457–460.

# Physiotherapy and Rehabilitation of Orthopedic Patients

# 15

**Learning Objectives**

You will be able to understand the following after reading this chapter:

- Principles of physiotherapy and rehabilitation
- Different techniques of physiotherapy like cryotherapy, thermotherapy, passive range of motion, massage, hydrotherapy, therapeutic exercise and other modalities
- Rehabilitation in chronic cases and muscular contracture
- Assessment and monitoring of patients undergoing physiotherapy and rehabilitation protocols

**Summary**

- The primary objective of rehabilitation following an orthopedic surgery is to reduce pain and inflammation, improve joint range of motion and muscle strength, reduce postoperative complications and thereby accelerate healing and functional recovery. Cryotherapy (application of cold or ice) in the early postoperative period can decrease the blood flow to the injured site and production of tumor necrosis factor alpha, reduce nerve conduction and thus help reduce pain, swelling, and inflammation.
- Heat therapy (moist or dry) is used to improve circulation to the affected area (after the acute inflammation subsides in 2–3 days post-surgery), which can help reduce pain and improve healing.
- Passive range of motion exercises performed by flexing and extending the joints (after the initial inflammation and swelling subsides) can prevent muscular contraction and joint stiffness, reduce pain and help early regaining of normal limb function.
- Swimming is the best form of hydrotherapy, which can help increase the joint range of motion and facilitate early limb use.
- Therapeutic or controlled weight-bearing exercises can encourage weight-bearing, increase muscle strength, improve range of motion and re-establish proprioception and balance.
- Neuromuscular electrical stimulation, laser therapy, therapeutic ultrasound, short wave diathermy and shockwave therapy are physiotherapy modalities

(continued)


H. P. Aithal et al., *Textbook of Veterinary Orthopaedic Surgery*,
https://doi.org/10.1007/978-981-99-2575-9_15

used to rehabilitate orthopedic patients; they are known to increase the tissue temperature and thus help increase blood flow, minimize inflammation and accelerate bone healing.

- Quadriceps muscle contracture is a serious consequence of prolonged immobilization of limb mostly in cases of femoral fractures, wherein the *vastus intermedius* muscle forms a fibrotic scar with the bony callus, causing inability to flex or extend the stifle; this condition can be prevented by providing stable fracture fixation along with encouraging early use of limb, passive range of joint motion and massage therapy.
- Rehabilitation should be an essential component of the recovery plan for successful outcome of orthopedic patients; however, protocols should be tailor-made for the individual patient, and rehabilitation protocol should be adjusted and modified as the condition of the patient changes.

Physiotherapy refers to the treatment of disease conditions and disorders by physical method, and rehabilitation is restoration of normal function of the affected part [1]. Physiotherapy and rehabilitation accelerate tissue healing by hastening normal physiological repair processes so that the functional normalcy of the affected part is restored faster.

Physical therapy and rehabilitation are relatively novel concepts in veterinary practice, and there is still a lot to learn about its proper applications and indications for orthopedic conditions in animals; the practice of physiotherapy in veterinary rehabilitation is largely based on the expertise developed in human medicine [2–8]. Many animal patients affected with orthopedic injuries, such as a fracture, may have difficulty in returning to their normal activity after treatment. Just like in human patients, animal patients subjected to physiotherapy and rehabilitation after surgery could recover more rapidly and completely than those not subjected to physiotherapy. Pain, swelling, and inflammation associated with an injury and surgical trauma can cause inhibition of muscular contraction leading to muscular atrophy and decreased muscle strength. Hence, the primary objective of rehabilitation following an orthopedic surgery is to reduce inflammation, pain, and swelling, improve the range of motion of joints and increase muscle strength by protecting the injured site and to reduce postoperative complications and thereby accelerate recovery. This can be achieved by application of a combination of carefully selected physiotherapeutic procedures in addition to an individualized and structured exercise protocol.

In orthopedic patients, rehabilitation protocol should commence as soon as possible after the surgical treatment, while the patient is still in hospital [9, 10]. In hospital settings, it is easy to perform and monitor any procedure as and when needed. Movement restriction immediately after surgical fixation of the bone (at least for 24–48 h) is very important, especially in unstable fractures and in heavy large animal patients. Initial pain and inflammation can be reduced by administration of analgesics and anti-inflammatory drugs along with the use of ice, compression and gentle movement, etc. Regaining of joint range of motion should be worked out gradually as pain and swelling decrease. Gentle massage away from the wound and passive movements, along with controlled weight bearing, should be started in the early postoperative period. Once the inflammation and associated pain and muscle inhibition are taken care of, muscle strengthening should be addressed. The exercise should be very light and done in controlled manner initially; the intensity then can be increased gradually to overload the muscle, allowing increased adaptation and strength. It has been seen that patients subjected to physiotherapy early after the orthopedic surgery achieved strength more rapidly and regained fast overall functional recovery.

## 15.1 Techniques

There is a plethora of rehabilitation procedures that can be applied following orthopedic surgery [11]. It can be as simple as administration of analgesic medication, application of passive range of motion exercises, cold or heat, massage or assisted standing and ambulation using a range of physical support devices such as slings. It can also be more complex such as swimming, land or underwater treadmill, and use of other physiotherapeutic modalities such as ultrasound, electromagnetic field, etc. Selection of these techniques may differ from animal to animal depending on the need of the case, and it must be individualized. In any case, animal owners' education, involvement and support are very critical for successful outcome.

### 15.1.1 Cryotherapy

Cryotherapy or application of cold or ice in the early postoperative period is known to decrease the blood flow to the injured site and minimize the tumor necrosis factor alpha production, reduce nerve conduction and thus help reduce pain sensation, swelling and inflammation and improve weight bearing on the treated limb [12–14]. Commercially available flexible ice packs can be used on the same day of surgery after the complete recovery of the animal from anesthesia. To preclude ice burns, the ice pack should be covered with a wet towel before placing over the affected site, and intermittent applications of about 10–20 min should be practised rather than continuous application. During the ice treatment, the animal should be continuously observed for skin redness or irritation to prevent an ice burn. Cryotherapy can also be provided by circulating ice cold water in a bladder wrapped around the limb using a compression system; it reduces tissue temperature as well as massages the limb. Ice treatment can be repeated several times a day during the first 48–72 h and can be continued for longer time in case swelling and oedema persist. It can be performed 2–3 times a day during the first postoperative week.

### 15.1.2 Thermotherapy

After the acute swelling and inflammation have subsided, that is, 2–3 days post-surgery, heat can be used to improve circulation to the affected area, which will help reduce pain and assist with healing. Heat can be given either as moist heat (also called as fomentation – it may be done using a cloth dipped in boiling water and squeezed) or as dry heat (given by heated sand or rice bran bundled in a cloth). The moist heat is generally preferred over the dry heat owing to its smoothening effect. Heat packs can be applied over the injured site or the animal may be allowed to sit on the warm pack for about 10 min 3–4 times a day prior to resuming passive range of motion exercises. Care should be taken not to cause thermal burns due to excessive heating. Warm water therapy can also be performed by placing the animal in a bathtub filled with warm water (90–95 °F). Special care should be taken to prevent drowning of the patient's head. Alternating cold and heat application can also be used after the initial swelling and inflammation has subsided to assist in reducing the swelling. Cold therapy will reduce the blood flow and subsequent heating will increase the blood flow to the area and thus help draining out the inflammatory exudates from the affected site. Heat and cold can be used alternatively for 10 min each, over a period of 50–60 min, 3–4 times a day.

### 15.1.3 Passive Range of Motion

Passive movements of the joints of the affected limb can be done after the initial inflammation and swelling has subsided. Movement exercises of the joint can be performed by flexing and extending the joints to a point of slight discomfort without traumatizing the healing tissues. It will help prevent muscular contraction (such as quadriceps contraction in femoral fractures) and joint stiffness, reduce pain and help regain normal ambulation. Extension and flexion of the joints should be performed within pain free range (should not be forced to painful level) so that the animals can tolerate. The joint is slowly flexed manually until the animal shows the signs of discomfort and then slowly extended until signs of discomfort are noticed again. Generally, 10–20 repetitions performed 3–4 times a day are sufficient, but the frequency can be decreased once the joints regain their near normal range of motion.

### 15.1.4 Massage

Massaging of soft tissues will help reduce oedema, adhesion formation, muscle tension and associated pain [15, 16]. Joint compressions will reduce joint effusion and thus help regain normal joint movements. In orthopedic patients, gentle massage of the major muscle groups of the affected limbs is recommended in the post-surgery period. Massaging in the direction of the flow of blood can help reduce the swelling and drain out the waste products from an immobilized area. Massaging should be done away from the surgical site without causing pain in the immediate postoperative period. Subsequently, gentle massage can be performed close to the surgical site. After the wound is completely healed, massaging of the scar tissue can be done at the wound site, which will help detach the scar from adhered underlying tissues.

### 15.1.5 Hydrotherapy

Hydrotherapy is an excellent method of rehabilitation of orthopedic patients [7, 17]. Hydrotherapy may be in the form of bath, effusion, lotion, douches, compresses, fomentation, poultices, or continuous irrigation. It should be started only after complete wound healing. Hydrotherapy allows unloading of painful joints and assist in reduction of limb oedema following surgery. Swimming is a good method of hydrotherapy and it can help increase the joint range of motion and facilitate early limb use. Some animals may be apprehensive to get into the water in the beginning; hence it is advised to acclimatize the animals to swimming slowly with small quantity of water and careful monitoring for the signs of distress, with gradual increase in quantity of water. Movement in water encounters greater resistance than that on the land because density of water is greater than that of the air, thus requiring greater levels of exertion and promoting muscular strength. Swimming increases joint flexion motion, with little effect on joint extension; thus aquatic treadmill therapy may be more beneficial for rehabilitation following stifle joint surgery. Underwater treadmill therapy allows gentle loading on the limbs (with reduced load at injured site), muscle strengthening with accelerated bone healing and return to function. Hydrotherapy is contraindicated in patients with open wounds (including in ESF), severe systemic disease conditions, respiratory compromise, skin irritations and ear infection.

### 15.1.6 Therapeutic Exercise

Therapeutic or controlled weight-bearing exercises by the patient (with the help of animal owner or a caregiver) are aimed at increasing weight-bearing, increasing muscle strength, improving range of motion and re-establishing proprioception and balance [7, 18]. Controlled weight bearing (increased mechanical load) following an orthopedic surgery can help prevent disuse muscle atrophy, increase bone healing and assist in the early return of limb function. Postoperative therapeutic exercise is an excellent tool to promote musculoskeletal metabolic and physiological functions. These exercises include postural activities (sit to stand), controlled leash walking, stair and obstacle negotiating, treadmill locomotion, playing with toys, reaching for food, dancing and wheel barrowing, etc. These exercises can be started following complete wound healing and bandage removal. The animals should be assisted to stand and bear the weight on the affected part to promote muscular function. Harness or slings can be used to assist the animal, if it is unable or reluctant to support its own weight.

Slow walking should be encouraged as early as possible during the early postoperative period. It can initially be for 5–10 min duration, 2–3 times a day, and then gradually increased depending on the condition of the animal until complete bone healing and regaining of limb function. In the early postoperative period, normal limb use may be promoted by restricting speed of walking as animals prefer holding the limb off the ground while running. The walking speed should be increased gradually as the animal regains near normal gait. To ensure that the animal bears weight on the affected limbs, it can be taken for walking on the slopes and climbing steps/stairs in a slow-controlled manner. The animal may be forced to use both limbs. Stair climbing needs a greater excursion of the limb segments than over-ground walking and encourages limb use in case of reluctance. Negotiating obstacles like rocks, boxes, or a ladder put on the ground may be effective methods of promoting use of the limb in orthopedic patients.

Treadmill walking can promote ambulatory function. Dogs generally adapt to treadmill locomotion very quickly, but a handler/assistant walking alongside can encourage the patient. The moving belt of treadmill can encourage the use of limbs that remain unused during over-ground ambulation. Further, the treadmill can control the velocity of the patient that promotes coordination, balance, and proprioception. The moving belt also provides passive extension of the limbs; hence range of joint motion does not occur as during over-ground locomotion.

Balancing exercises stimulate coordination and stability and also encourage the animal for weight bearing on the affected limb. Exercises like dancing and wheel barrowing can help in functional recovery of the limb. These exercises result in increased extension of the shoulders/hips and improved weight bearing on the two limbs touching the ground. If possible, the patient may be subjected to jumping exercises to further encourage limb strength.

In cases of fracture repair with external support (a splint or cast), therapeutic exercises may be delayed. The joints proximal to the cast may be subjected to passive motion exercises. Movement exercises and massage may help the animals with external skeletal fixator to retain mobility to some extent during the healing process. It is recommended to encourage weight bearing and limb use during the postoperative period to stimulate fracture healing and to reduce the likelihood of disuse limb atrophy.

### 15.1.7 Other Modalities

Other modalities used for rehabilitation of orthopedic patients include electrical neuromuscular stimulation, laser therapy, therapeutic ultrasound, short wave diathermy, shockwave therapy, acupuncture stimulation, etc. [7, 19–27]. The use of transcutaneous electrical nerve stimulation shortly after surgery has been found to reduce pain sensation, swelling and oedema and stimulate bone healing. Electrical stimulation can be administered for 30–60 min daily for 4–6 weeks. A low-level laser therapy has also been reported to have beneficial effects on healing following orthopedic surgery; it has been shown to increase the tissue temperature and thereby increase circulation at the site of injury. Low-intensity pulsed ultrasound can promote endochondral ossification during fracture healing and articular cartilage repair. About 15–30 min of ultrasound therapy can be used daily for 4–6 weeks as per the case to promote new bone formation and healing of non-union fractures. Short wave diathermy utilizes electromagnetic radio waves to generate deep heat. Exogenous heat is not applied to the skin, but the body itself generates its own heat from the waves produced by the diathermy machine. Diathermy can be used to treat pain from inflammatory diseases, as well as other painful conditions and muscle spasms or arthritis. The generated heat can minimize inflammation and accelerate healing by increasing blood flow. It can be applied for 20–30 min daily for 2–3 weeks. Extracorporeal shockwave therapy can also promote healing of tendons and bones (larger callus with more cortical bone); during shockwave therapy, it is advised to sedate the animal as the procedure may cause swelling or erythema and discomfort to the animal.

## 15.2 Rehabilitation in Chronic Cases and Muscular Contracture

In orthopedic patients having external support with a cast or splint, rehabilitation efforts may be hindered. It has been seen that if the limb is immobilized postoperatively, significant limb weakness will develop. Muscle atrophy due to immobilization of a limb may take a long time to recover (2–4 times the length of immobilization time). Immobilization of the limb has also been known to alter the articular cartilage physiology, disorganize the alignment of ligament collagen and their weakening and can cause permanent damage to the joints. Hence it is always recommended to keep the external support only for a minimum period of time to reduce complications and regain early functional recovery of the limb.

Quadriceps muscle contracture is a serious consequence of prolonged immobilization of limb mostly in cases of femoral fractures, wherein the vastus intermedius muscle forms a fibrotic scar with the bony callus, causing inability to flex and extend the stifle [28–31]. This condition can be prevented by providing stable fracture fixation along with encouraging for early use of limb, passive movement of the limb and massage therapy. If contracture develops, rehabilitation should be aimed at stretching the quadriceps manually to release the tissue from the bone and therapeutic ultrasound, promoting range of stifle motion and strengthening the hamstring muscles. Weight bearing should be encouraged, and therapeutic exercises, aquatic therapy and neuromuscular stimulation may be provided for several weeks.

In certain patients undergoing orthopedic surgery, even if rehabilitation has been initiated in the immediate postoperative period, prolonged therapy may be required to achieve full functional recovery. Therapeutic exercises in the chronic phase of healing should focus on attaining strength and improving proprioception and ability to perform the tasks. The use of elastic resistance bands to do eccentric exercises and flexion of the proximal limbs may help develop core strength and coordination. This band can be applied on a limb for about 10 min during a walk and then reversed onto the contralateral limb and the exercise continued for another 10 min. Balance and proprioception can be developed by making the animal stand on unstable surfaces like wobble boards or discs and performing body movement activities like sit-to-stands, turning the head, etc.

## 15.3 Assessment and Monitoring

Assessment of the animal patient is important before undertaking any rehabilitation program, which should include the type of surgery, treatments given, expected prognosis, condition of the animal owner, home environment, the nature of the animal prior to surgery, etc., which will help to develop tailor-made rehabilitation protocol and guide the animal owner for home exercise. The animal should also be monitored regularly during the treatment period for the response to treatment by assessing the lameness scores, observing the animal's posture and measuring the joint range of motion, extent of swelling and oedema, local reaction, etc. Some discomfort and/or inflammation after an exercise may be regarded as normal; however, overexertion during the therapeutic exercise leading to discomfort or exaggerated lameness for >2 h should be avoided. In cases of protracted discomfort, the intensity and duration of the therapy need to be reduced (most often by 50%) at the next session for at least a few days. If discomfort continues even after reducing the intensity and duration of exercise in the following session, the animal should be examined for any re-injury and fixation stability.

The owner should be properly advised to confine the animal in the immediate postoperative period to prevent complications of fixation failure. They should also be regularly enquired about the completion of the home exercise regimes as instructed, response to treatment and any other concerns. The animal should be periodically called for follow-up checkups and progress monitoring. Rehabilitation is an essential component of the postoperative care plan for successful outcome of orthopedic patients. Rehabilitation plan for orthopedic patients should be tailor made for the individual patient; one exercise or modality may work better for one patient than the others based on the condition and temperament [32]. Further, rehabilitation protocol should be adjusted and modified as the condition improves or changes.

## Chapter 15: Sample Questions

### Question No. 1: Mark the correct answer

1. Most of physiotherapeutic modalities help to increase blood circulation to the affected area, except for
   (a) electric stimulation (b) laser therapy (c) cryotherapy (d) thermotherapy
2. Which of the following is not true with respect to thermotherapy
   (a) can be started soon after surgery (b) improve circulation to the area (c) reduce pain (d) can assist in healing
3. In orthopedic patents, rehabilitation protocols should be started
   (a) immediately after surgery (b) after inflammation has subsided (c) one week after surgery (d) if lameness is persistent
4. Which of the following is not true for hydrotherapy
   (a) It should be started immediately after surgery.
   (b) It increases joint range of motion.
   (c) It helps in reduction of limb oedema.
   (d) It allows uploading of painful joints.

### Question No. 2: State true or false

1. Gentle passive motion, massage, and controlled weight bearing can all start in the early postoperative period.
2. Cryotherapy or application of cold or ice is not recommended in the early postoperative period.
3. Fomentation is a type of dry heat therapy used to increase circulation to the injured area.
4. Passive movements of the affected limb joints should only be done after the initial inflammation and swelling subsides.
5. Hydrotherapy is indicated in patients with open wounds.
6. Swimming can help increase the range of motion by increasing joint flexion, with little effect on joint extension.
7. Slow walking in the early postoperative period can prevent disuse muscle atrophy, increase bone healing and assist in the early functional recovery.

### Question No. 3: Fill in the blanks

1. The treatment of disease conditions by physical method is called ____________________, whereas restoration of normal function of the affected part is termed as ____________________.
2. The primary objectives of rehabilitation following an orthopedic surgery are to ____________________, ____________________, ____________________ and ____________________.

### Question No. 4: Write short note on the following:

1. Hydrotherapy for rehabilitation of orthopedic patients
2. Cryotherapy vs. thermotherapy
3. Role of therapeutic exercise in promotion of healing and functional recovery
4. Therapeutic ultrasound
5. Swimming vs. underwater treadmill

## References


1. Sharma, S.K., and V.K. Sobti. 2020. Physiotherapy. In *Ruminant surgery- a textbook of the surgical diseases of cattle, buffaloes, camels, sheep and goats*, ed. J. Singh, S. Singh, and R.P.S. Tyagi, 2nd ed., 533–539. New Delhi: CBS Publishers and Distributors Pvt. Ltd.
2. Alvarez, L.X., J.A. Repac, K.K. Shaw, and N. Compton. 2022. Systematic review of postoperative rehabilitation interventions after cranial cruciate ligament surgery in dogs. *Veterinary Surgery* 51: 233–243.
3. Baltzer, W.I. 2020. Rehabilitation of companion animals following orthopaedic surgery. *New Zealand Veterinary Journal* 68 (3): 157–167.
4. Colvero, A.C.T., M.L. Schwab, D.A. Ferrarin, A. Ripplinger, L.F.S. Herculano, M.R. Wrzesinski, J.S. Rauber, and A. Mazzanti. 2020. Physical therapy treatment in the functional recovery of dogs submitted to head and femoral neck ostectomy: 20 cases. CLINIC AND SURGERY • *Ciencia Rural* 50 (11). https://doi.org/10.1590/0103-8478cr20190545.
5. Henderson, A.L., C. Latimer, and D.L. Millis. 2015. Rehabilitation and physical therapy for selected orthopedic conditions in veterinary patients. *The Veterinary*

*Clinics of North America. Small Animal Practice* 45 (1): 91–121.
6. Millis, D.L. 2005. Physical rehabilitation: improving the outcome in dogs with orthopedic problems. https://www.dvm360.com/view/physical-rehabilitation-improving-outcome-dogs-with-orthopedic-problems.
7. Owen, M.R. 2006. Rehabilitation therapies for musculoskeletal and spinal disease in small animal practice. *EJCAP* 16 (2): 137–148.
8. Sharp, B. 2012. Feline physiotherapy and rehabilitation 2. Clinical application. *Journal of Feline Medicine and Surgery* 14: 633–645.
9. Millis, D.L., D. Levine, and M. Brumlow. 1997. A preliminary study of early physical therapy following surgery for cranial cruciate ligament rupture in dogs [abstract]. *Veterinary Surgery* 26: 434.
10. Shumway, R. 2007. Rehabilitation in the first 48 hours after surgery. *Clinical Techniques in Small Animal Practice* 22: 166–170.
11. Doyle, N.D. 2004. Rehabilitation of fractures in small animals: maximize outcomes, minimize complications. *Clinical Techniques in Small Animal Practice* 19: 180–191.
12. Freeden von, N., F. Duerr, M. Fehr, C. Diekmann, C. Mandel, and O. Harms. 2017. Comparison of two cold compression therapy protocols after tibial plateau leveling osteotomy in dogs. *Tierärztliche Praxis. Ausgabe K, Kleintiere/Heimtiere* 45: 226–233.
13. Kieves, N.R., M.S. Bergh, E. Zellner, and C. Wang. 2016. Pilot study measuring the effects of bandaging and cold compression therapy following tibial plateau leveling osteotomy. *The Journal of Small Animal Practice* 57: 543–547.
14. Martin, S.S., K.P. Spindler, J.W. Tarter, K. Detwiler, and H.A. Petersen. 2001. Cryotherapy: an effective modality for decreasing intraarticular temperature after knee arthroscopy. *The American Journal of Sports Medicine* 29: 288–291.
15. Deniox, J.M., and J.P. Pailloux. 1997. *Physical therapy and massage for the horse*. North Pomfret, VT: Trafalgar Square Publishing.
16. Hourdebaigt, J. 1997. *Equine massage: a practical guide*. New York: Hungry Minds, Inc.
17. Bertocci, G., C. Smalley, N. Brown, K. Bialczak, and D. Carroll. 2018. Aquatic treadmill water level influence on pelvic limb kinematics in cranial cruciate ligament-deficient dogs with surgically stabilised stifles. *The Journal of Small Animal Practice* 59: 121–127.
18. Millis, D.L., M. Drum, and D. Levine. 2014. Therapeutic exercises: joint motion, strengthening, endurance and speed exercises. In *Canine rehabilitation and physical therapy*, ed. D.L. Millis and D. Levine, 2nd ed., 506–525. Philidelphia, PA: Elsevier.
19. Busse, J.W., M. Bhandari, A.V. Kulkarni, and E. Tunks. 2002. The effect of low-intensity pulsed ultrasound therapy on time to fracture healing: a meta-analysis. *Canadian Medical Association Journal* 166: 437–441.
20. Draper, W.E., T.A. Schubert, R.M. Clemmons, and S.A. Miles. 2012. Low-level laser therapy reduces time to ambulation in dogs after hemilaminectomy: a preliminary study. *The Journal of Small Animal Practice* 53: 465–469.
21. Johnson, J.M., A.L. Johnson, G.J. Pijanowski, S.K. Kneller, D.J. Schaeffer, J.A. Eurell, C.W. Smith, and K.S. Swan. 1997. Rehabilitation of dogs with surgically treated cranial cruciate ligament-deficient stifles by use of electrical stimulation of muscles. *American Journal of Veterinary Research* 58: 1473–1478.
22. Lavery, P.H., and S.R. Mcclure. 2002. Initial experience with extracorporeal shockwave therapy in six dogs. Part 1. *Veterinary and Comparative Orthopaedics and Traumatology* 15: 177–183.
23. Levine, D., and B. Bockstahler. 2014. Electrical stimulation. In *Canine rehabilitation and physical therapy*, ed. D.L. Millis and D. Levine, 2nd ed., 342–358. Philidelphia, PA: Elsevier.
24. Levine, D., and T. Watson. 2014. Therapeutic ultrasound. In *Canine rehabilitation and physical therapy*, ed. D.L. Millis and D. Levine, 2nd ed., 328–341. Philidelphia, PA: Elsevier.
25. Zama, M.M.S., M.M. Ansari, M. Hoque, H.P. Aithal, S.K. Maiti, R. John, and G. Shakya. 2011. Clinical evaluation of ultrasound therapy in equine peripheral myopathy. *Indian Journal of Veterinary Surgery* 32: 133–134.
26. Zama, M.M.S., O.P. Gupta, G.R. Singh, and H.P. Aithal. 2001. Role of postoperative acupuncture therapy in the management of fracture of femur: radiological and ground bone section studies. *Indian Journal of Veterinary Surgery* 22: 26–28.
27. Zidonis, N., M. Soderberg, and A. Snow. 1999. *Equine acupressure: a working manual*. Larkspur, CO: Tallgrass Publishers, LLC.
28. Fries, C.L., A.G. Binnington, and J.R. Cockshutt. 1988. Quadriceps contracture in four cats; a complication of internal fixation of femoral fractures. *Veterinary and Comparative Orthopaedics and Traumatology* 2: 91–96.
29. Liptak, J.M., and D.J. Simpson. 2000. Successful management of quadriceps contracture in a cat using a dynamic flexion apparatus. *Veterinary and Comparative Orthopaedics and Traumatology* 13: 44–48.
30. Moores, A.P., and A. Sutton. 2009. Management of quadriceps contracture in a dog using a static flexion apparatus and physiotherapy. *The Journal of Small Animal Practice* 50: 251–254.
31. Taylor, J., and C.H. Tangner. 2007. Acquired muscle contractures in the dog and cat. A review of the literature and case report. *Veterinary and Comparative Orthopaedics and Traumatology* 20: 79–85.
32. Shaw, K.K., L. Alvarez, S.A. Foster, J.E. Tomlinson, A.J. Shaw, and A. Pozzi. 2020. Fundamental principles of rehabilitation and musculoskeletal tissue healing. *Veterinary Surgery* 49 (1): 22–32.

# Chapter-Wise Answers for Objective Questions

## Chapter 1: Sample Questions

**Q. No. 1: Mark the correct answer:** 1. (b); 2. (d); 3. (a); 4. (d); 5. (c); 6. (c); 7. (b); 8. (c); 9. (c); 10. (d).

**Q. No. 2: State true or false:** 1. (F); 2. (T); 3. (F); 4. (T); 5. (F); 6. (F); 7. (F); 8. (F); 9. (T); 10. (F); 11. (F) 12. (T); 13. (F); 14. (T); 15. (T); 16. (T); 17. (T); 18. (T); 19. (T); 20. (T); 21. (T).

**Q. No. 3: Fill up the blanks:** 1. cytoplasmic processes, canalicular; 2. acid phosphatase, collagenase; 3. type-1 collagen, proteoglycans, calcium phosphate (hydroxyapatite); 4. an osteon; 5. periosteum, articular/hyaline cartilage; 6. nutrient artery, nutrient foramen; 7. hyaline cartilage, connective tissue cells; 8. compression, tension; 9. inflammatory, reparative, remodeling; 10. stainless steel.

## Chapter 2: Sample Questions

**Q. No. 1: Mark the most appropriate answer:** 1. (a); 2. (b); 3. (c); 4. (d); 5. (c); 6. (c); 7. (c).

**Q. No. 2: State true or false:** 1. (T); 2. (T); 3. (F); 4. (T); 5. (F); 6 (T); 7 (F); 8 (T); 9 (T); 10 (F); 11. (T); 12. (T); 13. (T); 14 (F); 15 (T); 16 (F); 17 (T).

**Q. No. 3: Fill up the blanks:** 1. Velpeau, Ehmer; 2. normograde, retrograde; 3. 70–90%; 4. dynamic fixation, static fixation; 5. Locking compression, locking, non-locking; 6. less, more, less; 7. (full) cerclage wire, hemi-cerclage wire; 8. giving release incisions, pre-drilling pin holes, pouring of cold saline while drilling; 9. placement of any diameter pins at different directions, pins cannot be fixed under tension.

## Chapter 3: Sample Questions

**Q. No. 1: Mark the correct answer:** 1. (b); 2. (b); 3. (c); 4. (d); 5. (c).

**Q. No. 2: State true or false:** 1. (T); 2. (F); 3. (T); 4. (T); 5. (F); 6. (T); 7. (T); 8. (T); 9. (T); 10. (T); 11. (F); 12 (F); 13 (T).

**Q. No. 3: Fill up the blanks:** 1. knuckling; 2. radial, brachialis; 3. cranial; 4. femur, middle and distal third; 5. cranio-lateral, fascia lata, biceps femoris, vastus lateralis; 6. intercondylar fossa, cruciate ligaments; 7. normograde; 8. cranio-medial; 9. premolar, symphyseal; 10. reduce trauma to the tooth roots; 11. malocclusion; 12. vertebral body cross-pinning.

## Chapter 4: Sample Questions

**Q. No. 1: Mark the correct answer:** 1. (c); 2. (d); 3. (d); 4. (c); 5. (d).

**Q. No. 2: State true or false:** 1. (T); 2. (T); 3. (T); 4. (T); 5. (F); 6. (F); 7. (F); 8. (T); 9. (T).

**Q. No. 3: Fill up the blanks:** 1. bracialis, brachiocephalicus, brachialis, triceps brachi; 2. craniomedial, lateral; 3. lateral, cranial; 4. intercondylar fossa; 5. angular placement of the bone, heavy musculature around the



H. P. Aithal et al., *Textbook of Veterinary Orthopaedic Surgery*,
https://doi.org/10.1007/978-981-99-2575-9

stifle joint, conical shape of the limb; 6. circular, linear; 7. Wing of ilium.

## Chapter 5: Sample Questions

**Q. No. 1: Mark the correct answer:** 1. (d); 2. (d); 3. (a); 4. (b); 5. (d).
**Q. No. 2: State true or false:** 1. (T); 2. (F); 3. (F); 4. (T); 5. (T); 6. (F).
**Q. No. 3: Fill up the blanks:** 1. screw pullout/loosening; 2. hinder the widening of cortex, get trapped within the periosteal callus; 3. osteomalacia; 4. calcium, phosphorus; 5. disuse osteoporosis; 6. osteopetrosis; 7. IM pinning, plate osteosynthesis; 8. aspiration pneumonia, asphyxiation; 9. IM pinning.

## Chapter 6: Sample Questions

**Q. No. 1: Mark the correct answer:** 1. (a); 2 (b); 3 (a); 4 (d); 5 (d).
**Q. No. 2: State true or false:** 1. (T); 2. (T); 3. (F); 4. (T); 5. (T); 6. (F).
**Q. No. 3: Fill up the blanks:** 1. less soft tissue coverage; 2. extent of tissue damage, degree of contamination; 3. osteomyelitis; 4. control of infection, protection of soft tissues, providing stable fixation; 5. the separation of necrosed bone from the healthy part; 6. the persistence of infection; 7. removing the affected implants and bone fragments, rigidly stabilizing the bone using an alternate technique.

## Chapter 7: Sample Questions

**Q. No. 1: Mark the correct answer:** 1. (a); 2. (c); 3. (b).
**Q. No. 2: State true or false:** 1. (T); 2. (F); 3. (T); 4. (F); 5. (F); 6. (T); 7 (T).
**Q. No. 3: Fill up the blanks:** 1. osteoconduction; 2. isograft; 3. wing of the ilium; 4. poly L-lactic acid (PLA), poly glycolic acid (PGA), poly D, L-lactic acid-co-glycolic acid (PLGA); 5. extracellular matrix of bone, platelets; 6. stem cells; 7. haematopoietic, mesenchymal, mesenchymal stem cells.

## Chapter 8: Sample Questions

**Q. No. 1: Mark the correct answer:** 1. (c); 2. (b); 3. (c); 4 (d).
**Q. No. 2: State true or false:** 1. (T); 2 (F); 3. (T); 4 (F); 5 (T); 6 (T); 7 (T); 8. (F); 9. (F); 10. (T); 11 (T).
**Q. No. 3: Fill up the blanks:** 1. mechanical, biological; 2. viable nonunion, nonviable nonunion; 3. drainage, specific antibiotic therapy, stable fracture fixation; 4. fracture disease; 5. quadriceps contracture.

## Chapter 9: Sample Questions

**Q. No. 1: Mark the correct answer:** 1. (b); 2. (a); 3. (b); 4. (a); 5 (d).
**Q. No. 2: State true or false:** 1. (F); 2. (T); 3. (T); 4. (F); 5. (T).
**Q. No. 3: Fill up the blanks:** 1. nutritional secondary hyperparathyroidism (NSH); 2. rickets; 3. distal ulnar physis/growth plate; 4. joint laxity, joint degeneration/osteoarthritis; 5. hip dysplasia.

## Chapter 10: Sample Questions

**Q. No. 1: Mark the correct answer:** 1. (d); 2. (c); 3. (d); 4. (b).
**Q. No. 2: State true or false:** 1. (T); 2. (T); 3. (F); 4. (T).
**Q. No. 3: Fill up the blanks:** 1. antebrachium; 2. 85%, 70%, growth abnormalities.

## Chapter 11: Sample Questions

**Q. No. 1: Mark the correct answer:** 1. (c); 2. (d); 3. (d); 4. (a); 5. (d).

**Q. No. 2: State true or false:** 1. (F); 2. (T); 3. (F); 4. (T); 5. (T); 6. (T); 7. (F); 8. (T); 9. (F); 10. (F).

**Q. No. 3: Fill up the blanks:** 1. joint luxation/ dislocation, subluxation; 2. transposition of the biceps brachii tendon; 3. medial, medially, lateral; 4. the antebrachiocarpal; 5. craniodorsal; 6. trauma, joint degeneration; 7. trochleoplasty.

## Chapter 12: Sample Questions

**Q. No. 1: Mark the correct answer:** 1. (a); 2. (b); 3. (a); 4 (d).

**Q. No. 2: State true or false:** 1. (T); 2. (F); 3. (F); 4. (F); 5. (F); 6. (T); 7. (T).

**Q. No. 3: Fill up the blanks:** 1. haematogenous spread; 2. umbilical infection/ navel ill; 3. synovial fluid analysis; 4. joint lavage, arthrotomy/arthroscopy; 5. residual antigenic bacterial fragments, antigen-antibody deposition; 6. hyaluronic acid, glycosaminoglycan; 7. methotrexate, hydroxychloroquine; 8. idiopathic, erosive.

## Chapter 13: Sample Questions

**Q. No. 1: Mark the correct answer:** 1. (a); 2. (b); 3. (c); 4. (a); 5. (c).

**Q. No. 2: State true or false:** 1. (T); 2. (F); 3. (T); 4. (F); 5. (T); 6. (T).

**Q. No. 3: Fill in the blanks:** 1. tendons, ligaments; 2. Achilles; 3. racing/exercise, laceration injuries by farm machinery; 4. carpal, fetlock; 5. arthrogryposis; 6. cranial drawer sign (excessive cranial laxity of the proximal tibia), increased internal rotation of tibia.

## Chapter 14: Sample Questions

**Q. No. 1: Mark the correct answer:** 1. (c); 2. (b); 3. (a); 4. (b).

**Q. No. 2: State true or false:** 1. (T); 2. (F); 3. (F); 4. (F); 5. (T); 6. (T); 7. (F); 8. (T).

**Q. No. 3: Fill in the blanks:** 1. dogs, osteosarcoma; 2. Scottish Deerhound; 3. hypertrophic osteopathy; 4. sunburst appearance; 5. Analgesics, radiation therapy, limb amputation, chemotherapy; 6. Narcotic.

## Chapter 15: Sample Questions

**Q. No. 1: Mark the correct answer:** 1. (c); 2. (a); 3. (a); 4. (a).

**Q. No. 2: State true or false:** 1. (T); 2. (F); 3. (F); 4. (T); 5. (F); 6. (T); 7. (T).

**Q. No. 3: Fill in the blanks:** 1. physiotherapy, rehabilitation; 2. reduce pain and inflammation, improve joint range of motion and muscle strength, reduce postoperative complications, accelerate recovery.

MIX
Papier aus verantwortungsvollen Quellen
Paper from responsible sources
FSC® C105338

If you have any concerns about our products,
you can contact us on
**ProductSafety@springernature.com**

In case Publisher is established outside the EU,
the EU authorized representative is:
**Springer Nature Customer Service Center GmbH**
**Europaplatz 3, 69115 Heidelberg, Germany**

Printed by Libri Plureos GmbH
in Hamburg, Germany